Cardiology for Veterinary Technicians and Nurses

Cardiology for Veterinary Technicians and Nurses

Edited by

H. Edward Durham, Jr.
University of Missouri
Columbia
USA

WILEY Blackwell

This edition first published 2017

Registered Office
John Wiley & Sons, Inc., 111 River Street, Hoboken, NJ 07030, USA

Editorial Office
111 River Street, Hoboken, NJ 07030, USA

For details of our global editorial offices, customer services, and more information about Wiley products visit us at www.wiley.com.

Wiley also publishes its books in a variety of electronic formats and by print-on-demand. Some content that appears in standard print versions of this book may not be available in other formats.

Library of Congress CataloginginPublication Data

Names: Durham, H. Edward, Jr., editor.
Title: Cardiology for veterinary technicians and nurses / edited by H. Edward Durham, Jr.
Description: Hoboken, NJ : Wiley-Blackwell, 2017. | Includes bibliographical references and index. |
Identifiers: LCCN 2017012641 (print) | LCCN 2017014919 (ebook) | ISBN 9781119357414 (pdf) | ISBN 9781119357421 (epub) | ISBN 9780813813530 (paperback)
Subjects: | MESH: Heart Diseases–veterinary | Animal Technicians
Classification: LCC SF811 (ebook) | LCC SF811 (print) | NLM SF 811 | DDC 636.089/612dc23
LC record available at https://lccn.loc.gov/2017012641

Cover images: black dog – courtesy of Judy Heim; scans on black background – courtesy of H. Edward Durham, Jr.
Cover design by Wiley

Set in 10/12pt WarnockPro by Aptara Inc., New Delhi, India

10 9 8 7 6 5 4 3 2 1

FSC
www.fsc.org
MIX
Paper from responsible sources
FSC® C013604

To my wife Meredith, who supported me with a constant stream of encouragement and the patience of Job through this process; to my parents who supported all my life endeavors; and in memory of Kenneth L. Jeffery DVM who first introduced me to Veterinary Cardiology. Finally, thanks be to God for giving me such an amazing organ to learn and teach.

Contents

List of Contributors

Kathryn J. Atkinson, DVM, MS, DACVIM (Cardiology)
Cardiologist
Heart of Oregon Veterinary Cardiology
Lake Oswego, Oregon, USA

June A. Boon, MS
Clinical Instructor/Echocardiographer
Colorado State University
Veterinary Teaching Hospital
Fort Collins, Colorado, USA

Barbara P. Brewer, BA, BS, CVT, VTS (Cardiology)
New England Veterinary Specialists
Framingham, Massachusetts, USA

H. Edward Durham, Jr., CVT, RVT, LATG, VTS (Cardiology)
Senior Veterinary Technician (Cardiology)
University of Missouri
Veterinary Health Center
Columbia, Missouri, USA

Deborah M. Fine, MS, DVM, DACVIM (Cardiology)
Alii Veterinary Hospital
Kailua Kona, Hawaii, USA

Mark W. Harmon, DVM
Cardiology
University of Missouri
Veterinary Health Center
Columbia, Missouri, USA

Shari Hemsley, LVT, VTS (Cardiology)
Cardiology Technician
Cornell University Hospital for Animals
College of Veterinary Medicine
Ithaca, New York, USA

Kristin Hohnadel, BS, CVT, VTS (Cardiology)
Cardiology Department
University of Minnesota Veterinary Medical Center
Saint Paul, Minnesota, USA

Stacey Leach, DVM, DACVIM (Cardiology)
Assistant Professor
University of Missouri
Veterinary Health Center
Columbia, Missouri, USA

Anna McManamey, DVM
University of Missouri
Veterinary Health Center
Columbia, Missouri, USA

Anne Myers, RVT, VTS (Cardiology)
Veterinary Specialty Hospital of the Carolinas
Cary, North Carolina, USA

Robert J. Schutrumpf III, DVM, DACVIM (Cardiology)
VCA Northwest Veterinary Specialists
Portland, Oregon, USA

Foreword

The last 50 years have delivered tremendous advancements to veterinary medicine. Foremost has been the development of veterinary specialties and subspecialties, which have brought higher standards of knowledge and care to our companion animals. However, such specialization has also generated more complexity in the practices of veterinary technicians and nurses, who play a pivotal role in patient- and client-care. This situation has fostered a parallel development of specialization among some veterinary technician-nurses. One of the leaders of this movement is Mr H. Edward Durham, Jr., who has guided this textbook from an experience that includes more than 15 years as a focused, cardiology specialist in an academic teaching hospital. I consider this first edition of *Cardiology for Veterinary Technicians and Nurses* a landmark publication for the continuing growth of cardiology care in both general and specialty veterinary practice. Mr Durham has collaborated with other veterinary technical specialists as well as practicing veterinary cardiologists with whom he has worked. The result is a view of our specialty that is accessible, comprehensive, and practical.

Ed Durham is one of the first registered veterinary technician specialists in the field of cardiology and a leader in educating and training other veterinary technicians in the subject of cardiovascular disease. I had the privilege of working with him on a daily basis for over four years during my tenure at the University of Missouri. I can attest to Mr Durham's subject knowledge, technical expertise, and patient experience. These skills, combined with his enthusiasm for the subject and passion for teaching veterinary technicians and veterinarians in training, has resulted in this wonderful guide to the technical management and nursing of our patients with cardiovascular diseases.

Quality patient care involves more than procedures and physical tasks, and the modern veterinary technician-nurse increasingly wants to understand not only the "how?" but the "why?" of diagnostic and therapeutic management decisions. *Cardiology for Veterinary Technicians and Nurses* offers answers to both questions. The reader is provided with the theoretical framework for decision-making in diagnosis and treatment along with detailed explanations of specific procedures used for basic to advanced cardiac care. As with most practicing veterinarians, the vast majority of veterinary technicians and nurses are "generalists" who deliver diagnostic and therapeutic procedures across a variety of organ systems. Any textbook focused on the technician and nurse must first address the do-everything technician in private veterinary practice. Ed Durham started his career as a generalist in medicine and surgery, and this textbook effectively serves that audience. *Cardiology for Veterinary Technicians and Nurses* constitutes must-reading for the entry-level, technician-nurse who seeks guidance in day-to-day cardiology procedures. The text also functions as an excellent reference for the technician with more experience; that person wanting to understand the work better, develop advanced procedural skills, or even prepare for technician-specialist certification.

Cardiology for Veterinary Technicians and Nurses delivers on multiple levels. The prerequisite concepts and facts necessary to understand the management of cardiology patients are offered in the first two chapters; these focus on pertinent cardiac anatomy and physiology. The pillars of the clinical cardiac evaluation – history and clinical examination, electrocardiography, radiography, echocardiography and blood pressure measurement – are addressed in Chapters 3 to 7. These are foundational chapters that also relate to monitoring of cardiac patients, an essential task of technicians and nurses. The emerging issues related to systemic hypertension are also considered in Chapter 7. The diagnostic evaluation is completed with a discussion of angiography and cardiac biomarkers contained in the next two chapters. Although angiography is mostly confined to referral centers, cardiac biomarkers have become routine diagnostic tests in general practice. Chapters 10 to 12 deliver a summary of important congenital and acquired heart diseases affecting dogs and cats, with Chapter 13 addressing the pivotal syndrome of heart failure. The latter sets up Chapters 14 and 15 that deal with the sometimes-confusing topics of cardiac drugs and treatment approaches to patients with heart disease and failure. The reader can obtain a clear overview of these important topics, which can facilitate discussing therapy and patient follow-up care with clients. These chapters on diseases and therapy will increase the technician-nurse's accuracy and confidence during rounds, client meetings, and when administering or monitoring prescribed therapies. Additionally, Chapter 15 reviews approaches to cardiac arrhythmia management and as well as the control of pulmonary hypertension, an important emerging disorder in dogs. Chapter 16 is a microcosm of the entire volume. Multiple contributors deliver a chapter carrying the somewhat imposing title of "Interventional Therapies", and this moniker is apt, considering catheter-based closure of PDA, balloon valvuloplasty of pulmonary stenosis, and cardiac pacing are reviewed. However, Chapter 16 begins with the commonplace, detailing the procedures of abdominocentesis, pericardiocentesis, and thoracocentesis. For each procedure – whether basic or advanced – there is a clear delineation of the role of the technician along with listings of the equipment needed for a successful outcome. The final two chapters review important heart diseases of large animals. These discussions will be especially helpful to technicians still in school, those working in mixed- or large-animal practices, technicians in academic practice, and those individuals preparing for specialty technician examinations. Cardiology is one of those specialties that crosses species very well and perhaps even the technician in small animal practice might find the comparative large-animal aspects interesting.

Cardiology can be a difficult subject to learn, but the organization, delivery, and practical hints found within this volume make the topic quite approachable. Each chapter contains numerous illustrations and tables in support of the text. These are further supported by off-line content such as videos. In short, *Cardiology for Veterinary Technicians and Nurses* delivers an all-in-one-place compendium on the subject. The volume will be useful to students in the midst of their technical and nursing education as well as those working on the front lines of patient and client care. Even veterinarians might find utility in the procedural details and equipment lists. This textbook should find a place on every veterinary hospital bookshelf, and I am pleased to advance this brief foreword to such an important work.

John D. Bonagura, DVM, MS, DACVIM (Cardiology & Internal Medicine)
Cardiologist, Cardiology and Interventional Medicine Service at
the Ohio State University Veterinary Medical Center
Professor Emeritus of Veterinary Clinical Sciences at The Ohio State University
College of Veterinary Medicine
Columbus, Ohio, USA

veterinary hospital bookshelf, and I am pleased to advance this brief foreword to such an important work.

John D. Bonagura, DVM, MS, DACVIM (Cardiology & Internal Medicine)
Cardiologist, Cardiology and Interventional Medicine Service at the Ohio State University Veterinary Medical Center
Professor Emeritus of Veterinary Clinical Sciences at The Ohio State University College of Veterinary Medicine
Columbus, Ohio, USA

List of Abbreviations

1HB/2HB/3HB	First/second/third degree heart block
2-D/3-D	Two- and three-dimensional
ABP	Arterial blood pressure
ACDO	Amplatz Canine Ductal Occluder
ACE	Angiotensin-converting enzyme
ACEI	Angiotensin-converting enzyme inhibitors
ACh	Acetylcholine
ACT	Activate clotting time
ACVIM	American College of Veterinary Internal Medicine
ADH	Antidiuretic hormone
ADP	Adenosine diphosphate
AF	Atrial fibrillation
AIVR	Accelerated idioventricular rhythm
AM	Atypical myocarditis
ANP	Atrial natriuretic peptide
AO	Aorta
APC	Atrial premature complex
APVC	Anterior portion of the caudal vena cava
APVC	Anterior caudal vena cava
ARB	Aldosterone receptor blockers
ARVC	Arrhythmogenic right ventricular cardiomyopathy
AS	Aortic stenosis
ASD	Atrial septal defect
ATE	Aortic/arterial thromboembolism
ATP	Adenosine triphosphate
AV	Aortic valve/atrioventricular
AVN	Atrioventricular node
BCS	Body condition score
BNP	Brain natriuretic peptide
BP	Blood pressure
bpm	Beats per minute

cAMP	Cyclic adenosine monophosphate
CBC	Complete blood count
CFM	Color-flow mapping
cGMP	Cyclic guanosine monophosphate
CHF	Congestive heart failure
CK-MB	Creatinine kinase muscle/brain
CO	Cardiac output
CRI	Constant rate infusion
CS	Coronary sinus
cTI	Cardiac troponin
CVA	Cerebrovascular incidents
CVC	Caudal vena cava
CVP	Central venous pressure
CW	Continuous wave
DA	Ductus arteriosus
DAO	Descending aorta
DAP	Diastolic arterial pressure
DCM	Dilated cardiomyopathy
DV	Dorsoventral
ECG	Electrocardiogram
EDHF	Endothelial-derived hyperpolarizing factor
EDV	End diastolic volume
EF	Ejection fraction
EOL	End of life
EPSS	End point to septal separation
ESPVR	End systolic pressure-volume relationship
ESV	End systolic volume
ET	Ejection time
FON	Furosemide, oxygen, nitroglycerin
FS	Fraction shortening
GFR	Glomerular filtration rate
HBM	Heart-based mass
HCM	Hypertrophic cardiomyopathy
HDO	High definition oscillometry
HOCM	Hypertrophic obstructive cardiomyopathy
HR	Heart rate
ICR	Implantable loop recorder
IVR	Isovolumic relaxation
IVS	Interventricular septum
IVCT	Isovolumic contraction time
JPC	Junctional premature complex

LA	Left arm/Left atrial/Left atrium
LAFB	Left anterior fascicle
LBB	Left bundle branch
LBBB	Left bundle branch block
LCA	Left coronary artery
LL	Left leg
LV	Left ventricle/ventricular
LVID	Left ventricular internal diameter
LVOT	Left ventricular outflow tract
LVPW	Left ventricular posterior wall
MAP	Mean arterial pressure
MEA	Mean electrical axis
MR	Mitral regurgitation
MV	Mitral valve
MVD	Mitral valve dysplasia
NE	Norepinephrine
NO	Nitric oxide
NT-proANP	N-terminal pro-atrial natriuretic peptide
PA	Pulmonary artery
PDA	Patent ductus arteriosus
PE	Pericardial effusion
PFO	Patent foramen ovale
PG	Pressure gradient
PHT	Pulmonary hypertension
PMI	Point of maximal intensity
PPVC	Posterior portion of the caudal vena cava
PRF	Pulse repetition frequency
PS	Pulmonic stenosis
PSS	Portosystemic shunt
PTE	Pulmonary thromboembolism
PV	Pulmonic valve
PVC	Posterior vena cava
PW	Pulsed wave (Doppler)
RA	Right arm/right atrial/right atrium
RAAS	Renin-angiotensin-aldosterone system
RBB	Right bundle branch
RBBB	Right bundle branch block
RCA	Right coronary artery
RCM	Restrictive cardiomyopathy
RL	Right leg
RV	Right ventricle/ventricular
RVOT	Right ventricular outflow tract

SA	Shortening area
SAM	Systolic anterior motion
SAN	Sino atrial node
SAP	Systolic arterial pressure
SAS	Subaortic stenosis
SNS	Sympathetic nervous system
SSS	Sick sinus syndrome
ST	Sinus tachycardia
SV	Stroke volume
SVR	Systemic vascular resistance
SVT	Supraventricular tachycardia
TEE	Transesophageal echocardiography
TGC	Time gain compensation
TN-C	Troponin C
TN-I	Troponin I
TN-T	Troponin T
TOF	Tetralogy of Fallot
TR	Tricuspid regurgitation
TV	Tricuspid valve
TVD	Tricuspid valve dysplasia
UA	Umbilical artery
UCM	Unclassified cardiomyopathy
UV	Umbilical vein
VD	Ventrodorsal
VEB	Ventricular escape beat
VF	Ventricular fibrillation
VMD	Veterinary Medical Database
VPC	Ventricular premature complex
VSD	Ventricular septal defect
VT	Ventricular tachycardia

Introduction: Why Animals have a Circulatory System

> I have endeavored to make the following tract as plain and as intelligible as I can; and if it should appear prolix to those who are already acquainted with the subject, I must beg leave to observe, that it was not written for their information; but if any of those who were unacquainted with it before should from hence gain any useful knowledge, my end will be answered, and I shall be very much pleased
>
> Percivall Pott: *Observations on That Disorder on the Corner of the Eye Commonly Called Fistula Lachrymalis*, London, 1759

The world of veterinary cardiology has undergone a rapid expansion in the last 50 years. Starting in the early 1960s with Drs. Patterson, Detweiller and Buchanan, who first began looking at congenital disease in dogs, and blossoming in the last few years with four-dimensional echocardiography, electrocardiographically gated computed tomography and new genetic testing research. At no other time has more been understood about the function and dysfunction of the cardiovascular system. As the state of the art grows, so does the need for highly trained paraprofessionals to assist the doctors who are pushing back the frontiers of veterinary cardiology and those putting their discoveries into practical application.

The field of veterinary cardiology has grown so rapidly that each year approximately 10 veterinarians specialize in cardiology. There are so many boarded cardiologists in the USA that there is shortage of highly trained specialized veterinary technicians. It is the hope of the author that this text will be a launch point for those veterinary technicians and nurses who wish to pursue specialization in veterinary cardiology, as well as for veterinary technical students and veterinary students, to explore this fascinating and expanding world. It should be stated at the beginning that this textbook is not designed to be an exhaustive tome of all cardiovascular knowledge, but rather a summary of many other outstanding textbooks, formulated into an easily manageable text to give the reader fundamental knowledge that will prepare them for deeper study into the subjects that interest them. The author also hopes that this text will be a quickly accessible resource to aid in answering common clinical questions faced by the cardiology veterinary technician specialist. The interested reader is encouraged to dig deeper into the particular areas of veterinary cardiology that interest them by accessing the textbooks cited in the references and bibliographies.

Cardiology for Veterinary Technicians and Nurses, First Edition. Edited by H. Edward Durham, Jr.

Cardiovascular medicine continues to advance and the current horizons will soon be distant memories as new knowledge of the circulation system evolves. As we explore this new world of veterinary cardiovascular medicine we can begin with basic questions.

Why have circulatory systems? How does a circulatory system aid the species? Why is it so complicated? I'd like to think that I was the first to ask these questions, but I know better. These are questions that have been asked by great physicians going back to Hippocrates or earlier. However, Dr Alan C. Burton made quite a delightful description in his classic book *Physiology and Biophysics of the Circulation* [1] with the invention of the Celestial Committee on the Design of a Mammalian Circulation (CCDMC). This imaginary committee would of course be charged with the task of designing the mammalian circulatory system.

If such a committee was to exist, they would be faced with several daunting tasks. First let us consider the definition of circulation. The CCDMC has put forth the following: "*The function of the circulation is to supply oxygen, metabolic fuels, vitamins and hormones, and heat to every living cell of the organism and also to remove metabolic end products (carbon dioxide, water etc.) and heat. The amount of circulation should be in accordance with the needs of each cell.*"

So an answer to the first question of WHY comes forth. Put in a very simplistic way, if you are a very simple animal, say an amoeba, then diffusion is an acceptable way to move nutrients in and waste material out of the organism. *Diffusion,* of course is the passive transfer of molecules from an area of high concentration to low concentration across a permeable or semipermeable barrier. Unfortunately, if you are a very large animal, say a horse, then it is much more difficult to move enough nutrients in and waste out by diffusion alone. Diffusion is not efficient enough to work over long distances and multiple cell layers seen in complex organisms. A circulatory system allows the organism to carry nutrients to the cell directly where diffusion can work at the local cellular level and will pick up waste products from the cells and carry them to a disposal area to be eliminated from the body. By use of a circulatory system to move a viscous fluid (blood) to improve diffusion and heat exchange, large and biologically diverse organisms can be sustained.

With this definition as a starting point, we can begin to elaborate some of the challenges that would need to be overcome. How much flow does each tissue need? What determines these requirements? Do the needs of a tissue group change over time? What are the possible methods of making circulation work and what are the physical limitations? What methods are available for controlling the circulation? Of course the answers to these questions are interlocking.

The first thing to consider are the individual needs of the different tissues. It makes sense that different tissues need different amounts of nutrients, and/or waste removal at different times. At the same time, it is inefficient to simply supply the same amount of blood to all the tissues as required by the neediest. Consequently, some form of control or regulation is required. Certain tissues, like the brain and the heart that have critical functions, need some priority so that their blood supply remains constant at all times. Other tissues have varying requirements and different times. For example, during exercise the skeletal muscles would need more perfusion than the gut; after eating the reverse is true. Also we cannot forget the need to balance heat, as indicated in our definition of a circulatory system previously. Muscles and organs under work generate heat that must be removed from the body, to maintain the core body temperature. Temperature also has a large impact on metabolism. Remember that at higher temperatures, metabolism increases and decreases with a reduction in temperature. Maintaining the optimal temperature for cellular metabolism becomes crucial for proper function of the organs.

Another consideration is the function or task of the organ in question. Lungs and kidneys for example are organs that eliminate waste (in the case of the lungs, to pick up nutrients also). Their individual metabolic requirements are actually quite small, but if they do not receive a large amount of flow then they cannot effectively rid the blood of waste products. Although the critical importance of the organ alone is insufficient for dictating its required blood flow, the ability of an organ to continue its work in the face of diminished or even a terminated supply of nutrients or its "functional reserve" also plays into the equation. Tissues such a skin or skeletal muscle can continue to function in a state of "oxygen debt" and are said to have a high functional reserve. They will continue to function on anaerobic metabolism, allowing necessary blood to be shunted to organs with less of a functional reserve, like the brain, which has a low functional reserve. It becomes clear that a system that can change the volume of flow to a specific area at any given time is needed.

One of the limitations is that the tissues require a constant supply of nutrients, which means that the system must also function continuously. A second limitation is the physical properties that govern the movement of fluids. The most important of these is *Darcy's Law of Flow.* Darcy's Law states that flow (Q), that is volume of liquid moved over a period of time, is equal to the difference in pressure from one space to another in which it moves (P_1-P_2) divided by the resistance (R) to that flow (expressed mathematically: $Q= P_1-P_2/R$). This rule of physics is fundamental to regulating flow in all environs. There are other factors that affect flow, such as viscosity, but an in-depth discussion of these factors is beyond the scope of this text. With these concepts in mind, we can see that a simple solution to these problems is to provide a constant perfusion pressure. This means keeping the P_1 and the P_2 of Darcy's Law at the same pressure no matter the volume of blood moving to a tissue. By keeping the maximal flow the same to all tissues at all times, a constant perfusion pressure could be maintained, but we have already stated that as inefficient. So how can one provide the right amount of perfusion to the areas in need and yet maintain a constant perfusion pressure throughout the system?

The answer to this question involves two components: a pump and a series of conduction tubes to move the fluid to the cells. The heart in its essence is a very elaborate pump; actually two pumps in parallel. It has the ability to change its rate of pumping (*chronotropy)* and how hard it pumps (*inotropy*) providing sufficient output to maintain a constant flow of blood to the whole body or reducing flow when at rest to conserve energy. Additionally the heart has some stretch ability that allows it to increase the volume it will hold and consequently pump out changing volumes (*stroke volume*).

The conduction tubes are a complex system of arteries to carry blood away from the heart and use a similar system of veins to return blood to the heart. These veins and arteries are possessed of smooth muscle in places that can serve to open or close the vessels. In doing so, the arteries and their relative degree of openness constitute the resistance the heart pumps into. This total peripheral resistance is the "R" of Darcy's Law. The pressure difference across the capillary bed can be maintained by controlling either the flow or the resistance.

The pump is controlled by two mechanisms: first by the nervous system and second by humoral vasoactive substances. The sympathetic nervous system can directly increase heart rate while the parasympathetic system slows it. Hormones like adrenalin, thyroxine or angiotensin can also increase heart rate.

Similarly, the vasculature can be affected at large by the nervous system and hormonal influences. Fine control of perfusion pressure can be accomplished by allowing some local control of the dilation or constriction of vessels. This allows organs in immediate need to have some influence over their own blood flow. Waste products like carbon dioxide, nitric oxide and lactic acid can have direct vasodilatory effects on the surrounding tissue allowing tissue to increase their own amount of perfusion.

All in all, what we are dealing with is a sophisticated pumping and transport system that meet the requirements of the CCDMC's definition, which is energy efficient, allows for some local control, can dramatically increase performance based on need and will run for an extended period of time. In this overly simplified description, we can begin to see the fascinating underpinnings of cardiology. It is hoped that the reader will gain not only valuable knowledge from this text but also an appreciation of the intricate workings of the heart and how it carries out its mission. Of all the organ systems, the heart alone must work for a lifetime without a holiday or if all the other systems fail. It is truly a remarkable organ indeed.

Reference

1 Burton, A.C. (1972) *Physiology and Biophysics of the Circulation.* Chicago Year Book Medical Publishers Inc., Chicago.

Section I

Cardiac Anatomy and Physiology

1

Cardiac Anatomy

H. Edward Durham, Jr.

Fetal Circulation and Transition to Adult Circulation

Any study of cardiology begins with a complete and thorough understanding of the anatomy of the heart and its physiology. Understanding the arrhythmias, the cardiac disease process, congenital heart conditions and mechanisms of treatment all stem from a working knowledge of the cardiac anatomy and physiology. The general arrangement of the circulatory system is two circuits in series; two separate circulatory paths where the end of one feeds into the beginning of the other. However, the circulation did not start out this way.

In the fetus, circulation is a double circulation in parallel or two circulatory paths that cross over each other at strategic areas to incorporate placental blood flow and bypass the unused lungs (Figure 1.1). As highly oxygenated blood enters the fetus from the placental vein (*vein* because it carries blood toward the heart), it passes through the liver where it mixes with the deoxygenated blood of the lower body. From here it travels to the right atrium and is shunted almost directly into the left atrium. At this point, there is very little mixing with deoxygenated blood from the head and forelimbs due to the anatomic proximity of the posterior vena cava to the fossa ovalis, which channels the blood almost directly into the left atrium. This blood is still highly oxygenated and travels to the left ventricle and out of the aorta. At this stage, further mixing occurs, with some highly oxygenated blood travelling to the head and some mixing with deoxygenated blood from the right ventricle via the pulmonary artery and then the ductus arteriosus. This mixed blood then travels to the lower body and to the placenta to be remixed into the maternal circulation. It still carries enough oxygen to supply the lower extremities with all the nutrition that is needed. The highly oxygenated blood from the left ventricle flows directly to the head and forelimbs to ensure a highly oxygenated blood supply to the developing brain. Deoxygenated blood from the head and forelimbs then returns to the right atrium of the fetal heart and out of the pulmonary artery to mix as previously described. The circulation continues in this manner until birth.

During the last phases of cardiac development, as the atrial septum develops, the fossa ovalis transforms into the foramen ovale (Figure 1.2). The foramen ovale develops as a one-way valve through the interarterial septum that allows oxygenated blood to pass from the right atrium to the left, as the fossa ovalis did. The valve eventually closes to stop blood from shunting from the left atrium to the right in the adult.

Cardiology for Veterinary Technicians and Nurses, First Edition. Edited by H. Edward Durham, Jr.

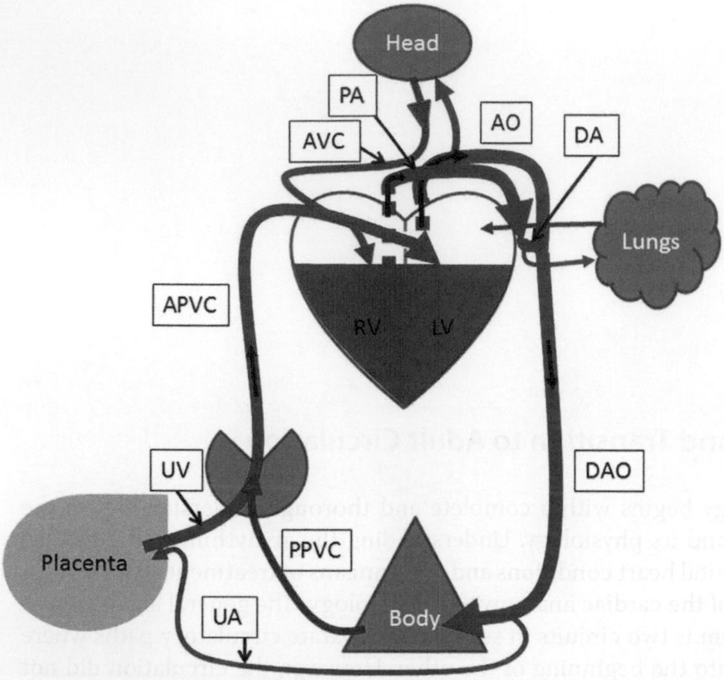

Figure 1.1 A simplified schematic of circulation in the fetus. Oxygenated blood enters the fetal circulation from the *umbilical vein* (UV) via the *ductus venosus* into the anterior portion of the *caudal vena cava* (APVC) in the liver. The oxygenated blood travels to the *right atrium* where the majority is shunted through the *foramen ovale* to the *left atrium* then into the *left ventricle* (LV). A small portion mixes with venous blood returning from the head, then travels to the *right ventricle* (RV). During fetal cardiac systole, the mixed oxygenated/deoxygenated blood from the right ventricle is pumped into the *main pulmonary artery* (PA) through the *ductus arteriosus* (DA) and into the descending *aorta* (DAO). A very small portion of this mixed blood bypasses the ductus arteriosus and enters the pulmonary arterial system (PA) to provide oxygen to the lung tissue and returns to the left atrium though the *pulmonary veins*. Simultaneously, the fully oxygenated maternal blood is pumped from the left ventricle into the aorta (AO), up the carotid arteries to the cranial fetus, as well as to the caudal portion of the fetus. The blood delivered to the cranial fetus has the most oxygen content; while the blood delivered to the caudal fetus carries less oxygen because of the mixing that occurs in the descending aorta distal to the ductus arteriosus. Although this blood has less oxygen than the cranial blood, it will still deliver sufficient oxygen to the caudal fetus to nourish the tissue before passing through the caudal capillary vessels and returning though the posterior portion of the caudal vena cava (PPVC) to the liver. Blood from the fetus is returned to the placenta through the umbilical artery (UA), which exits the fetal circulation at the iliac arteries. Red, fully oxygenated blood. Purple, mostly deoxygenated blood. Red–Purple, mixed oxygenated/deoxygenated blood. AVC, anterior caudal vena cava.

It is at parturition and shortly thereafter that two systems in series finally develop. This process starts with the first breath, which drops pulmonary vascular resistance dramatically. Simultaneously, the placental circulation is removed, which increases systemic vascular resistance and reverses the blood flow through the ductus arteriosus to move blood from the aorta to the pulmonary artery. The tissue of the ductus arteriosus is highly sensitive to oxygen. When exposed to the increased oxygen content of the arterial blood in the aorta, the musculature of the ductus arteriosus constricts and closes

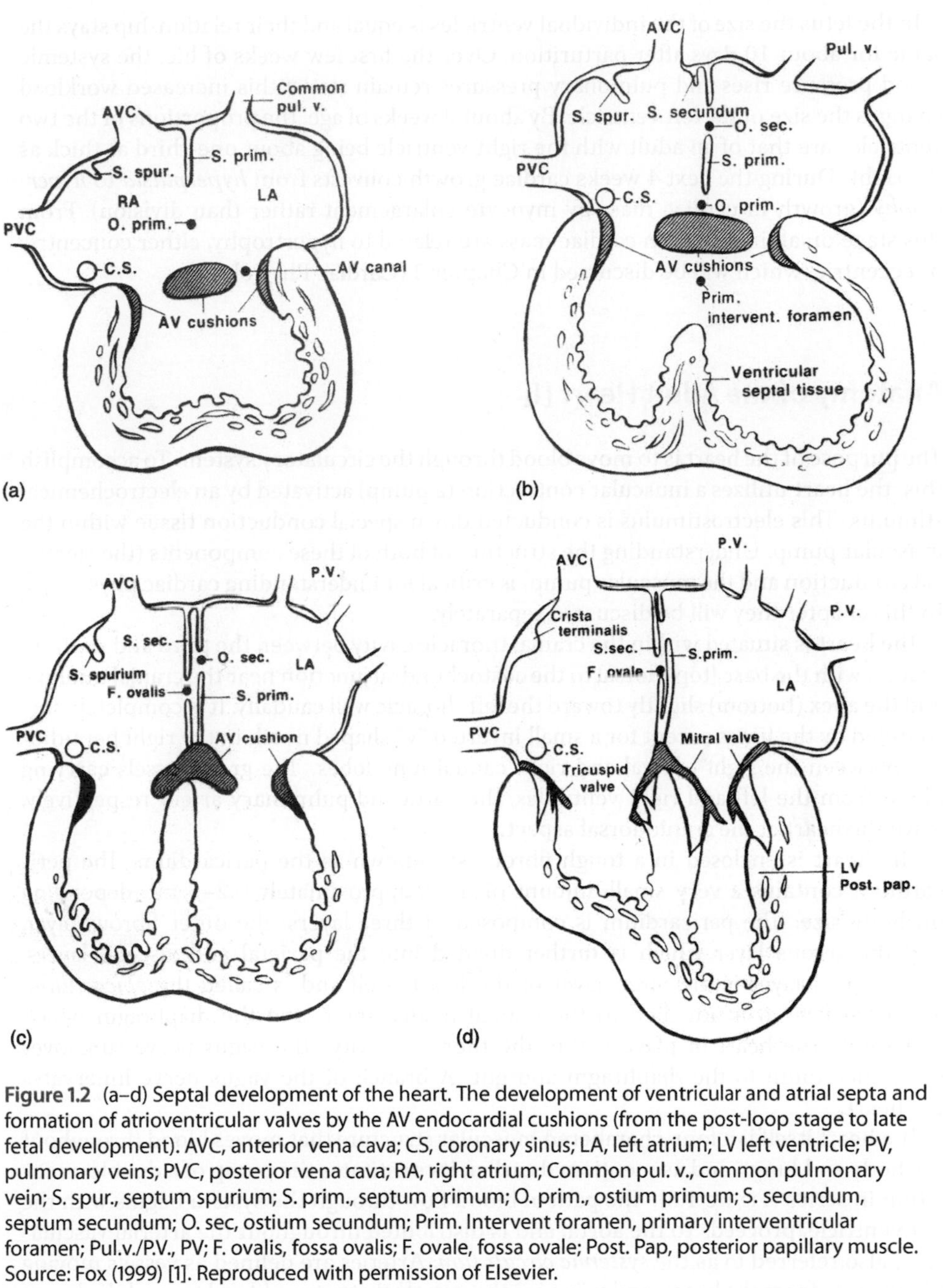

Figure 1.2 (a–d) Septal development of the heart. The development of ventricular and atrial septa and formation of atrioventricular valves by the AV endocardial cushions (from the post-loop stage to late fetal development). AVC, anterior vena cava; CS, coronary sinus; LA, left atrium; LV left ventricle; PV, pulmonary veins; PVC, posterior vena cava; RA, right atrium; Common pul. v., common pulmonary vein; S. spur., septum spurium; S. prim., septum primum; O. prim., ostium primum; S. secundum, septum secundum; O. sec, ostium secundum; Prim. Intervent foramen, primary interventricular foramen; Pul.v./P.V., PV; F. ovalis, fossa ovalis; F. ovale, fossa ovale; Post. Pap, posterior papillary muscle. Source: Fox (1999) [1]. Reproduced with permission of Elsevier.

the communication. The net effect of these changes is to decrease the volume of blood flowing through the right side of the heart and increase it in the left. These changes cause the pressure in the left atrium to increase which functionally closes the foramen ovale and finally separates the two circulations.

In the fetus the size of the individual ventricles is equal and their relationship stays the same for about 10 days after parturition. Over the first few weeks of life, the systemic blood pressure rises and pulmonary pressures remain static; this increased workload changes the size of the left ventricle. By about 2 weeks of age, the proportions of the two ventricles are that of an adult with the right ventricle being about one-third as thick as the right. During the next 4 weeks cardiac growth converts from *hyperplasia* to *hypertrophy* (growth in cardiac mass by myocyte enlargement rather than division). From this stage on all increases in cardiac mass are related to hypertrophy, either concentric or eccentric, which will be discussed in Chapter 2 (Cardiac Physiology).

Anatomy of the Adult Heart [1]

The purpose of the heart is to move blood through the circulatory system. To accomplish this, the heart utilizes a muscular contraction (a pump) activated by an electrochemical stimulus. This electrostimulus is conducted down special conduction tissue within the muscular pump. Understanding the structure of both of these components (the electrical conduction and the muscular pump) is critical for understanding cardiac physiology. In this chapter they will be discussed separately.

The heart is situated within the cranial thoracic cavity between the third and sixth rib spaces, with the base (top) dorsal to the costochondral junction near the cranial midline, and the apex (bottom) slightly toward the left thoracic wall caudally. It is completely surrounded by the lungs except for a small inverted "v" shaped notch in the right hemithorax between the right cranial and right caudal lung lobes. The great vessels carrying blood from the left and right ventricles, the aorta and pulmonary artery respectively, leave the heart at the craniodorsal aspect.

The heart is enclosed in a tough fibrous sac known as the pericardium. The pericardium contains a very small amount of fluid; approximately 0.2–5 mL depending on body size. The pericardium is composed of three layers: the outer fibrous layer, and the serous layer which is further divided into the parietal and visceral layers. The visceral layer is the outer layer of the heart itself and is called the *epicardium.* The pericardium is attached to the cranial mediastinum and the diaphragm which helps hold the heart in place within the thoracic cavity. The vagus nerve runs over the pericardium to the diaphragm and gut. A branch of the vagus nerve innervates the heart.

The heart itself is a four-chambered muscular structure that moves blood throughout the body and lungs, and as mentioned earlier, it constitutes the pump of a double circulation in series (Figure 1.3). The path of blood flow through the system begins with the left ventricle, proceeds to the aorta, and is distributed throughout the arterial vasculature, also referred to as the *systemic circulation.* Arteries are defined as vessels moving blood away from the heart, and veins are the vessels that return blood toward the heart. Blood then moves into progressively smaller arteries, arterioles and eventually into the capillaries to transfer nutrients and oxygen to the tissues. Also in the capillary system, waste byproducts of metabolism are collected and transported away from the tissues. The blood is then moved into venous capillaries, venules and finally to larger veins to be carried back to the heart through systemic veins.

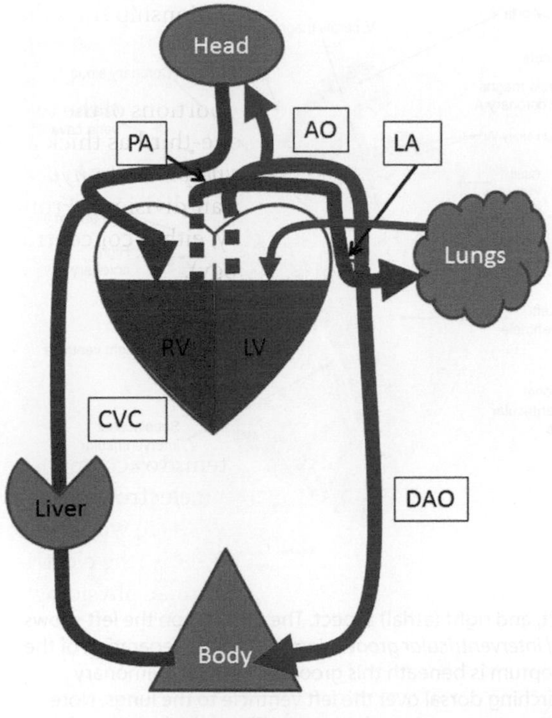

Figure 1.3 Post-parturition circulation. Starting in the left ventricle (LV), blood is ejected past the aortic valve and into the ascending aorta during ventricular systole. This oxygenated blood is distributed to the organs and tissues through the branching of the systemic arterial system from the aorta (AO). The first branches off the aorta are the left subclavian and common carotid arteries, exiting at the aortic arch, in most mammalian species. The other arteries exit the aorta from the descending aorta (DAO). As the oxygenated blood distributes through the body it passes through the arterioles then finally into the capillaries of each individual tissue. In the capillaries, oxygen is delivered and carbon dioxide is taken up. The blood then travels back toward the right atrium via the venous capillaries, venules and eventually veins, which drain in the venae cavae. There are two venae cavae in mammals; the cranial vena cava, and the caudal vena cava (CVC), which both return deoxygenated blood to the right atrium. During ventricular diastole, the deoxygenated blood passes through the tricuspid valve into the right ventricle (RV). From the right ventricle the blood is pumped into the lungs through the pulmonary artery (PA) where carbon dioxide is released through the blood–gas barrier in the alveoli and oxygen is taken up. After parturition the ductus arteriosus closes becoming the ligamentum arteriosum (LA), allowing blood to circulate through the pulmonary vasculature. The newly oxygenated blood is returned to the left atrium through the pulmonary veins. Blood then moves from the left atrium to the left ventricle past the mitral valve during ventricular diastole, to start the cycle anew.

The heart is divided along its long axis by two septa, the *interventricular*, that divides the ventricles or pumping chambers and the *interatrial* that divides the atria, the receiving chambers. The heart is additionally divided transversely by two valves that direct flow from the atria to the ventricles.

In viewing the exterior of the heart, multiple structures can be readily identified. From the ventral surface the auricular appendages are pointing at the observer. The right atrial appendage is more prominent than the left since the right atrium is positioned more to the dextrolateral aspect of the heart and the left is positioned more to the posterior. The

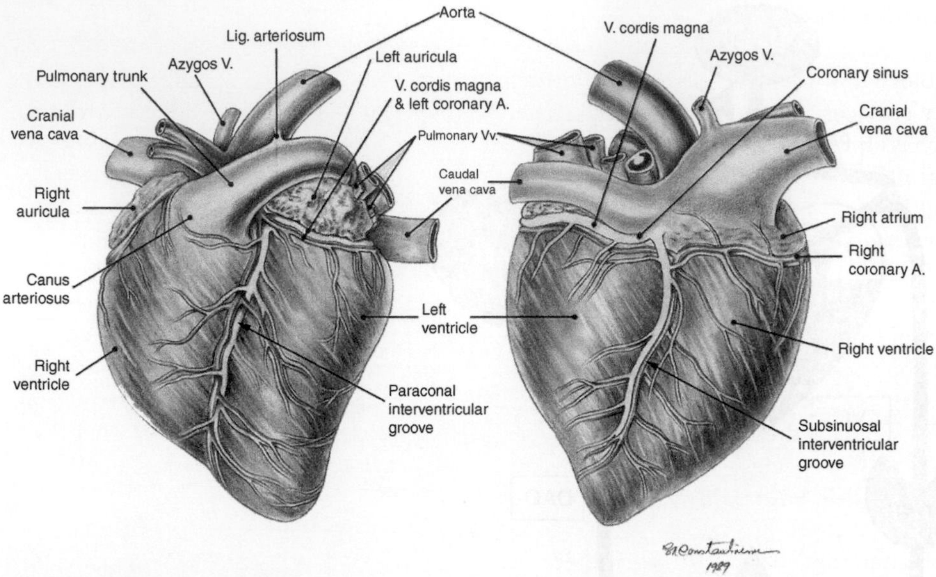

Figure 1.4 A horse heart: left (auricular) aspect, and right (atrial) aspect. The drawing on the left shows the ventral surface of the heart. The *paraconal interventricular groove* demarcates the separation of the right and left ventricles. The interventricular septum is beneath this groove. The main pulmonary artery can be seen exiting the right ventricle arching dorsal over the left ventricle to the lungs. Note the *ligamentous arteriosum* connecting the pulmonary artery and the aorta. This is the location of the *ductus arteriosus* in the fetus. The illustration on the right depicts the dorsal aspect of the heart. Notable features include the cranial and caudal vena cavae, and the coronary sinus. Azygos V., azygos vein; Lig. arteriosum, ligmentous arteriosum; V. cordis magna and left coronary A., vena cordis magna and left coronary artery; Pulmonary Vv., pulmonary veins; V. cordis magna, vena cordis magna; Right coronary A., right coronary artery. Source: courtesy of Constantinescue (1991) [3].

left coronary artery is apparent coursing toward the apex of the heart in the paraconal groove separating the right and left ventricles (Figure 1.4). Several smaller branches of the left coronary artery can also be appreciated. The cardiac apex consists of the bottom portion of the left ventricle divided from the right ventricle along the paraconal groove. Running parallel with the left coronary artery is the great coronary vein. Cranial to the paraconal groove is the right ventricular outflow tract leading to the pulmonary artery. The aorta exits the heart at the central cranial aspect.

From the dorsal surface the other coronary arteries can be seen, including the circumflex branch of the left coronary artery and the subsinousal interventricular branch. The cranial and caudal vena cava can be identified entering the right atrium. The four pulmonary veins returning blood from the lungs entering the left atrium are also noted just above the coronary sinus as it traverses the heart bringing blood from the left ventricle to the right atrium (Figure 1.4). From this view the left auricle is seen beneath the pulmonary trunk, as well as the posterior portion of the right atrium as it extends laterally then anteriorly.

Internal Structure

Histologically, the heart is made up of three layers: the *endocardium,* which lines the inner surfaces, the *myocardium* which is the muscular portion, and the *epicardium* which is also the visceral pericardium. The heart has a fibrous "skeleton" that helps form the structure at the base of the heart and insulates the atrial tissue from ventricular tissue electrically. In doing so, all supraventricular electrical impulses are directed into the atrioventricular (AV) node of the conduction system which will be discussed on p. 17. The fibrous skeleton also forms the framework from which the valves are attached. The formation of the *AV fibrous rings, aortic fibrous ring* and the *pulmonic fibrous ring* create the annulus for each valve, to which the valve leaflets are attached (Figure 1.5).

At the top of the heart, cranial to the valves, are the right and left atria. The atria function as the collecting chambers that hold blood during ventricular systole to fill the ventricle during the next ventricular diastole. Both atria are thin walled (0.5–2 mm thick depending on species and breed) and have auricular appendages that project ventrally which are lined with pectinate muscles.

The left atrium receives oxygenated blood returning from the pulmonary circulation via the pulmonary veins of which there are typically four to six. The inflow to the left

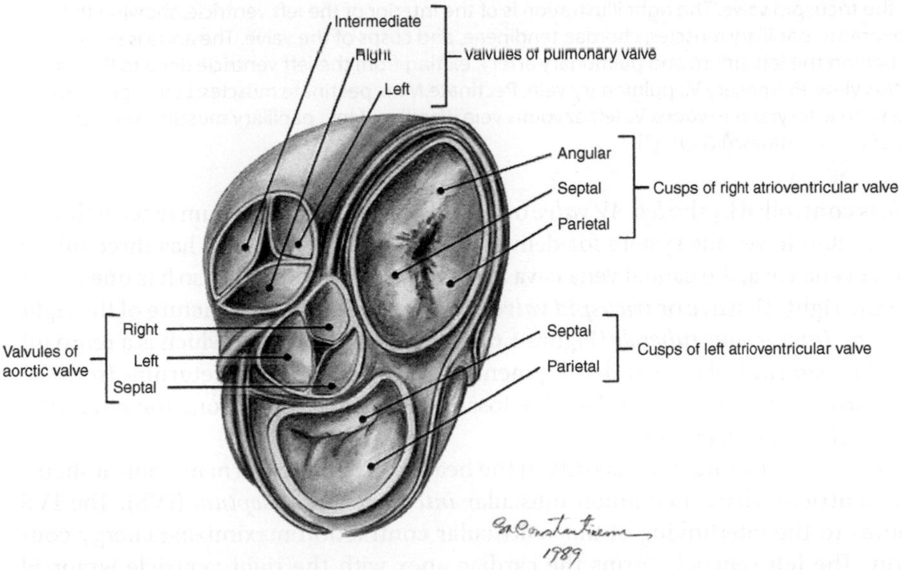

Figure 1.5 A horse heart: atrioventricular and arterial valves and the individual cusps of the four cardiac valves. This view of the heart shows the dorsal aspect of the ventricle, with the atria removed at the level of the valve orifices. Using the clock face analogy: the tricuspid valve is at 6 o'clock, the pulmonic valve is at 9 o'clock to 10 o'clock, the mitral valve runs from around 1 o'clock to around 3 o'clock. The aortic valve is situated in the middle. The inlet and outlet of the right ventricle are further apart than the inlet and outlet of the left ventricle, which are in extreme proximity. Individual leaflets or *cusps*, of the valves are labeled. The coronary arteries can be seen exiting from the near aortic valve; the *right main* coronary artery coming off at ~9 o'clock, and the *left main* coronary artery from ~12 o'clock. Source: courtesy of Constantinescu (1991) [3].

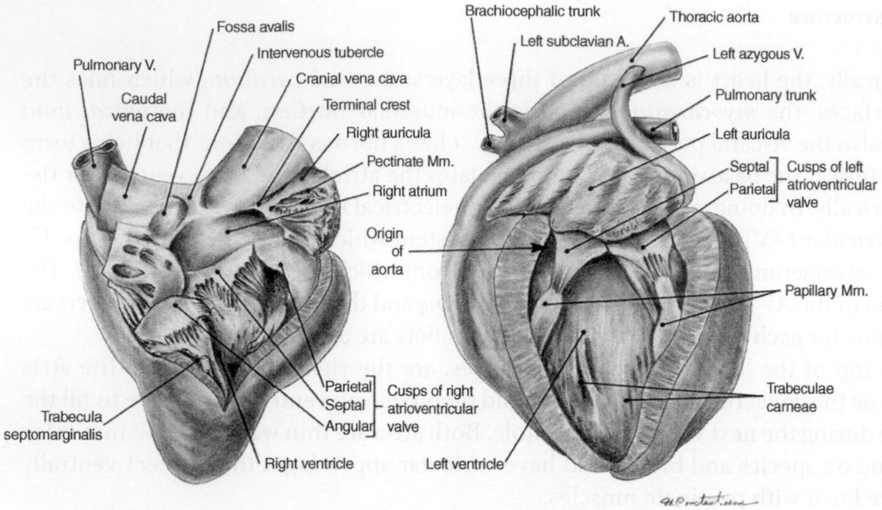

Figure 1.6 Interior of a pig heart with the right ventricle opened, and left ventricle opened. The left image shows the right ventricle open to reveal the interior structures. The right atrium is also open to show the interior of the right atrium and vena cavae. The individual features are labeled including the cusps of the tricuspid valve. The right illustration is of the interior of the left ventricle, showing the mitral apparatus; papillary muscles, chordae tendineae, and cusps of the valve. The aorta is seen running behind the left atrium and pulmonary artery, exiting from the left ventricle deep to the mitral valve in this view. Pulmonary V., pulmonary vein; Pectinate Mm., pectinate muscles; Left subclavian A., left subclavian artery; Left azygous V., left azygous vein; Papillary Mm., papillary muscles. Source: courtesy of Constantinescu (1991) [3].

ventricle is controlled by the *left AV valve* or *mitral valve.* The right atrium receives blood from the systemic venous system for delivery to the right ventricle. It has three inlets: the cranial vena cava, the caudal vena cava and the coronary sinus. It also has one outlet through the right *AV valve* or *tricuspid valve.* Another noteworthy structure of the right atrium is the *intervenous tubercle* (Figure 1.6); a small ridge of tissue which is a remnant of the *septum spurium* of cardiac development and helps direct blood returning from the vena cava toward the tricuspid valve. The fossa ovalis can be seen along the interatrial septum, on the right atrial side.

The ventricles constitute the majority of the heart and together form its conical shape. The two ventricles share a common muscular *interventricular septum* (IVS). The IVS contributes to the interlinking of the ventricular contraction maximizing energy consumption. The left ventricle forms the cardiac apex with the right ventricle wrapped around it. The left ventricle normally has the greater mass. The left ventricular inflow and outflow tracts are in extreme proximity with the anterior leaflet of the mitral valve separating the two during diastole making a cone like configuration; in contrast to the right ventricle in which the inflow portion and the outflow tract are at opposite ends of the "U" shape of the ventricle, creating a crescent shaped chamber "wrapping around" the left ventricle. The left ventricle is situated caudodorsal to the right.

The left ventricle is the high pressure system of the two circulations as it moves blood from the low pressure of the pulmonary system to the relativity high pressure of the systemic circulation. The free wall is approximately two-and-a-half to three times the thickness of the right ventricular free wall; left ventricular diastolic wall thicknesses range from 0.5 cm in small breed dogs to 1.0 cm or more in giant breeds. The left ventricle contains, within its lumen, papillary muscles with attached *chordae tendineae* leading to the mitral valve (Figure 1.6). Two papillary muscles are most common, but split or triple papillary muscles are not uncommon. The papillary muscles project from the apical portion of the ventricle toward the AV valves. The chordae tendineae are fibrous strands that attach the papillary muscles to the mitral valve leaflets. Blood flow into the ventricle enters via the mitral valve and exits out of the aorta. Forward flow is maintained by closure of the mitral valve during systole and closure of the aortic valve during diastole. The area immediately leading to the aortic valve narrows, forming a funnel shape, and is known as the left ventricular outflow tract.

The right ventricle pumps blood from the systemic venous circulation to the lungs. Along the inner surface of the right ventricle are muscular ridges known as *trabeculae carnae,* which are not typically present in the left ventricle. Papillary muscles and chordae tendineae are also attached to the tricuspid valve from the apex of the right ventricle. Additionally, *trabecilae septomarginalis* or moderator bands may at times be seen traversing the right ventricle. These thin bands of tissue often contain conduction tissue and can lead to the free wall or papillary muscles. They can also be present in the left ventricle.

The four cardiac valves (Figure 1.5) control the direction of blood flow through the heart. The right and left AV valves are also known as the tricuspid and mitral valves respectively. *Semilunar valve* is a term sometimes used to refer to the ventricular outflow valves collectively due to the half-moon shape of their cusps. The left ventricular outflow valve is the *aortic valve,* and the right ventricular is the *pulmonic valve.*

The AV valves are more accurately a valve apparatus, consisting of several components. The valve annulus is the anchor point for the valve leaflets or *cusps* and is part of the fibrous skeleton of the heart. The leaflets physically retard blood flow when they are closed. The cusps are attached on their ventricular surface to papillary muscles by the chordae tendineae. During systole, the papillary muscles contract, tightening the chordae tendineae and keeping the cusps closed against the rising ventricular pressure. If any of these components are damaged then the function of the valve may be compromised.

The mitral valve is the more robust of the two AV valves, and unless diseased is able to remain competent under pressures over 200 mmHg. It is sometimes referred to as the *bicuspid* valve since it has two leaflets: an anterior leaflet that is nearly contiguous with the aortic valve and a posterior leaflet attached near the left ventricular free wall. During systole the mitral valve prevents blood from the left ventricle flowing into the left atrium. This also protects the pulmonary venous circulation from the relatively high pressures of the left ventricle during systole.

The tricuspid valve of the right heart is similar to the mitral valve in that it also has two leaflets. The term “tricuspid” is borrowed from human medicine to indicate the right AV valve; although in some dogs an extra smaller cusp of tissue can be appreciated. The tricuspid valve is suitably strong to withstand normal right ventricular pressure (25–35 mmHg systolic) but will often become incompetent at pressures much above this.

Semilunar valves have a fibrous annulus and three cusps, but do not have associated chordae tendineae or papillary muscles. In the pulmonic valve the cusps are named *right, left* and *septal semilunar* cusps; for the aortic they are called *right coronary, left coronary* and *non-coronary* cusps (Figure 1.5). They are operated by the flow of blood through their associated vessels. As blood is ejected from the ventricle the valves open, then as flow ceases and the residual pressure in the great vessels allows blood to flow backward toward the ventricle, the valves close from this pressure. This closure stops the blood from returning to the ventricle and in doing so maintains a diastolic pressure in the circulation necessary for a pressure gradient across the capillary bed while allowing left ventricular pressure to fall to zero or below.

The great vessels carry blood from the heart beyond the semilunar valves. The aorta transports blood from the left ventricle to the systemic circulation of the body. The pulmonary artery carries blood from the right ventricle to the lungs or pulmonary circulation. The aorta leaves the cranial aspect of the ventricle from the center of the heart (*ascending aorta*) and arches (*aortic arch*) toward the caudal body running down the length of the torso along the spine (*descending aorta*). Branches exit the aorta along the arch to supply blood to the head and forelimbs. The number and configuration of these branches varies among species, but typically a *left subclavian trunk* and *brachiocephalic* branches are typically the first two major arteries to exit the aorta (Figure 1.7). Proximal

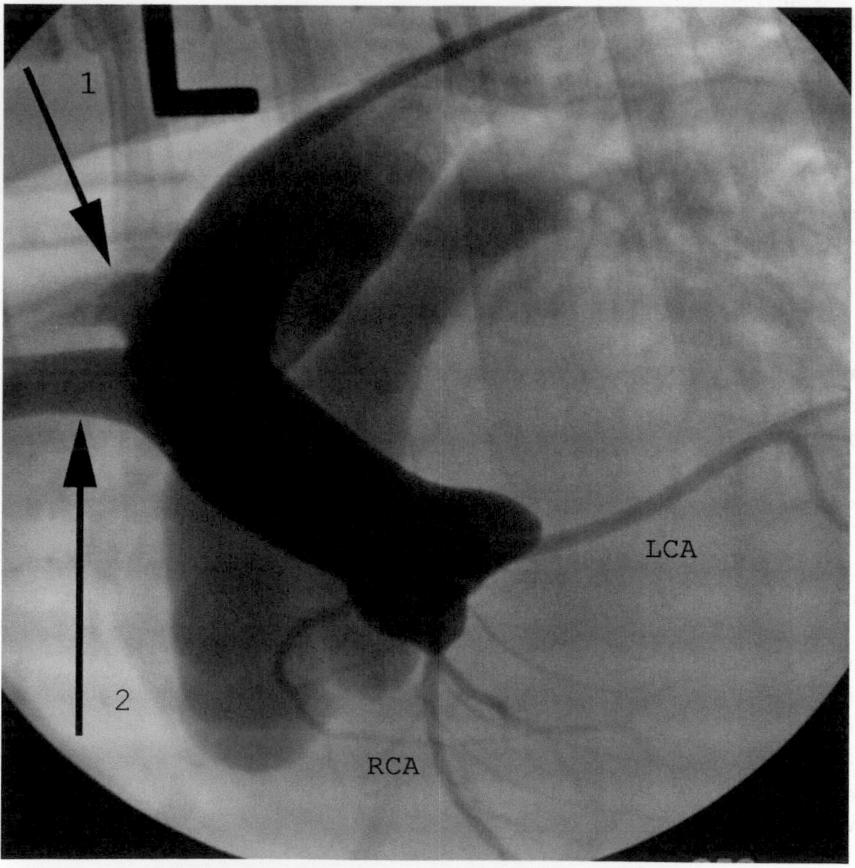

Figure 1.7 A contrast angiogram of the proximal aorta and its arteries. The left subclavian artery (arrow 1) and brachiocephalic trunk (arrow 2) bifurcate from the aorta at the craniodorsal aortic arch. The left coronary artery (LCA) and the right coronary artery. (RCA) can be seen exiting the aortic sinuses, demarcating the outer edge of the respective ventricles.

to the arch, the aorta widens just distal to the valve itself forming the *aortic sinuses* from which the coronary arteries arise (Figures 1.5 and 1.7).

The pulmonary artery exits the right ventricle on the craniodorsal aspect of the heart and branches into two large arteries that carry blood to the right and left set of lungs (Figure 1.4). The section from the pulmonic valve to the bifurcation is called the *main pulmonary artery* and each branch is named for which lung group it feeds; the *right pulmonary artery* or *left pulmonary artery.* Just proximal to the bifurcation the *ligamentum arteriosum* can be seen attached to the aorta, where these two vessels cross at nearly right angles. This structure is the remnant of the *ductus arteriosus* seen in the fetal circulation.

Cardiac Conduction System

An important part of cardiology and cardiac anatomy is the electrical conduction system of the heart (Figure 1.8). This specialized tissue within the heart allows for very rapid yet controlled depolarization of the myocardium. The cells that make up the

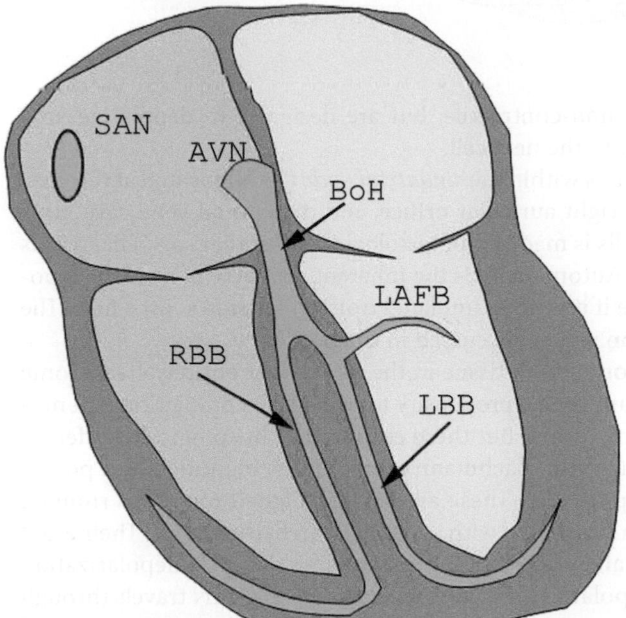

Figure 1.8 The cardiac conduction system. The sinoatrial node (SAN) is located in the right atrial wall. This cluster of cells has the fastest automaticity and generally drives the intrinsic heart rate. The SA node is innervated by both the sympathetic and parasympathetic nervous systems. The atrioventricular node (AVN) is located at the posteroventral region of the interatrial septum near the opening of the coronary sinus. This location puts it very close to the ventricle. The depolarization impulse is transferred through the fibrocardiac skeleton via the bundle of His (BoH). The bundle of His then divides into the right bundle branch (RBB) and the left bundle branch (LBB), which further splits off to a left anterior fascicle branch (LAFB) and a left posterior fascicle (not shown). Image courtesy of Virginia Luis-Fuentes, MRCVS, DACVIM.

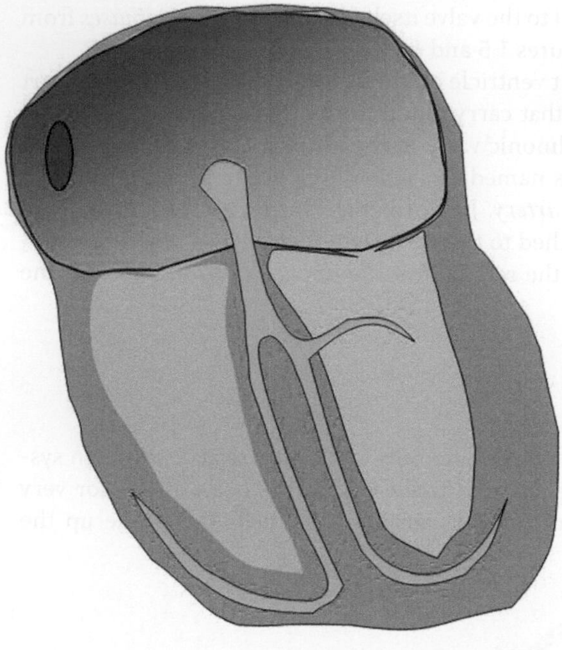

Figure 1.9 Atrial depolarization, showing the atria in red as the depolarization waves move from the sinoatrial node across the atrial wall and toward the atrioventricular node. Image courtesy of Virginia Luis-Fuentes, MRCVS, DACVIM.

cardiac conduction system are non-contractile, but are designed to depolarize very rapidly, transmitting the current to the next cell.

Cardiac depolarization originates within the *sinoatrial node* (SAN) located at the confluence of the right atrium, the right auricular orifice, and the cranial vena cava. This small wedge-shaped group of cells is made up of histologically discreet specialized cells that demonstrate *automaticity*. Automaticity is the inherent property of a cell to depolarize itself over a period of time if it is not stimulated from an outside source first. The exact mechanism of this function will be discussed in Chapter 2.

The presence of specialized conduction tissue in the atria is not entirely clear. Some cells within the atrial myocardium have a propensity for electrical conduction and may serve as functional conductive pathways, but these cells are not histologically different than the other atrial myocardium. The Bachmann's Bundle was identified as a potential interatrial conduction group of cells. These are parallel aligned myocytes running between the atria, and have been associated with some atrial arrhythmias [2]. Their exact role and function is controversial, but they may assist moving the SAN depolarization through the atrial tissue. The depolarization wave generated by the SAN travels through the atrial myocardium spreading outward throughout the tissue and is re-concentrated at the AV node (Figure 1.9).

The ventricles have a complex conduction system that begins with the AV node (Figure 1.10). The AV node is situated just at the top of the ventricles in the intra-atrial septum, as it attaches to the ventricles. This mass of Purkinje cells conducts the depolarization wave somewhat slower than the rest of the conduction system. This allows for all the depolarization waves of the atria to collect in the AV node before passing through the fibrous skeleton to the faster conduction of the *bundle of His* or *common AV bundle*. The bundle of His then divides into the bundle branches near the top of the inner ventricular

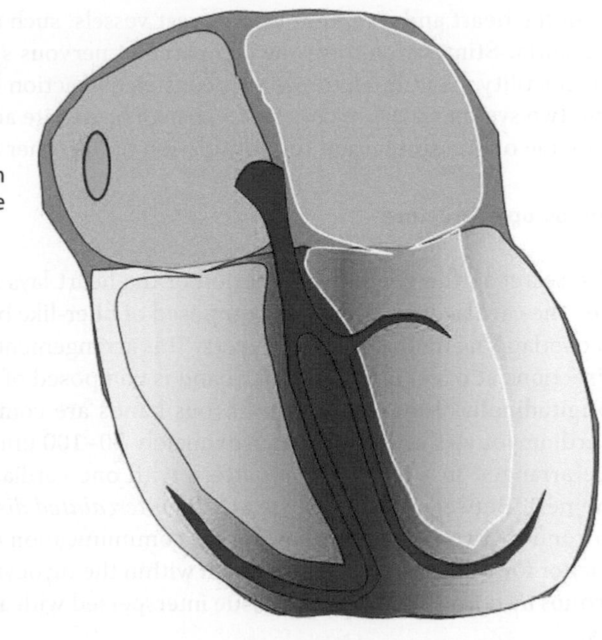

Figure 1.10 Ventricular depolarization, showing the depolarization of the bundle branches in red as the impulse is conducted out of the bundle branches to the ventricular Purkinje fibers, then to the myocytes. The sinoatrial node rests in the right atrium awaiting its next depolarization. Image courtesy of Virginia Luis-Fuentes, MRCVS, DACVIM.

septum. The right and left bundle branches can be identified and both run just beneath the subendocardium. The left further divides into posterior, anterior, and septal fascicles as it cascades toward the left ventricular apex finally spreading to the ventricular myocardium; each fascicle innervating a different portion of the left ventricle. The right bundle branch courses down the IVS subendocardially fanning out into the right ventricular free wall. Toward the ends of the bundle branches they become finer Purkinje fibers, finally terminating in the endocardium. The cardiac conduction system allows for rapid depolarization and contraction of all the myocytes nearly simultaneously.

Control of cardiac rate is accomplished with both sympathetic and parasympathetic innervations. The vagal nerves originating in the medulla oblongata provide the parasympathetic stimulation. Sympathetic stimulation is from nerves arising from the lateral reticular formation of the vasomotor center of the brain and relays signals through the central nervous system and thoracic ganglion exiting the spinal column between the first and fourth thoracic vertebrae.

A small ganglion between the pulmonary veins and the two vena cava is present near the SAN that the right-sided vagal nerve enters. Fibers from this ganglia innervate the SAN and when stimulated slow heart rate. The left vagal nerve courses to a corresponding fat pad ganglia near the AV node and slows AV nodal conduction when stimulated; however, there is overlap of these two nerves and one side of the vagal nerve does not innervate only one portion of the heart. Other parasympathetic innervations can be seen in the atrial myocardium. The ventricular myocardium itself has only a very small parasympathetic connection, but the ventricular conduction is heavily parasympathetically innervated.

Sympathetic nerves leading to the heart contain both afferent and efferent fibers. The afferent fibers carry signals from the heart itself back to the brain. The efferent fibers return impulses to the heart which are actually modified reflexively by afferent input from the heart and receptors in the great vessels, such as the baroreceptors located in the aorta. Stimulation from the sympathetic nervous system increases heart rate and contractility, in addition to the vasoconstrictive action exhibited on the blood vessels. The two systems work in concert to change heart rate and cardiac function by the suppression of one system and the stimulation of the other to maintain blood pressure.

Microscopic Structure

The secret to the contractile function of the heart lays in its specialized striated muscle. The cardiac myocardium is composed of fiber-like bands of muscle tissue arranged in overlapping multidirectional layers. This arrangement allows for contraction in three directions at once. Each muscular band is composed of many fibrous strands arranged longitudinally. These branching fibrous bands are composed of individual myocytes. Cardiomyocytes are tubular, approximately 50–100 μm long and 10–25 μm wide, and are arranged in a longitudinal pattern with one cardiac cell abutted end to end with the next. Between each myocyte are the *intercalated discs.* The intercalated discs serve to connect two myocytes, allowing for communication of two cells and establishing an anchor for the contractile mechanism within the myocytes. The cells are held as fibrous groups by collagen connective tissue interspersed with a high concentration of capillaries.

Within the myocyte, a high number of mitochondria can be found along with the nucleus and other organelles. The functional unit of the cardiac myocyte and of contraction is the *sarcomere.* The sarcomere is a segment of contractile fibers bordered by transverse discs, known as *Z-bands,* within each myocyte. There are many sarcomeres inside each myocyte, with individual sarcomeres stacked end to end and circumferentially to form a "cable effect" within the cell.

Each individual sarcomere is made up of thin actin bands attached to the Z-bands and a thick myosin band that sits between the actin fibers. The myosin fibers extend from the Z-band about two-thirds of the way towards the center of the sarcomere; the actin fibers are positioned between the myosin fibers, extending from the center outward, but not fully to the Z-bands, bridging the gap between the actin fibers from each end of the

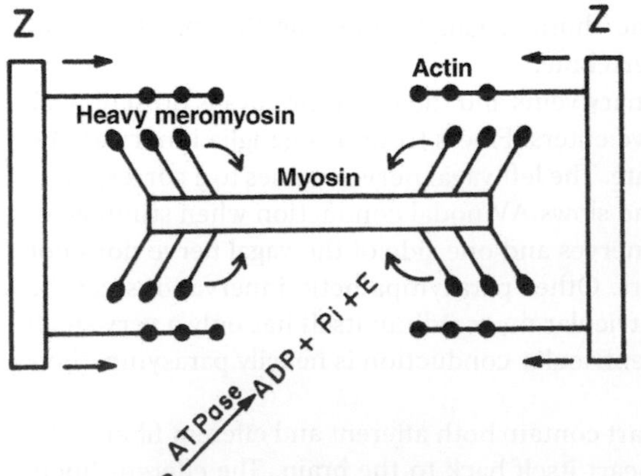

Figure 1.11 An individual sarcomere: the myosin molecule in the center is stationary. Contraction occurs when the heavy meromyosin and the actin react to depolarization; the heavy meromyosin pulls toward the center, shortening the cell, and draws the Z-bands closer together. When coupled with millions of other sarcomeres depolarizing rapidly, the heart contracts in unison. Source: Fox (1999) [1]. Reproduced with permission of Elsevier.

sarcomere (Figure 1.11). When the cell is depolarized, proteins along the length of the actin and myosin fibers shift position causing the fibers to slide along each other, pulling the Z-bands closer together and making the overall length of the sarcomere and thus the cell shorter and thicker. When done in unison, the overall effect will reduce the internal dimensions of the ventricle by 50%.

References

1 Fox, P.R., Sisson, D. and Moïse, S.N. (1999) Cardiac anatomy, in *Textbook of Canine and Feline Cardiology: Principles and Clinical Practice* (eds P.R. Fox, D. Sisson and S.N. Moïse), 2nd Edition. W.B. Saunders Company, Philadelphia.

2 van Campenhout, M.J.H., Yaksh, A., Kik, C. *et al.* (2013) Bachmann's bundle: a key player in the development of atrial fibrillation? *Circulation: Arrhythmia and Electrophysiology*, **6**, 1041–1046.

3 Constantinescu, G.M. (1991) *Clinical Dissection Guide for Large Animals.* Mosby-Year Book, St Louis.

2

Basic Cardiac Physiology

June A. Boon and H. Edward Durham, Jr.

Introduction

Cardiac muscle cells are specialized in that they can initiate their own electrical activity. When they generate their own action potential, resting membrane potential becomes less negative until a threshold is reached which initiates an influx of Na^{+} into the cell. At threshold an "all or none" phenomenon occurs; which means that a series of electrical and mechanical events occur that cannot be stopped and results in the cell depolarization. No further increases in electrical activity are necessary for the cell to completely contract. Cardiac muscle contraction allows blood to be pumped from the heart and adequate stroke volume and blood pressure are required to meet the body's metabolic needs. The following sections elaborate upon the electrical and mechanical activity in the heart and cardiovascular system.

Electrical Activity in the Heart

The Action Potential

The cardiac action potential represents the activity in the cell during contraction (systole) and relaxation (diastole). Every cell has a membrane potential, meaning they have an electrical voltage gradient between the inside and the outside of the cell. This exists because of ion concentration differences between the inside and the outside of the cell membrane. The ions involved in this membrane potential are primarily Na^{+}, K^{+}, and Ca^{++}. During diastole, Na^{+} and Ca^{++} are found in higher concentrations outside the cell, while K^{+} is found in higher concentrations inside the cell [1, p. 12]. These ions move across the cell membrane through channels that are specific for each ion (Figure 2.1). A channel is either open or closed and ions can move through their particular channels only at certain times, meaning they are gated. The number of channels that are open or closed at any given point in time for a specific ion is regulated by voltage. Therefore, as voltage changes during depolarization, repolarization and at rest, the channels specific for each ion open or close depending upon the voltage requirement of the channel. Each phase of the action potential has a membrane potential that activates or inactivates each type of channel [1, pp. 12–14].

Cardiology for Veterinary Technicians and Nurses, First Edition. Edited by H. Edward Durham, Jr.

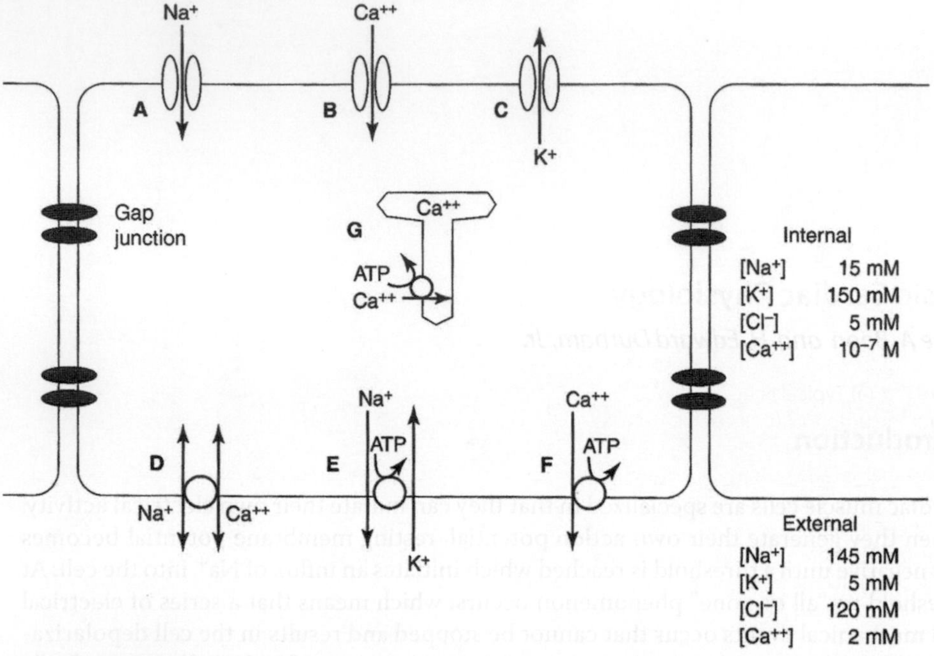

Figure 2.1 Ion channels, cotransporters and active transporters of the myocyte. **A**, Sodium entry through the fast sodium channel is responsible for the rapid upstroke (phase 0) of the action potential in non-pacemaker cells. **B**, Calcium enters the cell through the slow calcium channel during phase 2 of the Purkinje fiber and muscle cell action potential, and is the main channel responsible for depolarization of pacemaker cells. **C**, Potassium exits through a potassium channel to repolarize the cell during phase 3 of the action potential, and open potassium channels help maintain the resting potential (phase 4) of non-pacemaker cells. **D**, Sodium-calcium exchanger helps maintain the low intracellular calcium concentration. **E**, Sodium-potassium ATPase pump maintains concentration gradients for these ions. **F**, Active calcium transporters aid removal of calcium to the external environment. **G**, Active calcium transporters aid removal of calcium to the sarcoplasmic reticulum. ATP, adenosine triphosphate. Source: Lilly (2007) [1]. Reproduced with permission of Lippincott Williams and Wilkins.

The basic action potential is the same for all the cells in the heart with slight variations depending on the type of cell. Figure 2.2 shows a fast and a slow action potential. Fast action potentials occur within myocardial cells and the Purkinje fibers, while slow action potentials occur in the specialized conduction tissue of the sinoatrial node (SAN) and atrioventricular node (AVN). This allows cardiac muscle to depolarize quickly for coordinated and effective contraction [1, pp. 12–14].

Fast Action Potentials

Phase 4: Resting Cells

The resting cell membrane (phase 4) exists in an environment of high K^+ inside the cell and high Na^+ and Ca^{++} outside the cell (Figure 2.1). Potassium constantly moves out of the cell with its concentration gradient through voltage gated K^+ channels. Negative anions (proteins) are left inside the cell creating a negative environment. Potassium

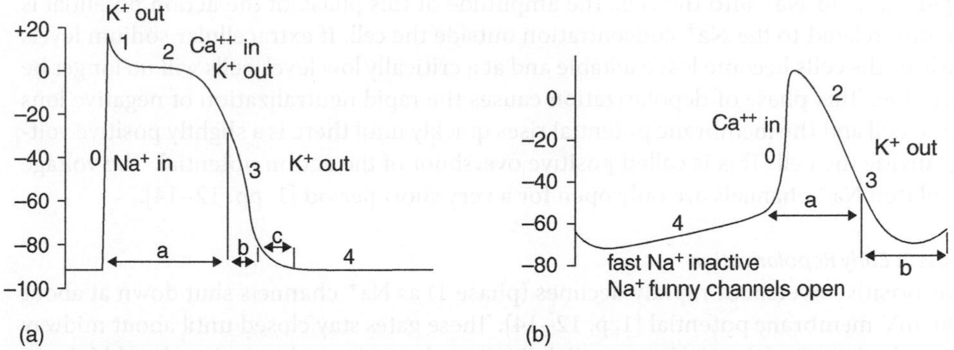

Figure 2.2 (a) Typical action potential (in millivolts) recorded from muscle cells in the heart. At resting membrane potential (phase 4) Na^+ and Ca^{++} channels are closed. As the membrane becomes less negative, sodium channels open and there is a rapid influx of Na^+ (phase 0). After the overshoot into a positive membrane potential, movement of K^+ out return the membrane to about 0 mV. Phase 2 of the action potential involves continued movement of K^+ out and Ca^{++} into the cell. Phase 2 ends as Ca^{++} movement in slows down and K^+ movement out exceeds Ca^{++} influx. Continued movement of K^+ out brings the membrane back to its resting potential of approximately −90 mV. (b) Typical action potential of pacemaker cells in the sinoatrial and atrioventricular nodes. These cells have a resting membrane potential that is less negative than contractile cells. This less negative level keeps the fast Na^+ channels closed. Phase 4 of the pacemaker cell cannot maintain a resting potential and is constantly moving toward the less negative level. This is caused by Na^+ into the cell through "funny current" channels. Phase 0 is slower because this phase is dependent upon Ca^{++} moving into the cell instead of rapid Na^+ channels. Calcium channels are inactivated and K^+ moves out of the cell during phase 3 as they do in ventricular and atrial muscle cells. **a**, effective refractory period; **b**, relative refractory period; **c**, super normal period.

is then lured back into the cell based on the electrical gradient. When the movement of K^+ out of the cell and the movement of K^+ back into the cell are in balance, there is no net movement and the membrane potential is at equilibrium at about −90 mV [1, pp. 12–14].

Although the membrane permeability to Na^+ is low at −90 mV [1, p. 12], this ion will move into the cell with its concentration gradient. Counteracting this flow of Na^+ into the cell is a Na^+/ K^+ pump that pumps three Na^+ ions out for two K^+ ions in. This is an energy (adenosine triphosphate – ATP) requiring exchanger [1, p. 12]. In order to maintain the resting membrane potential at −90 mV, this pump works faster when Na^+ concentrations are high. If potassium levels outside the cell are high, then diffusion out of the cell is reduced and the membrane becomes less negative, making it more excitable and susceptible to arrhythmia [1, p. 19].

Phase 0: Depolarization

The initial upstroke (phase 0) represents depolarization of the cell. When the resting membrane potential becomes less negative and reaches −65 mV, an action potential can be generated [1, pp. 12–14]. The membrane potential required for depolarization to start is called the threshold potential and anything that elevates the resting membrane potential to threshold will cause depolarization to start. This is an all or none phenomenon, in that once threshold is reached, depolarization is initiated and cannot be prevented. At threshold potential, fast Na^+ voltage regulated channels are activated, resulting in a rapid influx of Na^+ into the cell. The amplitude of this phase of the action potential is directly related to the Na^+ concentration outside the cell. If extracellular sodium levels are low, the cells become less excitable and at a critically low level, cells will no longer be excitable. This phase of depolarization causes the rapid neutralization of negative ions in the cell and the membrane potential rises quickly until there is a slightly positive voltage inside the cell. This is called positive overshoot of the action potential. The voltage regulated Na^+ channels are only open for a very short period [1, pp. 12–14].

Phase 1: Early Repolarization

This positive overshoot rapidly declines (phase 1) as Na^+ channels shut down at about $^+30$ mV membrane potential [1, p. 12–14]. These gates stay closed until about midway through phase 3 of the action potential. Because these channels are closed and Na^+ can no longer enter the cell until at least midway through phase 3, this period is referred to as the absolute or *effective refractory period* (Figure 2.2). No new action potential can be initiated. Potassium moves out of the cell with the electrical gradient (positive inside, negative outside) that now exists [1, p. 20; 2, pp. 18–22].

Phase 2: Contraction

Phase 1 is very brief and is followed by a long slow phase of maintained depolarization (phase 2) while Ca^{++} moves into the cell during systole. These calcium channels are voltage regulated and become active only as membrane potential becomes positive during phase 0. These Ca^{++} channels deactivate very slowly and are called L type channels (for long lasting). Overall cell membrane permeability to K^+ is reduced but this plateau phase is maintained because K^+ moves out of the cell through a small number of channels. There is an equal charge moving in and out of the cell, maintaining the membrane potential for the duration of contraction. Calcium channel blocker drugs close these L type channels and decrease the time the cell is in phase 2. The Ca^{++} that moved into the cell is the Ca^{++} that is used in excitation coupling of contraction. Calcium influx and Ca^{++} channel activity is enhanced by catecholamines. Catecholamines interact with ß-adrenergic receptors on the cell membrane that increases intracellular cyclic adenosine monophosphate (cAMP) which enhances the Ca^{++} L type channel activity, moving Ca^{++} into the cell [1, p. 20].

Phase 3: Repolarization

Phase 3 represents repolarization and the return to a resting membrane potential of −90 mV. Potassium moves out of the cell making the return to a more negative membrane potential rapid. Ca^{++} channels start turning off early in the plateau of phase 2 and K^+ channels which are actually slowly turned on during phase 1, remain on. This process is so slow that the effect is not felt until phase 3 and this efflux of K^+ actually initiates phase 3, ending the plateau and contraction phase. Two types of K^+ channels are active during this phase; a slow and a fast channel. Different cardiac tissues have greater concentrations of one or the other. Atrial muscle and endocardial tissue for instance have fast channels and thus have shorter plateau lengths (Figure 2.2). Epicardial muscle cells, however, have slow channels giving them a longer contraction time. By the end of phase 3, K^+ ions moving out of the cell exceed Ca^{++} ions moving in. This causes the membrane potential to rapidly approach −90 mV. Na^+ channels slowly start to open about halfway through phase 3 and the effective refractory period ends. Now, if a stimulus is strong enough, depolarization can occur again and this time period is referred to as the *relative refractory period.* Ca^{++} that moved into the cell during phase 2 is removed by a Na^+/Ca^{++} exchanger that moves two Na^+ ions in for every Ca^{++} ion out. There is also a Na^+/K^+ pump that pushes two K^+ back into the cells in exchange for three Na^+ out. The overall effect of these ion pumps is to restore the negative membrane potential to that of phase 4 [1, p. 20].

Slow Action Potentials

The slow response fibers of the specialized conduction tissue have a much slower initial rise during depolarization (phase 0), less of an overshoot into positive inside voltage (phase 1), and a less distinct plateau phase during systole (phase 2) (Figure 2.2). This is because there are no fast Na^+ currents in the SAN and AVN nodes. At threshold this slow influx of Na^+ creates the slow rise of this action potential. Phase 2 and 3 merge with each other. Phase 4 of the slow response action potential in conduction tissue is relatively unstable and not flat like the fast action potential. Because the resting membrane potential of conduction tissue is less negative than that of the myocytes, fast Na^+ channels remain closed. Slow Na^+ channels (called "funny channels") allow Na^+ to continuously move into the cell making phase 4 of the slow action potential drift toward a less negative point. At threshold an influx of Ca^{++} results in phase 0 of the action potential, initiating the electrical activity that moves through the rest of the heart [1, pp. 20, 21].

Contraction and the Action Potential

Electrical activity in the heart occurs before any mechanical activity (contraction). Phase 0 involves a rapid influx of Na^+ which depolarizes the cell (moves from negative to positive) and is completed before actual contraction (systole) of the muscle starts. Peak contraction occurs as the cell completes phase 3 of the action potential while muscle relaxation (diastole) occurs during phase 4 of the action potential.

Mechanical Activity in the Heart

Sinus Node and Conduction System Activation

The Cardiac Cycle

Muscle cells within the heart are a syncytium, meaning they are connected by the intercalated discs and once depolarized, the action potential spreads rapidly to the adjacent cell through the disc. Once the adjacent cell depolarizes, its electrical activity spreads to the next cell. In this manner, the entire heart contracts. For effective function of the heart, the chambers must contract in sequence and with a coordinated effort. The specialized conduction fibers of the heart are different from the rest of the cardiac muscle in that they contain less mitochondria and a smaller number of myofibrils. They have lost the ability to contract and their role is to conduct the electrical impulse in sequence throughout the heart.

The sinus node initiates the heart beat because it has the lowest threshold and the greatest excitability of all the specialized conduction tissue. This is because it has decreased permeability to K^+ and cannot maintain a resting potential during phase

4 for any length of time relative to the other components of the conduction system. Once a threshold potential of about −65 mV is reached an action potential is initiated [1, pp. 22, 23].

The electrical impulse travels in all directions through the atrial chambers via the syncytium of cells. Electrical activity converges at the AVN because the impulse cannot travel across the connective tissue located around the annular rings of the mitral and tricuspid valves. The speed of conduction through the AVN is slow allowing the atria to fill the ventricular chambers before ventricular contraction begins. This decrease in conduction speed is primarily due to decreased permeability to Na^+ and the action potentials of these cells have a much slower acceleration rate (slope). The bundle of His at the bottom of the AVN is the electrical bridge to the ventricular chambers [1, pp. 22, 23].

Conduction through the bundle of His is faster and it carries the electrical impulse to the ventricular septum. At the top of the ventricular septum, the His bundle splits into the right and left bundle branches which end in the network of Purkinje fibers. These fibers and the bundle branches conduct electrical activity very quickly relative to the rest of the conduction system. Coordinated contraction of the ventricular chambers involves contraction of the septum and papillary muscles first, closing the mitral and tricuspid valves, then subendocardial contraction of the ventricular chamber and lastly epicardial contraction. Contraction of the ventricular muscle increases pressure within these chambers and once pressure reaches systemic and pulmonary artery pressures, the aortic and pulmonary valves open respectively. Overall contraction of the ventricular chambers occurs from apex to base allowing effective emptying of the chambers into the aorta and pulmonary artery [1, pp. 22, 23].

Electrocardiography and Mechanical Events of the Heart

The electrocardiogram is the surface recognition of electrical activity as it travels through the heart (Figure 2.3). Typically the SAN controls the hearts rate (*chronotropy*) and initiate the cascade of events in a heart beat. The P wave representing electrical activity spreading through the atrial chambers occurs during the latter part of diastole causing the atrial chambers to contract pushing blood through open mitral and tricuspid valves into the ventricular chambers. By the end of atrial contraction, electrical activity has traveled through the AVN (*dromotropy*-rate of AVN conduction) and into the ventricular chambers. The time period from the P wave to the QRS complex represents the time delay within the AVN. The QRS complex represents the electrical activity as it travels through the ventricular chambers. The time from electrical activation of the ventricular muscle (the beginning of the QRS complex) to when the aortic and pulmonary valves open is the isovolumic contraction time. No change in volume has occurred, all valves are closed and the ventricles are merely building up pressure. The aortic and pulmonary valves open when ventricular pressure reaches systemic and pulmonary vascular pressures respectively. Contraction of the ventricles (*inotropy*) and a corresponding increase in ventricular pressure causes the atrioventricular valves to close. While the ventricular chamber is contracting and the atrioventricular valves are closed, the atrial chambers fill with blood. As ventricular contraction ceases, pressure declines within the right and left ventricles, and when pressure becomes lower than systemic and pulmonary pressure, the aortic and pulmonary valves close. A period of isovolumic relaxation starts during which time all valves are closed again and pressure declines while the muscle relaxes. The T wave of the electrocardiogram represents repolarization of ventricular muscle. Once ventricular pressure is less than intra-atrial pressure, the atrioventricular valves

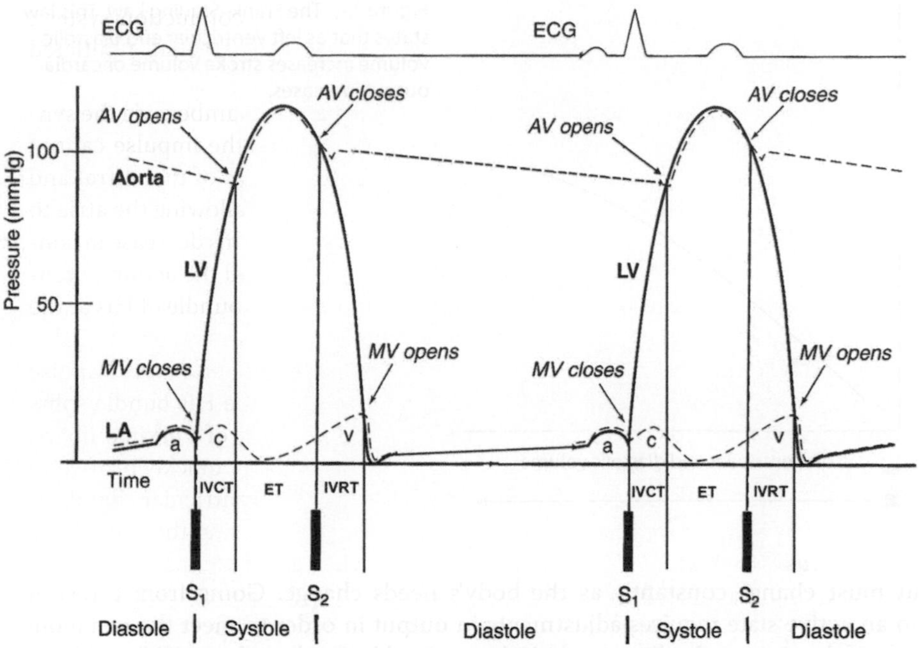

Figure 2.3 The normal cardiac cycle. During diastole, the mitral valve (MV) is open so that the left atrial (LA) and left ventricular (LV) pressures are equal. In late diastole, LA contraction causes a small rise in pressure in both the LA and LV (the a wave). During systolic contraction the LV pressure rises; when it exceeds the LA pressure, the MV closes, contributing to the first heart sound (S_1). As LV pressure rises above the aortic pressure, the aortic valve (AV) opens, which is a silent event. The time between MV closure and AV opening is called the isovolumic contraction time (IVCT): no valves are open as pressure builds. As the ventricle begins to relax and its pressure falls below that of the aorta, the AV closes, contributing to the second heart sound (S_2). The time the aortic valve remains open is the ejection time (ET), the portion of systole when blood flows out of the LV chamber. As LV pressure falls further, below that of the LA, the MV opens, which is silent in the normal heart. The time between AV closure and MV opening is called the isovolumic relaxation time (IVRT); no valves are open and pressure declines. In addition to the a wave, the LA pressure curve displays two positive deflections: the c wave represents a small rise in LA pressure as the MV closes and bulges toward the atrium, and the v wave is the result of passive filling of the LA from the pulmonary veins during systole, when the MV is closed. Source: Lilly (2007) [1]. Reproduced with permission of Lippincott Williams and Wilkins.

open and blood flows rapidly into the ventricular chambers with the pressure gradient. This is referred to as the early diastolic filling phase or the rapid ventricular filling phase (*lusitropy*-rate of myocardial relaxation). Pressure within the ventricular chambers rise secondary to this early filling phase and flow decreases as a result. Toward the end of diastole, the atrial chamber contracts again and the entire cardiac cycle repeats.

Cardiac Output

The ability of the heart to pump blood effectively to the body depends upon several factors including: the time available to fill between contractions, the volume within the chambers (stretch on the myofibers), the load the myofibers must contract against, contractility of the muscle, and proper conduction of electrical impulses through the heart. Cardiac output (CO) refers to the amount of blood the heart pumps each minute.

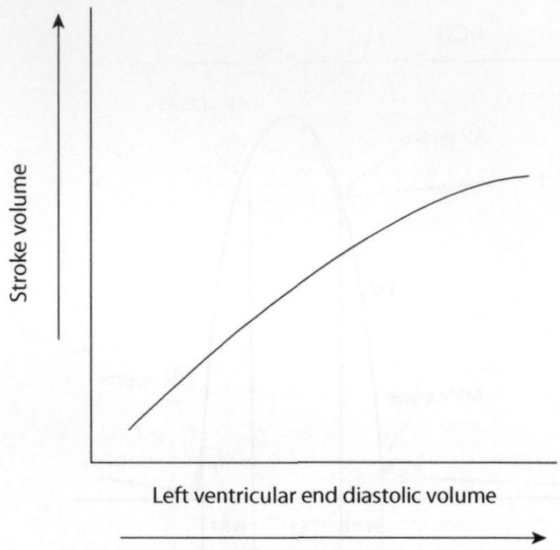

Figure 2.4 The Frank–Starling Law. This law states that as left ventricular end diastolic volume increases stroke volume or cardiac output increases.

Output must change constantly as the body's needs change. Going from a resting state to an active state requires adjustments in output in order to meet the metabolic demands of the tissues. Cardiac output is determined by stroke volume (SV) and heart rate (HR):

$$CO = SV \times HR \tag{2.1}$$

Heart rate is affected most by sympathetic and parasympathetic stimuli at the SAN. Stroke volume is influenced by preload, afterload and contractility. The ideas of preload and afterload may be confusing to some. To state it simply, preload is the volume available to fill a ventricle during diastole; afterload is the pressure or load a ventricle must contract against.

Effect of Preload on Stroke Volume: Frank–Starling Law of the Heart

In the early 1900s, several men including Otto Frank and Ernest Starling discovered that the heart contracts with greater force when it is filled to a greater degree. This discovery led to the Frank–Starling Law of the Heart which states that stroke volume increases as left ventricular volume increases (Figure 2.4). All other things being equal, increased preload stretches the myofibers, increasing the fiber length, allowing for more shortening as the thin and thick filaments slide over each other. This property of the heart is also shown in the pressure volume loop shown in Figure 2.5. A pressure volume loop shows the events of the cardiac cycle as a continuous loop of changing volume and pressure. The loop in Figure 2.5 shows that at a constant systolic pressure (blood pressure) and normal contractility, as volume (preload) increases within the heart, there is an increase in stroke volume.

Effect of Afterload on Stroke Volume

The degree that a cardiac muscle can shorten is directly related to the load that it must contract against. There is a linear relationship between end systolic fiber length and the tension ventricular muscle must shorten against. This relationship is shown in Figure 2.6

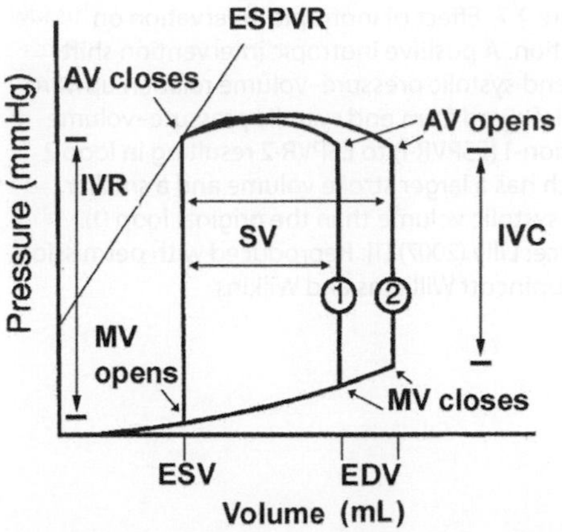

Figure 2.5 The normal pressure volume loop. The mitral valve (MV) opens and volume increases within the left ventricular chamber (line 1). The MV closes at end diastole. The left ventricle builds up pressure until it reaches systemic blood pressure and the aortic valve (AV) opens. The left ventricle rejects its blood and volume decreases. At end systole the AV closes and pressure declines. Pressure declines until it is less than atrial pressure at which point the MV opens and diastolic filling starts again. The time from MV closure to AV opening is the isovolumic contraction (IVC) phase where all valves are closed and left ventricular pressure is increasing. The time from AV closure to MV opening is the isovolumic relaxation (IVR) period when all valves are closed and left ventricular pressure declines. The end systolic pressure volume relationship line (ESPVR) defines the relationship between afterload (systolic blood pressure) and end systolic volume. When arterial blood pressure (afterload) and contractility are held constant but end diastolic volume (EDV) (preload) increases line 2, there is a higher stroke volume (SV) (per Frank Starling's Law) but a constant end systolic volume (ESV).

where for a given muscle fiber length it shows how much shortening can occur at any given tension (afterload). Therefore, cardiac myofibers cannot shorten as much when the load they must contract against increases. It also shows that at lower loads the muscle can shorten to a greater degree. This is referred to as the end systolic pressure–volume relationship (ESPVR). The ESPVR line represents the length tension relationship within the heart.

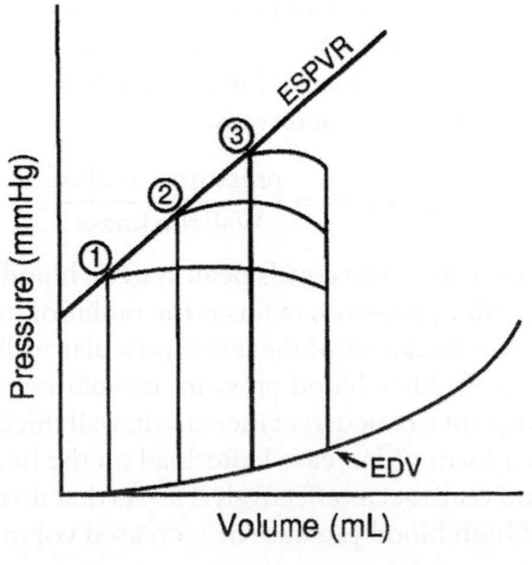

Figure 2.6 Effects of increased afterload on function. When the preload (end diastolic volume, EDV) and contractility are held constant, sequential increases (points 1, 2, 3) in arterial pressure (afterload) are associated with loops that have progressively lower stroke volumes and higher end systolic volumes. There is a nearly linear relationship between the afterload and end systolic volume (ESV), termed the end systolic pressure–volume relation (ESPVR). Source: Lilly (2007) [1]. Reproduced with permission of Lippincott Williams and Wilkins.

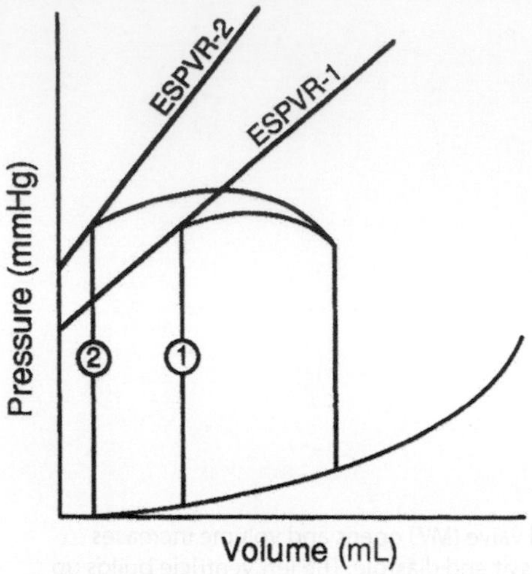

Figure 2.7 Effect of inotropic innervation on function. A positive inotropic intervention shifts the end systolic pressure–volume relation upward and leftward from end systolic pressure–volume relation-1 (ESPVR-I) to ESPVR-2 resulting in loop 2 which has a larger stroke volume and a smaller end-systolic volume than the original loop (1). Source: Lilly (2007) [1]. Reproduced with permission of Lippincott Williams and Wilkins.

Effect of Contractility on Stroke Volume

When the peak tension a muscle fiber can generate is increased, it is said to have increased contractility. This means that the peak length tension relationship changes (Figure 2.7). Increased contractility means that the ESPVR line moves to the left, where for any starting fiber length the peak tension it can develop is increased. When contractility is decreased the length tension relationship line shifts to the right.

The biggest determinant of contractility is the amount of norepinephrine (NE) available to the cell. Increased levels of NE increase heart rate but also allow muscle fibers to generate more tension for any given starting length. Norepinephrine mediates contractility by interacting with the β_{1}-adrenergic receptors. This activates cAMP-protein kinase A, allowing phosphorylation of Ca^{++} channels, increasing inward flow of Ca^{++} allowing more actin and myosin cross bridges to form [3].

Wall Stress

Wall thickness increases in a heart with normal myocardium depending upon the load against which it must contract. The normal heart muscle will increase in thickness (hypertrophy) whenever either a pressure or a volume overload is present. Wall stress must remain normal for the cardiac muscle fibers to effectively shorten. Laplace's Law for spherical structures is:

$$\text{wall stress} = \frac{\text{pressure} \times \text{radius}}{\text{Wall thickness}} \tag{2.2}$$

where pressure equals peak systolic blood pressure (also equal to peak systolic left ventricular pressure), radius is the radius of the left ventricular chamber, and wall thickness is the thickness of the left ventricular wall (Figure 2.8). Using this equation, we can see that if either blood pressure or volume within the left ventricular chamber increases without a concurrent increase in wall thickness, wall stress will increase. High wall stress is a form of increased afterload on the heart and the muscle will not be able to shorten and contract as effectively. Hearts that do not hypertrophy appropriately in the presence of high blood pressure or increased volume will fail.

$$\text{Wall stress} = \frac{P \times r}{h}$$

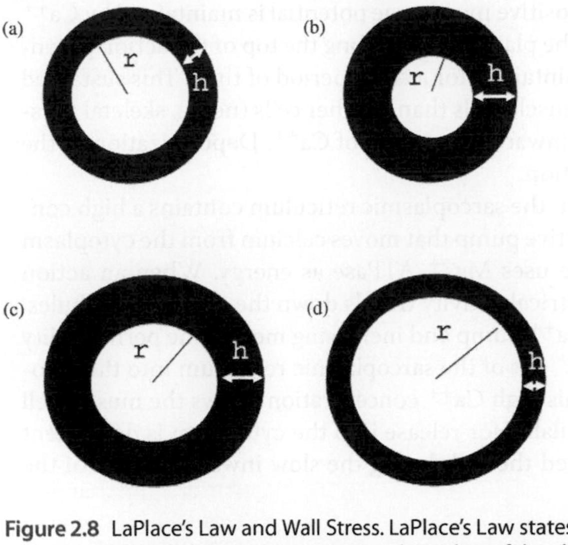

Figure 2.8 LaPlace's Law and Wall Stress. LaPlace's Law states that wall stress is dependent upon pressure the heart must contract against, the radius of the chamber and the thickness of the ventricular walls. In the normal heart (a) the wall thickness and radius are appropriate and wall stress is normal. If pressure increases (b) the heart will respond with hypertrophy that allows the relationship between wall thickness and chamber size (radius) to maintain normal wall stress. This is a concentric hypertrophy pattern, increased wall thickness and normal to decreased chamber size. When heart volume increases (c), wall stress is normalized by hypertrophy also. The relationship of wall thickness to radius is just enough to normalize wall stress. This is called an eccentric hypertrophy pattern. When the left ventricular muscle fails, the heart dilates in an effort to maintain normal cardiac output (d). Hypertrophy does not develop and because the wall thickness to chamber radius is not adequate wall stress is high. This is a form of high afterload within the left ventricular chamber and the muscle cannot contract effectively against this load.

A heart with increased volume and compensatory hypertrophy to normalize wall stress is eccentrically hypertrophied, which means that thick walls exist secondary to an increase in chamber size. A heart that hypertrophies in response to increased blood pressure is concentrically hypertrophied, which means that chamber size is not increased but wall thickness is. Both types of hypertrophy are compensatory responses in an effort to maintain normal wall stress.

Mechanisms of Contraction: Function of the Sarcomere

In the resting cardiac cell, there is a flux of ions into and out of the cell by electrical gradients and active transport systems. The net result is that the interior of the cell has less positive ions (because of diffusion and the active pump) creating the negative resting membrane potential. The resting membrane potential for the Purkinje fibers is about −90 mV and that of the AVN is about −60 mV [4].

When the cardiac muscle cells are electrically activated, it is called an action potential. Na^+ permeability of the cell membrane increases resulting in a rapid flow of Na^+ into the cell while the flow of K^+ remains unchanged. The resting membrane potential becomes positive (it decreases). This creates a rapid positive spike on the action potential diagram. Na^+ permeability decreases but the positive membrane potential is maintained by Ca^{++} movement into the cell. This creates the plateau shape along the top of the action potential diagram and depolarization is maintained for a short period of time. This sustained action potential is longer in cardiac muscle cells than in other cells (nerve, skeletal muscle) because of this maintained slow inward movement of Ca^{++}. Depolarization of the cardiac cell results in muscle contraction.

While a cardiac muscle cell is at rest, the sarcoplasmic reticulum contains a high concentration of Ca^{++} secondary to an active pump that moves calcium from the cytoplasm into the reticulum. This active pump uses Mg^{++}-ATPase as energy. When an action potential is initiated, the wave of electrical activity travels down the transverse tubules, depolarizing the cell, inhibiting the Ca^{++} pump and increasing membrane permeability to Ca^{++}. This causes an efflux of Ca^{++} out of the sarcoplasmic reticulum into the cytoplasm surrounding the myofibrils. This high Ca^{++} concentration allows the muscle cell to contract. The amount of Ca^{++} available for release into the cytoplasm is dependent upon the amount of Ca^{++} that entered the cell during the slow inward current of the preceding action potential.

Cross Bridge Formation

Contraction itself occurs when the thick and thin filaments slide over each other resulting in myofiber shortening (Figure 2.9). The length of the thick and thin filaments does

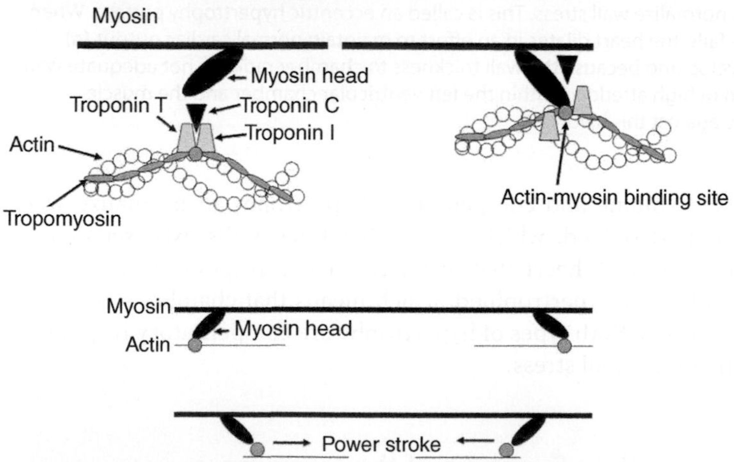

Figure 2.9 Contraction. The actin–myosin binding site is covered by tropomyosin and is not exposed until troponin subunit C binds with Ca^{++}. Once Ca^{++} is bound to the C subunit, the troponin I subunit is inhibited causing tropomyosin to change conformation. This exposes the actin–myosin binding site. The myosin head binds to actin and pulls the thin filament toward the center of the sarcomere (power stroke), resulting in muscle shortening. This shortening process and muscle contraction continues until the rise of cytosolic calcium comes to an end as the waved of excitation passes, no more calcium is admitted from the extracellular space, and release of calcium from the sarcoplasmic reticulum stops.

not change, but the length of the myofiber does. The overlap of the thin and thick filaments is facilitated by cross bridges that form between actin and myosin (actinomyosin interaction). Myosin, the thick filament, has globular heads that contain the binding sites for actin and the ATPase necessary to generate energy during contraction. Each thin actin filament has active sites that interact with the sites on the thick myosin filament. Tropomyosin is a protein that covers the actin binding sites until the muscle is ready to contract. Troponin is a complex of three subunits that are bound to the actin. Each subunit plays a role in contraction or relaxation of the muscle cell. Troponin T (TN-T) helps bind the entire troponin molecule to tropomyosin. Troponin I (TN-I) inhibits ATPase activity on actinomyosin. Troponin C (TN-C) is the Ca^{++} binding site on the tropomyosin molecule [5]. Calcium release from the sarcoplasmic reticulum into the cytoplasm during phase 2 of the action potential binds to TN-C. This removes the inhibitory TN-I protein from the tropomyosin complex, exposing the actin binding sites for myosin and making cross bridge formation possible. This is an active process requiring ATP which is released by the myosin. The energy released during the conversion of ATP to adenosine diphosphate (ADP) by the ATPase is also necessary for the cross bridges to form pulling actin toward the center of the sarcomere. The cross bridges act like a ratchet where they change their orientation and swing toward the center of the filament pulling actin with them [5]. Each cross bridge must be broken and the globular head of myosin swings back to its original orientation in order for it to attach to a new binding site and continue to pull in the thin filament. During relaxation, actin is again inhibited from binding with myosin by troponin and tropomyosin. This continuous ratcheting of the cross bridges continues during the plateau phase of the action potential until Ca^{++} levels fall in the sarcoplasm. Ca^{++} uptake by the sarcoplasmic reticulum and Ca^{++} removal from the sarcoplasm through active pumping channels exceed Ca^{++} inflow by the end of phase 2

Force of Contraction

The force of contraction is dependent upon the number of cross bridges formed and the degree of overlap between thick and thin filaments. During optimal overlap, all of the actin and myosin binding sites are aligned for cross bridge formation. When enough stretch (preload) is imposed upon the muscle that there is little or no overlap of the actin and myosin, then binding is not possible and no contraction is possible. When there is not enough stretch on the muscle fiber, then the overlap is excessive and the overall force that can be generated becomes less effective.

The number of cross bridges depends upon the availability of Ca^{++} and the duration of the contraction depends upon the length of time that Ca^{++} is available to the cell. Therefore, increasing Ca^{++} can increase the strength of a contraction or lengthen the duration of contraction. Contractility is defined as the potential for the cardiac muscle to shorten and is changed by increasing or decreasing the amount of Ca^{++} available to the cell. Remember that NE is the biggest determinant of increased Ca^{++} availability to the cell. Activation of β-adrenergic receptors activates membrane-bound adenylate cyclase. This in turn allows conversion of ATP to cAMP. Cyclic AMP determines how many Ca^{++} channels are open during the plateau phase of the action potential. The availability of more cAMP results in increased Ca^{++} concentration available in the sarcomere and increased contractility. Cyclic AMP also phosphorylates phospholamban, a protein kinase in the muscle cell. Phospholamban increases the uptake and release of Ca^{++} by the sarcoplasmic reticulum.

Relaxation begins once Ca^{++} levels within the cell drops. This occurs by active uptake of Ca^{++} by the sarcoplasmic reticulum, active uptake of Ca^{++} by the mitochondria in exchange for H^{+}, and removal of Ca^{++} from the cell via the Na^{+}/Ca^{++} pump.

Blood Pressure Regulation

Blood moves with pressure. It can only flow from high to low pressure. Pressure within the left ventricular chamber is high during systole as it drives blood into the aorta. This is equal to systolic blood pressure which is about 120 mmHg. As blood moves through the body it moves through vessels with lower and lower pressure. By the time blood moves through the venous circulation and back to the right atrium, pressure is almost 0 mmHg.

Pulsatile Flow

The systemic circulation distributes blood to the various tissues of the body. The heart pumps rhythmically and of course intermittently. The entire stroke volume is pumped into the aorta with every contraction and during systole, pressure within the arteries of the body are at their highest. Much of the stroke volume is held in the very distensible arteriole system of the systemic circulation. Known as the *windkessel effect:* Elastic recoil of the arteriolar walls during diastole after the aortic valve closes, moves blood through the capillary system. During diastole, arteriolar pressure is at its lowest. Mean arterial pressure is the pressure in the large arteries of the body averaged over time. It fluctuates between systolic and diastolic pressure and is affected by cardiac output and compliance (elasticity) of the large arteries. Pulse pressure is the difference between systolic and diastolic pressures. Blood pressure is determined as follows:

$$BP = CO \times SVR \qquad (2.3)$$

where BP, blood pressure; CO, cardiac output; and SVR, systemic vascular resistance.

There are instantaneous adjustments made via reflex mechanisms when blood pressure changes from normal. These mechanisms adjust stroke volume and peripheral vascular resistance in an effort to maintain normal blood pressure for short periods. Hormonal adjustments are made to manage elevations or decreases in blood pressure over the long term.

Resistance Vessels

The arteries and arterioles have small diameters but thick smooth muscular walls. They are able to change the resistance to blood flow by actively contracting and changing diameter of their lumens. This regulates blood flow to the organs, increasing blood flow to actively working organs and restricting blood flow to areas that are not metabolically active. Systemic vascular resistance is the sum total of all resistance in the arterioles. As resistance increases in one vascular bed, it must decrease in others for systemic vascular resistance and arterial pressure to remain stable. Arterioles govern the degree of flow entering the capillary beds, which is determined by the metabolic needs of the organ that the bed perfuses. More volume entering the capillary bed stimulates more capillaries to open up for diffusion into the tissues.

Capacitance Vessels

The walls of veins contain collagen, elastin and smooth muscle. Smooth muscle contraction and relaxation changes the capacity of these vessels. Increasing distension allows the veins to hold more blood volume while decreasing distension pressure moves blood forward toward the heart. Venous capacity to hold blood volume is about 85% greater than that of the arterial system. Changing peripheral vascular resistance in the venous system controls the amount of blood volume returning to the right atrium with resulting effects on left atrial and ventricular filling pressure. Blood within the thoracic cavity within the vena cava and the right atrium is referred to as the central venous pool. As this pool volume increases or decreases secondary to changes in vascular resistance within the venous system, it alters filling of the heart and stroke volume.

Venous Tone

Veins have no basal resting tone and are relatively unaffected by circulating vasodilators. Mechanical contraction of the muscles surrounding veins affects venous return to the heart. High forces of contracting muscle force blood to move forward through the venous system. The more vigorous the muscle contraction the more blood is moved from the peripheral venous pool to the central venous pool. This plays a large role in venous return to the heart and cardiac output. There is sympathetic innervation of veins, however, and epinephrine acting on the α_1-receptors cause vasoconstriction as it does in arterioles, resulting in increased movement of blood to the central venous pool and increased stroke volume.

Short Term Blood Pressure Regulation

The vessels of the arterial and venous system are composed of smooth muscle whose fibers are arranged circumferentially around the vessels. Larger arteries have multiple layers of fibers while arterioles have only a single layer of smooth muscle fibers. A layer of endothelial cells lines the vessel and this endothelial layer has projections into the smooth muscle of arterioles creating myoendothelial junctions. Thin and thick filaments exist in this smooth muscle and the action potential develops slowly creating a slow long-maintained contraction. There are no fast Na^+ channels in the smooth muscle of the vascular system. Instead, Ca^{++} comes into the cell during direct electrical stimulation via voltage-regulated channels or receptor-mediated channels (pharmacological).

Pharmacological mechanisms that initiate mechanical coupling of the cross bridges are typically hormonal without any electrical activation of the cell. Agonists are the major mechanism for initiating contraction in smooth muscle (Figure 2.10). These substances include catecholamines, histamines, acetylcholine, serotonin, angiotensin, adenosine, nitric oxide, and prostaglandins among others. Agonists at the smooth muscle receptors activate phospholipase C via G proteins. This causes phosphatidyl inositol biphosphate to hydrolyze to diacylglycerol and inositol triphosphate resulting in Ca^{++} release from the sarcoplasmic reticulum. Calcium binds with calmodulin, which activates the cross bridge formation and smooth muscle contraction. The vascular system

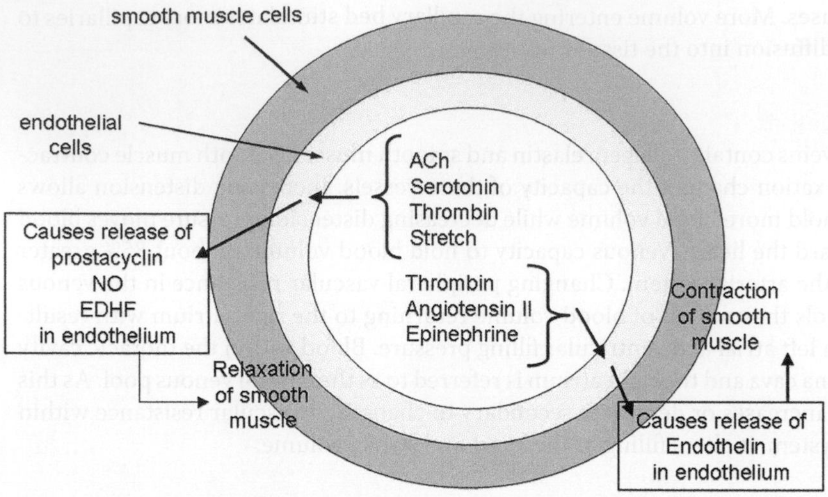

Figure 2.10 Vasoactive substances at vascular smooth muscle. Agonists which release endothelial-derived vasodilators and vasoconstrictors are shown. ACh, acetylcholine; EDHF, endothelial-derived hyperpolarizing factor; NO, nitric oxide.

is highly innervated by sympathetic nerves. When activated either electrically or pharmacologically they cause vasoconstriction. Parasympathetic nerves cause vasodilatation but are found in few vascular beds.

Endothelial Influences on Blood Pressure

Endothelial cells lining the vessels of the body release substances that cause vasodilatation in response to local conditions. The most common and important substance is nitric oxide (NO) (previously called endothelial-derived relaxing factor) which causes instant vasodilation. Nitric oxide is produced in response to increases in intracellular Ca^{++} through several agonists like acetylcholine and bradykinin, but probably the most common thing that stimulates NO production is stretch on the smooth muscle secondary to increased flow. This is one reason why flow increases in actively contracting muscles. There are several other less understood substances produced by endothelial cells that cause vasodilation including endothelin, prostacyclin, and endothelial-derived hyperpolarizing factor.

Arteriolar Baroreceptor Reflex

Reflex systems require a sensory receptor, an afferent path to the central nervous system, and an efferent pathway to an organ. Baroreceptors are the sensory receptors regulating blood pressure in the autonomic nervous system. They are found along the aortic arch and at the bifurcation of the carotid arteries in the neck. They are mechanical receptors that sense the stretch related to blood pressure on the smooth muscle in the artery walls. The baroreceptor increases its depolarization rate in response to increased stretch on the aorta or carotid arteries. Their afferent pathway leads to the medulla where vagal or sympathetic input regulates blood pressure. Increased mean arterial pressure increases baroreceptor activity while low blood pressure decreases baroreceptor response. The efferent pathways from the medulla controlling blood pressure are the sympathetic and parasympathetic nerves. When baroreceptors are activated secondary to increased blood pressure, vagal stimulation to the heart increases and sympathetic input to the heart and vessels decreases. The result is vasodilation of the arteries of the skin, splanchnic bed, kidneys, and muscle while venous dilation increases the venous pool and decreases the blood volume returning to the heart. Vagal influence also reduces heart rate. Low blood pressure, or decreased stretch on the vessels, decreases vagal input and increases sympathetic input to the heart and vessels. This results in increased systemic vascular resistance as vessels in the muscles, kidneys, splanchnic bed, and skin vasoconstrict. The splanchnic veins vasoconstrict as well which increases venous return to the heart, increasing left ventricular filling pressure and stroke volume. The increase in sympathetic activity also increases heart rate and contractility. These receptors adapt to increased pressure and over the course of a short period of time (days) the depolarization rate has a new set point. This reflex system is the most important modulator of minute-to-minute control of arterial blood pressure.

There are many mechanoreceptors at the caval atrial junction and along the pulmonary veins and many diffuse receptors within the walls of the atria and ventricles. The receptors located at the entrance to the atrial chambers are influenced by atrial filling and contraction. Distension of the vena cava or pulmonary veins increases sympathetic tone to the sinus node resulting in increased heart rate. These receptors also decrease sympathetic signals to the kidney causing increased water excretion (usually in conjunction with hormonal influences). The receptors in the atrial and ventricular chambers are activated when the pressure in these chambers rise. The result is similar to the aortic and carotid baroreceptors in the heart; sympathetic input decreases and vagal influence increases pressure. When pressure within these chambers falls, these receptors are turned off and blood pressure increases secondary to increased systemic vascular resistance modulated by increased constriction of splanchnic vessels.

Chemoreceptors

Chemoreceptors are found in conjunction with the baroreceptors at the aorta and carotid arteries. These sense changes in oxygen and carbon dioxide tension (PO_2, PCO_2) as well as hydrogen ion (H^+) concentration in the blood. Increases in PCO_2 or decreases in PO_2 or pH send information to the medulla. The frequency of the action potentials generated in this response is directly proportional to the alteration from normal. While PO_2 has to decrease from a normal level of about 95 mmHg to less than 80 mmHg for afferent activity to start in the chemoreceptors, PCO_2 and pH need only change slightly from normal to initiate impulses [6]. The result is an increase in respiratory rate until these parameters are again normal. Additionally, central chemoreceptors in the brain help maintain cerebral blood flow and homeostasis. Vagal stimulation decreases heart rate and coronary arteries dilate. There is vasoconstriction of the resistance vessels in the splanchnic bed and kidneys secondary to sympathetic tone, and there is vasodilation of the vessels in the skin secondary to sympathetic inhibition. The end result is an increase in blood pressure and coronary vasodilation which maintains cerebral and cardiac levels of oxygen, carbon dioxide and pH at normal levels.

Sympathetic and Parasympathetic Nervous System Influences on Blood Pressure

The heart has automaticity and can initiate an electrical impulse and ensuing contraction without any external innervation. It does, however, have an extensive network of nerve inputs, both sympathetic and parasympathetic. All parts of the heart have input from adrenergic sympathetic fibers. These release NE. The effects of NE on β-receptors in the heart increase heart rate, increase the action potential, increase the rate of contraction, and increase the force of contraction (contractility). Parasympathetic inputs via the vagus nerve are found at the SAN, the AVN and atrial muscle. Parasympathetic innervation releases acetylcholine at muscarinic receptors resulting in decreased HR by its effect on the SAN and decreased rate of conduction through the AVN.

Resistance and capacitance blood vessels and systemic veins have a large supply of sympathetic nerve endings. Adrenergic stimulation (NE release) results in strong vasoconstriction. The exceptions are coronary arteries, vessels in the brain and lungs, and vessels draining the large muscles. These have little sympathetic innervation in an effort to maintain critical functions of cerebral and cardiac vessels where vasoconstriction would limit the oxygen supply and and pulmonary function where vasoconstriction would hinder alveolar oxygen exchange. Large skeletal muscles contain a large portion of the body's fluid and vasoconstriction would potentially cause transudation out of the vasculature creating peripheral edema. The overall effect of adrenergic stimulation then is to increase heart rate, increase contractility, and increase systemic vascular resistance, all of which will increase blood pressure. There is very little parasympathetic innervation in the peripheral vasculature but where found it decreases systemic vascular resistance.

Long Term Blood Pressure Regulation

Ultimately, blood pressure is what is necessary to maintain a balance between fluid intake and fluid excretion. Increases in arterial pressure will cause increased fluid excretion in order to decrease the peripheral venous pool, causing decreased central venous pressure and decreased left ventricular stroke volume with resulting decreases in blood pressure. The opposite occurs when blood pressure decreases. Fluid retention increases the peripheral venous pool, the central venous pressure and stroke volume causing blood pressure to increase. These hormonal mechanisms do not happen instantaneously as baroreceptors and circulating catecholamines do but they are long lasting and they overshadow all other mechanisms of blood pressure control.

Circulating Catecholamines

Adrenal glands release catecholamines during activation of the sympathetic nervous system. These activate cardiac adrenergic receptors, which increases heart rate and contractility. Moderate levels of increased epinephrine act at vascular β_2-adrenergic receptors causing vasodilation while high levels of catecholamines act at the less sensitive vascular α_1-receptors to cause vasoconstriction.

Renin Angiotensin Aldosterone System

Renin is released by the kidney in response to increased renal sympathetic stimulation via β_1-adrenergic receptors and in response to lowered glomerular filtration rate (Figure 2.11). The increase in sympathetic innervation is in response to low cardiac output and low blood pressure. Sympathetic tone causes vasoconstriction of renal arterioles,

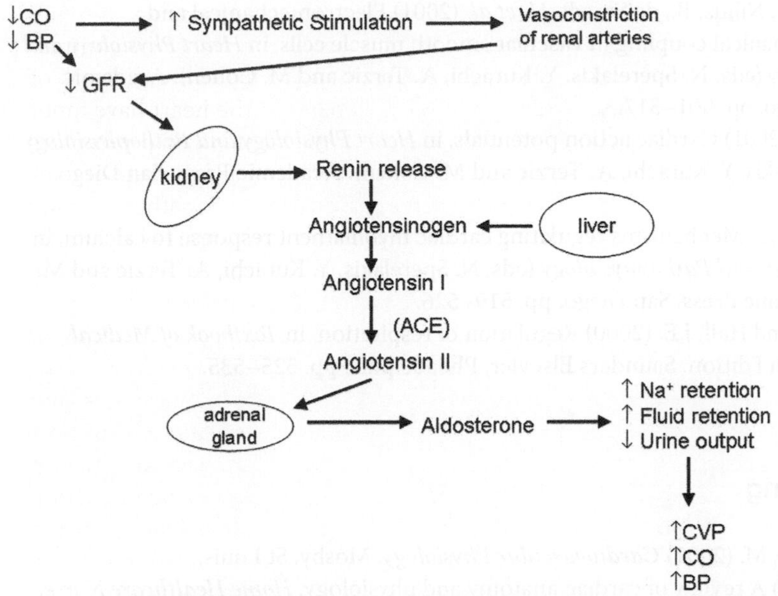

Figure 2.11 The renin angiotensin aldosterone system. The response to decreased cardiac output (CO) or low blood pressure (BP) is shown. ACE, angiotensin-converting enzyme; CVP, central venous pressure; GFR, glomerular filtration rate; Na^+, sodium.

which in turn decreases glomerular filtration pressure and filtration rate. Renin is an enzyme that initiates angiotensin I formation from angiotensinogen, a circulating protein. Angiotensin I rapidly converts to angiotensin II by angiotensin-converting enzyme which is found in endothelial cells. This conversion primarily takes place in the lungs. Angiotensin II acts on the adrenal glands to release aldosterone. Aldosterone promotes Na^+ retention in the renal tubules. This increases renal tubular fluid re-absorption, which decreases urinary output. Increased fluid retention by the kidneys increases blood volume, central venous pressure, left ventricular cardiac output and maintains blood pressure.

Vasopressin

Decreased baroreceptor activity influences the hypothalamus and pituitary gland to release vasopressin. Vasopressin is released by the pituitary gland when blood pressure falls. It acts in the collecting system of the kidneys and decreases water excretion. Permeability changes in the renal tubules secondary to vasopressin promote fluid reabsorption and decreased urine production. Increased water retention increases blood volume in an effort to maintain normal cardiac output and blood pressure.

References

1 Lilly, L. (ed.) (2007) *Pathophysiology of Heart Disease*. Lippincott Williams and Wilkins, Baltimore.
2 Berne, R. and Levy, M. (2001) *Cardiovascular Physiology*. Mosby, St Louis.

3 Droogmans, G., Nilius, B., de Smedt, H. *et al.* (2001) Electromechanical and pharmacomechanical coupling in vascular smooth muscle cells, in *Heart Physiology and Pathophysiology* (eds, N. Sperelakis, Y. Kurachi, A. Terzic and M. Cohen). Academic Press, San Diego. pp. 501–517.

4 Wahler, G.M. (2001) Cardiac action potentials, in *Heart Physiology and Pathophysiology* (eds, N. Sperelakis, Y. Kurachi, A. Terzic and M. Cohen). Academic Press, San Diego. pp. 199–211.

5 Solaro, R.J. (2001) Mechanisms regulating cardiac myofilament response to calcium, in *Heart Physiology and Pathophysiology* (eds, N. Sperelakis, Y. Kurachi, A. Terzic and M. Cohen). Academic Press, San Diego. pp. 519–526.

6 Guyton, A.C. and Hall, J.E. (2000) Regulation of respiration, in *Textbook of Medical Physiology*, 10th Edition. Saunders Elsevier, Philadelphia. pp. 525–535.

Further Reading

Berne, R. and Levy, M. (2001) *Cardiovascular Physiology.* Mosby, St Louis.

Flanigan, M. (2004) A review of cardiac anatomy and physiology. *Home Healthcare Nurse,* **22.**

Fox, P.D., Sisson, D.D. and Moise, N.S. (eds) (1999) *Textbook of Canine and Feline Cardiology: Principles and Clinical Practice.* W.B. Saunders, Philadelphia.

Gavaghan, M. (1998) Cardiac anatomy and physiology: a review. *Association of Registered periOperative Nurses,* **67**, 802–822.

Kittleson, M. (1994) Left ventricular function and failure - part I. *Compendium for Continuing Education for Practicing Veterinarians,* **16**, 287–308.

Kittleson, M. (1994) Left ventricular function and failure - part II. *Compendium for Continuing Education for Practicing Veterinarians,* **16**, 1001–1017.

Knowlen, G.G, Olivier, N.B. and Kittleson M.D. (2008) Cardiac contractility: a review. *Journal of Veterinary Internal Medicine,* **1**, 188–198.

Lilly, L. (ed.) (2007) *Pathophysiology of Heart Disease.* Lippincott Williams and Wilkins, Baltimore.

Mohrman, D. and Heller, L. (2003) *Cardiovascular Physiology.* Lange Medical Books/McGraw Hill, New York.

Olivier, N.B., Kittleson, M.D. and Knowlen, G.G. (1987) Cardiac preload: physiology and cardiac implications. *Journal of Veterinary Internal Medicine,* **1**, 81–85.

Shepherd, J. and Vanhoutte, P. (1979) *The Human Cardiovascular System: Facts and Concepts.* Raven Press, New York.

Smith, J. and Kampine, J. (1980) *Circulatory Physiology: The Essentials.* Williams and Wilkins, Baltimore.

Sperelakis, N., Kurachi, Y., Terzic, A. and Cohen M. (eds) (2001) *Heart Physiology and Pathophysiology.* Academic Press, San Diego.

Section II

Diagnostics

3

History and Physical Examination

H. Edward Durham, Jr.

Patient History

In evaluating the cardiac patient, a complete and thorough history, and physical examination are essential. Detailed information about the clinical signs is critical for creating a complete picture of the patient's current condition. The observations made during the history and physical examination will guide all diagnostics throughout the patient's care. Therefore, the importance of a thorough history and physical examination cannot be overemphasized.

In the non-emergency situation, a history is taken with the patient in the examination room. This will allow the patient to acclimatize to the environment and allow for important observations of the patient as part of the physical examination. Good listening skills are critical when taking a medical history. It is important to filter what the client relates into an accurate and complete summary that can be included in the medical record. Often clients will give more information than is truly relevant. It is up to the veterinary professional to extract the salient features. One method is to allow the client tell "their story" uninterrupted. This can give you a good feel for the clinical signs they are seeing at home and the level of anxiety caused by these clinical signs. Usually during this time the client will tell you what they think is the problem. After they have expressed all their concerns, more targeted questions can be asked.

Identified early in the history is the patient's species and breed, age, gender and reproductive status. Congenital heart defects are often first noted in young animals, and certain congenital cardiac defects have breed predispositions and defects, such as patent ductus arteriosus (PDA) which is more common in female patients. Acquired diseases such as valvular insufficiency, or myocardial disease, are noted in middle-aged to geriatric patients. Small breed dogs are more prone to chronic valvular degeneration whereas large breed dogs are more prone to myocardial failure.

It is also relevant to ascertain if the patient has an "occupation". Is the patient a house pet, or is it a show or breeding animal? Some patients are working animals and the ability to return to work may be part of the therapy goal. This may be especially true in equine cardiology, but may also include service or herding dogs.

The medical history should start with the presenting complaint or the reason the client felt the need to bring the animal to the veterinary cardiologist. The client is the best judge of abnormal behavior. Often there are no overt clinical signs of heart disease, but

Cardiology for Veterinary Technicians and Nurses, First Edition. Edited by H. Edward Durham, Jr.

a murmur or arrhythmia may be auscultated during a routine examination, prompting a visit to the veterinary cardiologist. The client may present the animal for coughing, exercise intolerance or poor performance, rapid breathing or other abnormal breathing patterns such as open mouth breathing in cats. Occasionally there may be a complaint of abdominal distension. Follow-up questions should be targeted to learn specific information and should only be directed at one aspect of the patient's health. Asking question with a "yes" or "no" answer will help direct the client to give limited responses. Questions about previous or concurrent medical conditions are an appropriate place to start. This area of questioning should include a vaccination history, previous illnesses or surgeries, parasite testing and prevention. Inquiring about the patient's diet and other animals in the house with the patient will help establish the home environment. Information such as whether the animal is housed indoors, outdoors, or both should not be forgotten. In addition to asking about the diet, it is important to ask about the patient's appetite and any apparent weight gain or loss. Fluid retention will increase body weight. Ascites may make the patient appear "fat" in the abdomen to the owner. Anorexia can lead to weight loss or cachexia.

Vomiting and diarrhea are not typically signs of heart disease, but may be seen with heart failure or indicate a concurrent disease condition, intolerance to current medication, or may affect the ability of the patient to take oral medications. Questions about the duration and frequency of vomiting and diarrhea should be asked.

During the interview, any medications the patient may be taking should be listed. When collecting the medication history, the veterinary technician should endeavor to learn the name of the medication, the strength of the dose and the frequency of administration. From this, the veterinary cardiologist can determine the dose and if there is room for adjustment. When the medication was started and how easily the patient can be medicated should also be ascertained. All current medications should be listed, including heartworm prevention and the last heartworm test.

Although pain is not typically associated with heart disease or failure, determining if the patient exhibits any signs of pain is part of a complete history. Pain may be perceived as difficulty lying down or rising, or more obvious signs such as limping or crying out when touched may be noted. With cats, limb paresis is a common sign of thromboembolic disease and is extremely painful.

Information about exercise can be useful in assessing overall cardiovascular function. Often the presenting complaint for a patient with cardiac disease may be exercise intolerance, which may manifest as a decreased ability to exercise or a complete lack of desire to be playful. Some clients notice that during a walk, the patient may have to stop and rest when it had not done so previously. Identifying exercise intolerance in cats can be more difficult and often manifests as decreased play time or open mouth breathing after play.

Respiratory effort and character provides important clues to the status of cardiac disease. Determination of how the patient breaths at home can be very important, especially when the patient is asleep, as rapid or labored breathing are common signs of congestive heart failure (CHF). Some dogs with CHF will demonstrate *orthopnea* or positional breathing. Animals showing orthopnea assume a standing or sitting position with elbows abducted and neck extended. Movement of the abdominal muscles that assist ventilation is often exaggerated. Orthopnea may be seen as reluctance to lay in lateral recumbency, preferring to stay sternal to ease breathing. The animal may also extend their neck to facilitate breathing and increase oxygenation. Sleeping habits can be an indicator of respiratory effort. One subtle sign of orthopnea is difficulty finding a "comfortable position". If the client reports the patient seems to have difficulty sleeping through the night, or is restless during sleeping hours, the patient may be experiencing difficulty breathing.

In cats, tachypnea is a more common sign than orthopnea, which may be seen as the cat sitting sternally with the head and neck extended. Coughing is rarely associated with heart failure in cats and is more indicative of respiratory disease.

Coughing in dogs is a common clinical sign of CHF. Coughing is also a clinical sign of respiratory disease and differentiating the two can be challenging. Careful inquiry into the nature of coughing is helpful. Differentiation between respiratory disease and heart disease can be difficult since many dogs with chronic myxomatous valvular degeneration may have concurrent respiratory disease, such as collapsing trachea. Determining if the cough is productive or dry will help define CHF. A moist or productive cough is more likely associated with heart failure, where dry hacking coughs are more indicative of disease of the respiratory system. The time of day the coughing occurs can also be important. In CHF, coughing is often more pronounced in the morning. One should also ask if the coughing is worse after exercise or activity. The duration of the cough is also important. Cough due to heart disease is usually slow to onset then progresses with time. Occasionally, other signs may be associated with the cough such as *syncope*.

Syncope, a temporary loss of consciousness, can occur for many reasons in patients with heart disease. A cough can increase vagal tone and cause a temporary sinoatrial node arrest leading to syncope. Poor cardiac output, profound atrial or ventricular arrhythmias, pulmonary hypertension or simple CHF can all lead to syncope. Clients will usually mention syncopal episodes as fainting, but one should always ask specifically if it occurs when collecting historical information. One challenge is to determine if the events reported by the owner are syncope or seizures. Syncope typically only lasts 10–15 seconds and afterward the patient is fully alert. There may be paddling motions though as the patient attempts to right themselves which can be misleading. In cases of seizure, the patient usually has a postictal phase during which they seem disoriented or weak for several minutes. Urination or defecation can occur, but are not commonly seen with syncope, which makes these signs non-specific.

A body system review with the client can yield important information the client may have failed to mention in the main interview. Simply asking if there has been any discharge from the eyes or nose, any hair loss or skin issues, any limping, or discharge from the reproductive organs, any difficulty urinating or defecating, or frequent urination can uncover forgotten details of the patient's current health status. Lastly the veterinary technician should ask if there is any other information the client wishes to share.

Physical Examination

Introduction

In patients that present with a history or clinical signs indicative of cardiovascular disease, the physical examination is an irreplaceable tool in the diagnostic process. The approach to the physical examination should be systematic. Some clinicians start at the head of the patient, others at the tail; either is acceptable providing that examination is performed the same way every time to minimize potentially overlooking an important sign. This chapter will present the physical examination from head to tail, focusing on the indicators of cardiovascular disease. Any abnormal findings should be reported.

Observing the Patient

Begin the physical examination by simply observing the patient when it is relaxed and breathing undisturbed. Noting the respiratory pattern and rate is best done before you begin handling the patient as stress can elevate respiratory rate. Pay particular attention to the breathing pattern, coughing, muscle wasting, or abdominal distention. Always record the rate, depth, and effort of respiration. The normal respiratory rate in small animals is approximately 18–30 breaths/minute. Several standard terms are used to describe breathing patterns in patients with cardiac disease. *Tachypnea* is an increase in the respiratory rate, but no increase in effort. *Dyspnea* is defined as distressed and labored breathing that may be tachypnic, but not always. Care must be given to uses these terms correctly. Dyspnea is divided into *inspiratory dyspnea* and *expiratory dyspnea.*

Inspiratory dyspnea is characterized by a prolonged, labored inspiratory effort, and a quicker, easier expiratory phase. Inspiratory dyspnea usually indicates an upper airway disorder. *Stertor* and/or *stridor* frequently accompany inspiratory dyspnea and an upper airway obstruction may be present. Stertor is a low-pitched snoring noise; this is often heard in bulldogs and other brachycephalic breeds; while stridor is a high pitched, harsh, wheezing noise. This is the sound made by dogs with laryngeal paralysis.

Expiratory dyspnea is characterized by a prolonged, labored expiratory effort and indicates an intrathoracic airway disorder such as chronic bronchitis, pulmonary edema due to CHF, and/or a restrictive disorder as seen with pleural effusion. Intrathoracic airway disease will frequently cause both inspiratory and expiratory dyspnea. This is a good time to be observant for orthopnea. As mentioned above, orthopnea is a term applied to respiratory distress that is exacerbated or relieved by recumbency.

An important indication of the patient's overall health is the body condition score (BCS). The body condition score gives a numerical number score from 1–10 based on the patient's percent body fat based on the impression of the observer. Charts for rating body condition score are readily available. In general, patients that are underweight will score low and those that are obese will score high. The ideal score is a BCS of 4. As with humans, obesity is associated with increased morbidity. Cachexia may be seen in patients with late stage heart failure, especially right heart failure. Cachexia is also seen with other serious health conditions such as neoplasia.

Head and Mucous Membranes

Although this text has a cardiovascular focus, it is important to examine the whole animal. Observation of other body systems will provide information about concurrent disease in addition to providing clues about cardiovascular disease. The examination of the eyes, ears and nares should begin the physical examination. Often respiratory disease is mistaken for CHF, so any nasal discharge should be noted. Ocular examination should be both external and internal, using an indirect lens, which may reveal abnormal fundic vessels due to venous congestion or polycythemia. Feline patients with taurine deficiency may demonstrate characteristic retinal degeneration, and the hypertensive patient may have torturous retinal vessels or retinal detachment. Aural health should be noted, since ear infections may be one reason for lethargy in the patient. Examination of the oral cavity can show dental or periodontal infection that could be a source of infection for bacterial endocarditis. Palpation of the neck in cats should be performed to identify possible functional thyroid tumors. Hyperthyroidism is a common cause of cardiac hypertrophy.

Mucous membranes should be examined to allow assessment of hydration, cardiac output, and oxygenation. The gingiva is the most common place to evaluate mucous membrane color, but in the pigmented patient, other sites may be warranted. Mucous membrane color can also be assessed at the vulva in females, or the prepuce in males. Normal mucous membranes are pink and moist, with a capillary refill time of less than two seconds.

Pale (*pallor*) mucous membranes indicate anemia, but may also be present with decreased cardiac output due to sympathetically induced peripheral vasoconstriction. Peripheral vasoconstriction occurs with hypothermia, poor cardiac output, and shock. Prolonged capillary refill time indicates peripheral vasoconstriction and is helpful in determining if the pallor is due to anemia or vasoconstriction. Anemic patients will be pale but have normal capillary refill times. *Plethora* is the term for brick red mucous membranes and indicates polycythemia or profound vasodilation as might be seen with septic shock.

Mucous membranes that are blue-colored are termed *cyanotic* which indicate an increase in the concentration of deoxygenated hemoglobin; approximately 5 mg/dL of desaturated hemoglobin. Cyanosis can be either central or peripheral [1, p. 48]. Central cyanosis is classified as having low arterial partial pressure of oxygen. Central cyanosis is seen with right-to-left shunting cardiac defects (such as tetralogy of Fallot), severe respiratory disease secondary to any disorder impairing oxygenation, or CHF related to concurrent pulmonary edema also impairing oxygenation. With right-to-left shunting defects, central cyanosis may be exacerbated by exercise as the muscles demand more oxygen and increased systemic vasodilation. Systemic vasodilation leads to decreased systemic vascular resistance thereby increasing the amount of right-to-left shunting.

Peripheral cyanosis is defined as having a normal arterial partial pressure of oxygen but decreased tissue oxygen content. Peripheral cyanosis is seen with marked hypothermia, arterial obstruction, or conditions creating low cardiac output such as dilated cardiomyopathy. In states of reduced perfusion, like dilated cardiomyopathy, the tissues extract more oxygen from the blood to compensate for the decreased perfusion. This in turn desaturates the venous blood more than usual exhibiting a cyanotic appearance to the observer.

A unique presentation of cyanosis is "differential" cyanosis which describes patients whose oral mucous membranes are normal colored, but genital mucous membranes are cyanotic. This finding is characteristic of a right-to-left shunting PDA, sometimes called a "reversed" PDA. Differential cyanosis occurs because the PDA is in the descending aorta or "downstream" to the brachiocephalic trunk in the aortic arch which supplies the head. The desaturated pulmonary blood shunts through the PDA and flows to the caudal body (See Chapter 10).

Examination of the Jugular Veins

Evaluation of the jugular veins can yield a wealth of information about disease of the right heart. Assessment of the jugular veins is often overlooked, especially in cases with peripheral edema or cavitary effusions. It is often necessary to wet or clip the hair coat over the area of the jugular veins to visualize jugular pulsations or jugular distention, although persistent jugular distention can frequently be palpated. Persistent jugular distention is an important indicator of right heart failure. It is commonly seen with pericardial effusion and tamponade, but also occurs with other causes of right-sided CHF (e.g. dilated cardiomyopathy), volume overload, or less commonly, cranial vena caval tumors or caval syndrome due to heartworm disease.

Normal jugular vein pulsation extends approximately one-third of the way up the neck. It occurs with normal atrial contraction. The head should be held in a "normal" position with the mandible parallel to the floor for this evaluation. A bounding carotid pulse may sometimes be mistaken for a jugular pulse. Differentiation may be made by gently holding off the jugular vein at the thoracic inlet. True jugular pulses will vanish but underlying carotid pulses will remain visible.

A jugular pulse that extends a distance greater than one-third of the neck is abnormal [1, p. 49]. Jugular pulsations may indicate tricuspid regurgitation, created by retrograde volume crossing the tricuspid valve during systole. The sudden increase in right atrial (RA) pressure combined with atrial contraction generates a pulse wave that is reflected up the neck. A jugular pulse may also be present in patients with atrioventricular (AV) asynchrony, such as complete AV block or ventricular tachycardia. In this instance the atria and ventricle are contracting simultaneously, the tricuspid valve is closed and the atrial blood cannot move to the ventricle. The resulting jugular pulse is termed a *canon a-wave* [1, p. 50].

Jugular pulses may occasionally be seen in patients with a poorly compliant right ventricle (RV). Right ventricular hypertrophy as seen with pulmonic stenosis is an example of decreased right ventricular compliance. As the right atrium contracts into the stiff RV the lack of compliance causes the atrial pulse wave to travel up the neck generating the so called *giant a-wave.*

The *hepato-jugular reflux* is a simple test to uncover elevated RA pressure in patients with right heart failure. To perform this test, observe the jugular veins while simultaneously compressing the cranial abdomen. In the normal patient no change in the jugular veins will be seen, because the right atrium has plenty of compliance to receive the additional volume displaced cranially by compressing the liver. In patients with elevated RA pressures and decreased RA compliance, the jugular veins distend following liver compression as the additional volume is displaced into the jugular veins. Elevated RA pressures are often associated with right ventricular dysfunction.

Evaluation of the Arterial System

Palpation of arterial pulses provides much information about cardiovascular function. The femoral artery is usually the most convenient to locate in small animals. In a patient with a normal rhythm, the heart rate and pulse rate will be equal. Pulse deficits indicate the presence of an arrhythmia. Pulses are characterized in terms of rate, rhythm, and quality. It is important to remember that palpation of the pulse does not estimate the blood pressure, as you are merely palpating the difference in systolic to diastolic pressure known as the *pulse pressure.* This will feel hyperkinetic when the difference is great or hypokinetic when the difference is small, but palpation alone gives no information about blood pressure. Arterial blood pressure measurement is described in detail in Chapter 7. Some variability may be noted in the pulse quality with sinus arrhythmia. After a long pause the next beat may demonstrate a stronger pulse when compared to the other pulses. This is due to the Frank–Starling law of the heart (see Chapter 2) and a prolonged diastolic period.

A hyperkinetic pulse is the result of a wide pulse pressure. These can occur in states of increased cardiac output such as anemia. Hyperkinetic pulses are a classic physical examination finding for left-to-right shunting PDA and may also be present for cases with significant aortic regurgitation. Sometimes referred to as a "water hammer pulse", these two examples are a result of the diastolic pressure in the aorta dropping as blood is shunted off to another chamber (the pulmonary artery or left ventricle [LV], respectively). Typically the systolic blood pressure is normal, but the diastolic pressure is low generating a dramatic difference between the systolic and diastolic blood pressures.

Hypokinetic pulses are those that are weak. This occurs with poor cardiac output as seen in conditions such as subaortic stenosis. Weak pulses do not mean the blood pressure is low, only that the pulse pressure is narrow.

The term variable (or sometimes unequal) is used to describe pulses that vary in strength from one beat to the next. Variable pulses are the hallmark of some tachyarrhythmias such as atrial fibrillation. Any arrhythmia can change the diastolic period of each beat. The variable filling period causes differences in stroke volume creating the variability in pulse pressure.

Pulsus alternans and *pulsus paradoxsus* are uncommon in veterinary medicine but will occur occasionally. Pulsus alternans will be felt as alternating strong pulses and weak pulses. Pulsus alternans may be felt in patients with myocardial dysfunction. Pulsus paradoxsus is an increase in the pulse during expiration and a decrease during inspiration. Although this phenomenon is actually normal, it generally cannot be appreciated on palpation unless it is exaggerated by conditions such as cardiac tamponade [1, p. 63].

Another feature of pulse palpation common with arrhythmias is *pulse deficits.* Premature depolarization of the heart results in a shortened diastolic period in which little or no flow actually leaves the LV. A heart sound may be heard but no pulse felt on palpation. To fully appreciate this, one must perform cardiac auscultation and palpate the femoral pulse simultaneously. It is not possible to tell if the premature depolarization is of ventricular or atrial origin without an electrocardiogram.

Auscultation

Introduction

The technique of auscultation of the thorax is as old as recorded medicine, as far back as Hippocrates. The sounds of the thorax, however, were not well appreciated until 1816 when René-Théophile-Hyacinthe Laennec invented the first stethoscope. Although it took almost 100 years for cardiac auscultation to be accepted as standard medical practice, auscultation and a stethoscope are now widely recognized as symbols of medicine.

Auscultation of the thorax provides information regarding the heart rhythm, movement of blood through the heart, abnormal function of the lungs and the presence of intrathoracic fluid. A firm command of the normal heart and lung sounds will make identifying abnormal sounds much easier.

Murmurs are the most common abnormal heart sound reported and can imply serious cardiac abnormalities. Murmurs are the sound of turbulent blood flow in the hemocardiac structures. In the normal heart, blood flow moves in a laminar fashion and is silent. That is, all the blood moves in a smooth unidirectional motion. Turbulence is created when the blood moves in multiple directions at varying velocities all at once. This turbulence creates vibrations which can be heard with a stethoscope or in extreme cases felt with the fingers (a *thrill*). The turbulence can be created as a result of high velocity outflow, septal defects or regurgitation backward through a valve. The intensity of the murmur is often not correlated with the severity of disease. Radiographs and echocardiograms are necessary for a complete diagnosis and prognosis; however, accurate isolation and identification of the murmur can limit the list of differentials.

Most murmurs are detectable by a veterinary technician. There is no reason why as part of the initial temperature, pulse and respiration assessment, the veterinary technician should not auscultate for and characterize any murmurs or abnormal heart sounds detected. This information should be relayed to the doctor in an organized and concise fashion. Standard nomenclature has been developed to simplify the process, which includes a grading scale for rating murmur loudness (Table 3.1), descriptors of murmur quality and timing (Figure 3.1), and names for transient cardiac sounds. Understanding these terms can be confusing, and they are often misused.

A top quality stethoscope is essential for good cardiac auscultation. Most cardiac sounds are outside the range of human hearing (Figure 3.2). The old adage "You get what you pay for" is true when purchasing a stethoscope. Select a reputable manufacturer and a top quality model. Features of a good stethoscope include short (25 inches, 63.5 cm or less) double lumen tubing, a brass or high quality steel head with both large (approximately 1.75 inches, 4.4 cm) and small diaphragms (approximately 1 inch, 2.5 cm) and a bell. For very small animals such as cats, kittens or puppies a neonatal stethoscope is indispensable. The ear pieces of quality stethoscopes point forward to align with the ear canals for optimal acoustics. The ear pieces should be comfortable with an adjustable

Table 3.1 Grading scale of heart murmur loudness.

Grade 1	A murmur sufficiently soft that it takes an experienced listener several minutes to hear under ideal conditions
Grade 2	A soft murmur that can be heard in only one valve location
Grade 3	A murmur easily heard that radiates to more than one valve area but has an identifiable point of maximal intensity
Grade 4	A loud murmur that is easily heard anywhere on the thorax, has no palpable thrill and can be difficult to locate the point of maximal intensity
Grade 5	A loud murmur that can be heard anywhere in the chest with a palpable thrill
Grade 6	A very loud murmur, with a thrill, and can be heard with the stethoscope raised off the body wall

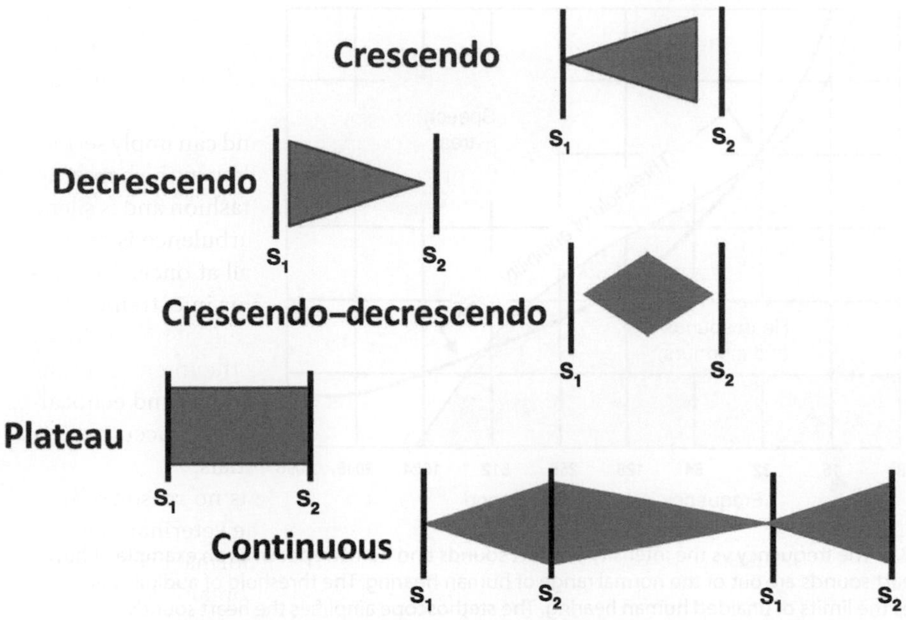

Figure 3.1 The relative timing of various murmurs in relation to the first and second heart sounds and their acoustic quality. The crescendo systolic murmur begins at S_1 and gets louder over systole ending near S_2. The decrescendo systolic murmur begins at S_1 and become softer as it ends near S_2. A crescendo–decrescendo (aka diamond shaped) systolic murmur begins at S_1, increases in intensity to mid-systole and then decreases until it ends near S_2. These three murmur sounds are most often associated with ejection murmur of ventricular outflow tracts. The plateau-shaped murmur begins at S_1 and remains the same intensity throughout systole. The continuous murmur occurs through all of systole and diastole with no interruption in the murmur.

tension yoke. The diaphragm side of the stethoscope head is best for hearing high frequency sounds such as murmurs.

A separate bell side seems to be more useful in veterinary medicine than a combined diaphragm/bell side due to the patient's hair coat. The bell side of the stethoscope head is best suited for hearing low frequency sounds such as gallops (discussed later). When using the bell, soft pressure must be used since too firm a touch will tense the skin making it perform like a diaphragm, obviating the low frequency acoustics. Electronic stethoscopes are also available, some with very useful features, but their cost is prohibitive for most veterinary technicians. No one stethoscope is perfect in all instances, and a variety of stethoscopes should be available.

During auscultation, the listener should be completely focused on the heart sounds. The most important part of the stethoscope is the "bit between the earpieces". Concentrate on isolating the heart sounds from the lung sounds; then identify the first and second heart sounds as an indicator of cardiac timing. Timing will be discussed in greater detail later in the chapter. Also take plenty of time to listen. Rushing will virtually guarantee missing subtle sounds. Other tips for acquiring the best auscultation include listening in a quiet room, controlling any panting or sniffing, positioning the patient in a standing position and placing the ear pieces pointed forward. In some cases, distracting

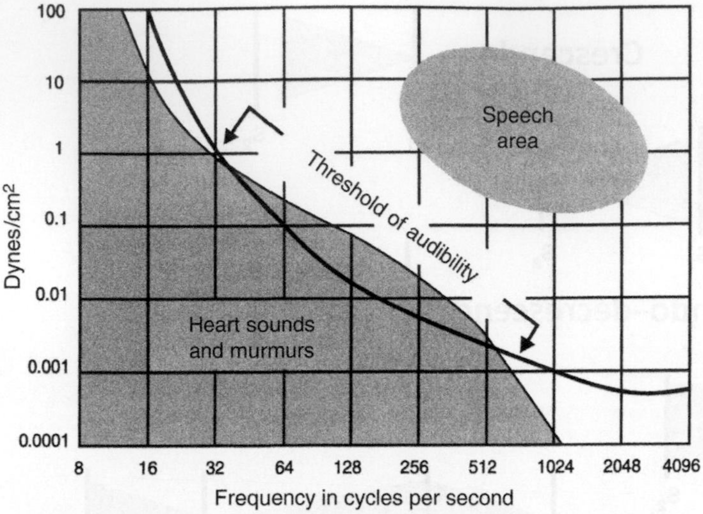

Figure 3.2 The frequency vs the intensity of heart sounds and human speech as an example of how most heart sounds are out of the normal range of human hearing. The threshold of audibility line indicates the limits of unaided human hearing. The stethoscope amplifies the heart sounds as they pass through the thorax wall allowing for evaluation of the heart sounds. Source: Fox, Sisson and Moïse (1999) [1]. Reproduced with permission of Elsevier.

the patient with a squeaky toy or running water will allow the listener to gain adequate restraint in anxious or fidgeting animals. Running water or an alcohol swab under the nose is particularly effective for controlling purring in cats.

Heart sounds can be divided into two groups: transient sounds and murmurs. Transient sounds are short in duration and low frequency. This category includes the normal heart sounds (S_1, S_2) as well as some abnormal sounds such as split sounds and gallops. Murmurs are typically longer in duration and higher in frequency.

Murmurs are characterized by their *location, timing,* and loudness or *grade.* A scale for cardiac murmur grade has been established that is widely used. The scale grades the loudness of a murmur from one to six, with six being the loudest. Some subjectivity is allowed in the system based on the listener's skill and hearing capabilities. This subjectivity should be of little concern, as the general idea is still transmitted, that a grade 5 murmur is very different than a grade 2.

The term *point of maximal intensity,* or *PMI,* is used to describe the location of the greatest intensity of a murmur. Murmur PMI is either right or left hemithorax and by valve area as detailed in the next section. A simplified method of describing PMI location is to identify a murmur ventral to the costochondral junction (the mitral valve area) as *apical*; the term *basilar* is applied to murmurs dorsal to the costochondral junction, near the aortic and pulmonic valves. Correct recognition of the PMI and pattern of radiation can be very helpful in identifying the specific cardiac abnormality.

The timing is related to the phase of the cardiac cycle: systolic or diastolic. The periods of the cardiac cycle are identified by the normal heart sounds commonly called the *lub* and *dub*, or more correctly as S_1 and S_2 respectively. The S_1 sound indicates the closing of the AV valves and signals the acoustic beginning of systole. S_1 is loudest at the left apex of the heart and is slightly lower pitch and longer than S_2. The S_2 sound occurs with the closing of the semilunar valves, marks the end of systole and is heard loudest at the left base of the heart. It is slighter higher pitched than S_1. The period between S_2 and the next S_1 is diastole.

Murmurs that occur between the first and second heart sounds are termed systolic and those which last the entire duration of systole are *holosystolic.* Holosystolic murmurs may mask S_1 and S_2 if they are very loud. Diastolic murmurs occur between S_2 and the next S_1 but are very rare in small animals. Continuous murmurs are almost always due to a left-to-right PDA, and are heard with no break in the sound during systole and diastole. Continuous murmurs peak in intensity near S_2 (Figure 3.1). Very rarely, a murmur will be heard in both systole and diastole but with a break between the two phases. These are called combination murmurs or "to-fro" murmurs.

When describing a murmur to the veterinarian include all three components. For example a moderately loud murmur heard best over the mitral valve during systole would be described as "left apical grade 3 systolic"; a murmur associated with a PDA might be described as a "left basilar grade 5 continuous" murmur.

Auscultation Process

Cardiac auscultation must be systematic and complete. Ideally, the animal should be standing during auscultation to maintain the normal anatomic position of the various valve areas of auscultation. If standing is not possible then sternal recumbency will suffice. Palpation of the thorax is the first step to an accurate auscultation. Thoracic palpation allows you to assess the strength and location of the apex beat. The *precordium* is the part of the thoracic wall directly over the heart on both sides. The apex beat is the point on the chest where you feel the heart beating the strongest against your hand. The apex beat or *apical impulse* is sometimes incorrectly referred to as the point of maximal intensity.

The left ventricular apex is the most muscular part of the heart and is located closest to the thoracic wall. The apex beat is normally found at or just below the costochondral junction in the left fourth to sixth intercostal space. There is variability with breed and conformation. Deep-chested dogs like Doberman pinchers, and greyhounds tend to have an apical impulse more cranial than bulldogs or corgis. A caudally displaced apex beat may indicate cardiomegaly, or a cranial mediastinal mass causing caudal displacement of the heart. An apical impulse stronger on the right side of the thorax may indicate right-sided cardiomegaly, or a mass displacing the heart to the right. A hypokinetic apex beat suggests decreased contractility but may be the result of obesity or pericardial effusion diminishing the precordial impulse.

During palpation, note any vibration felt over the heart. This vibration is known as a palpable *thrill,* and is associated with turbulent blood flow in the heart. A thrill is felt when the turbulence of the murmur can be felt through the chest wall. A thrill on palpation may be the first indication that a murmur is present. The presence of a thrill is part of the loudness grading scale for murmurs and therefore palpation is important in the grading process. The sensation is quite characteristic and feels like a high frequency buzzing on your fingers. One must be careful to distinguish a strong apex beat from a true thrill, especially in a thin animal.

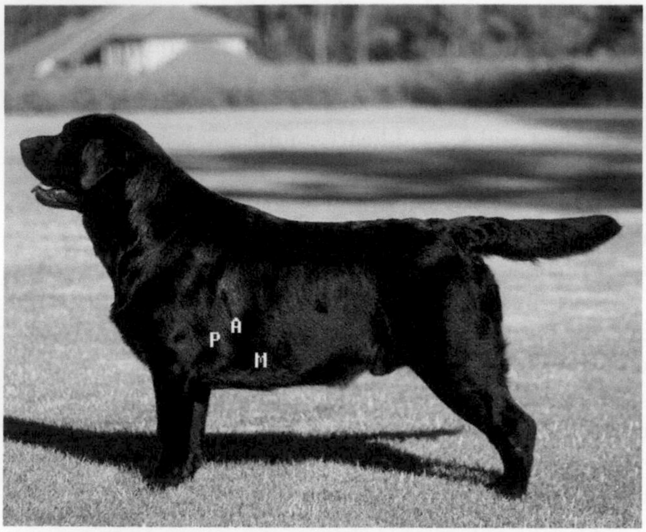

Figure 3.3 A view of the left lateral aspect of a dog showing the valve areas for auscultation of the left hemithorax: M, mitral valve; A, aortic valve; P, pulmonic valve. The extreme axillary base of the heart is the location for continuous murmur associated with patent ductus arteriosus. This is located cranial to the aortic valve and dorsal to the pulmonic valve. Source: courtesy of Judy Heim; Grand Ch. HySpire Singular Sensation "Single" owned and bred by HySpire Labradors.

Murmurs associated with the mitral valve are best heard at the fifth to sixth intercostal space on the left hemithorax (see Figure 3.3). However, due to breed differences the exact location may be variable. The apical impulse is a convenient "landmark" for the mitral valve area auscultation in normal animals. A murmur of mitral regurgitation will be heard best over the apex beat on the left side of the thorax. From there, moving the stethoscope cranially approximately one intercostal space and dorsally one intercostal space (left fourth intercostal space) will locate the aortic valve. Murmurs associated with the aortic valve will best be heard in this location. Move approximately one intercostal space cranially and ventrally (left third intercostal space) to locate the pulmonic valve where the murmur of pulmonic stenosis is best heard. This is the classic P-A-M scheme of auscultation on the left hemithorax [1, pp. 52,53].

Before proceeding on to the right hemithorax, listen deep in the left axillary region, another intercostal space cranial and dorsal, where the great vessels cross. This area is the best site for hearing the continuous murmur of PDA.

The tricuspid valve is located on the right hemithorax directly across from the left apical impulse. This will allow for the best auscultation of tricuspid regurgitation. Lastly, move the stethoscope to the cranial dorsal region of the heart on the right side of the chest for the murmur of ventricular septal defects (VSD) or a murmur radiating within the aortic blood column such as can occur with aortic outflow tract obstructions.

Auscultation of the cat is slightly different than in dogs. The heart of the cat tends to have more sternal contact than in dogs. An effective method for feline auscultation starts with the stethoscope head placed directly in the central ventral thorax over the sternum where the apical impulse is palpated. The stethoscope is then moved just off the left lateral sternum. From this position most feline murmurs of mitral regurgitation or gallop sounds may be heard; then the stethoscope is moved approximately 1 inch (2.5 cm) cranial. The process is repeated for the right sternal border where the murmur of VSDs is loudest. In some cats a right cranial sternal border murmur may be appreciated as a result of turbulence in the aortic arch associated with hypertrophic obstructive cardiomyopathy.

During auscultation the heart rate should be counted. Normal heart rate for the dog ranges from 70 beats/min in larger dogs to as high as 220 beats/min in puppies. Normal heart rates for cats and kittens range from 140 to 240 beats/min [1, p. 75]. A slower than normal heart rate is termed a *bradycardia,* and a faster than normal rate is termed a *tachycardia.* Abnormalities in heart rate or rhythm must be identified and characterized. There are two normal rhythm variations in the dog. Normal sinus rhythm has a regular beat with a normal rate. A normal sinus arrhythmia has a normal to slow heart rate, and is characterized by cyclic increase and decrease in heart rate. This is sometimes specifically associated with respiration, and results in an increase in heart rate during inspiration and a decrease in heart rate with expiration. Respiratory sinus arrhythmia is common in dogs, but very uncommon in the cat. Sinus arrhythmias are associated with increased vagal tone, and are usually a sign of a healthy heart. However, a much exaggerated sinus arrhythmia can occur secondary to other disease processes, the most common of these being chronic gastrointestinal disease, chronic pulmonary disease, increased intracranial pressure, and increased intraocular pressure.

Arrhythmias can usually be heard during the auscultation. Pauses, skips, bursts, rapid changes in rate, or asynchrony are indicative of arrhythmias. Arrhythmias such as atrial fibrillation are so completely asynchronous they are distinctive and can be practically diagnosed by auscultation alone.

A number of recognizable patterns of arrhythmias can be described. Beats that occur prematurely, and are associated with pulse deficits are termed *extrasystoles.* They may be atrial and ventricular premature complexes. Bursts or runs of extrasystoles are termed *paroxysmal tachyarrhythmias* such as with paroxysmal atrial and ventricular tachycardia. As already mentioned, a remarkably irregular tachyarrhythmia is termed a *chaotic* tachyarrhythmia, as occurs with atrial fibrillation. A persistent regular tachycardia may be seen with a continuous supraventricular or ventricular tachycardia. A persistent regular bradycardia is typical with complete AV block. An electrocardiogram is always indicated if any arrhythmia is appreciated other than sinus arrhythmia. No other diagnostic is as useful for defining the exact nature of a suspected arrhythmia.

At some point during auscultation, it is important to simultaneously palpate the pulses. Pulses should be synchronous with cardiac auscultation. During this phase of the exam, the examiner should palpate an arterial pulse in the patient to detect any *pulse deficits* created by any arrhythmia. A pulse deficit is detected when a heart sound is heard but no corresponding pulse is felt, as with extrasystoles. The femoral pulse is most easily accessible in dogs and cats. A facial artery can be used in large animals.

Next, the lungs are auscultated. The animal should be standing and relaxed when you perform auscultation of the respiratory system. To acquire a good respiratory auscultation, the patient should not be panting. If necessary, the animal's mouth must be gently held shut during auscultation. The entire thorax should be systematically auscultated. One method is to mentally divide the lung fields into four quadrants on each side of the thorax and listen to each individually. In very large dogs, further dividing the quadrants into smaller sections may be needed. Normal breathing should be almost silent. Several abnormal lung sounds are recognized. The following terminology is used to describe abnormal lung sounds.

Rales, or more commonly called crackles, are short snapping sounds usually heard during inspiration. They are frequently described as course or fine. The sound of crackles has been compared to crinkling plastic food wrap near your ear. Rales are caused by various pulmonary disorders such as chronic bronchitis or pulmonary edema, in which some of the smaller airways are collapsed during the early phase of inspiration, and then suddenly open with a crackling sound as inspiration progresses. Crackles occurring with a low to normal heart rate suggest primary pulmonary disease. The low heart rate is related to increased vagal tone caused by the pulmonary disease. Crackles with an elevated heart rate are suggestive of CHF due to increased sympathetic tone. It is not correct that the presence of crackles always equals "wet lungs" [2, pp. 70, 71].

Wheezes, which may be further classified as high-pitched and low-pitched are continuous musical or whistling sounds generated by air passing through narrowed airways. Intrathoracic tracheal collapse is a common cause of wheezes. Wheezes that arise from intrathoracic disorders are usually more pronounced during expiration. Expiratory wheezes are commonly heard in cases with bronchoconstriction like asthma or smoke inhalation [2, pp. 71, 389, 482].

Stertor is a low pitched noise that is similar to the sound of snoring in humans. This can commonly be heard in brachycephalic breeds. *Stridor* is a high pitched noise heard on inspiration. This is the sound commonly heard with disease of the larynx or upper trachea such as laryngeal paralysis.

Muffled breath sounds may occur with conditions such as pleural effusions. With pleural effusion, careful auscultation of your patient in the standing position will frequently reveal a fluid line – normal breath sounds in the dorsal lung fields, and muffled or absent breath sounds in the ventral lung fields. Thoracic percussion can also help confirm the presence of a fluid line. By placing one hand flat on the patient then tapping it briskly with two fingers of the other hand a difference in resonance can be appreciated between the ventral fluid-filled portion and the dorsal air-filled portion of the thorax.

Bronchovesicular sounds are the sound of increased air movement. It can be a normal finding in an animal breathing heavily, or may be a sign of early pulmonary abnormalities such as bronchitis.

Murmurs

When discussing murmurs, it is often helpful to characterize the pitch and quality of the murmur. Pitches are usually described with terms such as high, low, musical, rumbling, or whooping. The quality of the murmur refers to the changes in tone over time. The quality of murmurs can be displayed with a phonocardiogram that can show the "shape" of the tone. These shapes are the plateau, crescendo, decrescendo, and the crescendo–decrescendo (Figure 3.1).

Some murmurs have characteristic sounds such as subaortic stenosis which commonly has a crescendo or crescendo–decrescendo quality at the left heart base. These murmurs are sometimes referred to as "ejection" murmurs and tend to start slightly after the onset of systole or stop just before the end. Pulmonic stenosis will have a similar sound and may be indistinguishable from subaortic stenosis in some breeds.

The murmur of mitral regurgitation is typically a low harsh plateau shape when recorded by phonocardiogram. This feature can be helpful when it is difficult to determine if the murmur is apical or basilar.

Murmurs can be classified into two groups: *organic* and *physiologic*. Organic murmurs are present due to a change or abnormality in the architecture of the cardiac structures. Physiological murmurs exist in the presence of a structurally normal heart. Also known as *functional*, or *innocent*, these murmurs are not related to heart disease at all. Physiologic murmurs are best heard on the left hemithorax over the aortic valve as they are usually created by a small amount of turbulence in the left ventricular outflow tract. These murmurs are of ejection quality, medium to low intensity, typically a grade 3/6 or less. As the underlying condition that creates the murmur is treated then the murmur may diminish or even disappear completely.

Functional or physiologic (these terms are interchangeable) murmurs can be heard in patients with fever, anemia, and/or metabolic high output conditions, such as hyperthyroidism or in patients of advanced athletic training. Anemic patients presenting with hematocrits of less than 22–25% [1, p. 59] have a low enough viscosity of the blood to make it more easily turbulent. Athletic dogs, those with fevers, or hyperthyroidism have physiological murmurs related to the hypervigorous contraction of the heart. Female dogs in estrus, pregnant, or lactating can also have physiologic murmurs due to increased cardiac output.

Innocent murmur is a term mostly used for soft murmurs heard in puppies or kittens less than 16 weeks of age, which they normally outgrow. The exact cause of an innocent juvenile murmur is not clearly understood. Contributing factors are thought to be the lower hematocrit of juveniles and/or a mismatch in the aortic to LV size that corrects as the puppy or kitten grows. When evaluating puppies or kitten that present with murmurs, some guidelines are useful for determining if the murmur is innocent or pathologic. Three criteria seem to be the most useful:

1) The murmur is soft; graded 3 or less.
2) The murmur is completely resolved by 16 weeks of age.
3) The murmur gets softer over time.

A murmur in a puppy that is continuous or loud is unlikely to be innocent. Also, if the murmur gets louder over the course of the vaccination schedule or persists beyond the rabies vaccination, then it is unlikely to be innocent.

Of the organic murmurs, mitral regurgitation is the most commonly heard. Mitral regurgitation is extremely common in small breed dogs and cats. This murmur is best heard over the left apex of the heart although a loud murmur will radiate over other areas of the thorax. The grade of the murmur does not correspond well with the severity of disease. An echocardiogram and thoracic radiographs are required to fully assess these dogs. Mitral regurgitation can be caused by chronic myxomatous valvular degeneration (endocardiosis), endocarditis, volume overload, or valve dysplasia.

Tricuspid regurgitation is almost identical to mitral regurgitation in quality, pitch, and timing. Tricuspid murmurs are loudest in the right hemithorax. If mitral regurgitation is present it is often difficult to tell if the murmur in the right is mitral regurgitation radiating to the right or if it is tricuspid regurgitation. In some cases a subtle difference in pitch or quality can be a clue to true tricuspid regurgitation, but an echocardiogram is the best diagnostic for conformation.

Murmurs of subaortic and pulmonic stenosis are also important murmurs. The difficulty can be separating the two by auscultation alone. The valves are in close proximity and distinguishing the difference can be difficult even for an experienced listener. Although some breed predilections are known, a Doppler-echocardiogram is required to determine the exact valve in question and the severity of the obstruction. The murmur of both subaortic stenosis and pulmonic stenosis are heard at the left heart base and are ejection quality murmurs. In this case, the grade of the murmur correlates better with the severity of disease. A severe stenosis will usually present with a louder murmur than a mild stenosis.

As previously stated, in the extreme left axillary region over the great vessels, the continuous murmur of a PDA is best heard. The continuous murmur is distinct in that it occurs in both systole and diastole with no pause in between. The sound of the murmur is always present. Patients with PDA routinely have moderate to severe amounts of mitral regurgitation. A murmur of mitral regurgitation combined with the systolic portion of the PDA can make it is easy to miss the diastolic portion of the murmur without careful auscultation of the left axillary region. When a continuous murmur is heard in the left axillary region, a PDA is virtually assured. Again an echocardiogram is used to confirm the diagnosis, guide the treatment options and assess any long-term damage to the heart.

In VSDs, typically a loud grade 4–6/6 right basilar systolic murmur is heard. The VSD is an instance in which the grade of the murmur is inversely related to the severity of disease. The loud murmur implies normal ventricular chamber pressures and systolic function and thus carries a better prognosis. As the heart starts to fail, the murmur actually grows softer.

Sometimes in the presence of a VSD a fairly loud (grade 3–4/6) left basilar murmur may also be heard. This murmur is known as *a murmur of relative pulmonic stenosis* and sounds similar to a murmur of pulmonic stenosis. This is the sound of an increased volume of blood passing through a normal-sized orifice. The blood shunting through the VSD from the left to the RV is added to the normal volume of blood returning from the right atrium. Together these represent an increased volume trying to pass through the pulmonic valve. Since the amount of time the heart has to move this extra volume remains unchanged, it must increase the blood velocity thereby creating turbulence and a murmur. In the case of an atrial septal defect, the shunt itself does not create a murmur, but if the volume of the shunt is sufficient to create a relative pulmonic stenosis, a murmur is heard.

Transient Sounds

Transient heart sounds are very short sounds of the heart and include the normal S_1 and S_2 (Figure 3.4). In large animal species additional sounds can normally be heard (see Chapter 17). These sounds, identified as S_3 and S_4, are associated with early ventricular filling and atrial contraction during the diastolic period, respectively. In small animals, however, S_3 and S_4 are always considered abnormal. In small animals, these sounds are commonly referred to as *gallops* and are associated with cardiac disease. Gallops can be difficult to hear, particularly at high heart rates, such as those normal for small animals. It is even harder to distinguish whether it is S_3 or S_4.

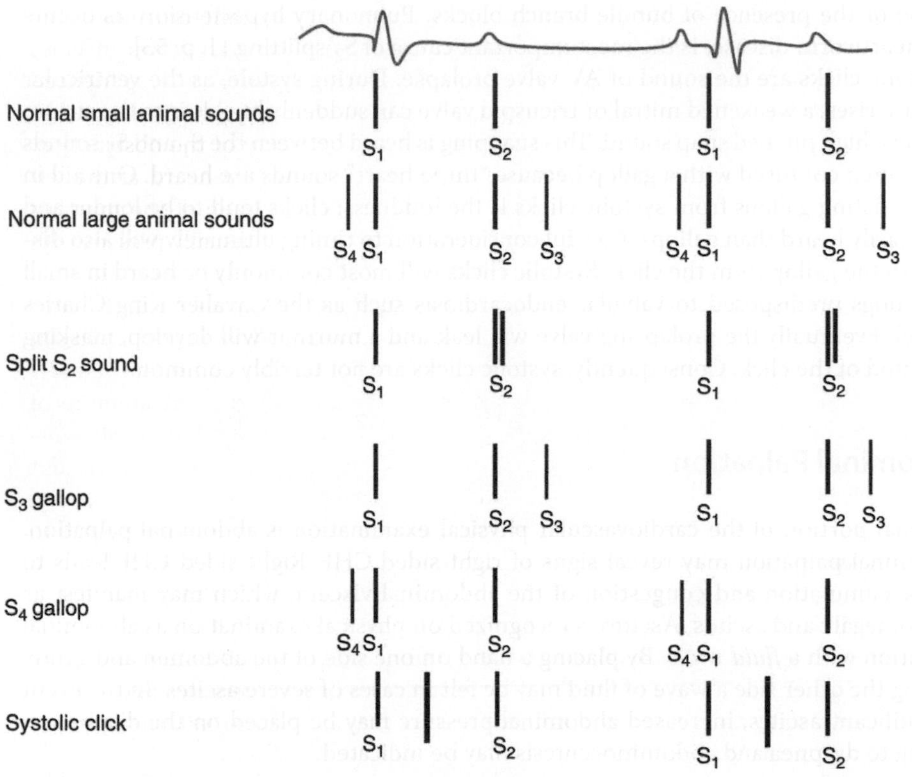

Figure 3.4 A diagram of various abnormal transient heart sounds. An electrocardiogram runs across the top to indicate timing. S_1 occurs with the QRS complex and S_2 occurs at the end of the T wave. The thickness of the vertical bar indicates the relative loudness of the sound indicated. S_3 and S_4 are typically soft sounds indicated by the thinnest bars; systolic clicks tend to be loud as indicated by the thick bar. The normal heart sounds for all mammals are S_1 and S_2. Large animal species may have all four heart sounds present or a combination of three, but S_1 and S_2 are always present. Gallop sounds are soft and occur during systole either before the QRS as with S_4 or after the T-wave as with S_3. The systolic click occurs between S_1 and S_2.

Fortunately, since there are no normal gallops in small animals, differentiating between the two gallops is not necessary; simply identifying the abnormal sound is sufficient to warrant additional diagnostics. As a general rule, S_3 is more commonly associated with dilated cardiomyopathy in dogs and S_4 is associated with hypertrophic cardiomyopathy in cats. A *summation gallop* is heard when at very high heart rates, S_3 and S_4 are summated on top of each other because the atrial are contracting simultaneously with the ventriclular relaxation [1, p.57]. This is commonly heard in cats with hypertrophic cardiomyopathy.

Other transient sounds which can be heard include *split sounds* and *systolic clicks*. Usually, the AV valves close almost simultaneously, so that only one heart sound (S_1) is heard. Similarly, the semilunar valves close nearly simultaneously producing a single S_2. Split sounds are heard when the two valves (either the AV valves or the semilunar valves) close at slightly different times. Split S_2 is more commonly heard in veterinary medicine then a split S_1 sound. A split second heart sound may be due to pulmonary disease or the presence of bundle branch blocks. Pulmonary hypertension, as occurs with heartworm disease, is the most important cause of S_2 splitting [1, p. 55].

Systolic clicks are the sound of AV valve prolapse. During systole, as the ventricular pressure rises, a weakened mitral or tricuspid valve can suddenly buckle into the atrium causing a high pitched snap sound. This snapping is heard between the S_1 and S_2 sounds and is often confused with a gallop because "three heart" sounds are heard. One aid in differentiating gallops from systolic clicks is the loudness; clicks tend to be louder and more easily heard than gallops. Careful consideration to timing ultimately will also distinguish the gallop from the click. Systolic clicks will most commonly be heard in small breed dogs predisposed to valvular endocardiosis such as the Cavalier King Charles Spaniel. Eventually the prolapsing valve will leak and a murmur will develop, masking the sound of the click. Consequently, systolic clicks are not terribly common.

Abdominal Palpation

The final portion of the cardiovascular physical examination is abdominal palpation. Abdominal palpation may reveal signs of right-sided CHF. Right-sided CHF leads to fluid accumulation and congestion of the abdominal viscera, which may manifest as hepatomegaly and ascites. Ascites is recognized on physical examination as abdominal distention with a *fluid wave.* By placing a hand on one side of the abdomen and gently tapping the other side a wave of fluid may be felt in cases of severe ascites. In the event of significant ascites, increased abdominal pressure may be placed on the diaphragm leading to dyspnea and abdominocentesis may be indicated.

References

1 Fox, P.R., Sisson, D. and Moïse, N.S. (eds) (1999) *Textbook of Canine and Feline Cardiology: Principles and Clinical Practice*, 2nd Edition. W.B Saunders Company, Philadelphia.

2 King, L.G. (2004) *Respiratory Disease in Dogs and Cats.* Saunders Elsevier, St Louis.

4

Electrocardiography

Shari Hemsley

Introduction

Electrocardiography is the study of the heart's electrical activity [1], fascinating generations of researchers, clinicians, and technicians. The instrumental device that detects and records the activity, known as the electrocardiograph, is based upon the string galvanometer modified by Willem Einthoven [1]. An electrocardiogram (ECG) is the recorded tracing produced by the electrocardiograph [2] giving rise to the familiar and beloved waveforms, PQRST.

History – the Highlights

The evolution of electrocardiography is rich in history. Throughout the centuries, many were eager to pursue the subject of electricity and its effects on tissue. Observations, theories, and inventions were varied. Only a few of the notables are mentioned here.

Luigi Galvani, an Italian anatomist, studied the effects of electricity on animal tissues in the 1780s [3, p. 20]. Galvani's name is given to the galvanometer, which is an instrument for measuring and recording electricity [4].

In the 1880s British physiologist, Augustus Waller, published the first electrocardiograms in man by using the capillary electrometer [1]. He would often demonstrate his technique on his dog, Jimmy, who stoically stood with paws plunged into jars of saline [5] (Figure 4.1). The saline acted as electrodes on the body surface rather than contact electrodes in use today.

In 1895, a Dutch physiologist known as Willem Einthoven, used an improved electrometer and a correction formula to distinguish five deflections which he eventually named P, Q, R, S, and T [2]. Even with refinement the capillary electrometer showed tracings of diminished intensity and limited high-frequency response [3, p. 59]. The mathematical formula of differential equations that he devised contained more detailed waves and allowed for compensation of the mercury's inactivity and friction inside the electrometer's tube [2; 6, p. 24]. Theories vary widely as to the labeling of the peak deflections; was it simply an arbitrary choice or due to Einthoven's mathematical training, reflecting Descartes' Cartesian coordinate system influences [2; 5; 6, p.25; 7; 8]? Regardless of the naming debate these five derived deflections were labeled with the second

Cardiology for Veterinary Technicians and Nurses, First Edition. Edited by H. Edward Durham, Jr.

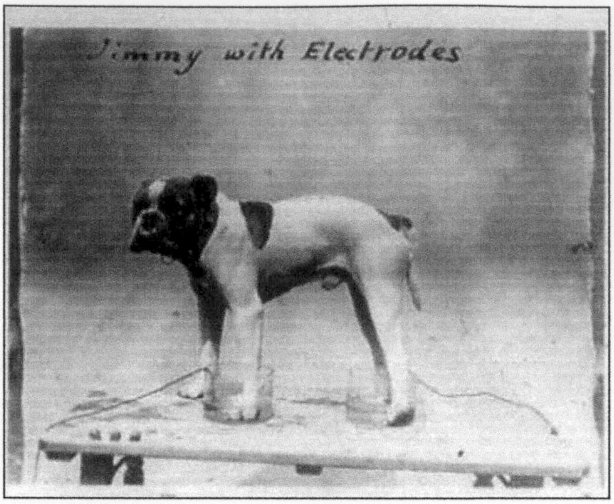

Figure 4.1 Augustus Waller's dog, Jimmy, helped him in his research amid controversy. The photo shows Jimmy standing with his paws in containers of saline solution. Waller believed the body itself conducts electricity and that the limbs act as cable extensions of the heart. Source: Besterman [5]. Reproduced with permission of West Indian Medical Journal.

half of the alphabet to differentiate them from the four deflection labels previous to the correction formula (A, B, C, D). Einthoven's desire to show the difference between the uncorrected tracing, ABCD, and the mathematically corrected and transformed tracing, PQRST, led to the labeling change [2; 7].

In 1899, Karel Wenckebach published a paper on the analysis of irregular pulses describing impaired atrioventricular (AV) conduction [9]. This impairment led to progressive lengthening and then blocking of AV conduction in frogs later called the Wenckebach phenomenon or Mobitz type I block [9].

Einthoven refined the string galvanometer, invented in 1897 by Clement Ader, and in 1901 he described his work [1; 10, p. 118]. The instrument's sensitivity surpassed older instruments. Einthoven was able to produce electrocardiograms in 1902 using the modified string galvanometer [2]. The increased sensitivity of this device produced higher quality tracings than earlier versions of the capillary electrometer, resulting in precise stellar recordings with five waveforms, PQRST, that validated his earlier correction formula work [2]. And then, in 1924, he was awarded the Nobel Prize for his discovery of the mechanism of the ECG [2]. The string galvanometer has since developed into the electrocardiograph we know today (Figure 4.2).

The ECG – A Great Tool to Have in Your Cardio Kit

The ECG is a dynamic, exciting tool that can provide insight into the heart's rhythm and rate, but like many tools, it has limitations. Used thoughtfully and well, the ECG can aid the clinician in the animal's final diagnosis in conjunction with other diagnostic tests and observations.

As a technician, learn how to obtain the best ECG possible under normal and various limiting circumstances. Aim for a steady baseline, artifact-free waveforms, and publish worthy tracings while keeping the patient comfortable. To help you accomplish this feat, arm yourself with ECG knowledge. Be able to identify waveforms as well as artifacts so that problems in obtaining an ECG can be resolved. Know your machine and its settings. Measure waveforms, segments, and intervals accurately and then compare the

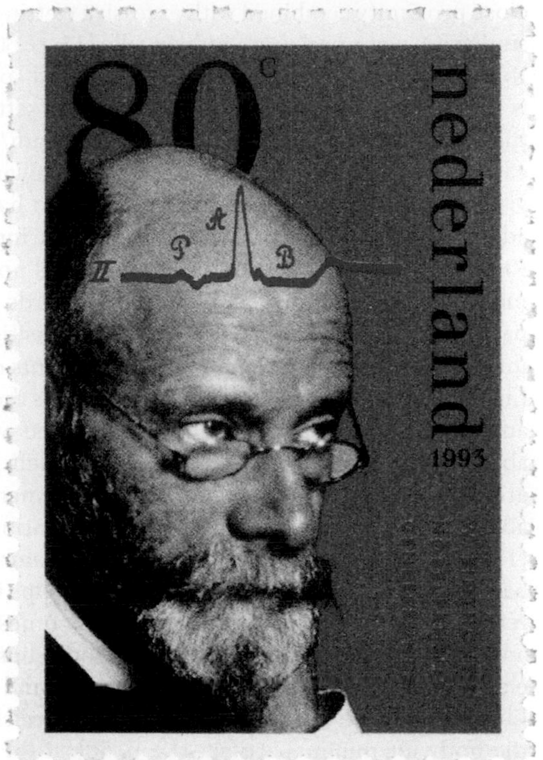

Figure 4.2 Dutch stamp issued in 1993 by the Royal Post Office of the Netherlands commemorating the first recording of a modern electrocardiogram by Willem Einthoven (1860–1927), 1924 Dutch Nobel Laureate. Source: Reproduced with permission of Royal PostNL.

measurements to reference tables of known species and breed values (see Table 4.3). Detailed descriptions are discussed later in this chapter.

Here are some tips to guide you when obtaining an ECG:

- Properly grounded equipment is important in reducing electrical interference known as 60-cycle artifact, an interference of the alternating current that creates a thick horizontal ECG line with an up-and-down wave pattern [11, pp. 60, 61]. Use of an insulator beneath the patient, such as a rubber mat or blanket, and a dedicated ECG machine outlet aid in decreasing electrical interference [11, pp. 60, 61].
- Flattened alligator clips provide patient comfort. Adhesive electrode patches may be used during prolonged monitoring [12, p. 50].
- Fit electrode clips tightly to the attachment cables to prevent any loose connections [13, p. 33].
- Achieve good contact and low resistance between the skin and the electrode clips with isopropyl alcohol or conducting gel: too dry and there will be no contact communication; too wet and there might be electrical interference [11, p. 60]. Interestingly, if an animal is soaking wet from a recent bath or rain shower, this can also cause electrical interference and conductivity problems. Use clean electrode clips since poor contact could be caused by dry gel build-up on the clips. Be careful not to touch the electrode clips or allow the clips to touch each other during acquisition as this could cause electrical noise artifact [11, p. 60]. Use care when wetting chest electrodes. Their

close proximity combined with excessive wetting may cause an unhappy result of lead similarity; wet or gel them individually [11, p. 60].

- Know your ECG machine settings. Standard speed is 50 mm/s. Standard sensitivity is 10 mm = 1 mV [12, p. 51]. Adjust these settings for each patient or situation. If the heart rate is fast, slow the speed to 25 mm/s in order to see the rate trend more easily at a glance. If R waves are extremely tall and running into another lead making visibility difficult, decrease the sensitivity to half so that 5 mm = 1 mV. Take these adjustments into consideration when measuring amplitudes and durations.
- Right lateral recumbency is the conventional position for dog and cat ECG measurements using limb lead technique with regards to detection of cardiac enlargement patterns. If the patient is in distress other positions will at least give rate and rhythm information, although standard measurements cannot be obtained [11, pp. 26, 27].
- Limb lead placement is typically just above the olecranons for the right arm (RA) and left arm (LA) electrode clips (color coded white and black, respectively) and just above the stifles for the right leg (RL) and left leg (LL) electrode clips (color coded green and red, respectively), although attachment just below these sites is also acceptable in patients with heavy or rapid respiration to lessen or avoid motion artifact [13, p. 27]. A mnemonic device for right lateral recumbency limb lead placement based on the above color-coded electrode clips is "snow and grass are on the ground; read the morning paper first; Christmas comes at the end of the year", where snow and grass refer to white and green electrode clips, newspaper refers to black and white electrode clips, and Christmas refers to red and green electrode clips.
- Limbs should be extended, separate yet parallel to each other and perpendicular to the body for minimal artifact [12, p. 50]. If the patient is breathing rapidly and the elbows are tucked in and touching the thorax, ECG artifact is likely. Keep the cables and electrode clips, or the patient, or both, as still as possible during acquisition.
- Standing is the conventional position for horse, cow, and other farm animal ECG measurements using base apex technique [11, p. 27] (see Chapter 17; Figure 17.2).
- Base apex lead placement is typically as follows: the negative electrode placed in the right jugular groove one-third up the neck and the positive electrode placed at the heart apex near the left elbow of the sixth intercostal space [14]. The ground is placed anywhere. The base apex technique is a single lead only and modifies the electrodes from one of the bipolar standard limb leads (I, II, or III) allowing the largest QRS deflections [14]. Lead I: positive LA/negative RA; Lead II: positive LL/negative RA; Lead III: positive LL/negative LA [13, p. 12] (Table 4.1).
- A soothing atmosphere is best for minimal baseline and muscle tremor artifacts. Bring on your Zen maneuvers; a quiet voice, a calm hand on their chest wall, a soft blowing or light tapping on the nose, or perhaps an ear rub will produce an artifact-free baseline, at least for several beats. Keep in mind that while some arrhythmias are observed when the patient is calm and resting, others are elicited when the patient is excited.

The ECG is an outstanding tool in characterizing rhythms and arrhythmias, monitoring treatment therapy and pacemaker function, and in identifying certain electrolyte disturbances and drug toxicity changes [13, p. 21]. It provides information about normal and abnormal heart conduction. It is also helpful in monitoring the patient during anesthesia and surgery as well as the critically ill patient in the intensive care unit. However, the ECG is not as sensitive in cardiac enlargement detection [15, p. 73]. In this

Table 4.1 The two types of ECG limb leads: bipolar and unipolar. Bipolar limb leads use a single positive and negative electrode, and includes leads I, II, and III. Unipolar limb leads use a single positive electrode and a combination of the other two electrodes that serve as the negative electrode, and includes leads aVR, aVL, aVF. Together the bipolar and unipolar limb leads create the hexaxial reference system and view the electrical activity of the heart in the frontal plane while the precordial chest leads, another type of unipolar lead, view the heart's activity in the transverse plane.

Bipolar leads: standard limb leads I, II, II	
I	+ Left arm; – Right arm
II	+ Left leg; – Right arm
III	+ Left leg; – Left arm
Unipolar leads: augmented limbs leads aVR, aVL, aVF	
aVR	+Right arm; – Left arm and Left leg
aVL	+Left arm; – Right arm and Left leg
aVF	+Left leg; – Right and Left arms

a, augmented; V, vector; R, right arm; L, left arm; F, foot or leg.

area, there may be false positive and negative findings, but ECG enlargement patterns may have significance in context with other diagnostic findings [13, p. 22]. The echocardiogram is best at viewing heart structure and pumping function and the radiograph at overall heart size [12, p. 49].

Importantly, however calm a patient may appear in the hospital setting, heart rate can be unfavorably elevated due to stress levels. The ECG acquired in such a setting may give an inaccurate accounting of the patient's true heart rate. Improved arrhythmia frequency detection and review of treatment response management is achieved with longer recordings. In these situations, the hospital ECG is inadequate and a 24-hour ambulatory ECG recording, such as a Holter monitor, is ideal [15, p. 331]. Instructing the owner on how to count the heart rate is helpful in getting a general idea of the rate at home, as well as empowering the client in the care and management of their animal.

The digital era is here. Soon we will all have electronic ECG machines. Even now these are innovative and über-sophisticated and will only improve in the days ahead. Interpretative software tools such as on-screen calipers, zoom features, and efficient post-processing options are forward thinking and on trend. The ability to post process rate, amplitudes, and noise filters opens up new levels of interpretation. Viewing tachycardias at 100 mm/s that were acquired at 50 mm/s or increasing amplitudes to 20 mm/mV that were acquired at 10 mm/mV are possible. Storage and retrieval modes streamline file organization and will eventually eliminate the need for specialized ECG paper. The ability to email tracings quickly and conveniently to third parties is a great benefit. Many digital machines allow longer recordings at the highest sampling frequencies for better analyses; however, accuracy of the software diagnoses is not yet dependable until veterinary-specific software is improved.

Finally, ECG reading can be fun and interesting although often people avoid them, seeming tentative in their approach. If you approach them systematically, they will soon begin to make sense and reveal their mysteries.

Lead Systems Point the Way

It is ideal to view the electrical activity of the heart from several angles [16, p. 78]. Multiple views are better than one view, providing more information. The various lead systems and their orientations to the heart provide this benefit giving greater accuracy in ECG interpretation and axis determination, while sometimes aiding in localization of specific abnormalities [16, p. 78–80].

The bipolar leads record electrical potentials between a single positive electrode and a single negative electrode [16, p. 79]. It is a recording of the voltage differences between two electrodes during a cardiac cycle. The bipolar limb leads consist of I, II, and III [16, p. 79] (Table 4.1).

> **Tech Tip 1:** typical lead I is upright on the tracing [13, p. 61]. If you notice that it is negative, check lead placement first before assuming an ECG abnormality. If the left and right arm electrodes are reversed in placement on a normal dog, for instance, the polarity will be negative on the tracing. Another lead placement reality check involves the P wave. In the dog and cat, it is normally positive in leads I, II, III, and aVF and NEGATIVE in aVR [13, p.61]. Check lead placement if the polarity is positive in aVR on the tracing as this commonly indicates incorrect lead placement.

Unipolar leads have positive electrodes but no negative electrodes [16, p. 79]. The unipolar leads record electrical potentials between a single positive electrode and a combination of other electrodes which act as the negative electrode making augmentation necessary for improved signal strength [16, p. 79]. The positive electrode is termed the 'exploring' electrode and its electrical potential is compared with the sum average of the electrical activities at the other two limbs [13, p. 13]. The voltages detected at the two remaining electrodes are used to derive a reference point called the central terminal [16, p. 79]. The unipolar limb leads consist of aVR, aVL, and aVF, where 'a' refers to augmented, 'V' refers to vector, 'R' refers to right arm, 'L' refers to left arm, and 'F' refers to left foot or leg [3, p. 205] (Table 4.1).

> **Tech Tip 2:** the unipolar limb leads are an easy addition to the bipolar limb leads because they use the same electrodes as leads I, II, and III. If you apply **four** limb electrodes using the black, white, red, and green clips, **six** leads will be recorded with **six** different electrical views of the heart: I, II, III, aVR, aVL, and aVF leads.

The three standard limb leads when combined with the three augmented limb leads create the hexaxial reference system [15, p. 74] (Figure 4.3). The midpoints of the lead axes intersect and this reference system is used to calculate the heart's electrical axis in the frontal plane [13, p. 74].

Other unipolar leads are the precordial chest leads V1, V2, V3, V4, V5, V6, V10 where 'V' refers to voltage or potential [16, pp. 79–80]. These leads were introduced in 1944 by Frank Wilson and may provide additional information on rhythm or provide

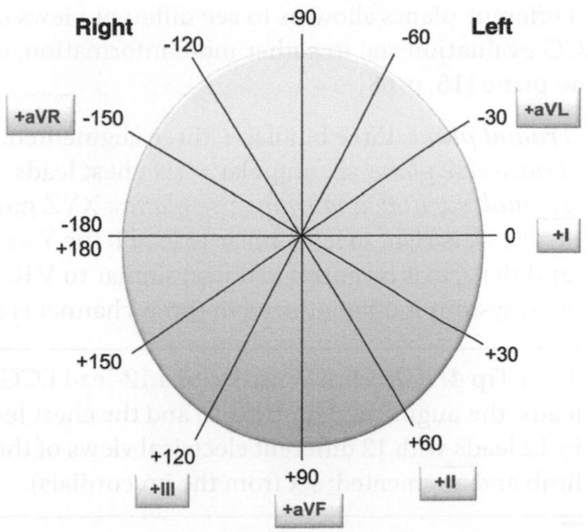

Figure 4.3 The mean electrical axis circle as a reference axis based on Einthoven's triangle and the hexaxial lead system. The circle is divided into wedges of conventional degrees with each lead labeled at its positive pole. Note that aVR and aVL's positive poles are on the *negative* sides of the circle. The calculation results may indicate conduction disturbances and/or ventricular enlargement patterns in conjunction with other ECG findings and diagnostics.

corroborative evidence of heart enlargement by referencing different ventricular areas [15, p. 70]. Due to their close proximity to the heart, augmentation is not necessary. Since the chest leads measure potentials close to the heart, they can be helpful in identifying P waves not discernible in the limb leads to rule out or rule in atrial fibrillation, for instance [15, p. 70]. They may also aid in identification of right and left heart enlargement not visible in the limb leads [15, p. 70]. Of course, whenever there is an arrhythmia, multiple simultaneous leads provide more information for specific identification [15, p. 70]. Chest leads are not meant to be intimidating, but informative in contributing other views when necessary. In the chest leads, the positive electrodes are the exploring surface electrodes at the ventral, lateral, and dorsal aspects of the heart that are then each compared with the RA, LA, and LL electrodes acting as the central terminal [16, p. 79]. Table 4.2 describes the placement for chest V leads [13, p. 12].

Tech Tip 3: not all ECG machines have V10. If this lead needs to be acquired, simply move V6 to V10's proper placement and note it on the tracing.

Table 4.2 Unipolar precordial chest leads and their placement on the chest wall: 'V' refers to voltage or potential.

V1	(CV5RL, also known as rV2): right fifth intercostal space near the sternum (lead at the fifth right lower)
V2	(CV6LL): left sixth intercostal space near the sternum (lead at the sixth left lower)
V3	Evenly spaced between V2 and V4 in the sixth intercostal space
V4	(CV6LU): left sixth intercostal space near the costochondral junction (lead at the sixth left upper)
V5	Evenly spaced upward and dorsal from V4 in the sixth intercostal space
V6	Evenly spaced upward and dorsal from V5 in the sixth intercostal space
V10	Over the dorsal process of the seventh thoracic vertebra

Different planes allow us to see different views of the heart on the ECG. To improve ECG evaluation and to gather more information, use more than one lead in more than one plane [15, p. 68].

- *Frontal plane:* three bipolar + three augmented unipolar = six limb leads
- *Transverse plane:* six unipolar = six chest leads
- *Frontal, sagittal, and transverse planes:* XYZ modified *orthogonal* leads, where the X lead axis is right to left similar to lead I, the Y axis is craniocaudal similar to lead aVF, and the Z axis is ventral to dorsal similar to V10 [15, p. 70]. This modified orthogonal lead system is often utilized in three-channel Holter monitoring systems.

Tech Tip 4: if the clinician asks for a 12-lead ECG, this will include the standard limb leads, the augmented limb leads, and the chest leads; 10 placed electrodes will result in 12 leads with 12 different electrical views of the heart (four from a combination of limb and augmented; six from the precordials).

Mean Electrical Axis – Poles Apart

Calculating the mean electrical axis (MEA) is an important tool in determining the summation of cardiac vectors that occur with ventricular depolarization in the frontal plane using the six limb leads. A negative and positive electrical charge causes a potential force to occur, called a dipole [15, p. 71]. In a vector model, the heart is an electric dipole located in the thorax [13, p. 7]. The dipole theory uses the concept of representing the electric forces from the heart by recording vector forces from the body surface [16, p. 78]. The depolarization wave begins; the myocardium then contracts [11, p. 8]. The wavefront advances with positive charges and trails with negative charges as it travels toward a positive electrode; the ECG will detect it as a positive potential [16, p. 77]. If the electrodes are reversed, the ECG will detect it as a negative potential.

Direction of the wavefront can be determined by comparing more than one lead [16, p. 77]. A parallel wavefront has the largest deflection. A perpendicular wavefront has little or no deflection. A combination wavefront has a deflection somewhere in the middle [16, pp. 77–78]. Vector represents direction and magnitude. There can be many forces and directions of depolarizations in the heart, but the ECG will show the average of the electrical forces [16, pp. 77–78].

Stimulus spreads through the heart in an overall direction. The mean direction of the QRS complex is typically estimated in the frontal plane [16, p. 86]. The MEA is the average direction of the total ventricular depolarization in the frontal plane [16, p. 81]. The QRS complex for each limb lead is shaped differently because the perspective of the depolarization is different. This aids in determining the direction of the wavefront most travelled [16, p. 81].

Tech Tip 5: heart position in the body can be a factor when determining MEA. For example, the vertical positioning of the heart in a deep-chested breed such as the Doberman pinscher will be perpendicular in the frontal plane; all leads equally positive and negative. The axis cannot be determined [16, p. 87]. Consequently, heart enlargement in these dogs may not exhibit tall or deep complexes due to the heart's position in the body.

When Einthoven conducted research on respiratory effects on the ECG, this led him to the idea of the equilateral triangle in considering the extremities as extensions of the electrodes [3, p. 124]. Einthoven's triangle refers to the hypothetical inverted equilateral triangle centered on the chest with the points acting as the standard leads on the arms and leg [16, p. 78]. Each standard lead is configured to look toward the positive pole. Lead I looks toward 0 degrees, the left arm. Lead II looks toward 60 degrees, the left leg. Lead III looks toward 120 degrees, the right leg. This scheme allows a view of the heart every 60 degrees [13, pp. 13–16; 16, p. 82].

However, it wasn't until 1942 that the development of the augmented lead system by Emanuel Goldberger allowed a view of the heart every 30 degrees [17]. The relatively smaller electrical signal of these leads made augmentation necessary [17]. The increased coverage increased the specificity in more accurately determining location of cardiac pathology [17] (Figure 4.3).

The augmented leads subdivide and alternate with Einthoven's leads. aVR looks over the right shoulder toward −150 degrees, aVL looks over the left shoulder toward −30 degrees, and aVF looks straight down toward +90 degrees [13, pp. 13–16; 16, p. 82]. Normal canine axis is +40 to +100 degrees while normal feline axis is 0 to +160 degrees [12, p. 53] (Figure 4.4).

In combination with other diagnostic tests, such as the echocardiogram and thoracic radiographs, determination of the MEA can be a powerful tool, aiding in establishing clinical significance of ventricular enlargement and conduction abnormalities [15, p. 76]. The axis tends to shift or deviate towards the hypertrophied ventricle in pathologically increased cardiac muscle mass [16, p. 87]. Primary conduction disturbances caused by changes in the sequence of ventricular activation can also cause axis shifts [16, p. 87].

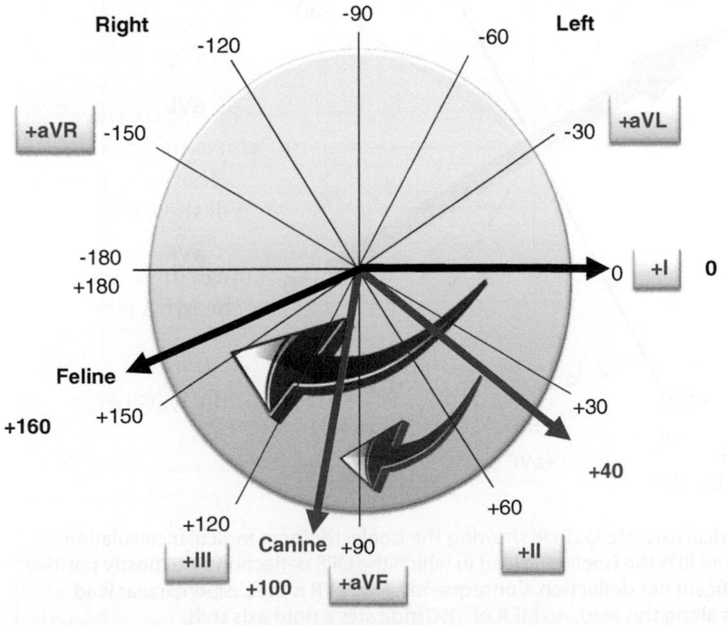

Figure 4.4 The mean electrical axis circle with normal ranges for dogs and cats. Normal canine axis: +40 to +100 degrees. Normal feline axis: 0 to +160 degrees.

Three typical methods in estimating the MEA are now described:

1) *Isoelectric and perpendicular.* To determine the MEA from the ECG, find the limb lead that is isoelectric (equally positive and negative QRS deflections, little or no net deflection) [16, p. 86]. Then find the limb lead that is perpendicular (90 degrees) to the isoelectric lead. The MEA lies along this perpendicular lead. Determine whether the perpendicular lead is mostly positive or negative and find it on the MEA circle (Figure 4.3). The MEA will be toward either the positive or negative pole of this lead depending on whether the QRS of the perpendicular lead is mostly positive or negative. This is a quick and easy method. If two leads are equally isoelectric, either of these leads can be used or the average of both calculations. However, when no isoelectric lead is obvious, one of the other methods can be used. In the event that all leads are isoelectric, such as in some deep-chested dogs (the Doberman pinscher's heart, for example, lies vertically within the thorax), then the electrical axis cannot be determined in the frontal plane [16, p. 87]

Tech Tip 6: while viewing the MEA circle, be careful to note that the positive poles of leads aVR and aVL have negative values. For example, if the MEA is toward the positive pole of aVR the axis is toward −150 degrees NOT toward +30 degrees (Figure 4.5).

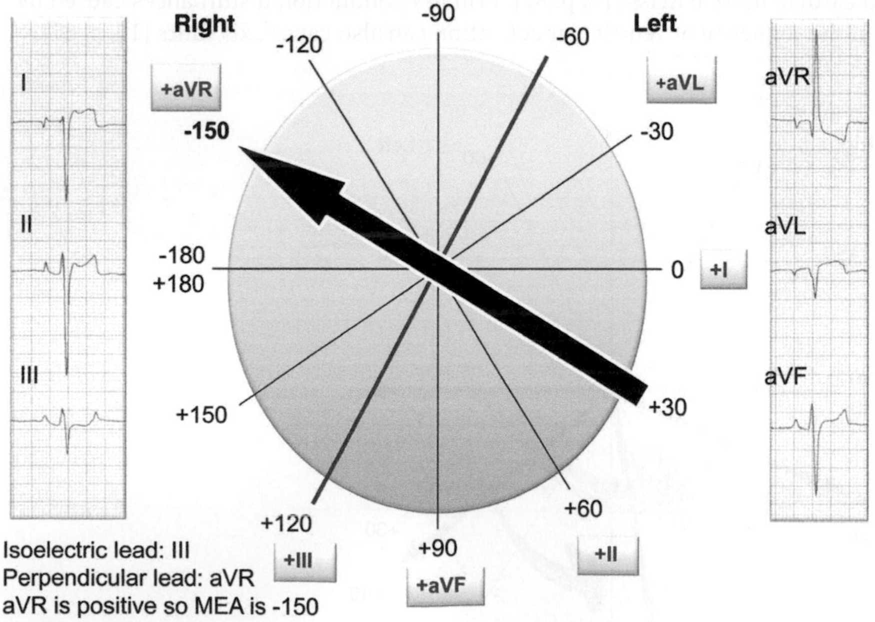

Figure 4.5 The mean electrical axis (MEA) circle showing the isoelectric/perpendicular calculation method. In this example, lead III is the isoelectric lead in which the QRS deflections are mostly positive and negative with no significant net deflection. Consequently, lead aVR is the perpendicular lead signifying that the MEA lies along this lead. An MEA of −150 indicates a right axis shift. Echocardiographic findings indicate severe pulmonic stenosis with right ventricular hypertrophy. Note the deep S waves in lead II.

2) *Largest net deflection.* To determine the MEA from the ECG, find the limb lead where the QRS complex has the largest net deflection. The net deflection of any lead is the algebraic sum of all the deflections of the QRS in that lead, positive or negative [16, p. 86]. For example, if the Q wave is three boxes below the baseline, the R wave is 10 boxes above the baseline, and the S wave is three boxes below the baseline, then the resulting net deflection is positive four (−3 +10 −3 = +4). The MEA will lie parallel along this lead. If the lead with the largest net deflection is positive, the MEA is toward the positive pole of this lead. If the lead with the largest net deflection is negative, the MEA is toward the negative pole of this lead. If two of the limb leads are equal in being the leads with the largest net deflection, the MEA will lie between them. As with all MEA methods, this is not a very precise method but it is a quick and simple general inspection method [16, p. 86].
3) *Vector plotting leads.* To determine the MEA from the ECG, the axis can be calculated by plotting the vectors of any two of the hexaxial limb leads on a graph grid [16, p. 87]. The positive and negative deflections for each lead are added and then plotted on the grid (Figure 4.6). The point at which the plotted values intersect indicates the MEA. This is a more meticulous method, and seemingly more precise, but there may be a false sense of accuracy using this method. If the patient shifts a leg during ECG acquisition, the MEA can change. Use this method with care.

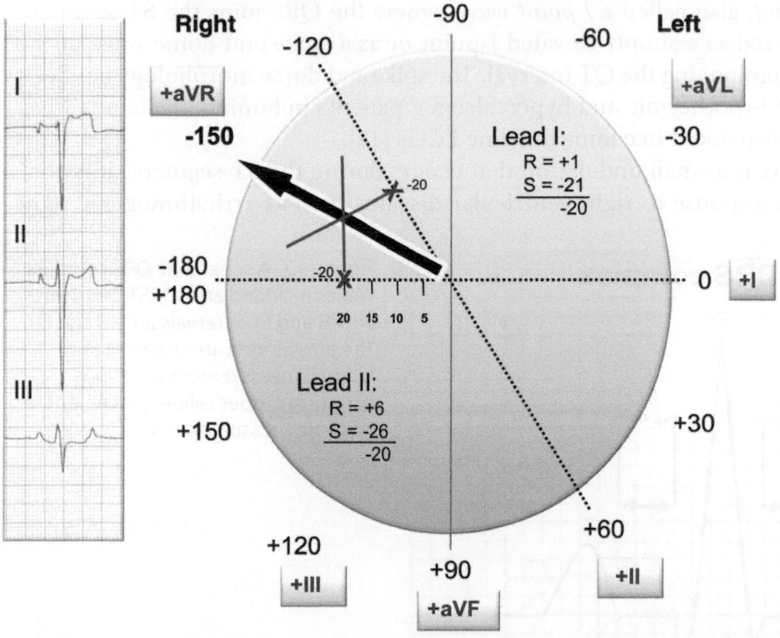

Figure 4.6 The vector plotting calculation method for mean electrical axis (MEA). In this example leads I and II are used to calculate the algebraic sum of the QRS deflections. Lead I is calculated as 1 box positive for R and 21 boxes negative for S; lead II is calculated as 6 boxes positive for R and 26 boxes negative for S. The algebraic sum of the QRS deflections is negative 20 in lead I as well as negative 20 in lead II. The sums are plotted on their frontal plane axes (red X). Perpendicular lines are drawn from their respective axes (blue lines). The black arrow is drawn through the center of the intersecting blue lines indicating the direction of the MEA.

Waveforms Deconstructed

The ECG complex is an electrocardiographic representation of the heart's electrical activity [16, p. 72]. Each wave generated depicts a segment of the sequence of events in depolarization and repolarization:

- *The P wave* depicts atrial muscle depolarization. Each cell depolarizes in turn causing the atria to contract [16, p. 80].
- *The QRS wave* depicts ventricular muscle depolarization. As the wave travels down along the conduction system ventricular contraction occurs, the steps organized like a dance beginning with the septum and then continuing with the left and right ventricular walls [16, p. 80].
- *The T wave* depicts ventricular relaxation, known as repolarization. Repolarization represents the recovery period, the resting state that occurs after the cells have discharged an action potential [15, pp. 70–72] (Figure 4.7).

Other waves for interested technicians:

- *The delta wave* is characterized by a short PR interval and initial slurring of the QRS upstroke. It is caused by pre-excitation of the ventricles through a bypass tract which is usually congenital [7].
- *The Osborn wave,* also called a *J-point wave,* where the QRS joins the ST segment. It can be observed as a simply elevated J-point or as a spike and dome wave of the QRS complex, prolonging the QT interval. The spike and dome morphology has been documented in hypothermic and hypercalcemic patients in human medicine [7,18]. J-points have been noted in canine baseline ECGs [18].
- *The epsilon wave* is a small undulation that occurs during the ST segment. It is considered to be a response to right ventricular diseases such as arrhythmogenic right

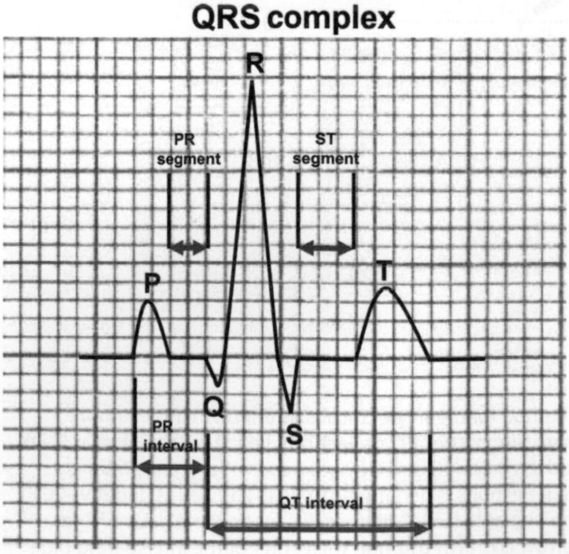

Figure 4.7 A schematic QRS complex. Waves included are PQRST. Segments are PR and ST. Intervals are PR and QT. The arrows indicate segment and interval measurement durations denoting proper caliper placement for accurate measurements.

ventricular dysplasia where myocytes are replaced with fat as the disease progresses causing a delay in myocyte excitation [7].

- *The U wave* follows the T wave and is typically small and not usually seen. The basis for the U wave has a variety of hypotheses and may either represent normal repolarization of the His-Purkinje system or could be due to a mechanical function in which stretch-induced delayed afterdepolarizations are caused by ventricular wall distension during rapid ventricular filling [18]. Abnormal U waves are large or inverted and are seemingly second components of interrupted T waves [18].

Conduction Sequence – A Cardiac Travelogue

The conduction system is composed of specialized tissues that are responsible for the organizational sequence of electrical events [16, pp. 8–9]. The following is a description of the conduction journey, highlighting electrical events, tissue locations, and the corresponding ECG waves, segments, and intervals.

Atrial Depolarization – SA node–P wave

During normal atrial activation, impulses begin in the sinoatrial node (SAN) [11, pp. 98]. The SA node contains specialized cells known as pacemaker cells that possess automaticity, allowing spontaneous discharge without an outside stimulus [11, p. 9] (See Chapter 2). The pacemaking cells in the SA node generate action potentials on their own, depolarize most rapidly, and set the pace of the inherent heart rate [16, p. 453]. Once the SA node fires, the electrical impulse spreads across the atria to the atrioventricular (AV) node; a P wave is produced [16, p. 80]. The shape and amplitude of the P wave depends on the origination of depolarization and the variation in impulse exit points [19, 20]. In a normal dog, the anatomical architecture of the SA node is complex with regional heterogeneity affecting morphology and pacemaker shifting [19, 20]. While the SA node has the most rapid rate of spontaneous discharge and sets the heart rate, other slower pacemaking cells are located in the AV node and the ventricular conducting system and can assume control of the heart rate if the SA node is impaired [16, p. 73]. The further the conducting site is from the SA node, the slower the heart rate.

Tech Tip 7: rates of depolarization in the dog – SA node fires at 60–180 beats per minute (bpm), AV node fires at 40–60 bpm, and Purkinje fibers fire at 20–40 bpm [16, pp. 73–74]. If for any reason the controlling depolarizing site is impaired, the next fastest site will assume pacing dominance of the heart rate [11, pp. 7–8].

AV Nodal Depolarization – AV node–PR segment and interval

The impulse then travels to the AV node where it is delayed; a PR segment is produced [21, p. 38]. The AV node lies between the atrial chambers in the septal wall of the right atrium [13, p. 8]. The voltage is normally small to isoelectric. This important delay allows completion of atrial contraction and ventricular filling before the impulse conduction continues [21, p. 11]. The PR interval represents both atrial depolarization and delay at the AV node [21, p. 38].

> **Tech Tip 8:** the PR interval encompasses the P wave and the PR segment with the measurement beginning at the onset of the P wave to the onset of the QRS complex, technically the PQ interval [21, p. 38] (Figure 4.7).

The bundle of His and the AV node lie within the AV junctional tissue and are considered supraventricular, or above the ventricles [15, p. 338]. After the nodal delay the impulse conduction emerges, speeding up as it rapidly follows the bundle of His to begin its journey into the ventricles via the bundle branches and Purkinje fibers [16, p. 80].

Ventricular Depolarization – Left and Right Bundle Branches, Purkinje Fibers–QRS complex

The bundle of His branches into three bundles: the right, the left anterior, and the left posterior bundle branches [13, pp. 8–9]. During normal ventricular activation, impulses are conducted down the left and right bundle branches on either side of the septum; the left bundle is activated first. This causes the septum to depolarize in a left-to-right direction, giving rise to the Q wave [16, p. 80]. Since the mean electrical vector is heading slightly away from the positive electrode the Q wave is recorded as a small negative deflection, although not always impressively visible (*Q wave-septal depolarization*) [16, p. 80]. Following the Q wave, the mean vector points downward toward the apex, and heads toward the positive electrode [11, p. 13]. Depolarization reaches the ventricular walls via the thin Purkinje fibers and occurs quickly at this point [11, p 13]. Normally the left ventricular heart mass is greater than the right, so the mean vector is toward the left, producing a tall, narrow, positive deflection in lead II characterized by the R wave (*R wave-early ventricular free wall depolarization*) [11, p. 13]. Following the R wave, the basal areas of the septum and posterior ventricular walls activate last [11, p. 13]. The wave of depolarization travels up along these areas, resulting in a slight negative deflection, negative because the mean vector now heads away from the positive pole; an S wave is produced (*S wave-late ventricular basilar depolarization*) [11, p. 13].

> **Tech Tip 9:** typically, atrial repolarization (T sub a or Ta) occurs during the QRS complex while the ventricles are depolarizing, but since it is smaller in magnitude, the QRS wave obscures it [22]. However, body surface mapping studies indicate involvement of Ta during the PR interval through amplification of very low signals during this time [23]. Ta waves are the opposite polarity of P waves so that prominent Ta evident during prolonged PR intervals causes the interval to appear depressed [11, pp. 92–93; 24, pp. 983, 1002]. Exaggerated Ta can extend through the QRS producing ST segment depression in some diseased myocardial states such as ischemia, atrial disease, or tachycardia [24, p. 1004; 12, p. 62].

End of Ventricular Systole before Repolarization – Ventricle–ST segment

Ventricular systole has occurred. The ST segment represents the period following the QRS and is normally isoelectric before repolarization begins [25, p. 44]. The atrial cells are relaxed while the ventricles are contracted and emptying; it is an electrically neutral time between ventricular depolarization and repolarization, therefore no electrical activity is visible [25, p. 44].

Ventricular Repolarization – Ventricle–T wave

This reflects the electrical activity produced when the ventricles are resting and recharging for the next contraction; it is an extremely vulnerable period [26, p. 21]. Electrical potentials of the myocardial cells are restored. Myocardial cells are refractory during and shortly after repolarization when they usually will not respond to a stimulus. An impulse no matter how strong that arrives during the *absolute* refractory period (onset of QRS to onset of T) will not initiate depolarization or affect the ventricular myocardium [21, p. 39]. However, during the *relative* refractory period (the interval which immediately follows the absolute period during ventricular repolarization) impulses can, under certain circumstances, get through this dangerously vulnerable period [21, pp. 39–40] (See Chapter 2).

> **Tech Tip 10:** during depolarization, the impulse wave activates from the endocardium to the epicardium. During repolarization, the impulse reverses this activation order and the myocardial cells recharge from the epicardium to the endocardium [16, pp. 76, 82].

To recap the normal sequence of events: the atria contract first, then the ventricles, followed by relaxation. The road most traveled: SA node–AV node–Bundle of His–Right and Left bundles and Purkinje fibers to the ventricular walls.

Complexes, Segments, And Intervals – Identify and Measure

The following is a guideline of measurement locations for each wave, deflection, segment, and interval with brief comments on enlargement patterns and indications (Figure 4.7). Remember to be consistent and measure from leading edge to leading edge, preferably with your trusty calipers, whether electronic or actual, but a straight edge will suffice. Durations are measured on the X-axis (Figure 4.8); amplitudes on the Y-axis (Figure 4.9).

With digital ECG software programs, electronic calipers automatically measure but can be inaccurate. Care is needed to reset the lines in the different leads. Also available are specific electronic caliper programs which claim to have pixel perfect accuracy and calibration options while interfacing with many formats and applications.

> **Tech Tip 11:** lead II is the standard lead for measuring the PQRST waveforms and is obtained in right lateral recumbency [12, pp. 50–51]. Heart rate, however, can be measured in any lead and in any position; standing or lateral [11, pp. 26–27].

Table 4.3 is a reference table of normal measurements for dogs and cats.

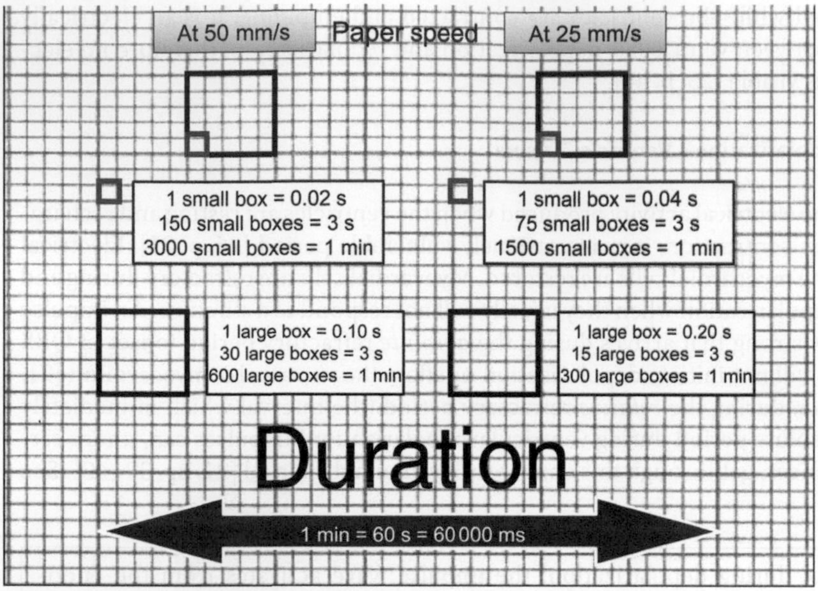

Figure 4.8 ECG duration. The left side values are at a paper speed of 50 mm/s; the right side is at 25 mm/s. The speed can be adjusted per patient depending on the ECG situation.

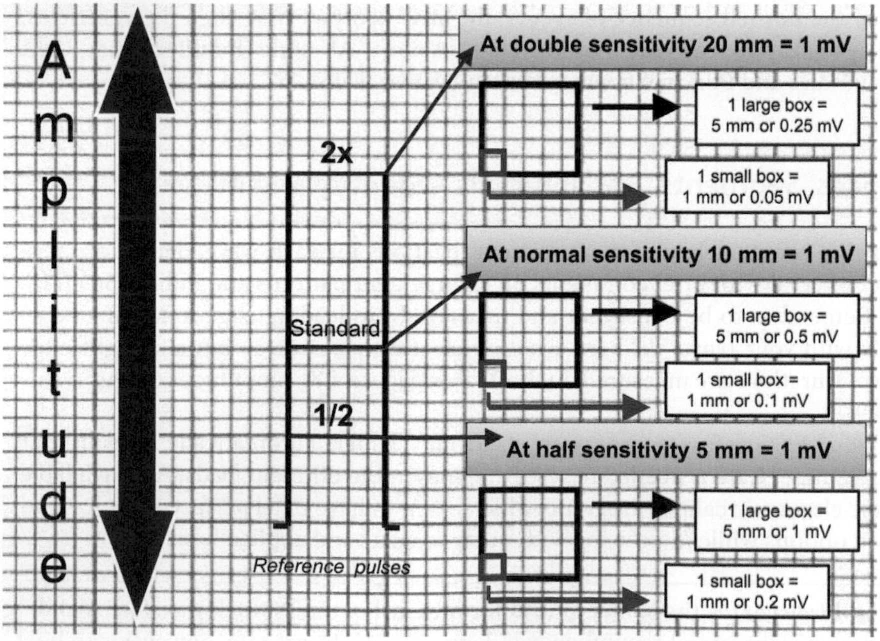

Figure 4.9 ECG amplitude. The reference pulse is an amplitude measurement of 1 mV. 'Standard' is normal sensitivity, 2 large boxes high; '1/2' is half sensitivity, 1 large box high; and '2×' is double sensitivity, 4 large boxes high. The sensitivity can be adjusted per patient depending on the ECG situation.

Table 4.3 Standard ECG measurements of the dog and cat.

	Dog		Cat	
	Duration Max. width (ms)	**Amplitude Max. height (mV)**	**Duration Max. width (ms)**	**Amplitude Max. height (mV)**
P wave	40 50 (giant breeds)	0.4	40	0.2
PR interval	60–130	N/A	50–90	N/A
QRS complex			40	0.9
Small breeds	50	2.5		
Large breeds	60	3.0		
ST segment	N/A		N/A	
No depression		0.2		0.1
No elevation		0.15–0.2		0.1
T wave	N/A	0.05–1.0	N/A	0.3
	Not greater than 25% of R wave height Positive, negative, or biphasic		Positive, negative, or biphasic	
QT interval	150–250	N/A	120–180 (range 70–200)	N/A
	At faster rates, shorter intervals At slower rates, longer intervals		At faster rates, shorter intervals At slower rates, longer intervals	
Rate: bpm In hospital Adults	60–160		140–240	
Puppies	up to 220 or greater when excited			
Rhythm	Normal sinus rhythm Sinus arrhythmia Wandering SA pacemaker		Normal sinus rhythm Sinus tachycardia in response to physiologic excitement	
MEA: degrees (frontal plane)	+40–+100		0–±160	

bpm, beats per minute. MEA, mean electrical axis. Sources: [11, 13, 15].

P Wave

P wave: first wave of the complex represents atrial depolarization.
Duration: beginning of the P to the end of the P [12, p. 56].
Amplitude: height of the P (if P waves vary in height, as with wandering pacemaker, use the tallest P wave) [12, p. 56].

P wave duration and amplitude can be affected by atrial enlargement. Technically, taller P shapes indicate right atrial enlargement (*P pulmonale*) while wider sometimes notched

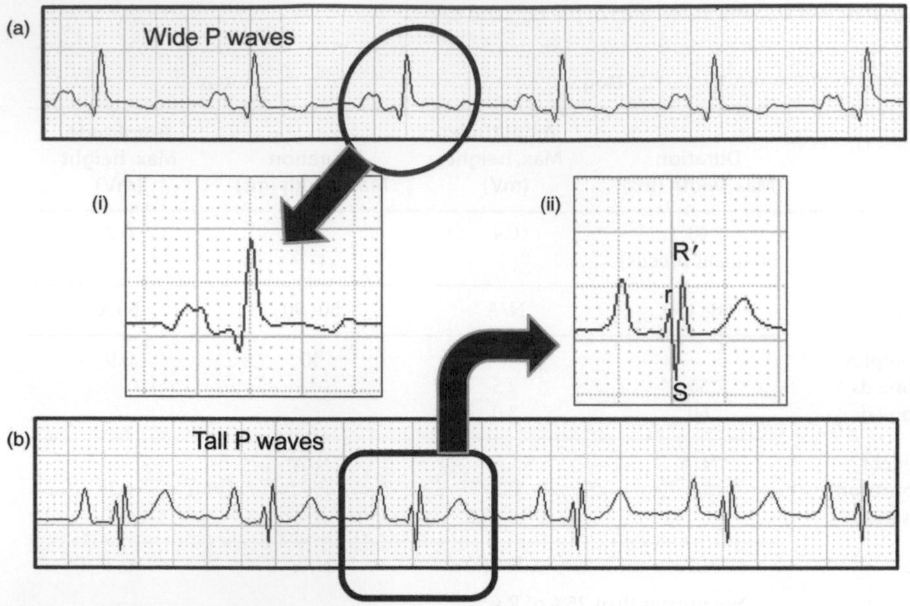

Figure 4.10 Lead II; 50 mm/s, 10 mm/mV. (a) Example of wide P waves in an 8-year-old boxer mix dog. (i) Enlarged example of a QRS complex from (a). The P wave measures 60 ms and is notched. This dog has a severely dilated left atrium and severe mitral regurgitation. Coincidentally, a large heart-base mass presses against the left atrium. (b) Example of tall P waves in a Labrador retriever puppy. (ii) Enlarged example of a QRS complex from (b). The P wave measures 0.5 mV. Note the rSR′ pattern. This dog has tricuspid valve dysplasia with a severely dilated right atrium and right ventricle as well as severe tricuspid regurgitation.

shapes indicate left atrial enlargement (*P mitrale*), since the right atrium depolarizes first, followed quickly by the left atrium [11, p. 93]. However, although this guideline may be true in some cases, it is often oversimplified. Either P wave shape change can generally be caused by either right or left atrial enlargement due to the summation of atrial depolarization [16, pp. 87–88]. If a P wave is too tall or too wide, consider that one or both of the atria may be enlarged (Figure 4.10).

PR Segment

PR segment: represents electrical activity traveling down toward the ventricles from the AV node to the other conducting fibers, albeit a brief reflection of the beginning of this path, not the whole journey, not the contraction; it is typically a straight isoelectric line indicative of atrial systole and ventricular diastole, although it may deviate in the presence of atrial injury [21, p. 38].

Duration: end of the P to the beginning of the QRS [12, p. 56].

Amplitude: not measured [112, p. 56].

However, depression of the PR segment may be seen as a result of prominent atrial repolarization, Ta, by possibly increased current generation associated with right atrial enlargement [11, pp. 92–93].

PR Interval

PR interval: represents the time between the onset of atrial depolarization and the onset of ventricular depolarization or the time the impulse travels across the AV node as it reaches the ventricles from the SA node; it is an indicator of AV node function [16, pp. 85].
Duration: beginning of the P to the beginning of the QRS; it includes the P wave and the PR segment [12, p. 56].
Amplitude: not measured [12, p. 56].

A prolonged PR interval can be due to slowed conduction and is called first degree heart block [12, p. 55] (Figure 4.11). Slowed conduction is caused by certain drugs such as digitalis and sotalol, for example, and by increased vagal tone, profound bradycardias, AV node conduction disease, or affected metabolic states such as hyperkalemia [11, pp. 100–102]. If the normal pathway is impaired or diseased, the impulse could travel down a faster accessory pathway resulting in a shortened PR interval as in pre-excitation syndrome [15, p. 86; 12, pp. 67–71] (Figure 4.11).

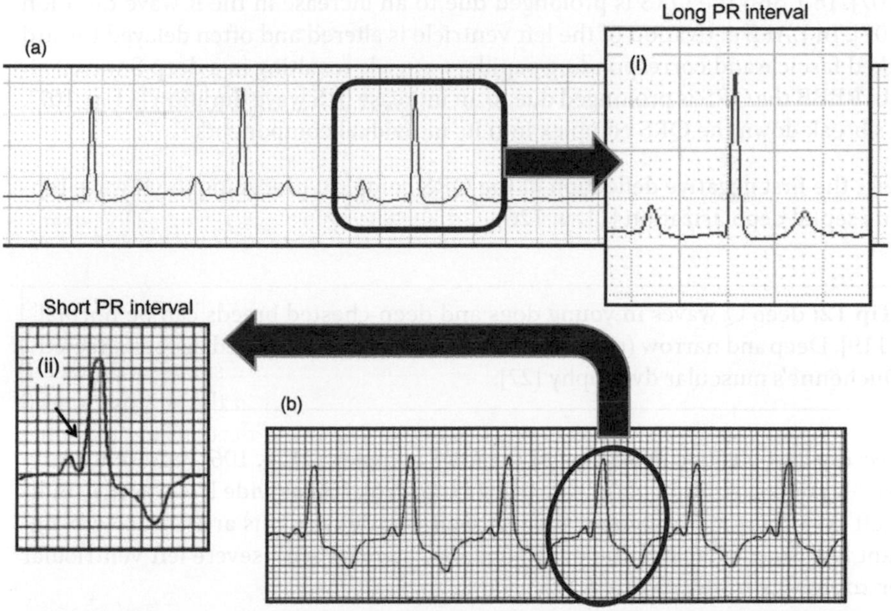

Figure 4.11 Lead II; 50 mm/s, 10 mm/mV. (a) Example of long PR intervals in a 4-year-old bull terrier. (i) Enlarged example of a QRS complex from (a). The PR interval measures 170 ms. This is an example of first-degree atrioventricular block. (b) Example of short PR intervals in a 7-year-old domestic short-haired cat. (ii) Enlarged example of a QRS complex from (b). The PR interval measures 40 ms. This is an example of pre-excitation. Pre-excitation occurs when impulses are conducted along an accessory pathway that bypasses the AV node, avoids the usual delay, and prematurely activates the ventricle. It is rare in cats but can be associated with acquired and congenital cardiac diseases as well as idiopathic diseases. In human literature this type of pathway is known to be a congenital bypass tract often referred to as the bundle of Kent, of which Wolff–Parkinson–White syndrome is an example. The black arrow indicates slurring of the initial part of the QRS complex, known as the delta wave. Also note the wide QRS at 60 ms.

QRS Complex

QRS complex: represents rapid ventricular depolarization and includes the waves Q, R, and S; waveform nomenclature is defined when discussing patterns in which the major deflections are represented by capital letters and the minor deflections by lower case letters, such as Qr pattern where the Q wave is larger than the R wave or rS pattern where the R wave is smaller than the S wave; additional components are called by various prime names when electrical changes lead to complexes with waves that change direction and cross the baseline such as R prime (R′) and S prime (S′) variations. An R′ wave would be a second positive deflection following the S wave as in an RSR′ or rSR′ pattern (Figure 4.10); an S′ wave would be a second negative deflection following the R wave [13, p. 49].

Duration: beginning of the Q to the end of the S [12, p. 56].

Amplitude: height of the R [12, p. 56].

Increased duration of the QRS complex can be caused by conduction delays or disturbances in the left bundles as in left bundle branch block (LBBB) and left anterior fascicular block (LAFB) or in the right bundle as in right bundle branch block (RBBB) [11, p. 107]. In LBBB the QRS is prolonged due to an increase in the R wave duration [11, p. 107]. In LAFB activation of the left ventricle is altered and often delayed toward the blocked fascicle and corresponding papillary muscle resulting in a deep S wave [11, p. 107]. In RBBB the QRS is prolonged due to an increase in S wave duration [11, p. 107]. Now let's break down the QRS complex into its individual components:

1) *Q wave*: the first negative deflection of the QRS complex, preceding the R wave represents septal depolarization [11, p. 126].

> **Tech Tip 12:** deep Q waves in young dogs and deep-chested breeds can be normal [11, p. 119]. Deep and narrow (not wide) Q waves have been observed in dogs affected with Duchenne's muscular dystrophy [27].

2) *R wave*: the first positive deflection of the QRS complex [11, p. 106] represents early ventricular depolarization of the free wall [11, p. 126]. Tall or wide R waves may indicate left ventricular enlargement such as seen in patent ductus arteriosus with significant left ventricular dilation or in subaortic stenosis with severe left ventricular hypertrophy [15, p. 79] (Figure 4.12).

> **Tech Tip 13:** remember the R wave is the first positive deflection of the QRS complex, even if a Q wave is not visibly present and even if the R wave is very short.

3) *S wave*: the first negative deflection following the R wave [11, p. 106] represents late ventricular depolarization of the basilar areas [11, p. 126]. Deep S waves may indicate right ventricular enlargement such as seen in pulmonic stenosis with severe right ventricular hypertrophy [15, p. 78] (Figure 4.5).

Following the QRS complex are the ST segment and T wave.

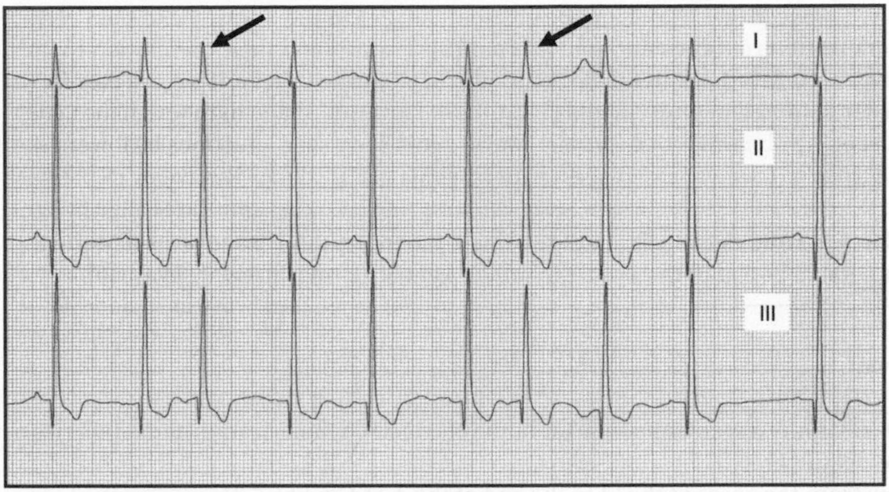

Figure 4.12 Leads I, II, and III; 50 mm/s, 10 mm/mV. Example of tall R waves in a 9-year-old mixed breed dog. The R waves measure 3.7 mV. This dog was diagnosed with severe dilated cardiomyopathy. Echocardiographic findings reveal severe left ventricular dilation with moderate mitral regurgitation. The black arrows indicate atrial premature contractions.

ST Segment

ST segment: represents the time in which the entire ventricle is completely depolarized and is a period of neutrality between ventricular depolarization and repolarization; the myocardium is in a contracted state as blood is ejected from the ventricles; normally isoelectric [25, p. 44].

Duration: end of the S wave to the beginning of the T wave; usually included in the QT interval measurement [12, p. 56].

Amplitude: above or below the baseline [12, p. 56].

Above the baseline values greater than 0.15 mV in the dog indicates elevation, below the baseline values greater than 0.2 mV indicates depression [13, p. 60]. Values other than zero are considered abnormal in the cat [13, p 100]. Changes in the ST segment are associated with ventricular muscle abnormalities and hypoxia [13, pp. 84–87]. Signs of elevation include hyperkalemia and pericardial effusion while signs of depression include hypokalemia and digitalis toxicity [113, pp. 84–87]. Slurring, sagging or coving of the segment can also occur in which the line slides into the T wave without distinction [13, pp. 84–87]. ST slurring in conjunction with wide QRS complexes can be an indicator of left ventricular hypertrophy [13, pp. 84–87].

T Wave

T wave: a positive or negative deflection following the ST segment [11, p. 115] represents ventricular repolarization and the vulnerable period when stimuli may affect the heart rhythm under favorable circumstances [26, p. 21].

Duration: beginning of the T to the end of the T [12, p. 56].

Amplitude: height of the T [12, p.56].

Generally, T wave height should not be greater than 25% of the R wave height but often this generalization rule does not hold [11, p. 115]. T waves and their orientation to the QRS are extremely variable in the dog and cat [16, p.82]. No exact criteria are currently available for standard measurements [11, p. 115]. However, shape may sometimes give clues to specific abnormalities. Wide T waves have been seen in myocardial hypoxia while tall, spiked T waves may suggest hyperkalemia [11, p. 115].

Tech Tip 14: avoid electrically cardioverting a patient on the T wave; a shock during this vulnerable period of the cycle can induce ventricular fibrillation! [21, p. 40].

QT Interval

QT interval: this represents the time for both ventricular depolarization and repolarization to occur [11, p. 117].
Duration: from the onset of the Q to the end of the T [12, p. 56].

The QT interval has an inverse relationship with heart rate and should be less than half of the preceding R–R interval [12, p. 62]. Increases are caused by slower heart rates such as bradycardias. Other causes of interval prolongation are ethylene glycol toxicity, central nervous system disturbances, hypokalemia, hypocalcemia, quinidine, and procainamide therapies [12, p. 63]. Shortening of the interval is evident in rapid heart rates such as tachycardias. Other causes of interval shortening are hyperkalemia, hypercalcemia, and digoxin treatment [12, p. 63].

Heart Rate Primer

Heart rate is measured as beats per minute (bpm) and usually refers to ventricular contractions [13, p. 44]. This applies when the ventricular and atrial rates are the same. However, there are times when the ventricular and atrial rates differ, such as in atrial tachycardia and second or third degree heart block, and determining both rates becomes important [13, p. 44].

P–P intervals are intervals between P waves: measuring these intervals will determine the atrial rate. R-R intervals are intervals between R waves: measuring these intervals will determine the ventricular rate [13, p. 44].

The heart rate is calculated along the horizontal x-axis of the ECG; the width/time axis. A few of the methods used for ventricular heart rate are now described along with some helpful facts [11, pp. 70–73;13, pp. 44–45; 15, p. 74;16, pp. 84–85] (Figure 4.8):

1) The quickest method is the pen method. Use a pen whose length measures 5 7/8 inches, or 150 mm. The time interval for this pen length is 3 s at 50 mm/s or 6 s at 25 mm/s. Lay down the pen on the ECG strip lengthwise. Count the number of beats along the pen length and multiply by 20 at paper speeds of 50 mm/s ($3 \times 20 = 60$ s); multiply by 10 at paper speeds of 25 mm/s ($6 \times 10 = 60$ s). Regardless of the pen type, know your personal pen length with its related time interval and adapt the instructions to suit.
2) A variant of the pen method is also quick; the 3- and 6-second rule. Some ECG paper has helpful indicators such as hatch tick marks or bolded lines indicating a

measure of time. Others do not. The indicators are 75 small boxes wide from one mark to another and are spaced at 1.5 s with paper speeds of 50 mm/s; 3 s with paper speeds of 25 mm/s. Count the beats between three marks or bolded lines. This will be 150 small boxes if counted; 3 s at 50 mm/s or 6 s at 25 mm/s. Now multiply the number of beats by 20 at paper speeds of 50 mm/s (3 × 20 = 60 s) or multiply by 10 at paper speeds of 25 mm/s (6 × 10 = 60 s).

3) In bradycardia with very slow rates, improve accuracy in heart rate calculations by widening the scope of counting. Take advantage of a longer rhythm strip and count beats within 300 small boxes. This equals 6 s at 50 mm/s or 12 s at 25 mm/s. Count the beats between five marks or bolded lines. Now multiply the number of beats by 10 at paper speeds of 50 mm/s (6 × 10 = 60 s) or multiply by five at paper speeds of 25 mm/s (12 × 5 = 60 s).
4) The R–R interval method. This method is best applied when the rate is regular. Numbers of boxes are counted rather than number of beats. Count the number of large boxes in one R–R interval. At 50 mm/s 600 large boxes equal 1 min (1 large box = 0.1 s, 10 large boxes = 1 s × 60 s = 600 large boxes/min). At 25 mm/s 300 large boxes equal 1 min (1 large box = 0.2 s, five large boxes = 1 s × 60 seconds = 300 large boxes/min). In summary, divide 600 (if 50 mm/s) or 300 (if 25 mm/s) by the number of large boxes in an R–R interval. For example: the number of large boxes between two beats (one R–R interval) is for, thus the time for one beat = four boxes. If 50 mm/s, 600 large boxes = 1 min, therefore the number of bpm = 600/4 = 150 bpm. If 25 mm/s, 300 large boxes = 1 min, therefore the number of beats per minute = 300/4 = 75 bpm.
5) Digital systems often use the R–R interval method but take the beat average of several, anywhere from four to ten beats. Many systems display heart rate trends graphically as tachograms, a beat to beat record of R–R intervals trending over time [28]. Investigate individual systems for the best calculation options and parameter minimal and maximal settings. It is also important that these systems algorithms are proficient in beat classification and identification. For example, are tall T waves identified falsely as QRS complexes? In this case the displayed heart rate may be twice the real rate.

Tech Tip 15: heart rates are often high when leads are first attached. More accurate rates can be obtained once the patient is calmer. Run a long rhythm strip and see how the rate is trending.

Heart Rhythm – Exploring Relationships and Arrangements

It is critical to identify complexes and recognize their relationships to each other since the arrangements of beats and the resulting patterns have impact on heart health. Consider the following questions as the clinician evaluates the rhythm [11, pp. 73–74;12, p. 64; 15, p. 74].

1) *Are there P waves?* Remember that P waves represent atrial contraction so their presence indicates that the rhythm has an atrial or supraventricular component and is sinus. Similar P waves indicate that only one pacemaker site is firing. Differing P waves could mean that the pacemaker shift is occurring within the SA node itself

resulting in different exit points [19, 20], or that additional pacemaker sites other than the SA node are firing (biphasic P wave) [11, p. 93], or that another wave from a preceding complex, such as the T wave, is occurring at the same time. In dogs it is normal for P waves to vary slightly in height due to vagal tone influence [16, p. 75].

Tech Tip 16: if P waves are difficult to identify it can be helpful to double the sensitivity to 20 mm = 1 mV. However, artifacts are magnified along with the waves and amplitudes, so be certain the tracing is as clean as possible. The chest leads may also aid in P wave detection when limb leads are inconclusive [13, p. 109].

2) *Is there a P wave for every QRS; a QRS for every P?* The association of P waves and QRS complexes comes into play. If there are a greater number of P waves or a greater number of QRS complexes, this indicates an arrhythmia is present [11, p. 109]. Determining if the P wave that precedes a QRS complex is responsible for the firing of that QRS will help in identifying normal beats, premature beats, or blocks. If P waves are associated with a QRS complex, then the rhythm is likely sinus. If P waves are obviously disassociated from a QRS complex, the rhythm is likely ventricular or junctional [12, p. 64].

Tech Tip 17: the rule of thumb is that relationships between P waves and QRS complexes help in distinguishing arrhythmias while wave shape and duration may indicate enlargement patterns.

3) *Are the QRS complexes narrow or wide?* Narrow complexes typically indicate supraventricular origin while wide complexes typically indicate ventricular origin [12, p. 64]. However, pay attention to the P wave relationship. If associated with a wide QRS, conduction disturbances should be considered, as in bundle branch blocks [12, p. 72].
4) *Does the PR interval vary or remain constant?* Prolongation indicates first degree AV block. Shortening of the interval can be seen with increased sympathetic tone or in accessory pathway scenarios such as pre-excitation [12, pp. 67, 71].
5) *Is the rate normal or abnormal; is the rhythm regular or irregular?* Compare rates with known species references to determine whether the rate is normal, slow, or fast. Arrhythmias may be classified according to their regularity or irregularity such as atrial fibrillation. Atrial fibrillation has a beat to beat irregularity and this often differentiates it from other forms of supraventricular arrhythmias such as atrial tachycardia [12, p. 66]. It should be noted, however, that some supraventricular and ventricular tachyarrhythmias can be either regular or irregular [15, p. 335].

Tech Tip 18: if an arrhythmia is present, run a long rhythm strip to gather more beat and rhythm information. Abnormal beats can look different in various leads, therefore it is important to acquire multiple leads when an arrhythmia is suspected to further define the abnormality.

Common Normal and Abnormal Rhythms

Sinus Rhythm

This is a normal rhythm with complexes originating from the SA node producing organized contractions and regular R–R intervals [12, p. 65]. The complexes occur consistently at regular intervals. The heart rate is within normal limits (Figures 4.13 and 4.14).

Sinus Arrhythmia

This can be a normal arrhythmia in dogs but usually uncommon in cats. Classified as an arrhythmia since the rhythm is not regular, sinus arrhythmia is characterized with slight variation in R–R intervals, evident with respiration. The rate increases with inspiration and decreases with expiration [12, p. 65; 15, p. 337]. Inspiration increases venous return by lowering intrathoracic pressure [29]. This arrhythmia is greatly influenced by high vagal tone and is often seen in brachycephalic breeds where vagal tone is increased by upper airway constriction [12, p. 65]. Profound respiratory sinus arrhythmias may be associated with chronic pulmonary disease [12, p. 65].

Sinus Tachycardia

This is a rapid sinus rhythm with regular or slight variation in R–R intervals and constant PR intervals, but the rate is above normal [15, p. 91]. P waves are present and

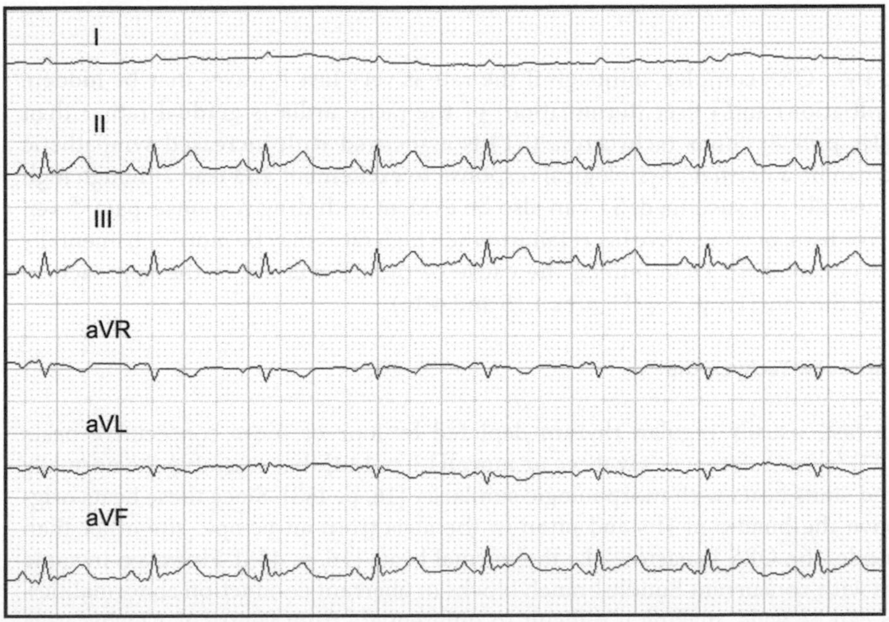

Figure 4.13 Leads I, II, III, aVR, aVL, aVF; 50 mm/s, 10 mm/mV. Normal feline recording from an adult domestic short-haired cat showing sinus rhythm. The HR measures 180 bpm.

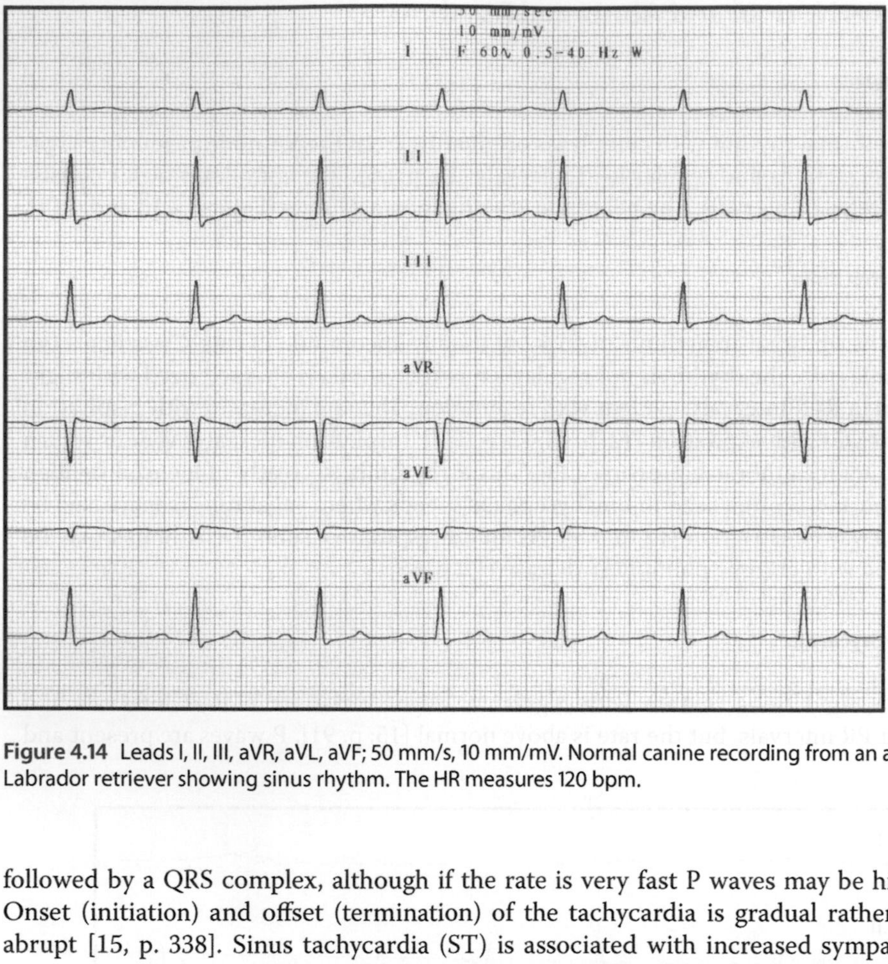

Figure 4.14 Leads I, II, III, aVR, aVL, aVF; 50 mm/s, 10 mm/mV. Normal canine recording from an adult Labrador retriever showing sinus rhythm. The HR measures 120 bpm.

followed by a QRS complex, although if the rate is very fast P waves may be hidden. Onset (initiation) and offset (termination) of the tachycardia is gradual rather than abrupt [15, p. 338]. Sinus tachycardia (ST) is associated with increased sympathetic tone and can be a normal physiological response to excitement and fear, although high rates are usually not sustained. ST can also be evident with drug response, pain, fever, hyperthyroidism, or congestive heart failure when high rates may be more detrimentally sustained [15, p. 338]. Determining the cause of the ST will aid in the approach to controlling the rate [12, p. 66] (Figures 4.15 and 4.16).

Supraventricular Tachycardia

This is a fast, usually regular, rhythm depicted by four or more consecutive beats [11, p. 177] (some references say three or more)[13, p. 142] that resemble the normally conducted sinus beats with morphologic similarity [16, p. 453]. Since these beats originate above the bundle of His and often in the atria from an ectopic site other than the SA node, the QRS is narrow like the normal beats [16, p. 453]. However, in some instances with concurrent bundle branch blocks or aberrant conduction abnormalities, the QRS can be wide, making it difficult to differentiate from ventricular tachycardia [16, p. 464]. Supraventricular tachycardia (SVT) can be a sudden intense burst that is brief and intermittent, starting and ending abruptly. This is known as paroxysmal SVT

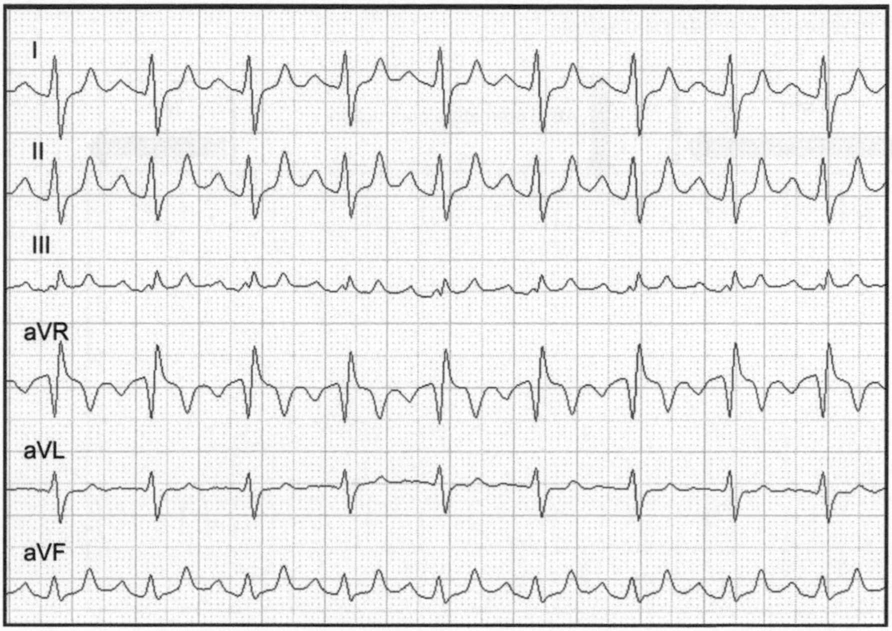

Figure 4.15 Leads I, II, III, aVR, aVL, aVF; 50 mm/s, 10 mm/mV. Example of sinus tachycardia in a 5-year-old St Bernard dog. The HR measures 190 bpm. Echocardiographic findings show moderate systolic dysfunction. The dog also experienced widespread systemic disease due to a splenic torsion.

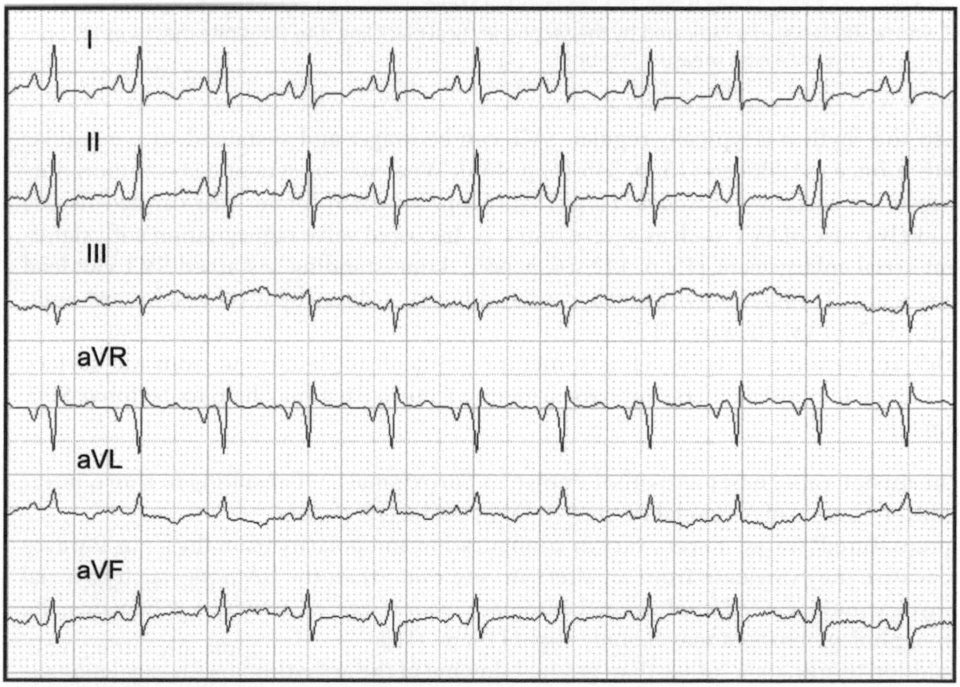

Figure 4.16 Leads I, II, III, aVR, aVL, aVF; 50 mm/s, 10 mm/mV. Six limb lead ECG from a 10-year-old domestic short-haired cat with hyperthyroidism prior to radio-iodine therapy. HR measures 240 bpm which is within the upper limits of normal for a cat. Echocardiographic findings show mild generalized hypertrophy with a normal left arm size. Post-therapy the HR dropped to the 180 bpm range which likely represents the normal range for this cat.

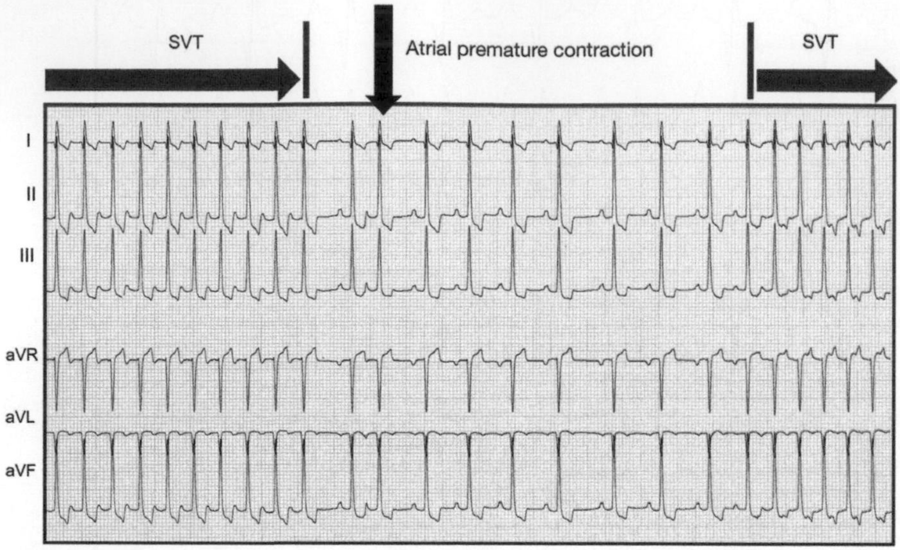

Figure 4.17 Leads I, II, III, aVR, aVL, aVF; 25 mm/s, 5 mm/mV. Example of supraventricular tachycardia in a 12-year-old cocker spaniel. The blue arrows indicate supraventricular tachycardia (SVT). The first blue arrow shows a run of SVT in mid-occurrence with a sudden cessation indicated by the first vertical black line. This is followed by a normal sinus beat, an atrial premature contraction (indicated by the black arrow), and seven sinus beats. The second blue arrow shows the beginning of a second run of SVT whose sudden start is indicated by the second vertical black line. The sinus rate measures 120 bpm while the tachycardia rates measure 200 bpm.

when the rhythm is typically regular. SVT can be longer and sustained with a regular rhythm once established [15, p. 345;16, p. 463]. Weakness or syncope is common during faster or sustained episodes [11, p. 184; 16, pp. 464–465]. Underlying cardiac disease is a likely cause of SVT such as severe mitral or tricuspid valve regurgitation with significant atrial enlargement [13, p. 142; 16, p. 465]. Long-standing sustained SVT can lead to myocardial failure known as tachycardia-induced cardiomyopathy or tachycardiomyopathy [15, p. 337] (Figure 4.17).

Differentiating SVT from ST is sometimes difficult to determine from the surface ECG, even for cardiologists, but here are some features that may help to decipher SVT from ST:

- an abrupt, rapid onset and offset known as paroxysmal SVT resulting in short, intermittent bursts of AV nodal re-entrant tachycardia [15, p. 345].
- premature P waves, if seen, vary in configuration and polarity from the sinus P waves because they originate from an alternate site other than the SA node, such as atrial myocardium, caused by abnormal automaticity or triggered activity mechanisms; the morphology changes may be only slight [15, p. 341].
- sudden termination rather than gradual slowing of the arrhythmia with vagal maneuvers that increase vagal tone such as appropriate ocular pressure or carotid sinus massage; this type of re-entrant SVT is dependent on sympathetic tone [13, p. 345].
- 24-hour Holter monitoring is helpful in correlating inappropriate heart rate and rhythm with activity in the home environment [30].

Tech Tip 19: classification of arrhythmias may be noted by origin or rate. (i) Origin classification – supraventricular beats originate from the atria or AV node; ventricular beats originate from the ventricle. (ii) Rate classification – brady refers to slow rhythms, tachy refers to rapid rhythms.

Atrial Fibrillation

This is a rapid and irregular rhythm characterized by disorganized fibrillatory *f* waves rather than organized P waves causing an undulating wavy baseline; P waves are absent [15, p. 343]. Unlike sinus arrhythmia, atrial fibrillation (AF) is typically highly irregular with no discernible pattern. The QRS complexes are upright and narrow in lead II unless a conduction abnormality is present, such as a bundle branch block. It is a common type of supraventricular arrhythmia, although rare in the cat [12, p. 66]. With a slower ventricular rate the presence of *f* waves is more pronounced. The fibrillatory waves may be fine or coarse [15, p. 345; 16, p. 471] (Figure 4.18). When the waves are saw tooth and regular they are flutter F waves, as in atrial flutter; this finding is rare [16, p. 469]. In AF, severe structural heart changes may be a contributing factor, such as dilated

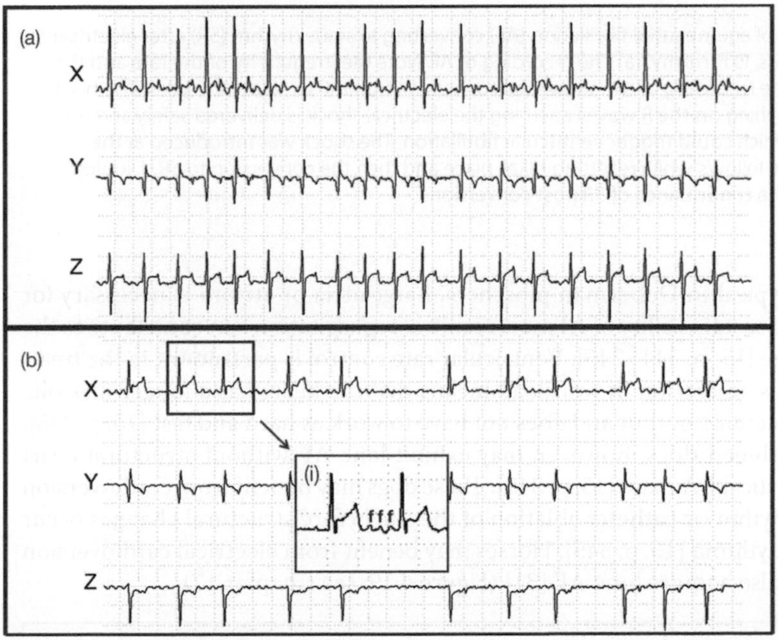

Figure 4.18 Leads X, Y, Z from Holter recordings; 25 mm/s, 10 mm/mV. Example of atrial fibrillation (AF) in a 9-year-old Newfoundland dog with dilated cardiomyopathy. (a) AF pre-treatment. The HR measures 162 bpm in this example but increased to 260 bpm during the 24-hour period. Note the rate irregularity. (b) AF post-treatment with diltiazem at 5 mg/kg. HR measures 100 bpm. The HR has slowed to a satisfactory rate post-treatment; the AF is controlled but still present. Note in (i) the enlarged example from channel X showing *f* waves, or fibrillatory waves, occurring between T waves and QRS complexes throughout the entire recording. Echocardiographic findings divulge a dilated left ventricle and atrium with mitral regurgitation.

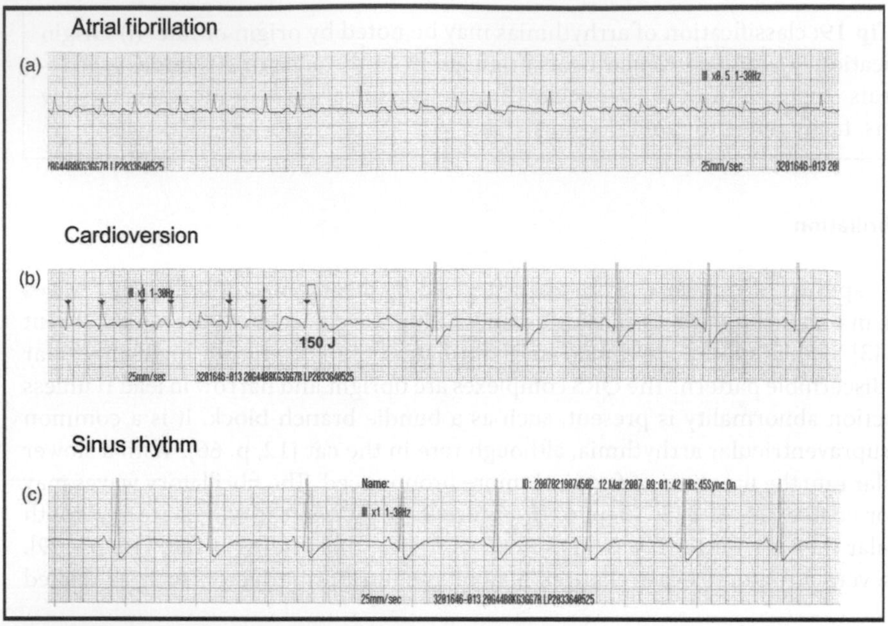

Figure 4.19 Example of equine atrial fibrillation (AF) converting to sinus rhythm (SR) after electrical cardioversion; 25 mm/s, 10 mm/mV. (a) The recording of AF. Note the irregularity of the rate and the lack of p waves. (b) The recording of the successful conversion from AF to SR at 150 joules. The black triangles indicate synching on the R waves ensuring the electrical shock is delivered safely and not during the T waves which could trigger ventricular fibrillation. The shock was introduced at the seventh beat. A pause follows while resetting takes place and then the conversion to SR. J, joules. (c) The recording of the continuance of SR post conversion.

cardiomyopathy typical in Doberman pinschers. Large atria or atrium is necessary for the generation and sustainability of AF; severe mitral regurgitation can contribute to the increased atrial size [15, p. 344–345]. Ventricular rate control is paramount in the treatment of these cases; reduction in workload means that the heart has a longer diastolic period increasing cardiac output and does not have to work as hard and fast [15, p. 345].

Large and giant-breed dogs, however, may exhibit lone AF without structural heart disease but with critical LA mass [15, p. 343]. These dogs may benefit from cardioversion to normal sinus rhythm or catheter ablation of the site before structural changes occur from the tachyarrhythmia [15, p. 345]. Horses may benefit from electrical cardioversion as well since they also acquire lone AF [31] (Figure 4.19; see Chapter 17).

Tech Tip 20: a wavy baseline is commonly misidentified as AF when it is, in fact, just a messy baseline. Improve the quality of the ECG by reducing this artifact; for example, stretch the legs so that elbows are not touching the chest wall and legs are parallel to each other. If P wave identification is difficult to determine, another tip is to either increase the amplitude or to apply the precordial chest leads. Since the chest leads are placed directly over the heart, indistinct P waves in the limb leads can be more noticeable in the chest leads if present [13, p. 293].

Sinus Bradycardia

This is a slow sinus rhythm with regular or slight variation in P–P intervals and constant PR intervals, but the rate is below normal [15, p. 91]. Large and athletic breeds can normally have a slower rate [12, p. 65]. Persistently slow rates that do not respond to exercise challenge, excitement stimulus, or atropine administration may point toward an underlying disease [13, pp. 133–134].

Atrial Standstill

This is a condition that can be persistent, temporary, or terminal [13, p. 166]. Skeletal muscle wasting and dystrophy, fibrous replacement of atrial muscle cells, myocarditis, and feline dilated cardiomyopathy are examples of persistent atrial standstill patients [13, p. 167; 15, p. 81; 16, pp. 341, 461]. Hyperkalemia is a common factor of temporary atrial standstill [13, p. 167; 15, p. 81]. A dying heart is an example of terminal atrial standstill [13, p. 166]. Persistent atrial standstill is commonly seen in English springer spaniels [15, p. 81]. There is sinus node function but impulses do not cause atrial depolarization [16, p. 461]. P waves are absent due to inactivation of atrial myocardium; heart rate is typically slow but regular (<60 bpm in the dog, <160 bpm in the cat) [15, p. 81; 16, p. 461]. Normal QRS complexes are seen with persistent atrial standstill [13, p. 166]. Wide QRS complexes are seen with temporary or terminal atrial standstill [16, p. 461]. Treatment will be determined based on the underlying condition such as lowering potassium concentration in the hyperkalemic patient or implanting a permanent ventricular pacemaker in the syncopal patient [16, p. 461].

Sinus Arrest

This is a failure of the SA node to form an impulse commonly due to high vagal tone or depressed automaticity of the SA node [16, p. 456; 15, p. 92]. A pause in the rhythm occurs and is greater than twice the preceding R–R interval [12, p. 65]. In dogs, this definition is flawed due to underlying sinus arrhythmia making determination of the cause in R–R interval variation difficult [15, p. 92]. It is also not possible to know from the surface ECG whether there is a failure of the SA node to fire or failure of the depolarization to exit the SA node into the atrial myocardium, as in SA block [16, p. 456]. Escape beats often follow long pauses when other pacemaker sites activate and pitch in to help the heart recover [12, p. 65]. Intermittent sinus arrest can be normal for brachycephalic breeds, but prolonged or frequent sinus arrest may result in episodic weakness, fainting, even death [13, p. 164]. Presenting signs can be syncopal episodes, seizures, or sudden weakness during exercise or excitement. Pacemaker implantation can benefit this patient [13, p. 164] (Figure 4.20).

Sick Sinus Syndrome

This is a rhythm abnormality caused by an impaired, erratic, or diseased SA node often involving one or more areas of the conduction system [15, p. 372]. Episodic weakness, lethargy, and syncope are the most common presenting clinical signs [15, p. 372]. The ECG is characterized by episodes of marked bradycardia with sinus arrest or block [13, 184]. Escape rhythms may be noted and are actually welcomed as a mechanism

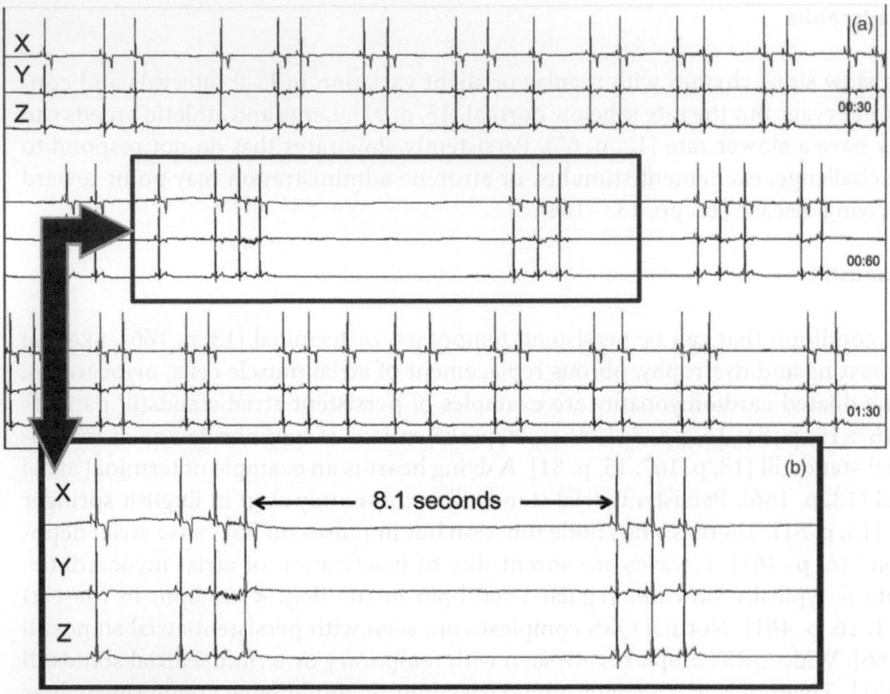

Figure 4.20 Leads X, Y, Z from a 24-hour Holter recording. Example of sinus arrest in a 6-year-old miniature schnauzer. In (a) leads X, Y, and Z are continuous for 1.5 min; each line equals 30 s in time. (b) is a zoomed in area of (a) showing an 8.1 s pause. This dog presented with a chief complaint of collapse while running uphill. The Holter recording over the 24 h shows multiple instances of sinus arrest with over 4000 pauses greater than 2 s. Pacemaker implantation was recommended for this patient.

to rescue the dangerously slow heart rhythm but syncope will result with pauses 8 s in length or longer [15, pp. 93, 373]. Long pauses may follow atrial premature contractions [13, p. 184]. Some ECGs also exhibit a pattern of marked bradycardia and intermittent sinus arrest alternating with periods of paroxysmal SVTs (sudden burst of transient supraventricular tachycardia) known as brady-tachy syndrome [12, p. 324–325]. Typical breeds are miniature schnauzers, west highland white terriers, cocker spaniels, and dachshunds [12, p. 324]. Often 24-hour Holter monitoring is necessary to characterize the intermittent arrhythmia [12, p. 324]. The most effective treatment for severe types of this arrhythmia is a permanent pacemaker; lead placement either in the right atrium with normal AV nodal function or in the right ventricle (or dual chambers) with AV nodal dysfunction [12, p. 324] (Figure 4.21).

Atrioventricular Heart Blocks

First Degree Heart Block

In first degree heart block (1HB), the PR interval is prolonged resulting from slowed conduction through the AV node [15, p. 81]. This type of block may occur in normal healthy animals or can be due to conduction system inflammation, secondary to drug administration, or increased vagal tone [15, p. 81–82] (Figure 4.11).

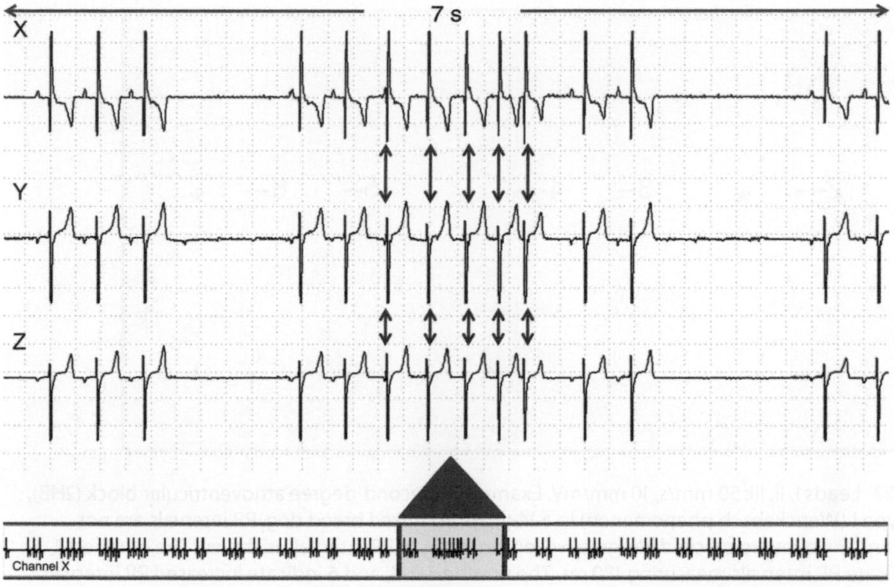

Figure 4.21 Leads X, Y, Z from a 24-hour Holter recording; 25 mm/s, 5 mm/mV. Example of sick sinus syndrome in a 12-year-old west highland white terrier. There is an alternating bradycardia tachycardia present. The 7-s strip shows a 1 s pause and a 1.5 s pause with a cluster of supraventricular tachycardia (SVT) indicated by the blue arrows. Below this there is a longer 60-s strip from channel X showing the rhythm in context. Note the alternating short bursts of paroxysmal SVT and pauses. This dog presented with a recent history of numerous collapse episodes and suspected bradycardia. Pacemaker implantation was recommended for this patient.

Second Degree Heart Block

In second degree heart block (2HB), there are some P waves without QRS complexes resulting from intermittent failure of atrial depolarizations to reach the ventricles; they fail to get through to their destination [15, p. 82]. There are two types of 2HB. In Mobitz Type I, also known as Wenckebach phenomenon, there is prolongation of the PR interval with successive beats until a P wave is actually blocked [15, p. 82]. The PR interval of the beat preceding the blocked beat is longer than the PR interval of the beat that follows the blocked beat [16, p. 488]. In Type I, the block is typically caused by a delay in the AV node with a normal QRS duration, although it may occur in the bundle of His [13, p. 232] (Figure 4.22).

In Mobitz Type II, the PR interval remains constant in all conducted beats yet may be normal or prolonged [15, p. 82]. QRS complexes can be wide if the block occurs below the His within the bundle branches [13, p. 232]. Escape rates can be slower and less stable [13, p. 232]. Type II is characterized by a sudden block while the PR interval of conducted beats remains unchanged and can occur due to disease in the His-Purkinje system [15, p. 82]. A block is considered low grade when there is 2:1 block (2 P waves to 1 QRS) and high grade when there is a 3:1 block or greater (3 P waves to 1 QRS) which has the added danger of morphing into complete AV block.[15, p. 82] (Figure 4.23). Pacemaker implantation is helpful when the patient exhibits syncopal episodes [15, p. 400; 16, p. 489].

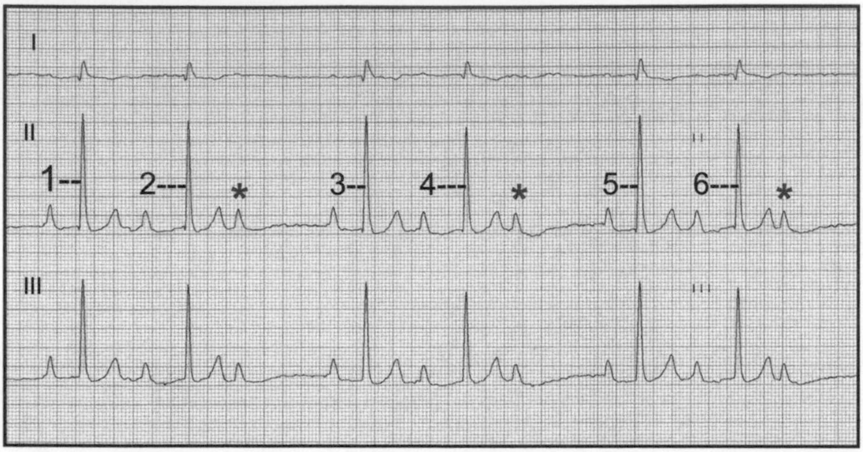

Figure 4.22 Leads I, II, III; 50 mm/s, 10 mm/mV. Example of second-degree atrioventricular block (2HB), Mobitz Type I (Wenckebach phenomenon) in a 14-year-old mixed breed dog. PR intervals are not constant and P waves are blocked. Progressive lengthening of PR intervals is shown. The numbers 1, 3, and 5 indicate PR intervals measuring 180 ms. The numbers 2, 4, and 6 indicate increased PR intervals measuring 240 ms. The red asterisks indicate P waves that have been blocked and are not followed by QRS complexes. The PR interval following a blocked beat is shorter than the preceding PR interval.

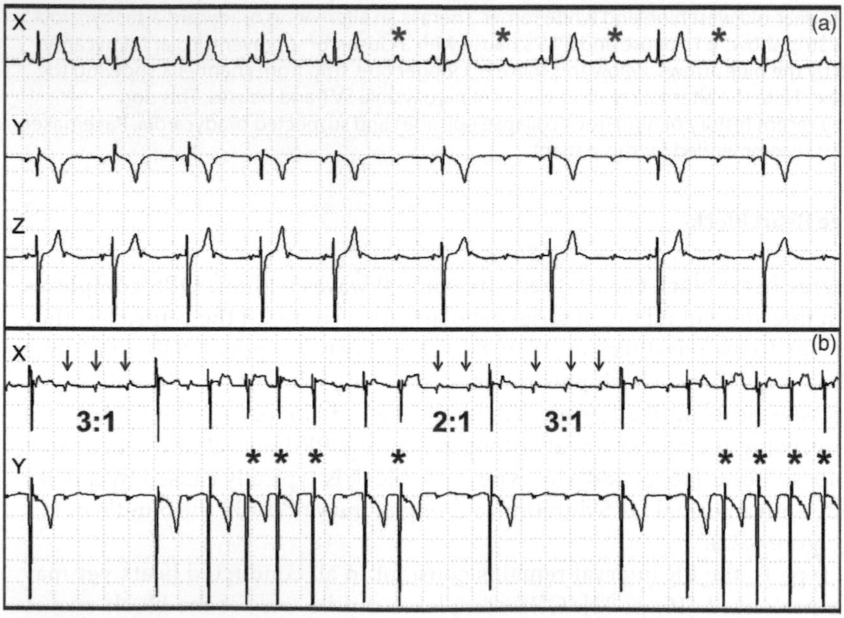

Figure 4.23 (a) Leads X, Y, Z from a 24-hour Holter recording; 25 mm/s, 10 mm/mV. Example of a low-grade second-degree atrioventricular block (2HB) in a 7-year-old shar-pei dog. The red asterisks indicate blocked P waves. PR intervals remain constant in conducted beats. (b) Leads X, Y from a 24-hour Holter recording; 25 mm/s, 10 mm/mV. Example of high grade 2HB in a 12-year-old cocker spaniel dog. The blue arrows indicate 3:1 blocks and 2:1 block, showing 3 or 2 P waves to 1 QRS complex. The blue asterisks indicate supraventricular beats: a triplet, a single, and a run of at least four beats are shown. PR intervals are not constant but there is the complicating factor of the supraventricular arrhythmia.

Third Degree Heart Block

In third degree heart block (3HB), there is complete block as in, no conduction between the SA node and the ventricles [15, p. 83]. There is absolutely no association between the P waves and the QRS complexes, known as *AV dissociation* [16, p. 489]. However, the P–P and R–R intervals usually remain constant [16, p. 490]. The P waves occur at their own rate from SA node depolarization while the QRS complexes occur at their own slower rate from either the AV node (normal QRS duration, supraventricular origin) or Purkinje fibers (wide QRS duration, ventricular origin) [16, p. 489]. Pacemaker implantation is the treatment of choice in patients with 3HB due to debilitating clinical signs, severe bradycardia, reduced cardiac output, and frequent collapse [16, p. 492] (Figure 4.24). Cats with 3HB normally do not exhibit clinical signs due to a faster ventricular rate and a less active lifestyle [16, p. 491].

Tech Tip 21: 1HB – prolonged or delayed conduction, 2HB – intermittent conduction, 3HB – no conduction.

Bundle Branch Blocks: Right or Left

This is an intraventricular conduction disturbance of the right or left bundle branches [15, p. 84]. The complexes are preceded by P waves, but the affected branch activates later and more slowly than normal causing a delay in ventricular depolarization

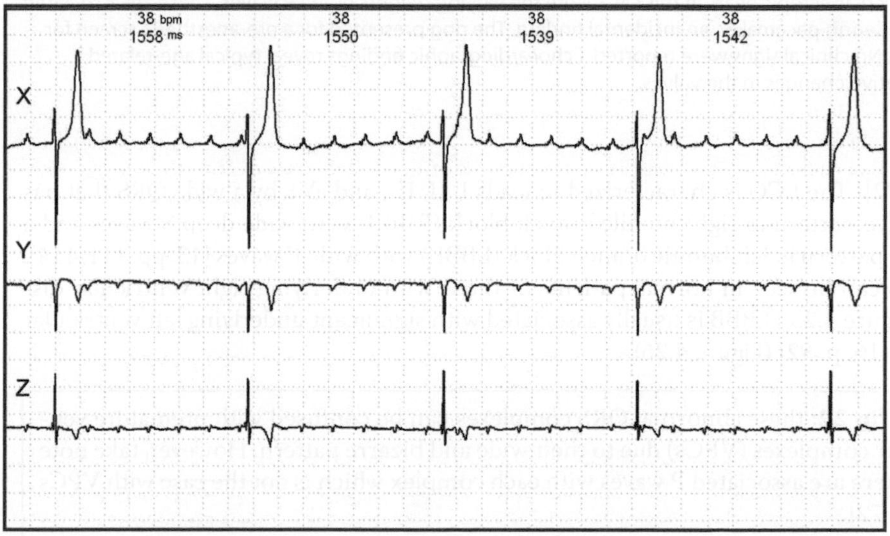

Figure 4.24 Leads X, Y, Z from a 24-hour Holter recording; 25 mm/s, 10 mm/mV. Example of third-degree atrioventricular block (3HB) in a 7-year-old shar-pei dog. Note the QRS complexes are ventricular with a ventricular escape rhythm at 38 bpm; the atrial rate appears to be 243 bpm. This is complete heart block in which the ventricles and atria are disassociated and occurring at their own relatively constant rates. The dog presented with collapse episodes. Auscultation revealed intermittent bradycardia. On the 24-hour Holter recording there was intermittent 2HB and 3HB. Pacemaker implantation was recommended for this patient.

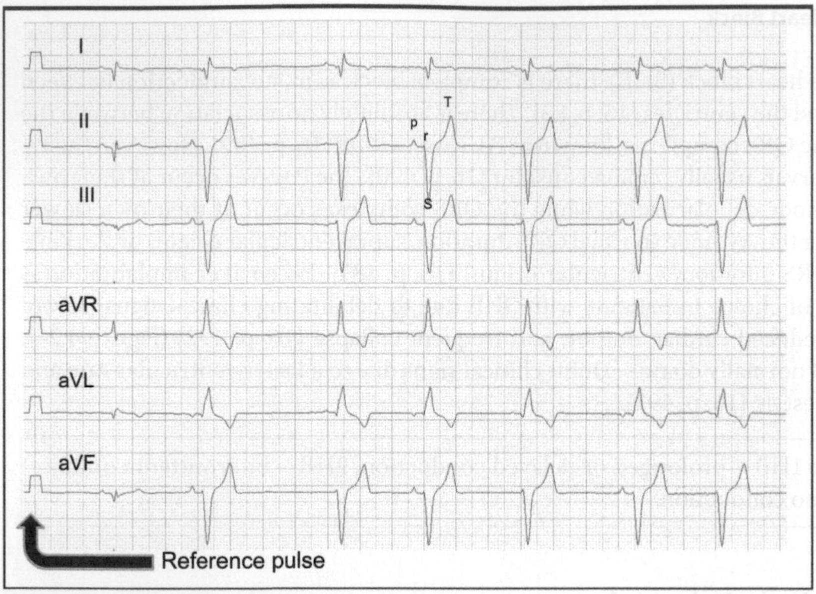

Figure 4.25 Leads I, II, III, aVR, aVL, aVF; 50 mm/s, 5 mm/mV. Example of right bundle branch block in an 8-year-old Pembroke Welsh corgi dog. The block appears to be intermittent. The first beat after the reference pulse is the dog's normal beat followed by six beats of right bundle branch origin. There is a negative pattern in leads II, III, and aVF as evidenced by the deep S waves of these abnormal beats that have widened the QRS complexes, measuring 70 ms. The mean electrical axis has shifted to the right. Although these beats appear wide and bizarre, the associated P waves and normal PR intervals rule out ventricular ectopic beats in this case. Note the varying heights of the P waves. These are associated with wandering pacemaker, an incidental finding. The dog presented for a pre-anesthesia screen for dentistry. No clinical signs were reported. Echocardiographic findings reveal typical age-related degenerative changes to the valves.

[12, p. 72]. The ECG is characterized in leads I, II, III, and aVF by a wide QRS that has a negative pattern in right bundle branch block (RBBB) with wide deep S waves and a positive pattern in left bundle branch block (LBBB) with wide R waves [13, pp. 111, 114].

RBBB can be seen in normal patients or those with underlying right ventricular disease (Figure 4.25); LBBB is usually associated with significant underlying left ventricular disease [16, p. 92] (Figure 4.26).

Tech Tip 22: these abnormal QRS complexes can be confused with premature ventricular complexes (VPCs) due to their wide and bizarre pattern. However, take note that there are associated P waves with each complex which is not the case with VPCs [12, p. 72].

Left Anterior Fascicular Block

This is an intraventricular conduction disturbance of the left anterior fascicle [15, p. 84]. The blocked fascicle causes a delay in ventricular conduction and the associated

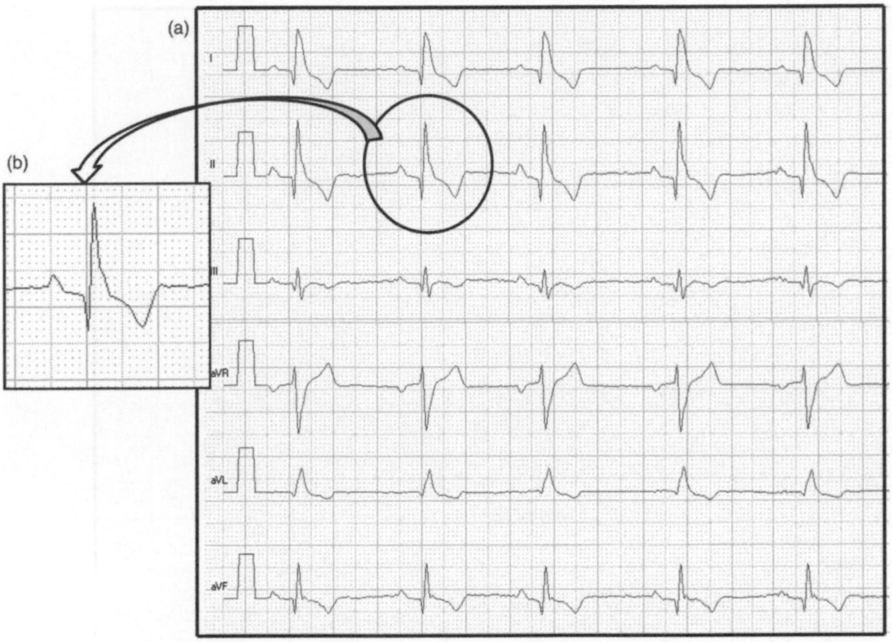

Figure 4.26 (a) Leads I, II, III, aVR, aVL, aV: 50 mm/s, 10 mm/mV. Example of left bundle branch block in a 10-year-old Doberman pinscher dog who presented for a pre-anesthesia workup for mandibular mass removal. There is a positive pattern in leads I, II, III, and aVF with wide QRS complexes due to wide R waves. This is consistent with marked conduction disturbance and slowing. Note the associated P waves and normal PR intervals. (b) Enlarged example of a QRS complex from (a). R wave measures 80 ms. Echocardiographic findings are consistent with dilated cardiomyopathy and include dilated left ventricular chamber along with dyskinetic and hypokinetic motion. The dog is at risk for general anesthesia.

papillary muscle [12, p. 72]. The QRS complexes remain normal in duration with a qR pattern in leads I and aVL; however, notable ECG findings are deep S waves in leads II, III, and aVF along with a marked left axis deviation [12, p. 72] (Figure 4.27).

Tech Tip 23: while uncommon in dogs, left anterior fascicular block is a very common abnormality seen in cats with hypertrophic cardiomyopathy; learn how to recognize it [12, p. 72; 16, p. 93].

Atrial Premature Contractions

Atrial premature contractions are supraventricular complexes that occur prematurely as singles, couplets, or triplets [15, p. 94]. The site of origin is typically from an atrial ectopic site other than the SA node [13, p. 140]. The complexes are usually narrow and appear 90% like the normally conducted sinus beats [15, p. 332]. There is an association of P waves to QRS complexes although the premature P waves are different in configuration from the sinus P waves [13, p. 140]. This difference can be slight or obvious.

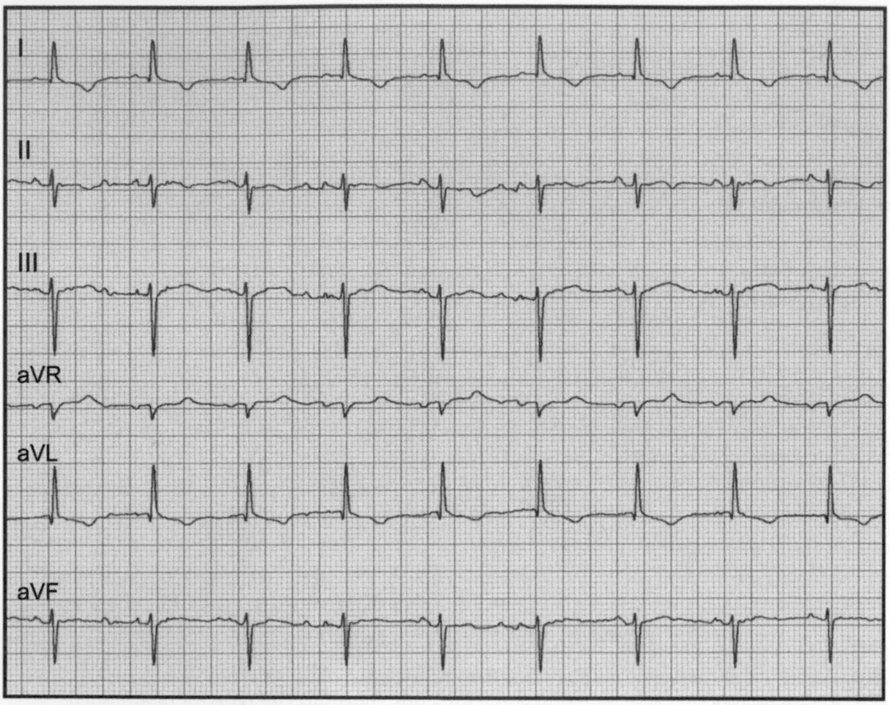

Figure 4.27 Leads I, II, III, aVR, aVL, aVF; 50 mm/s, 10 mm/mV. Example of left anterior fascicular block in a 9-month-old domestic short-haired cat. This is a common conduction abnormality in cats with hypertrophic cardiomyopathy (HCM). It is uncommon in dogs. Note the S waves present in leads II, III, and aVF. The mean electrical axis using method 1 (isoelectric/perpendicular method) is –30 indicating marked left axis deviation. Echocardiographic findings are classic for HCM.

The premature P waves may be positive, negative, somehow altered in morphology, or superimposed upon the preceding T wave [13, p. 140]. Although the QRS complex is premature as well, the P–R interval of this abnormal beat can be longer than the sinus P–R interval [13, p. 140]. By themselves, atrial premature contractions are not viewed as dangerous although there may be underlying atrial disease causing atrial enlargement or tissue bruising in the trauma patient [13, p. 140]. Other diagnostic tests should be pursued (Figures 4.12 and 4.17)

Junctional Premature Contractions

These complexes originate in the AV junctional area [12, p. 66]. Junctional premature contractions (JPCs) are considered supraventricular in origin since they occur above the ventricles. The P wave is often inverted and appears negative on the ECG and may occur before, during, or after the QRS depending on the origination site [12, p. 66]. QRS configuration is normal. An escape rhythm is a run of consecutive JPCs with a rate between 40 and 60 bpm, the inherent AV nodal rate [12, p. 74]. If the SA node is impaired, the AV node will take over as the pacemaker site [11, p. 7,8].

Tech Tip 24: junctional escape beats should not be suppressed; this rhythm aids in maintaining cardiac output. The SA node dysfunction needs to be addressed [12, p. 74].

Premature Ventricular Complexes

These are ventricular complexes that occur prematurely as singles, couplets, or triplets [15, p. 97] (Figures 4.28 and 4.29). The site of origin is typically from a ventricular ectopic site rather than the SA node [13, p. 154]. The complexes are usually wide and bizarre as the impulses travel slowly through the ventricular muscle; however, they can be narrow if the ectopic site is closer to the atria near the His bundle, for example [15, p. 335].

Tech Tip 25: remember to run multiple leads simultaneously while recording the ECG in order to gain insight as to the origination site of the complexes. For example, supraventricular beats look 90% like the normally conducted sinus beats in every lead; narrow ventricular beats can mistakenly be called supraventricular if only one lead is acquired. Narrow ventricular beats may look very different in other leads, maybe not wide and bizarre, but definitely not 90% like the normally conducted sinus beat [15, p. 333].

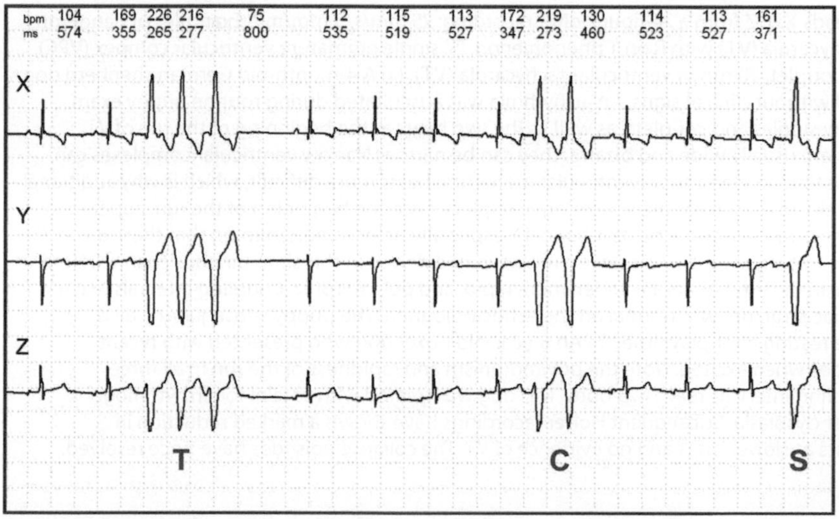

Figure 4.28 Leads X, Y, Z from a 24-hour Holter recording; 25 mm/s, 5 mm/mV. Example of premature ventricular complexes in a 9-year-old boxer dog. A triplet indicated by 'T' has a coupling interval of 226 bpm, the couplet indicated by 'C' has a coupling interval of 219 bpm and the single indicated by 'S' has a coupling interval of 161 bpm. They appear similar in morphology to each other, known as monomorphism. The dog diagnosed with arrhythmogenic right ventricular dysplasia is being treated with sotalol for ventricular arrhythmias.

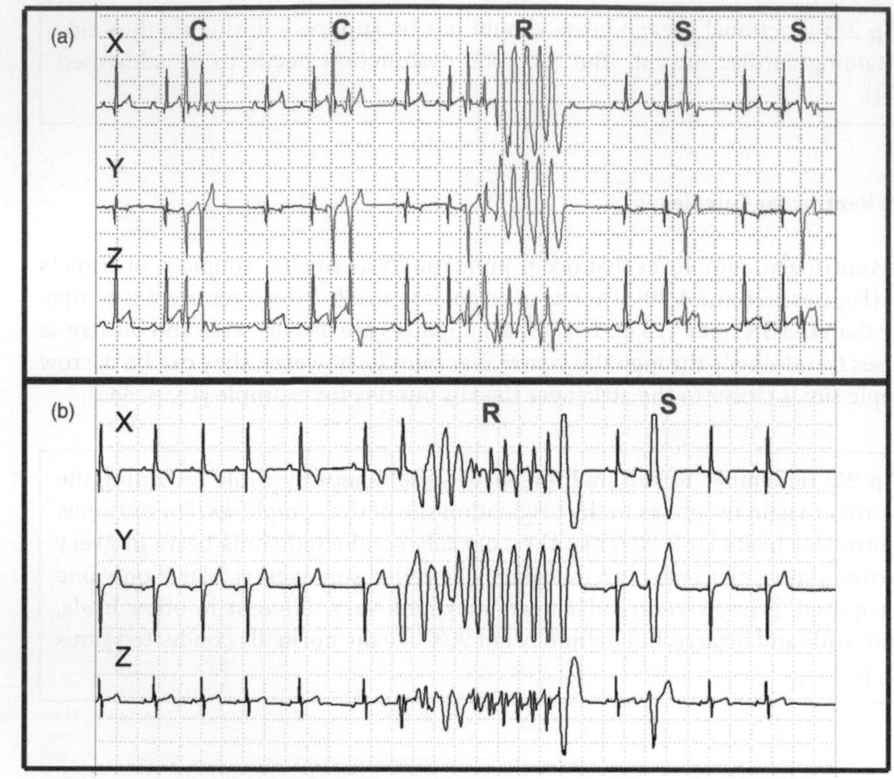

Figure 4.29 Leads X, Y, Z from a 24-hour Holter recording; 25 mm/s, 5 mm/mV. Examples of dangerous ventricular tachycardia (VT) with R on T phenomenon. 'S', single premature ventricular compex (VPC). 'C', ventricular couplet, 'R', run of ventricular tachycardia (VT). (a) A 4-month-old German shepherd dog who presented without clinical signs. An arrhythmia was auscultated during routine puppy exam. Note the narrow singles and couplets, as well as the two beats at the beginning of the run of VT. Although VPCs are usually wide and bizarre, they can be narrow. Narrow ventricular complexes can make differentiation between supraventricular premature beats more difficult, which is why additional channels can help. In channel X, the singles and couplets, even the beginning of the run, appear narrow and similar to the normal beats. Channel Y especially helps in determining that these are in fact, ventricular, not supraventricular since they are very different in this simultaneous channel. Note the rest of the run of seven beats are wider, more rapid, and polymorphic. Coupling intervals reach 600 bpm. Cardiac structure was normal on the echocardiogram. The puppy subsequently died suddenly while resting after play time. (b) An 8-year-old boxer dog who presented with recent collapse episodes when excited. Note the polymorphism and rapidness of the run in all three channels. Coupling intervals reach 425 bpm. This dog was treated with sotalol for arrhythmogenic right ventricular dysplasia. Subsequent Holter recordings have shown a marked reduction in ventricular beats at slower rates and no evidence of VT. The collapse episodes have since resolved.

VPCs are not associated with P waves [15, p. 332]. They are called uniform or monomorphic if the morphology of abnormal beats is similar; they are considered multiform or polymorphic if the morphologies differ [13, p. 154]. VPCs can be present in cases with traumatic myocardial injury, hemangiosarcoma, hypotension/shock, and gastric dilatation volvulus [15, p. 371]. The Doberman pinscher with dilated cardiomyopathy typically displays VPCs that are negative in lead II, an indication that the beat originates from a site in the left ventricle [16, pp. 476, 481]. The boxer with arrhythmogenic right ventricular cardiomyopathy typically displays VPCs that are positive in lead II, an indication that the beat originates from a site in the right ventricle [12, p. 369; 15, p. 368; 16, p. 477]. When the VPC is incredibly premature so that it occurs within the T wave of the preceding sinus beat during vulnerable repolarization it is called the R on T phenomenon [15, p. 357]. This is more dangerous, hemodynamically unstable, and may progress to ventricular tachycardia or ventricular fibrillation [16, p. 479].

Bigeminal pattern refers to a VPC occurring every other beat, *trigeminal* pattern refers to a VPC occurring every third beat or a normal sinus beat occurring every third beat [13, p. 155]. A *fusion beat* refers to the clashing of simultaneous activation from the SA node and the ventricular ectopic site [13, p. 155]. The complex will be a melding of both morphologies, normal QRS meets VPC. An *interpolated* VPC refers to a VPC occurring between two normal sinus beats in which the underlying rhythm is not disturbed or altered [13, p. 155]. A *ventricular escape beat (VEB)* does not occur prematurely but typically late and may actually help to rescue the heart from a severe bradyarrhythmia [13, p. 152].

Tech Tip 26: it is imperative that a ventricular escape rhythm not be suppressed since it is taking control over the heart rate at the inherent ventricular rate of 30–4 bpm during sinus node dysfunction or 3HB. Cardiac output is maintained with this safety mechanism [13, p. 152].

Ventricular Tachycardia

Ventricular tachycardia (VT) is a fast, usually regular, rhythm depicted by four or more consecutive beats [11, p. 177] (some references say three or more) [13, p. 156] originating from the ventricles. The severe forms of this arrhythmia carry an increased risk of collapse or sudden death [15, p. 357]. The complexes are typically wide and bizarre. P waves are not associated [15, p. 332]. VT may be sustained when a run lasts 30 seconds or longer or nonsustained when a run ends within 30 s, monomorphic or polymorphic, fast or slower [16, p. 481]. Those considered dangerous are typically polymorphic and fast and should be treated [13, p. 33]. Also dangerously noteworthy is a run of VT with R on T phenomenon in which the beats are practically on top of each other with the R waves occurring in the vulnerable T wave period which can degenerate into ventricular fibrillation [15, p. 357; 16, p. 479]. German shepherd dogs are known to die suddenly when they exhibit the severe form in inherited ventricular arrhythmia [15, p. 370; 32; 33] (Figures 4.29 and 4.30).

Accelerated Idioventricular Rhythm

Accelerated idioventricular rhythm (AIVR) is considered to be a relatively slow and benign ventricular rhythm between 60 and 100 bpm and is usually not considered dangerous and thus, not treated. AIVR is often associated with other systemic diseases, postgastric volvulus surgical procedures, and with neurologic diseases [16, p. 480–481].

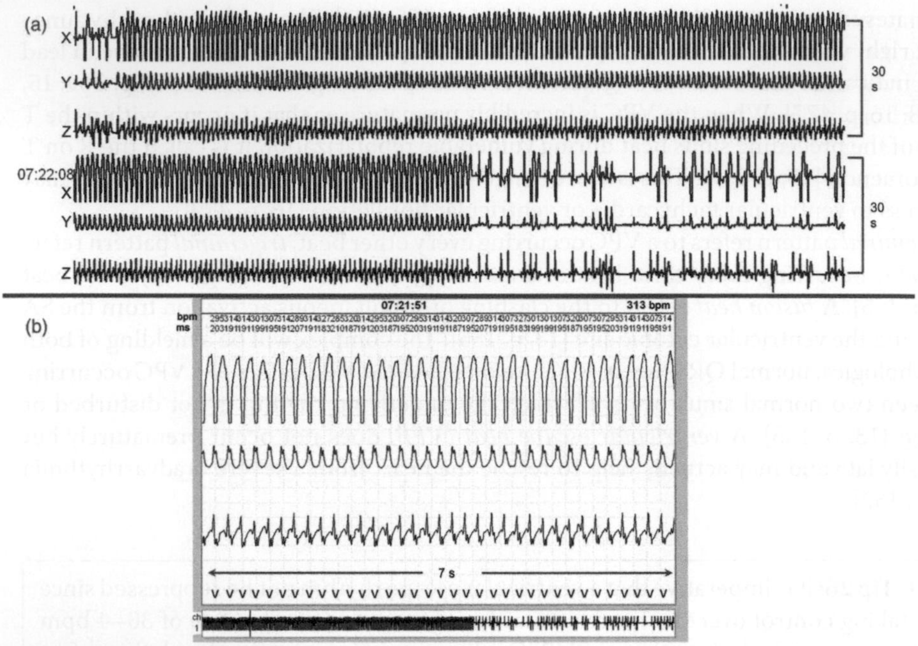

Figure 4.30 Leads X, Y, Z from a 24-hour Holter recording; 25 mm/s, 5 mm/mV. Example of a sustained run of ventricular tachycardia (VT) with dangerous R on T phenomenon in a 4-year-old Doberman pinscher. (a) A 1 min excerpt from the full disclosure showing all three channels simultaneously, beginning with approximately 45 s of sustained VT and finally breaking into sinus beats interspersed with ventricular arrhythmias. (b) An enlarged 7-s strip of all three channels from the full disclosure in (a) giving a dramatic look at the R on T phenomenon. Coupling intervals reach 320 bpm. This type of dangerous VT can degenerate into ventricular fibrillation. The dog is at great risk of sudden death. Below this there is a longer 60-s strip from channel X (ch 1) showing the beats in context. Echocardiographic diagnosis includes dilated cardiomyopathy and congestive heart failure. Medications were instituted to manage the congestion and a regimen of sotalol was started immediately to control the ventricular arrhythmias.

Ventricular Fibrillation

Ventricular fibrillation (VF) is an irregular rhythm in which there are no distinguishable P waves or QRS complexes and may be fatal [13, p. 160]. The baseline undulates chaotically with variable amplitudes. The activity in the ventricles is disorganized and there is no mechanical beating resulting in a severe drop in blood pressure and no cardiac output [12, p. 330]. Intervention in the form of immediate cardiopulmonary resuscitation and defibrillation is necessary and must be performed as soon as possible [13, p. 160].

Electrical Alternans

This refers to beat variation of the QRS complex (although it can refer to P and T waves as well) resulting in a pattern of changing amplitudes, alternating in height or direction [13, p. 188]. This is commonly seen with pericardial effusion when the heart is swinging within large quantities of abnormal fluid in the pericardial sac, the shifting movements forcing the heart closer to the electrodes and then further away [13, p. 188]. Other causes of electrical alternans are extremely rapid rates such as SVT and VT or in some types of bundle branch block due to alternating recovery rates [13, p. 188]. This is an interesting ECG finding, but treatment of the cause is of overriding importance [13, p. 188].

Low Voltage Complexes

Amplitudes of R waves are decreased in all leads [13, p. 82]. This ECG damping effect is typical in patients with pericardial and/or pleural effusion [13, p. 82]. Other causes are normal variation, obesity, hypothyroidism, or restrictive diseases [13, p. 82].

Wandering Pacemaker

This ECG finding is characterized by a gradual change in either the P wave amplitude or morphology or both, although the PR interval remains constant [13, p. 138]. The change is due to the impulse shifting to an alternate area of the pacemaker site within the SA node (the dog has a large SA node, up to 40 mm) [15, p. 334], or to differing excitation exit points perhaps along the peripheral borders of the SA node or the atrial myocardium surrounding the SA node [19, 20, 34]. It is associated with sinus arrhythmia and usually a normal interesting finding with no clinical significance [11, p. 93]. Vagal stimulation can cause a shift of the leading pacemaker site [16, p. 75]. The change in P wave can be associated with rate change [13, p. 138]. For example, when the heart rate slows the P wave amplitude is smaller than in previous beats. The P wave is positive if originating from the SA node, but will be negative if originating from the AV junction or very low in the SA node near the coronary sinus [13, p. 139] (Figure 4.25).

Other Monitoring Aids

Physiological monitoring of the critically ill patient often involves ECG devices that are set to monitor mode equipped with filter settings that eliminate artifacts and are appropriate in daily routine monitoring [35, p. 108]. Monitor mode set at a frequency of 0.5–40 Hz is more filtered but produces more distortion of complexes [35, pp. 107–108]. For increased diagnostic purposes, a diagnostic mode is preferred that allows more accurate readings for interpretation [35, p. 108]. Diagnostic mode set at a frequency of 0.05–100 Hz while less filtered is prone to more artifact visualization but less distortion of complexes [35, pp. 107–108].

Ambulatory ECG monitoring is an extremely valuable tool in a patient with a collapse or syncopal history whose resting ECG or long rhythm strip has inconclusive findings [15, pp. 102, 332, 338]. For rhythms or conduction abnormalities that are transient or infrequent, monitoring with an external loop event recorder, external nonlooping event recorder, Holter monitor, or new generation mobile real-time cardiac telemetry can help pin point the problem [15, pp. 102, 332, 338]. Several types are available for veterinary use.

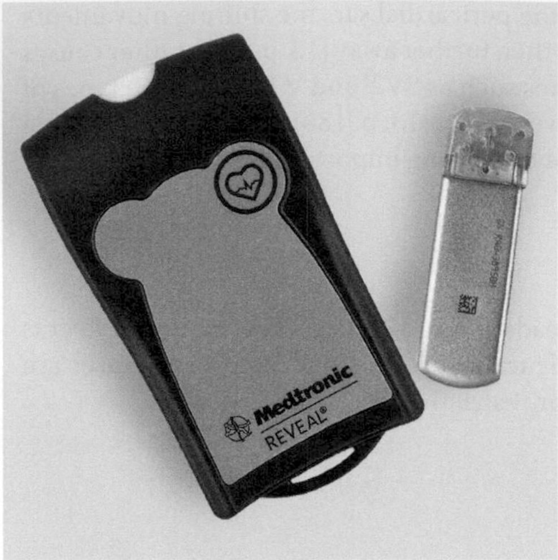

Figure 4.31 An implantable loop recorder (ILR) and the remote control device. The device is approximately 6 × 2 × 1 cm and has two exposed metal electrodes on the reverse side. The device is implanted with the electrodes toward the heart under the skin on the thorax. The remote control device allows the client to activate the "save" feature of the ILR should they notice a symptom by pressing the heart diagram on the upper right of the remote.

External Loop Event Recorders

These devices record continuously for several minutes at a time, then begin recording over again (looping) so that current ECG information constantly replaces past data [36]. It may be worn for an extended period, one to two weeks at a time or longer. Owner activation is required directly after witnessing an episode in order to save the ECG data associated with the event. Once activated, the ECG data prior to and following activation is stored in the memory [36]. Two external electrodes are usually required for one channel recording. Application duration may be a problem due to the inconvenience of frequent electrode replacement and protection of the unit from damage. Loop recorders are ideal for capturing brief, nonsustained rhythms in patients with intermittent but obvious clinical signs; however, owner participation is critical in capturing events [36]. An implantable loop recorder (ILR) is a better option for animal patients without obvious or very infrequent clinical signs as it is inserted subcutaneously, the ILR can be preprogrammed with specific parameters that will automatically save an ECG event that is later accessible and retrievable with an external interrogation device similar to those used for pacemaker programming. The ILR records a single ECG channel with two internal electrodes [36]. No external electrodes or owner activation are required. However, the owner can activate the save function with a handheld remote. Anesthesia or sedation is necessary for insertion and removal in subcutaneous tissue. The prolonged monitoring period increases the diagnostic yield in patients with infrequent syncope [36] (Figure 4.31).

External Nonlooping Event Recorders

These devices are less sophisticated postevent recorders, recording only when activated by the owner during an event [36]. It is temporarily held by the owner against the patient's chest wall and activated for a minute or two as it records the ECG. External electrodes are within the unit; therefore, skin electrode attachment is not required. One of the limitations of the device is that it typically does not show onset and offset of an arrhythmia and may even miss a brief arrhythmia altogether [36]. It is ideal for recording sustained rhythms in patients with infrequent but obvious clinical signs. However, again, owner participation is critical in capturing events.

Holter Monitors

Invented by biophysicist Norman J. Holter in the 1940s, these monitors record and store 24–72 hours or longer of continuous ECG data without owner activation [37]. Five to seven external electrodes are required for two- or three-channel recording (Figure 4.32). Impeccable skin preparation is necessary for low to zero artifact recordings as with any external electrode application process [30]. Inadequate skin preparation will result in varying degrees of signal artifact and dropout which could impair analysis [30]. The Holter is ideal for patients with frequent syncopal episodes or for arrhythmic patients without obvious clinical signs [15, p. 332]. Editing by a trained professional is necessary for detailed interpretation accuracy, although editing time will vary dependent upon the type of analysis software and the amount of artifact present [15, p. 332]. Consecutive monitorings are extremely useful for comparative studies of baseline Holters with subsequent recheck Holters [15, p. 332].

Other uses for the Holter monitor [30]:

- Quantify type and severity of arrhythmias.
- Assess rate and rhythm of average, maximal, and minimal heart rates, especially in the AF patient.
- Assess efficacy response or adverse reactions to drug therapy.
- Observe circadian variation of arrhythmic events.
- Evaluate onset and offset of arrhythmias, critical in arrhythmia interpretation.

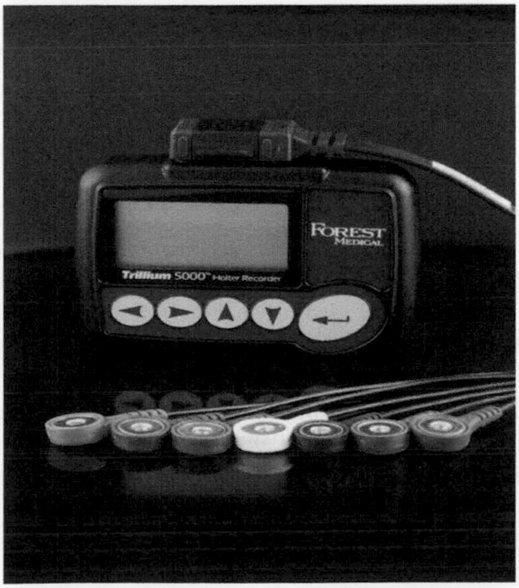

Figure 4.32 A digital Holter monitor with seven cable leads capable of three channel recording. Model is the Trillium 5000. Source: courtesy of Forest Medical, Syracuse, NY.

- Discern trends in heart rate and arrhythmic events during activities and in the home environment versus a hospital setting; a diary log kept by the owner of the patient's activities and medication times is especially useful with correlation of these trends.
- Assess pacemaker function.

Mobile Real Time Cardiac Telemetry

This is the newest generation of remote monitoring systems that include the latest mobile, cloud, and sensor technologies [36]. It is an evolving and most likely transformative era in human medicine that as always will involve creativity to adapt in the veterinary world. Some current examples include an iPhone snap-on electrode case with an application called the AliveECG Vet app and the BodyGuardian system by Preventice. The BodyGuardian is recently FDA approved for development. It is a small body sensor that attaches to the chest wall and transmits biometric data such as ECG, heart rate variability, and respiration rate through a smart cell phone to a monitor system.

Conclusion

This chapter is merely an introduction into the graphic world of ECGs. References, manuals, and textbooks are out there to further enhance your knowledge, honing your skills as a cardiology veterinary technician. Explore websites dedicated to ECG learning; many of the veterinary schools and universities have excellent modules available. The more you learn the better equipped you are as an essential cardiology team member.

References

1 Fisch, C. (2000) Centennial of the string galvanometer and the electrocardiogram. *Journal of the American College of Cardiology*, **36**, 1737–1745.

2 Kligfield, P. (2010) Derivation of the correct waveform of the human electrocardiogram by Willem Einthoven, 1890–1895. *Cardiology Journal*, **17**, 119–113.

3 Burch, G.E and DePasquale, N.P. (1990) *A History of Electrocardiography* (reprint: originally published by Yearbook Medical Publishers, Chicago, 1964). Norman Publishing, San Francisco.

4 Rivera-Ruis, M., Cajavilca, C., Varon, J. (2008) Einthoven's string galvanometer: the first electrocardiograph. *Texas Heart Institute Journal*, **35**, 174–178.

5 Besterman, E.M.M. (2005) The beginnings and development of the electrocardiograph. *West Indian Medical Journal*, **54**, 213–215.

6 Snellen, H.A. (1995) *Willem Einthoven (1860–1927): Father of Electrocardiography.* Kluwer Academic Publishing, Dordrecht.

7 Hurst, J.W. (1998) Naming of the waves in the ECG, with a brief account of their genesis. *Circulation*, **98**, 1937–1942.

8 Henson, J.R. (1971) Descartes and the ECG lettering series. *Journal of the History of Medicine and Allied Sciences*, **26**, 181–186.

9 Mendoza-Davila, N. and Varon, J. (2008) Karel Wenckebach: the story behind the block. *Resuscitation*, **79**, 189–192.

10 Fleming, P.R. (1997) *A Short History of Cardiology*. Editions Rodopi, Clio Medica 40, Amsterdam and Atlanta.

11 Edwards, N.J. (1993) *ECG Manual for the Veterinary Technician*. W.B. Saunders, Philadelphia.

12 Tilley, L.P., Smith Jr, F.W.K, Oyama, M.A. and Sleeper, M.M. (2008) *Manual of Canine and Feline Cardiology*, 4th edition. Saunders Elsevier, St. Louis.

13 Tilley, L.P. (1992) *Essentials of Canine and Feline Electrocardiography: Interpretation and Treatment*, 3rd Edition. Lea & Febiger, Malvern.

14 Jesty, S.A. and Reef, V.B. (2006) Evaluation of the horse with acute cardiac crisis. *Clinical Techniques in Equine Practice*, **5**, 93–103.

15 Fox, P.R, Sisson, D. and Moïse, N.S. (1999) *Textbook of Canine and Feline Cardiology: Principles and Clinical Practice*, 2nd Edition. W.B. Saunders, Philadelphia.

16 Kittleson, M.D. and Keinle R.D. (1998) *Small Animal Cardiovascular Medicine*. C.V. Mosby, St. Louis.

17 AlGhatrif, M. and Lindsay, J. (2012) A brief review: history to understand fundamentals of electrocardiography. *Journal of Community Hospital Internal Medicine Perspectives*, **2**, 4.

18 Antzelevitch, C. (2006) Cellular basis for the repolarization waves of the ECG. *Annals of the New York Academy of Sciences*, **1080**, 268–281.

19 Boyett, M.R., Honjo, H. and Kodama, I. (2000) The sinoatrial node, a heterogeneous pacemaker structure. *Cardiovascular Research*, **47**, 658–687.

20 Shibata, N., Inada, S., Mitsui, K. *et al.* (2001) Pacemaker shift in the rabbit sinoatrial node in response to vagal nerve stimulation. *Experimental Physiology*, **86**, 177–184.

21 Catalano, J.T. (2002) *Guide to ECG Analysis*, 2nd Edition. Lippincott, Williams & Wilkins, Philadelphia.

22 Bayès de Luna, A. (2012) *Clinical Electrocardiography: A Textbook*, 4th Edition. John Wiley & Sons, Ltd, Chichester. p. 43

23 Ihari, Z, van Oosterom, A. and Hoekema, R. (2006) Atrial repolarization as observable during the PQ interval. *Journal of Electrocardiography*, **39**, 290–297.

24 Topol, E. (2007) *Textbook of Cardiovascular Medicine*, 3rd Edition. Lippincott, Williams & Wilkins, Philadelphia.

25 Garcia, T.B. and Holtz, N. (2001) *12 Lead ECG: The Art of Interpretation*. Jones and Barlett, Sudbury.

26 Conover, M.B. (2002) *Understanding Electrocardiography*, 8th Edition. C.V. Mosby, St Louis.

27 Moïse, N.S., Valentine, B.A., Brown, C.A. et al. (1991) Duchenne's cardiomyopathy in a canine model: electrocardiographic and echocardiographic studies. *Journal of the American College of Cardiology*, **17**, 812–820.

28 Eleuteri, A., Fisher, A.C., Groves, D. and Dewhurst, C.J. (2011) An efficient time-varying filter for detrending and bandwidth limiting the heart rate variability tachogram without resampling: MATLAB open-source code and internet web-based implementation. *Computational and Mathematical Methods in Medicine*: Article ID 578785:1.

29 Pinsky, M.R. (2005) Cardiovascular issues in respiratory care. *Chest*, **128**(5 Supp 2), 592S–597S.

30 Charter, M.E. and Renaud-Farrell, S. (2004) Holter monitoring: it doesn't miss a beat. *Veterinary Technician*, **25**, 627.

31 McGurrin, M.K.J., Physick-Sheard, P.W. and Kenney, D.G. (2008) Transvenous electrical cardioversion of equine atrial fibrillation: patient factors and clinical results in 72 treatment episodes. *Journal of Veterinary Internal Medicine*, **22**, 609–615.

32 Moïse, N.S., Meyers-Wallen, V., Flahive, W.J. *et al.* (1994) Inherited ventricular arrhythmias and sudden death in German shepherd dogs. *Journal of the American College of Cardiology*, **24**, 236.

33 Moïse, N.S. (1999) Inherited arrhythmias in the dog: potential experimental models of cardiac disease. *Cardiovascular Research*, **44**, 37–38.

34 Federov, V.V., Schuessler, R.B., Hemphill, M. *et al.* (2009) Structural and functional evidence for discrete exit pathways that connect the canine sinoatrial node and atria. *Circulation Research*, **104, 915**, 919–920.

35 Hensley Jr, F.A., Martin, D.E. and Gravlee, G.P. (2008) *A Practical Approach to Cardiac Anesthesia*. 4th Edition. Lippincott, Williams & Wilkins, Philadelphia.

36 Zimetbaum, P. and Goldman, A. (2010) Ambulatory arrhythmia monitoring: choosing the right device. *Circulation*, **122**, 1629–1630.

37 Newby, R. (2008) From Norman Jeffris 'Jeff' Holter, a serendipitous life: an essay in biography. *Drumlummon Views*, pp. 226–227.

5

Thoracic Radiography

Deborah M. Fine

Introduction

There are many indications for obtaining thoracic radiographs, but the most common include evaluating for cardiac disease, determining the cause of a patient's respiratory distress, and evaluating for evidence of metastasis [1]. Follow-up radiographs are especially important for evaluating a patient's response to therapy or assessing for disease progression.

Radiography is an indispensable tool in evaluation of cardiac disease. Abnormalities in the cardiac silhouette are useful for suggesting enlargement of specific cardiac chambers, and the diagnosis of left-sided congestive heart failure can only be definitively established with radiographs.

How Radiographs are Generated

A brief review of radiographic technology is presented here. Gamma rays or "X-rays" are a form of electromagnetic radiation [2]. They are generated in a tube consisting of a cathode which produces electrons, and an anode. The cathode consists of a coiled wire filament that is negatively charged. When heated the cathode emits fast-moving electrons. The anode is a positive-charged target which attracts the electrons. The high-velocity electrons collide with the anode and give off tremendous energy. However only 1% of the energy is released as X-rays, the remainder is emitted as heat.

The temperature of the cathode filament is determined by the milliamperage (mA) setting. As the mA increases, the filament emits more electrons. The two factors of milliamperage and time (mAs) determine the total number of X-rays leaving the machine.

The electrical charge difference between the cathode and anode is responsible for acceleration of the electrons toward the anode. This charge difference is measured in kilovoltage. The kilovoltage peak (kVp) indicates the maximum energy available at a given kilovoltage setting. At higher kVp settings the electrons accelerate faster toward the anode which increases the energy of the X-rays produced. The increased energy shortens the X-ray's wavelength, and increases their penetrating power.

Cardiology for Veterinary Technicians and Nurses, First Edition. Edited by H. Edward Durham, Jr.

Higher kVp settings allow for shorter mAs settings, resulting in shorter exposure times. This is desirable for two reasons: it reduces personnel exposure to radiation, and decreases the potential for motion-associated artifact.

Technical Aspects of High-Quality Thoracic Radiographs

Meticulous attention to the technical aspects of high-quality radiographs is crucial. Failure to obtain a diagnostic-quality radiograph may result in misdiagnosis of a patient's condition by failing to visualize an abnormality, or by creation of an artifact that could be interpreted as pathology. Complete coverage of all of the technical aspects of thoracic radiography is beyond the scope of this chapter; however, certain aspects are worth emphasizing.

Ideally, thoracic radiographs are obtained at peak inspiration for maximum inflation of the lungs. A few specific exceptions to this include evaluation for collapsing trachea, and suspected mild pneumothorax. These conditions are sometimes more obvious on expiration. Observing the patient for several respiratory cycles can help time the exposure appropriately. In animals with normal-to-thin body condition, at peak inspiration the caudodorsal aspect of the caudal lung lobes should be caudal to T-12 on the lateral view. This increases the separation of the caudal cardiac silhouette and the diaphragm. On the dorsoventral/ventrodorsal (DV/VD) view the dome of the diaphragm should be caudal to the mid T-8 vertebral body and the caudolateral lung lobes should be caudal to T-10. Foam wedges and troughs should be used to straighten the patient if necessary. When a patient is straight, the rib heads and costochondral junctions align on the lateral, and the spine and sternum align on the DV/VD view.

Radiographic Density and Contrast

Density is a measure of the blackness of a radiograph. A properly exposed radiograph is of sufficient density that a viewer cannot see their hand held on the other side of a film in the non-patient exposed areas. A number of factors influence the density of a radiograph including mAs, kVp, developing time, and developer temperature. Increasing the mAs increases the total number of X-rays generated, and increasing kVp increases their penetrating power.

Film density is also influenced by the thickness of the body part being radiographed and the density of the subject tissues. Radiographic density is inversely proportional to tissue density. As tissue density doubles, the number of X-rays reaching the film will be halved. This is part of the basis for different technique charts for different body parts or regions.

Contrast describes the difference in density of adjacent areas on a radiograph. When there are large differences in density (i.e. the radiograph is mostly black and white), a radiograph is described as having a short scale of contrast. When a radiograph demonstrates many shades of grey and small differences in the density of adjacent areas, it is described as having a long scale of contrast.

Radiographic contrast is influenced by the density of the tissue of interest, the kVp level, scatter radiation, film type, and film fog. The subject area determines the degree of contrast appropriate. In general, a long scale of contrast is desirable for soft tissues, while bone and abdomen is better visualized with a short scale of contrast.

When the correct mAs is used, contrast depends primarily on kVp. However, if the mAs is too low then the contrast will be decreased because fewer X-rays reach the film. Overexposure by too much mAs increases overall density, with less effect on contrast. However, if kVp is too low the result is a light gray image with poor anatomic detail because of the low penetration.

To some extent the desired degree of contrast is dependent upon the preferences of the viewer. Many radiologists prefer a relatively long scale of contrast for viewing thoracic radiographs. This increases the likelihood of detecting subtle pulmonary nodules. However, many cardiologists prefer a shorter scale of contrast for thoracic radiographs. This increases the ability to detect changes in the vasculature and early pulmonary edema. In either instance, the key to successful interpretation is a thorough and consistent evaluation of every radiograph.

Trouble Shooting

If a film is too light, the viewer must determine if the patient was adequately penetrated. This is determined by seeing if the outlines of internal organs are visualized. If not, then the kVp should be increased by 10–15%. If the patient is adequately penetrated then the mAs should be increased by 30–50%. Obesity is another consideration. The kVp setting should be increased by 10–15% compared to an animal with a normal body condition of the same size.

If a film is too dark then either the kVp or the mAs is too high. If the bone is gray and there is not much contrast with the soft tissues, then the kVp should be reduced by 10–15%. If the contrast is appropriate (i.e. bone is white) then the mAs should be reduced by 30–50%.

Digital Radiography

Conventional film-screen radiography is still the most common form of image acquisition in veterinary medicine. However, digital radiography is becoming more common, and is likely to become the standard in the future.

Digital radiography is a form of X-ray imaging where digital X-ray sensors are used instead of traditional photographic film. The X-ray tube, generator, and peripheral hardware are essentially the same for conventional and digital radiography. The film cassette is replaced by an image receptor with an intensifying screen. The image receptor receives X-rays and exposes a "digital plate" that is then transformed to a latent electrical image.

The light emitted from the digital intensifying screens is an analog signal. Analog information is produced as a continuous waveform. In order for this information to be used by a computer it must be digitized. An analog to digital converter samples the waveform at a very high rate, and then transforms it to a representative digital signal.

All digital images are composed of tiny picture elements called pixels, which are arranged in a matrix of rows and columns. The actual pixel size is determined by the size of the image divided by the size of the matrix. Image quality is improved by increasing the number of pixels without changing the field of view. This decreases pixel size and increases the matrix size.

A computer stores information in a format known as bits (binary digits) which are a series of zeros and ones. Bit depth defines the amount of information (i.e. shades of gray) that an image can contain. A higher bit number will increase the number of shades that can be represented in an image. It has been recommended that digital radiographs should be obtained with a minimum of a 12-bit depth, which makes 4096 shades of gray available for viewing. Shades of grey are coded as digital numbers. The computer assigns one number to each pixel, and each pixel represents the intensity of the X-ray signal at a given location within the patient.

The quality of the display monitor is critical when viewing a digital image. A medical-grade gray-scale monitor will give the best quality image. Gray-scale monitors have a greater dynamic range and higher resolution than color monitors; however, they are quite expensive. A monitor for digital images should be greater than 2000 Í 2000 pixels, and should have very high brightness capabilities. Digital images can also be printed to film with the use of a special film printer.

Types of Digital Radiography

There are two types of digital devices suitable for thoracic radiography: computed radiography, and direct digital radiography which uses flat-panel detectors or charged coupling detectors.

Computed radiography is a digital imaging system that utilizes a phosphor detector screen. The thin, multilayer imaging sheet contains a layer of photostimulable crystals, and is stored in a cassette that appears nearly identical to a conventional cassette. The cassette can be used in a Bucky tray or on a tabletop. When X-rays strike the imaging plate, the electrons in the crystals are energized and then stored in electron traps. After being exposed the cassette is placed in a computed radiography reader, which extracts the plate. The plate moves through a processor and is scanned by a helium-neon laser. The laser stimulates release of the trapped X-ray energy as visible light. The light is converted to an electrical signal that is proportional to the light energy released from the plate. The electrical signal is then digitized and available to be viewed. The imaging plate is then exposed to a bright light, which erases any residual image and is ready to be reused.

Computed radiography plates must be processed in a fairly timely manner. The latent image is temporary and loses 25% or more of its energy within 8 hours. Additionally, the plates are sensitive to secondary radiation and must be carefully stored. The plates should always be erased before use if they have not been used for 24 hours or more. Stored plates may produce artifact and reduction in the quality of images due to spurious exposure.

Flat-panel detectors consist of an X-ray intensifying screen coupled to an amorphous silicon flat panel that serves as the light detector. Flat-panel detector systems are similar to conventional screen-film systems, but an electronic sensor layer replaces the X-ray film. The silicon detector matrix is composed of a large number of individual detector units. Each individual element is composed of a light sensitive area and a smaller area of electronics. Flat-panel detectors either convert X-ray energy directly to an electrical pulse, or first convert the X-ray energy into light which is then converted to an electrical signal.

Flat-panel detectors and computed radiography machines are available as portable and stationary units.

Digital Image Quality

Traditional photographic film requires fairly precise exposure factors in order to make a diagnostic image and small deviations may result in an over- or underexposed image. With digital radiography under- and overexposure are less problematic. Post-processing correction will fix many, but not all exposure errors. This is an important time saving feature as it decreases the number of retakes. Specific technique charts are required for digital systems because they have different exposure characteristics than screen-film systems. However, digital technique charts are much simpler than conventional ones because of the greater latitude in exposure factors.

Latitude is the range of exposures that results in a diagnostic image. With screen-film systems, only a narrow range of X-ray energy results in shades of gray. Most of the X-ray intensities result only in black or white, which is ineffective for tissue resolution. With digital radiography, the number of electrons "trapped" by the digital-image receptor during an exposure is linearly related to the intensity of the X-ray beam. Consequently, digital images have more shades of gray then film images. With post-processing manipulation a single exposure can display a diagnostic image with both high contrast, and long gray scales.

The ability of digital radiography to compensate for over and underexposure is a significant advantage over traditional radiography. However, this capacity is not infinite. Underexposure will reduce the capacity to detect low-contrast abnormalities, and severe underexposure results in a coarsely stippled image (quantum mottle) caused by too few photons striking the imaging detector. Overexposure impairs the image quality in thinner, soft-tissue regions. This problem is most common in large and deep-chested dogs. In order to penetrate adequately the thicker regions of these patients, the lungs or body wall may become overexposed.

Advantages and Disadvantage of Digital Radiography

In addition to manipulating the contrast and density of an image, the advantages of digital radiography include increased time efficiency by bypassing chemical processing and the ability to digitally transfer, review, and store images at a computer terminal. Images can be reviewed at any terminal in the hospital, and transmission to an outside viewer is usually very simple. Further, many software packages for image review include a variety of tools for on-screen measurements, and the ability to magnify a region of interest.

The initial cost of digital radiography can be considerable. However, efficiency is gained by reducing the number of retakes from exposure problems, and there is no film, developing equipment, or chemicals to be purchased. Further, a large amount of physical space is no longer needed for film storage.

Conventional radiography still performs better with regard to spatial resolution of side-by-side objects. This is due to the higher number of line pairs that are achievable with film radiography (5–15 line pairs/mm) versus digital radiography (2.5–7 line

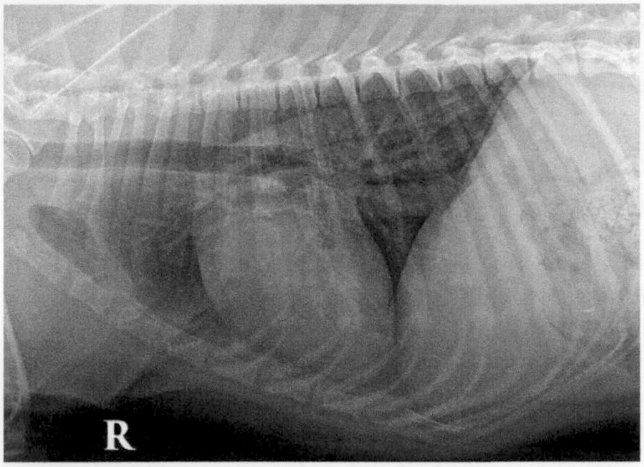

Figure 5.1 Normal right lateral radiograph of a dog. The features characteristic of this position include: apex of the heart near the sternum, parallel diaphragmatic crura, and the right crus is cranial to the left.

pairs/mm). However, the ability to manipulate contrast appears to makes up for this deficiency. Studies have shown that digital radiographs were equivalent or superior to conventional film in diagnostic quality for the thorax.

Manipulating the contrast of a digital image should be done with a degree of caution. Particularly in the thorax, it is quite easy to create "digital edema" and it is equally easy to administer "digital diuretics" and make actual disease disappear. It is very important to compare the manipulated images with the unprocessed ones.

Effect of Patient Positioning

There are differences in the appearance of the cardiac silhouette and lung fields based upon which view is obtained [3,4]. On the right lateral the cardiac silhouette is generally taller and more oval shaped, and the apex is closer to the sternum (Figure 5.1). The diaphragmatic crura are generally parallel, and the right crus of the diaphragm is usually cranial to the left. The caudal vena cava enters directly into the right crus.

On the left lateral the cardiac silhouette appears more rounded (Figure 5.2). In this position the apex of the heart falls away from midline, displacing the apex dorsally and

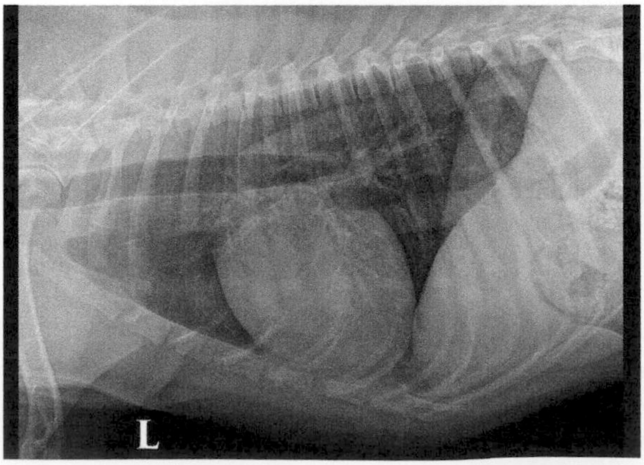

Figure 5.2 Normal left lateral radiograph of a dog. The features characteristic of this position include: apex is lifted off the sternum creating a more rounded appearance to the heart, the crura diverge at the center of the diaphragm, and the left crus is cranial to the right.

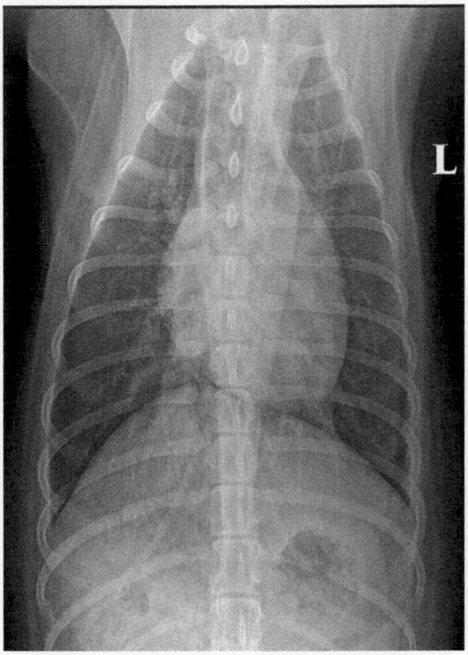

Figure 5.3 Normal dorsoventral radiograph of a dog. The apex of the heart is pointing toward the left side of the diaphragm. The diaphragm appears as a single smooth dome, and the peak of the dome is slightly to the right of midline.

creating a smaller cardiac profile. The right and left crura of the diaphragm diverge from one another at mid-diaphragm, and the left crus is usually cranial to the right. The caudal vena cava can be visualized traversing over the left crus to silhouette with the right. The right cranial lung lobe is seen best with the patient in left lateral recumbency. This is because in this position there is no compression of the lobe.

There are also differences in the appearance of the thoracic structures on the DV versus VD orientation. The DV view is recommended for evaluation of the cardiac silhouette and pulmonary vessels (Figure 5.3). In the DV position, the heart is suspended in its normal orientation and is closer to the sternum. The apex of the heart usually points toward the left crus of the diaphragm. The DV view also allows more easy visualization of the caudal lobar pulmonary vessels. There are a several reasons for this. With the patient in the DV position, the dorsal lung fields are more inflated and the air provides increased contrast with the vessels. Further, in this orientation the caudal vessels are more perpendicular to the X-ray beam, and the vessels are farther from the table top and are therefore more magnified.

On the VD view the shape of the cardiac silhouette is more variable than on the DV (Figure 5.4). The apex of the heart is not fixed, so positional changes can affect its orientation. The apex usually moves leftward, and the silhouette appears elongated compared with the DV view. The right heart may appear prominent, taking on a "reverse D" appearance. The viewer should be careful not to overinterpret this as right-heart disease. If in doubt, a DV view should be obtained.

The appearance of the diaphragm is distinctly different depending upon which orientation is obtained. This is due to the position of the X-ray beam relative to the diaphragm. On a VD view the X-ray beam is nearly parallel to the diaphragm. This results in the shadows of the cupula (central region) and crura projecting into the thorax, which gives

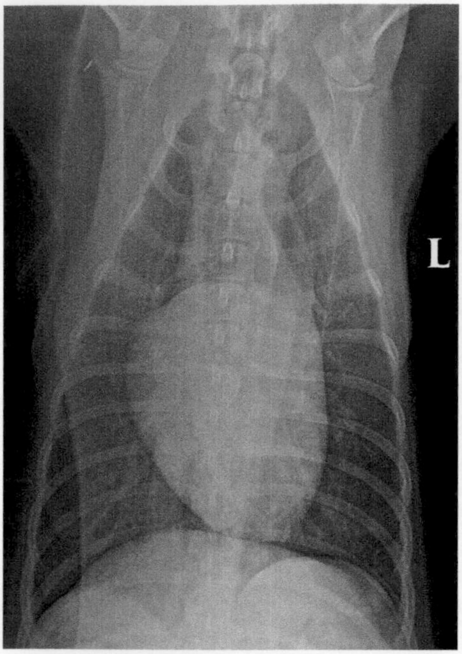

Figure 5.4 Normal ventrodorsal radiograph of a dog. The apex of the heart is close to midline, and the diaphragm demonstrates three distinct curves of the crura and cupula.

the diaphragm three distinct convex projections. On the DV view the X-ray beam passes through the diaphragm at approximately 45 degrees, causing the crura to superimpose over the liver. As a result, the diaphragm appears as a single curved dome with the peak laying slightly to the right of midline. However, if the X-ray beam is positioned caudally and centered over the mid-abdomen, three separate domes will also be seen on a DV projection.

The VD view is often preferred for evaluation of the lung fields and the cranial and caudal mediastinum. On the VD view the lungs appear larger, and the accessory lobe is better imaged. The accessory lobe is difficult to evaluate on the DV view due to the increased contact of the heart with the diaphragm. Magnification of the ventral lung fields on a VD view improves their evaluation. However, masses in the dorsal lung fields are more difficult to visualize on a VD view due to compression of the dorsal lungs in this position. For optimal visualization of pulmonary nodules, all four orthogonal views are necessary.

The VD view is usually preferred for evaluation of pleural effusion. When mild pleural effusion is present interlobar fissures may be the only abnormality observed (Figure 5.5). In the DV position, fluid accumulates along the sternum and does not readily enter the interlobar spaces. In the VD position, fluid seeps into the interlobar spaces and is more likely to result in overt fissure lines. However, there are occasional patients in which mild pleural effusion is actually more distinctly visualized from the DV orientation.

When a moderate to severe pleural effusion is present, the cardiac silhouette and lungs are also more accurately evaluated with a VD view. In the VD orientation the fluid accumulates in the dorsal thorax. The dorsal thorax has a larger volume of space compared to the ventral thorax. Since the effusion is distributed over a larger area the fluid level will not be as deep. As a result there is less likely to be border effacement with the

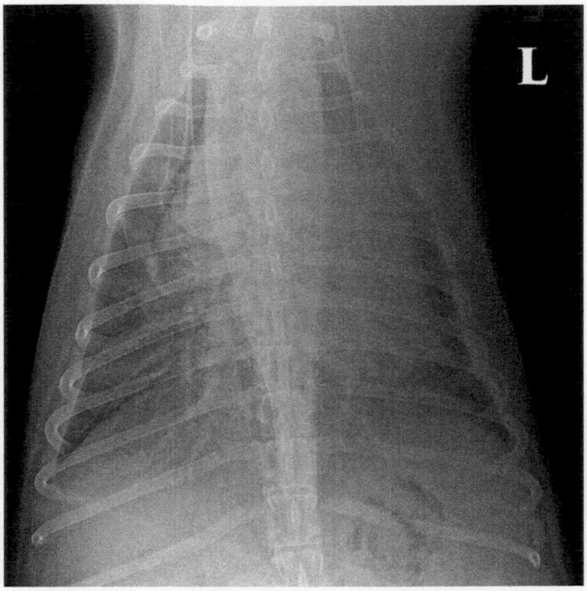

Figure 5.5 Ventrodorsal radiograph of a dog with mild pleural effusion. Pleural fissure lines delineate the right middle lung lobe between the cranial and caudal lobes.

cardiac silhouette and diaphragm. Further, the aerated lungs float upward and surround the heart with air which increases contrast. When the patient is in a DV position, the fluid accumulates to a greater depth in the narrower ventral thorax. This causes border effacement with the diaphragm, cardiac silhouette, and mediastinum.

It is often easier to obtain straight alignment of the patient using a VD view, particularly for deep-chested dogs. The VD position also allows for maximal inspiration. However, the DV orientation is less compromising for a patient with respiratory distress. The DV position also results in less compression of the airways in patients with mainstem bronchial disease.

Normal feline thoracic anatomy shows less marked positional changes compared to the canine thorax. In older cats the heart is often positioned more horizontally upon the sternum (Figure 5.6). It is also common for the aorta to demonstrate a bulge in the arch ("aortic knob") on the DV/VD view. The cause of this is uncertain, and does not appear to be associated with any overt disease such as hypertension or hyperthyroidism.

Interpretation of Thoracic Radiographs

A systematic approach to evaluation of thoracic radiographs is crucial to ensure accurate detection of abnormalities. The following areas should be evaluated with every thoracic radiograph: positioning and technique, size of the cardiac silhouette, pulmonary parenchyma, pulmonary vasculature, mediastinum and trachea, and extrathoracic structures.

Cardiac Anatomy

The canine and feline heart is slightly rotated along the base–apex axis. As a consequence, most of the right ventricle is actually cranial to the left. On the lateral view

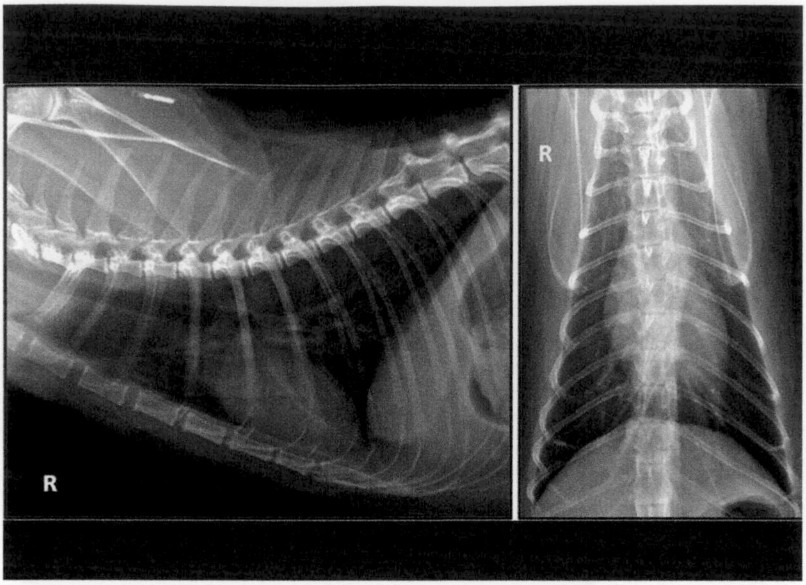

Figure 5.6 Normal thoracic radiographs of a cat. In older cats it is common for the heart to assume a relatively horizontal position on the lateral, and for the aorta to demonstrate a bulge on the dorsoventral view.

the cranial margin of the cardiac silhouette is composed of the right atrium and ventricle, and the caudal margin is made up of the left atrium and ventricle (Figure 5.7). The cranial dorsal region of the lateral cardiac silhouette includes several overlapping structures: the right atrium and vena cavae, the main pulmonary artery, and the ascending aortic arch. Consequently, enlargement of this region may be due to an abnormality in one or more of these structures. Therefore, evaluating the DV/VD view in conjunction with the lateral is critical to determining which structure is enlarged.

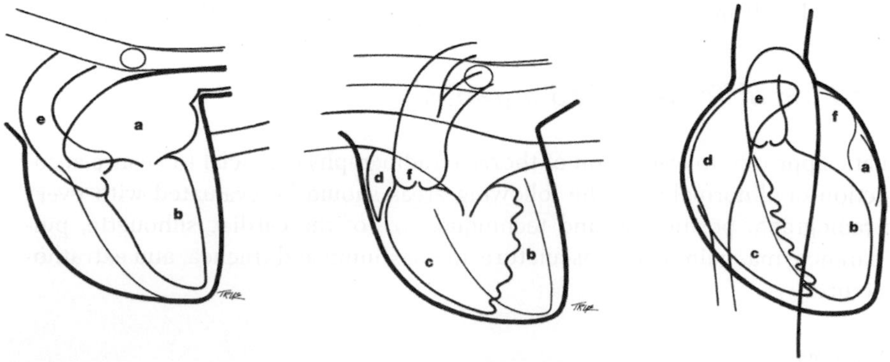

Figure 5.7 Diagrams demonstrating normal cardiac anatomy on the lateral and dorsoventral thoracic radiographs. Key: a, left atrium; b, left ventricle; c, right ventricle; d, right atrium; e, aorta; f, pulmonary artery. Source: Fox, Sisson and Moise (1999) [7]. Reproduced with permission of Elsevier.

It is common to use a clock-face analogy when identifying cardiac structures on the DV/VD view. The ascending arch of the aorta is positioned from approximately 11:00 to 1:00 o'clock, and the main pulmonary artery is from 1:00 to 2:00. The left auricle is from 2:00 to 3:00, and the left ventricle spans the region from 3:00 to 6:00. The right ventricle is from 6:00 to 9:00, and the right atrium is positioned from 9:00 to 11:00. The body of the left atrium is positioned centrally, just caudal to the bifurcation of the mainstem bronchi.

Evaluation of the Cardiac Silhouette

Although viewers often use the terms "heart" and "cardiac silhouette" interchangeably, it is important to remember that this structure on a radiograph simply represents the overall size of the pericardium and its contents [5]. If the cardiac silhouette is interpreted as enlarged, then the next question becomes "what is causing the enlargement"? An enlarged cardiac silhouette may be due to an actual increase in the size of the heart, presence of pericardial effusion, neoplastic mass, or herniation of abdominal contents into the pericardium (peritoneal pericardial diaphragmatic hernia). Frequently, additional imaging is necessary to make a final determination.

In order to assess accurately the size of the cardiac silhouette, it must be evaluated relative to the size of the thoracic space. The viewer must decide if the cardiac silhouette is truly enlarged, or if the thorax is actually small. As part of this determination, it is very important to take the patient's breed and body condition into consideration. The shape of a patient's chest can markedly affect the subjective impression of the size of the cardiac silhouette. Many small breed dogs (e.g. Boston terrier, Lhasa apso, etc.) have relatively shallow chests on the lateral view, but normal to barrel-shaped chests on the DV/VD view. This will cause the cardiac silhouette to appear enlarged on the lateral, but normal on the DV/VD view. Dogs with deep, narrow chests (e.g. Irish setter, greyhound, etc.) may have normal to small-appearing cardiac silhouettes on the lateral view and relatively enlarged cardiac silhouettes on the DV/VD view. Obese patients often have an enlarged-appearing cardiac silhouette. This is in part due to cranial displacement of the diaphragm by large deposits of intra-abdominal fat, decreasing the thoracic volume (referred to as Pickwickian syndrome). Further, these patients often have large deposits of pericardial fat which increases the size of the cardiac silhouette. Careful evaluation of the cardiac silhouette will sometimes allow the viewer to distinguish the pericardial fat from the soft-tissue density of the heart.

The age of the patient may also affect the interpretation of the heart size. The cardiac silhouette of younger patients often appears rounder subjectively, and this is sometimes interpreted as cardiomegaly.

A number of different measurements have been used to evaluate the overall size of the cardiac silhouette. On the lateral view, the cardiac silhouette should be no more than two-thirds of the total vertical height of the thorax when measured from the apex to the heart base at the carina. The width of the cardiac silhouette should be no more than 2.5 intercostal spaces in deep-chested dogs, and no more than 3.5 intercostal spaces in barrel-chested dogs. In cats, the width of the cardiac silhouette should measure between 2.5 and 3.0 intercostal spaces. On the DV/VD view the width of the cardiac silhouette at its widest point should be less than half of the width of the thorax at the ninth rib.

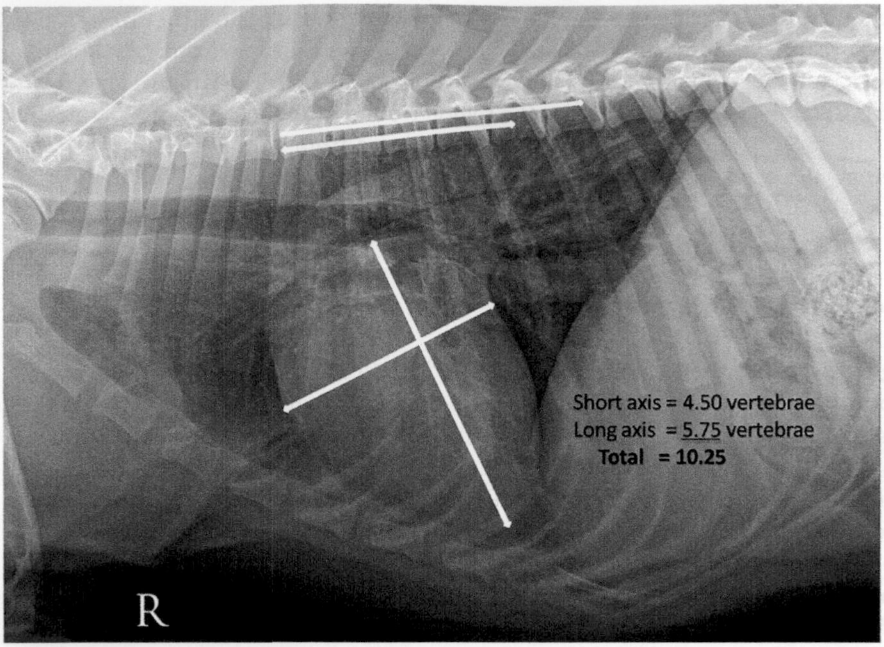

Figure 5.8 Right lateral radiograph demonstrating the method for calculating vertebral heart score. The long axis is measured from the ventral border of the carina to the apex of the heart. The short axis is measured at the widest point of the heart, perpendicular to its long axis. These two measurements are then superimposed over the thoracic vertebral bodies starting at T-4, and the long and short axes are summed.

A vertebral heart-scale system (also commonly known as the vertebral heart score) was developed in an attempt to provide a more objective determination of cardiac size (Figure 5.8) [6]. Using the lateral view, the long and short axes of the heart are measured. The long axis is measured from the apex to the base of the heart at the ventral border of the carina. If left atrial enlargement is present, the long axis is sometimes measured from the apex to the ventral edge of the elevated left bronchus. The short axis is measured perpendicular to the long axis, at the widest point in the cardiac silhouette. This is often just ventral to the caudal vena cava. The measurements are then superimposed over the vertebral column, both starting at the cranial edge of the fourth thoracic vertebra. The number of vertebral bodies covered by the long and short axes measurements is then summed. The normal range for the dog is 8.5–10.6. However, there is some breed variation in vertebral heart score. Dogs with relatively short thoracic vertebrae such as the miniature schnauzer and boxer can have a normal vertebral heart score up to 12. The normal range for the cat is 7.2–7.8.

One of the most useful applications of the vertebral heart score is assessing for changes in the cardiac silhouette over time, and is useful for monitoring progression of disease. In some patients the vertebral heart score will vary with the patient's recumbency. Therefore, it is recommended that the same recumbency should always be used when performing serial comparisons.

Hemivertebrae are very common in brachycephalic breeds such as bulldogs which confounds the utility of this measure in evaluating heart size in these dogs. In this instance the vertebral heart score is only useful for serial evaluations looking for changes in size over time.

No single measurement has been found to be completely superior. In instances where it appears that the cardiac silhouette is mildly enlarged, it is common to use several or all of these assessment techniques.

It is challenging to definitively diagnose specific chamber enlargement with radiographs because the heart actually twists around itself. As a consequence, several chambers and great vessels superimpose upon one another. Although changes on a radiograph can be interpreted as 'consistent with enlargement of a specific chamber', it is often necessary to obtain an echocardiogram to definitively diagnose the cause of an observed radiographic abnormality.

The exception to the previous statements is left atrial enlargement. In the dog, left atrial enlargement is easily appreciated on the lateral view. The left atrium sits at the caudal dorsal corner of the cardiac silhouette, and is not overlapped by any other structures (see Figure 5.7). As the left atrium enlarges, a distinct bulge appears in this region (Figure 5.9). On the DV/VD view, left atrial enlargement results in widening of the mainstem bronchi (sometimes referred to as the "cowboy sign" due to the bowlegged appearance of the bronchi). In the cat, left atrial enlargement is most obvious on the DV/VD view. This abnormality appears as an increase in the width of the heart base, particularly of the left heart. This appearance is sometimes referred to as a valentine-shaped heart (Figure 5.10).

It is challenging to distinguish left ventricular from right ventricular enlargement in the cat. However, the vast majority of feline heart disease is of left ventricular origin. In nearly all instances, the normally ovoid shape of the feline heart simply takes on more rounded and enlarged appearance (Figure 5.11). Therefore, the remainder of this discussion of chamber enlargement patterns will refer to the dog.

On the lateral view, left ventricular enlargement in the dog manifests predominantly as an increase in the vertical dimensions of the cardiac silhouette (Figure 5.12). This causes dorsal deviation of the trachea. Normally the trachea deviates approximately 15 degrees

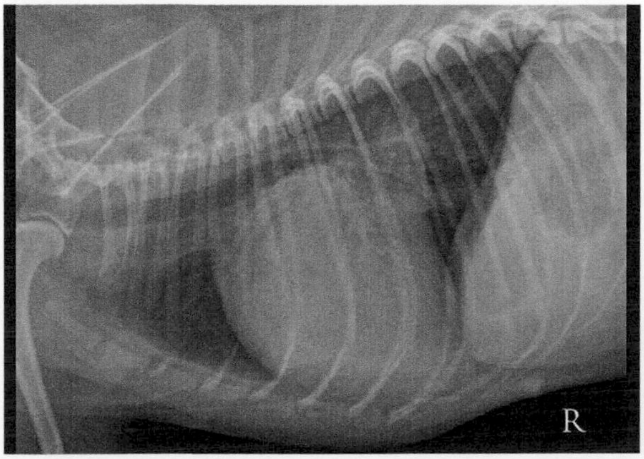

Figure 5.9 Radiograph of a dog with degenerative mitral valve disease demonstrating severe left atrial enlargement. The left atrium appears as a distinct bulge caudal to the carina and dorsal to the caudal vena cava. There is also evidence of left ventricular enlargement.

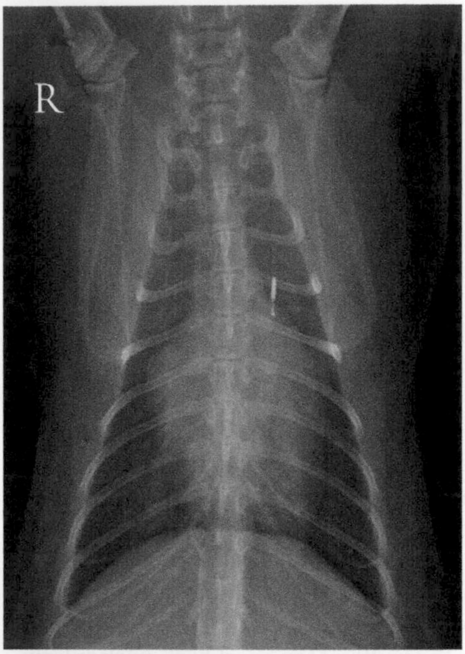

Figure 5.10 Radiograph of a cat with hypertrophic cardiomyopathy demonstrating severe left atrial enlargement. This results in a "valentine" shaped heart.

from the vertebral column. As cardiac enlargement progresses the trachea becomes parallel to the spine, and in some instances appears to almost press upon it. Left ventricular enlargement will also cause a mild increase in the width of the cardiac silhouette as well. The caudal vena cava normally maintains a horizontal course from the diaphragm to the cardiac silhouette, or in some instances it actually slopes ventrally from the diaphragm to the heart. With left ventricular enlargement the caudal vena cava may deviate dorsally from the diaphragm up to the heart. On the DV/VD view, left ventricular enlargement is manifested as rounding of the apex from 4:00 to 6:00 o'clock, and an increase in the overall width of the cardiac silhouette (Figure 5.13).

It is rare to have isolated right atrial or ventricular enlargement. These changes almost always occur together. On the lateral, right atrial enlargement appears as enlargement of

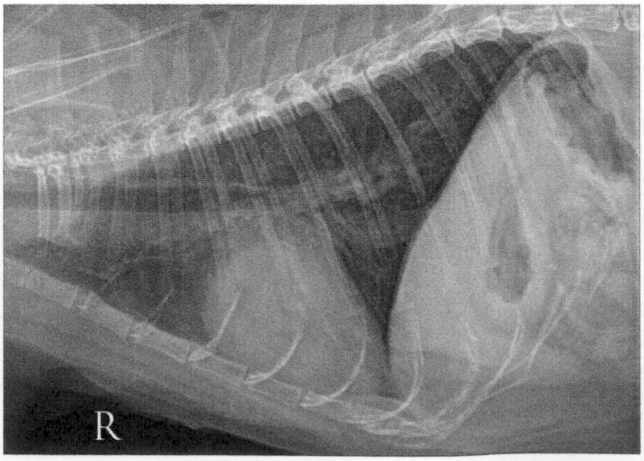

Figure 5.11 Radiograph of a cat with left ventricular enlargement. The width of the heart is approximately three intercostal spaces.

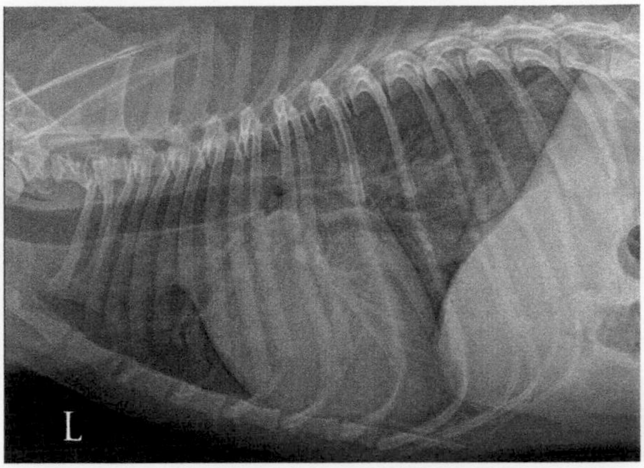

Figure 5.12 Radiograph of a dog demonstrating left ventricular enlargement. There is marked dorsal deviation of the trachea, and the width of the heart measures approximately four intercostal spaces.

the cranial dorsal region, with loss of the cranial cardiac waist. Right ventricular enlargement manifests as an increase in the cranial–caudal width with an increase in sternal contact (Figure 5.14). On the DV/VD, right-heart enlargement appears as rounding and bowing of the heart toward the right. In conjunction with the relatively straight left ventricle, this is sometimes referred to as a "reverse D" appearance (Figure 5.15).

Vascular Anatomy

On the lateral view, the pulmonary vessels are most easily visualized in the cranial lung lobes and are arranged from dorsal to ventral as artery, bronchus, and vein. On the DV/VD view, the vessels are most easily visualized in the caudal lung fields and are

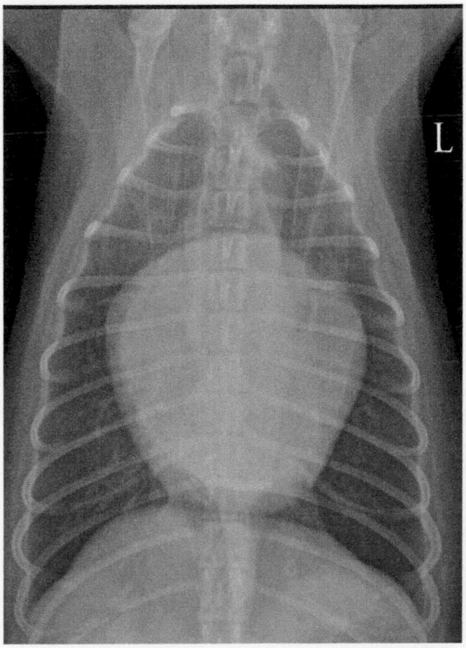

Figure 5.13 Left ventricular enlargement in a dog. The left ventricular apex is rounded, and the width of the heart is greater than half of the distance of the hemithorax at the ninth rib.

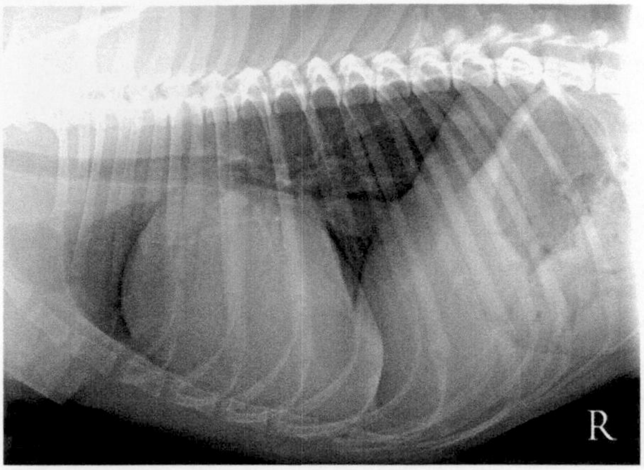

Figure 5.14 Radiograph of a dog with tricuspid valve dysplasia demonstrating severe right ventricular enlargement. There is a marked increase in sternal contact and the heart measures four intercostal spaces. Loss of the cranial cardiac waist is consistent with concurrent right atrial enlargement.

arranged from lateral to medial as artery, bronchus, and vein. A helpful mnemonic to remember this pattern is "veins are ventral and central"

Evaluation of Pulmonary Vasculature

Normal arteries and veins should be symmetrical in size. On the DV/VD view, the caudal pulmonary arteries and veins should be equal to the diameter of the ninth rib. On the lateral view, the cranial pulmonary arteries and veins should be equal to the diameter of the fourth rib. Where the vessels cross their corresponding ribs, the silhouette should make a box. If the vasculature is distended, the silhouette will make a fat rectangle. If the vasculature is underfilled, the silhouette will make a thin rectangle.

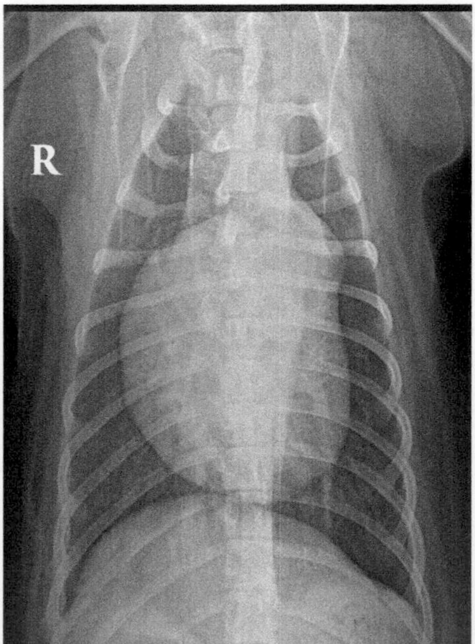

Figure 5.15 Right ventricular enlargement in a dog with pulmonic stenosis. The cardiac silhouette demonstrates a "reverse D" appearance, and there is a prominent bulge in the main pulmonary artery at the 1:00 to 2:00 o'clock position.

Enlargement of the pulmonary veins indicates an increase in the left atrial pressure. This is one of the hallmarks of left-sided congestive heart failure. Distention of the pulmonary arteries is indicative of pulmonary hypertension. In many regions, the most common cause of pulmonary hypertension is heartworm disease; however, primary pulmonary disease and left heart failure can also result in pulmonary hypertension. Symmetrical enlargement of the arteries and veins, particularly in a young animal, is very suggestive of a left-to-right shunting defect (e.g. patent ductus arteriosus, atrial septal or ventricular septal defect). In an older animal, this pattern is more likely due to a combination of left heart failure and pulmonary hypertension. Underfilled vasculature may be due to hypovolemia or sometimes secondary to a right-to-left shunting defect.

Diagnosis of Congestive Heart Failure

Heart failure is a syndrome characterized by activation of multiple neurohormonal systems including the renin angiotensin system and the sympathetic nervous system (See Chapter 13). These systems are designed to maintain arterial perfusion pressure to the vital organs. They do this by retaining sodium and water and constricting peripheral vasculature. When the increased plasma volume exceeds the vascular capacity, the fluid leaks out of the capillary beds. Pulmonary edema initially accumulates in the interstitial space, but as heart failure progresses the interstitium becomes saturated, causing the fluid to spill into the alveoli.

An interstitial pattern is recognized radiographically as an increase in the overall opacity of the affected lung fields. All of the normal structures are still visible, but the margins have a hazy quality (Figure 5.16). An alveolar pattern is characterized by complete effacement of the pulmonary vasculature, and the presence of air bronchograms. An air

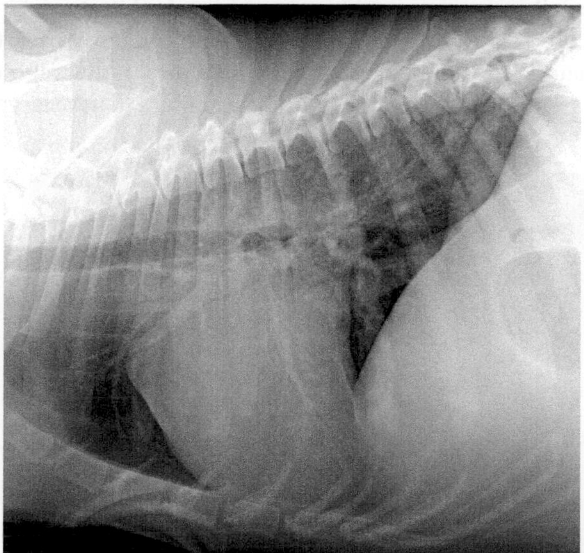

Figure 5.16 Radiograph of a dog with subaortic stenosis and congestive heart failure. There is a moderate interstitial pattern that is most severe in the perihilar and caudodorsal lung fields. Left atrial enlargement and pulmonary venous distention are also present.

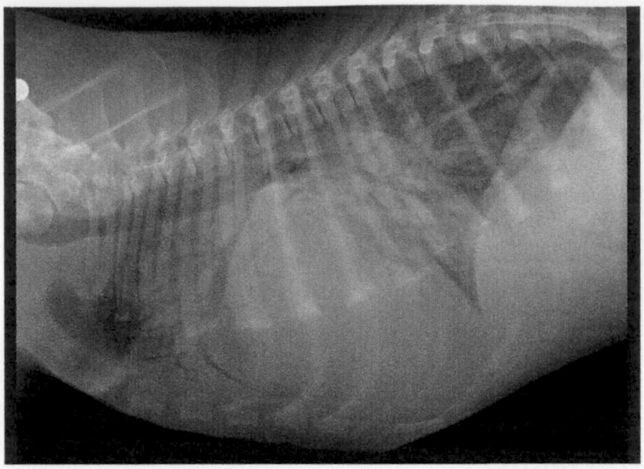

Figure 5.17 Radiograph of a dog with a patent ductus arteriosus and congestive heart failure demonstrating a severe alveolar pattern. A prominent air bronchogram is present in the cranioventral lung fields. There are also signs of severe left ventricular enlargement, including dorsal deviation of the trachea and a marked increase in the width of the heart.

bronchogram is caused by fluid or cells filling the terminal alveoli, which results in a uniform soft-tissue opacity surrounding the radiolucent bronchus (Figure 5.17).

Left-sided congestive heart failure is characterized by the presence of three radiographic findings: (1) left atrial enlargement, usually accompanied by left ventricular enlargement; (2) distention of the pulmonary veins; and (3) an interstitial to alveolar pattern in a location consistent with congestive heart failure. In order to make the diagnosis of heart failure, all three of these signs should be present.

In the dog, pulmonary edema due to heart failure is most prominent in the caudal dorsal and perihilar regions on the lateral view. On the DV/VD view pulmonary edema is normally bilaterally symmetrical and accumulates predominantly in the caudal lung fields. However, if an animal has been laterally recumbent for a prolonged period of time then the edema may accumulate more in the dependent lung fields.

In cats, the location of pulmonary edema is most commonly distributed in the cranial and caudal ventral lung fields on the lateral view (Figure 5.18). On the DV/VD view it usually appears as a diffuse generalized infiltrate.

It is relatively common for dogs with congestive heart failure to have a small volume of pleural effusion accompanying the typical radiographic signs of heart failure. However, it is uncommon for dogs with heart failure to have large volumes of pleural effusion. The

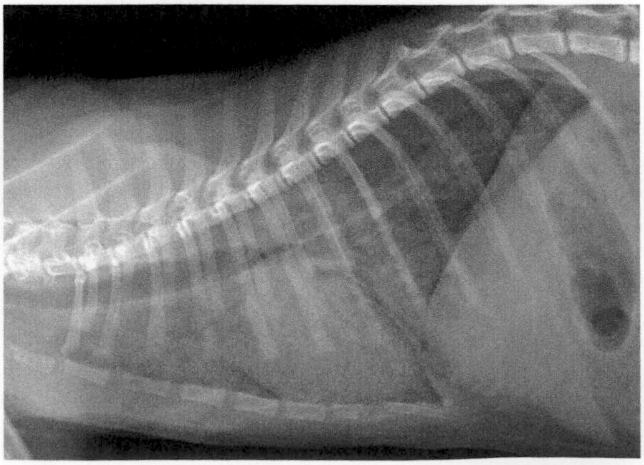

Figure 5.18 Radiograph of a cat with congestive heart failure secondary to hypertrophic cardiomyopathy. There is an alveolar pattern with air bronchograms in the cranial and caudoventral lung fields.

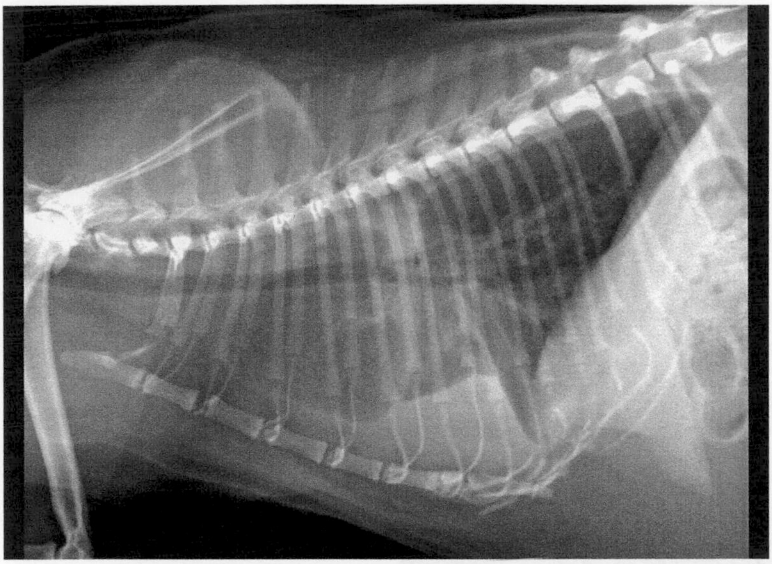

Figure 5.19 Radiograph of a cat with congestive heart failure and a moderate amount of pleural effusion. There is retraction and leafing of the lung lobes, and effacement of the cardiac silhouette.

presence of a severe pleural effusion in a dog should raise the viewer's index of suspicion for a non-cardiogenic cause. This observation is not true in cats. In fact, it is very common for cats with congestive heart failure to present with large volumes of pleural effusion (Figure 5.19). Often the cardiac silhouette and lung fields are partially or completely effaced by the effusion. Radiographs should be repeated following thoracocentesis to try to determine if the underlying cause is cardiac.

Early right heart failure is evident on the thoracic radiograph as an enlarged caudal vena cava and hepatomegaly due to passive congestion. Normally the caudal vena cava and aorta should be of approximately the same diameter. Advanced right heart failure includes the above signs and peritoneal effusion (ascites).

Pericardial Effusion

Pericardial effusion is the most common form of pericardial disease in the dog (See Chapter 12). It has a variety of causes; however, the most common are neoplasia and idiopathic pericarditis. Classically, pericardial effusion is characterized by an enlarged globoid cardiac silhouette on radiographs (Figure 5.20). However, the degree of enlargement is determined by the amount of pericardial effusion present. If only a mild to moderate amount of pericardial effusion is present, then changes to the cardiac silhouette may not be apparent.

In nearly all cases of pericardial effusion, the cause will not be apparent radiographically and requires echocardiography to diagnose the cause. The exception to this is heart base tumors. The term "heart-base tumor" refers to any neoplasm in this location. However, nearly all are chemodectomas. These tumors tend to grow to a massive size, and in some instances will be nearly as large as the heart (Figure 5.21). In most cases, dogs

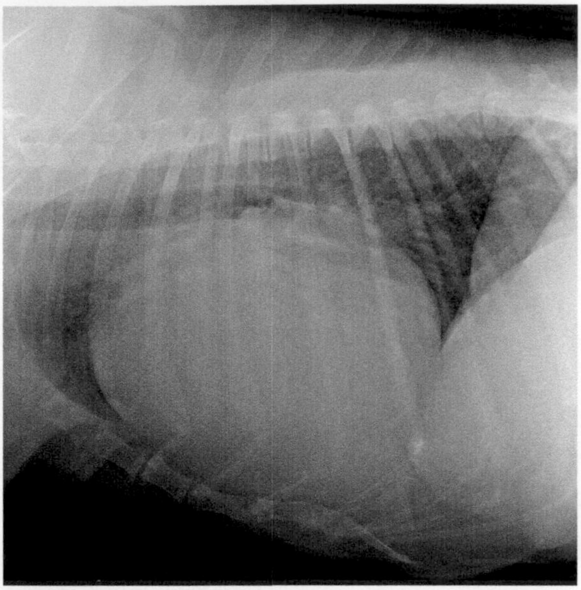

Figure 5.20 Radiograph of a dog with severe pericardial effusion. The cardiac silhouette is globoid and markedly enlarged.

with heart-base tumors will present with concurrent pericardial effusion. However, in some instances only the mass will be present.

Cats with congestive heart failure often have small volumes of pericardial effusion noted on echocardiogram. However, it is usually not of sufficient volume to cause clinical signs. Large volumes of pericardial effusion are rare in cats.

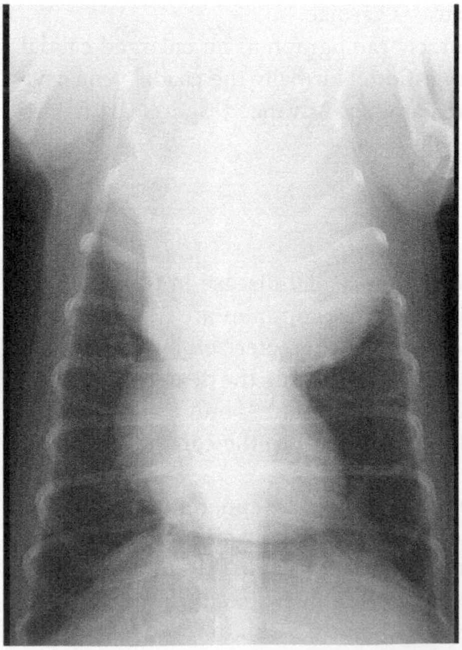

Figure 5.21 Radiograph of a dog with a massive heart-base tumor (diagnosed as a chemodectoma).

References

1 Thrall, D.E. (2007) *Textbook of Veterinary Diagnostic Radiology*. 5th Edition. Saunders, St Louis.
2 Lavin, Lisa M. (2007) *Radiography for Veterinary Technology*. 4th Edition. Saunders, St Louis.
3 Spencer C.P., Ackerman N. and Burt J.K. (1981) The canine lateral thoracic radiograph. *Veterinary Radiology Ultrasound*, **22**, 262–266.
4 Brinkman, E.L., Biller, D. and Armbrust, L. (2006) The clinical usefulness of the ventrodorsal versus dorsoventral thoracic radiograph in dogs. *Journal of the American Animal Hospital Association*, **42**, 440–449.
5 Poteet, B.A. (2001) Radiology of the heart, in *Manual of Canine and Feline Cardiology*, 4th Edition (eds L.P. Tilley, F.W.K. Smith, M.A. Oyama and M.M. Sleeper). Saunders, St Louis.
6 Buchanan, J.W. (2000) Vertebral scale system to measure heart size in radiographs, in *Veterinary Clinics of North America: Small Animal Practice: Clinical Radiology* (ed. B.J. Watrous). Saunders, Philadelphia.
7 Fox, P.R., Sisson, D. and Moise, N.S. (eds) (1999) *Textbook of Canine and Feline Cardiology: Principals and Clinical Practice*, 2nd Edition. WB Saunders, Philadelphia. p. 108.

6

Echocardiography and Doppler Study

Michelle St John and H. Edward Durham, Jr.

Introduction

Echocardiography is a noninvasive diagnostic tool that is used to image the heart and surrounding structures utilizing ultrasound technology. Echocardiography is used to evaluate systolic cardiac function, chamber size, wall thickness, and morphology of the valves. Hemodynamic information and diastolic cardiac function can be evaluated using Doppler echocardiography. Echocardiography is also useful in detecting fluid accumulation in the pericardial and/or pleural spaces, and can be helpful in visualizing tumors on or near the heart. Most patients tolerate an echocardiographic procedure well with gentle restraint or light sedation. An exception to this is transesophageal echocardiography where an ultrasound probe is inserted into the esophagus to image the heart from inside the patient. This technique requires general anesthesia.

The topic of cardiac ultrasound is very detailed and includes many concepts that are not suited to this text. This chapter will provide a brief overview of ultrasound technology and will also cover echocardiography is small animal patients only. The normal imaging planes, basic measurements, and fundamentals of the Doppler examination will be discussed. More detailed understanding of ultrasound physics, advanced echocardiographic studies, and advanced interpretation should be sought in ultrasound specific textbooks, such as those cited in the references [1, pp. 3–35].

There are three modalities of echocardiography that are frequently used: two-dimensional or B mode, motion mode, and Doppler evaluations. Doppler echocardiography will be discussed separately in this chapter. Two-dimensional (2-D) echocardiography displays images of the heart and surrounding structures on the monitor as an image that look like a heart. The normal structures are apparent to the untrained eye. This real time imagery allows for better appreciation of cardiac anatomy, physiology, and pathology.

Motion mode, commonly called M-mode, uses a single beam to transect a specific section of cardiac tissue. An image is displayed on the screen as a graph showing depth on the Y axis and time on the X axis. It is used to demonstrate how the cardiac tissue moves throughout the cardiac cycle.

Cardiology for Veterinary Technicians and Nurses, First Edition. Edited by H. Edward Durham, Jr.

Patient Preparation

Little preparation is needed prior to starting an echocardiogram. It is not necessary for the patient to fast unless general anesthesia is required. A dark quiet room is often helpful for making the patient feel more at ease. Loud startling noises tend to interrupt the examination. Shaving the thorax may be necessary to maximize contact between the transducer and the patient to improve image quality. If the hair coat is short, thin, or sparse, no shaving is necessary but a wetting agent (alcohol or water) should be used prior to applying the ultrasound gel. If the patient's hair coat is not moistened first, air will be trapped in the hair between the ultrasound probe and the patient when the ultrasound gel is applied, interfering with image quality.

If clipping is desired, the right hemithorax should be clipped from the third to the sixth intercostal space extending from the costochondral junction to the sternum. The left hemithorax should be clipped from the third to the seventh intercostal space along the thorax just lateral to the sternum, about one clipper blade width.

As with all ultrasonic examinations, coupling gel is used to eliminate air between probe and the patient. Air is not a good medium for ultrasound waves since they disperse easily. Air pockets will scatter the ultrasound beam resulting in poor image quality. In small patients, an ultrasound standoff may be used to enhance the image. Standoffs are flexible, gel-filled pads that enhance visualization of near field and superficial structures; by allowing the operator to have the ultrasound probe 2–3 cm from the target without creating an air artifact.

Images are best obtained with the patient in lateral recumbency. In this position, the heart will drop toward the chest wall creating an improved imaging window. Patients with dyspnea who cannot tolerate lateral recumbency, trauma cases, or fractious patients, may be imaged in sternal recumbency; standing on the table will often allow for an adequate examination. Giant breed dogs too large for the table can often be imaged standing on the floor.

The use of specially designed tables is necessary for obtaining studies on patients lying in lateral recumbency (Figure 6.1). There are many different styles of sonography tables but the basic concept is similar. These tables are designed with an opening situated such that when a patient is placed lateral recumbent on the table, these openings are directly under the precordium. The sonographer reaches up from underneath the table through the table openings with the transducer and performs the evaluation. Images from the right parasternal location will be better visualized with the patient's right forelimb slightly extended (Figure 6.2).

Ultrasound Technology

The ability to obtain diagnostic images depends on multiple technical factors such as transducer frequency, resolution, processor speed, beam width and angle, patient cooperation, and user experience. Cardiac ultrasound images are created by the use of high frequency sound waves. These sound waves are at a frequency not audible to the human ear, hence the term ultrasound. Sound waves are emitted from piezoelectric crystals into the patient's body. A piezoelectric crystal is made of quartz or ceramic. They possess a

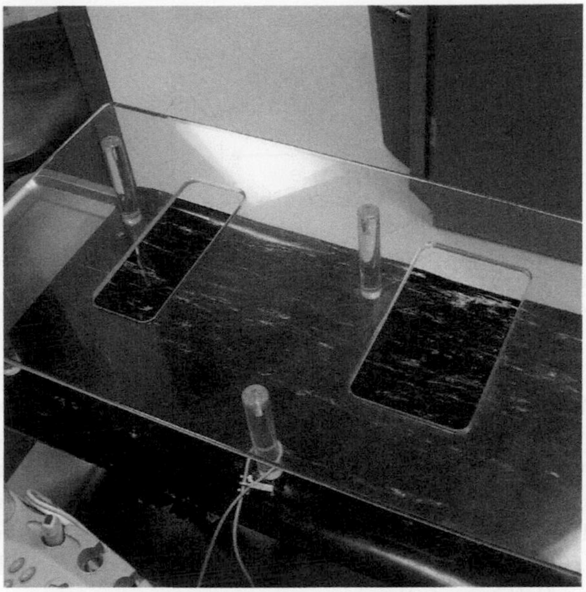

Figure 6.1 Echocardiography table: one style of small animal echocardiography table shows the two varying sized openings to reach under the animal to access the thoracic wall with the ultrasound probe. The smaller opening is sized for small dogs and cats, while the larger opening works well for larger dogs. A pad with corresponding openings can be added for patient comfort.

special property in that when they are stimulated by an electrical charge they generate an ultrasonic wave. Once the sound waves make contact with tissue, they are reflected back and received by more piezoelectric crystals which convert the ultrasound waves back into an electrical signal. The ultrasound machine then takes this reflected "echo" information and using a computer processor, the information is converted into a 2-D gray scale image which is displayed on a monitor screen.

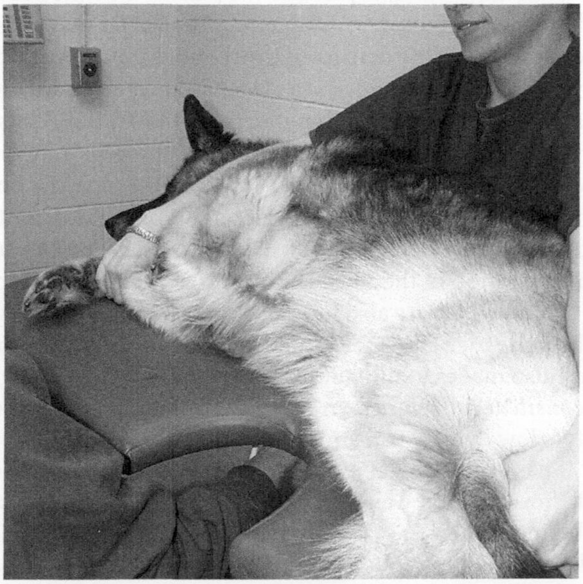

Figure 6.2 A patient during an echocardiogram showing the typical position of the patient. The ultrasonographer can be seen reaching under the patient to access the right lateral thorax from underneath the patient through a hole in the echocardiographic table. The assistant can stand at the dorsal aspect of the patient to allow for easy restraint.

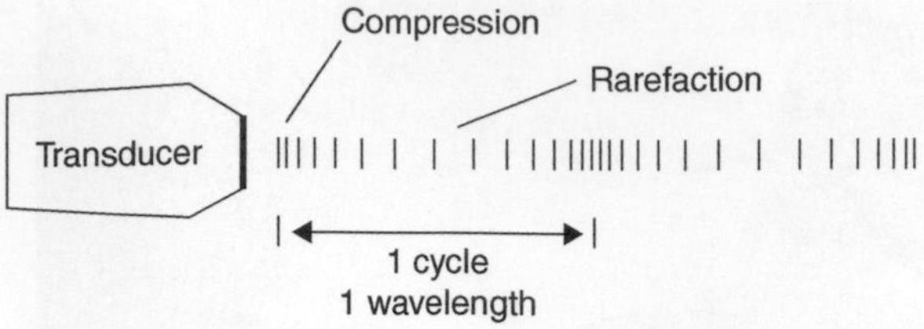

Figure 6.3 Ultrasound wavelength: the compression and rarefication that sound waves undergo traveling through a medium. The distance from one rarefication to the other is one wavelength or *cycle*. Source: Data from Boon, J (2011) Veterinary Echocardiography, 2nd Edition. Wiley-Blackwell, Ames.

It is useful to understand basic sound wave physics to make the most effective use of ultrasound diagnostic imaging. When an ultrasound wave is generated, it travels through a medium, in this case the patient's body, in a linear path. Along its path, the molecules encountered are repeatedly compressed and spread apart. The process of compressing and spreading these molecules apart is called *compression* and *rarefaction* [1, pp. 3–35]. The time it takes to complete one compression and rarefaction is known as a *cycle*. The distance the sound wave traveled to complete one cycle is the cycle's *wavelength* (Figure 6.3).

Frequency is the number of cycles the sound wave will complete each second; and is expressed as cycles per second called a *hertz* (Hz). One hertz equals one cycle per second; one kilohertz (kHz) equals 1000 cycles per second. One megahertz (MHz) equals 1 000 000 cycles per second. A high frequency ultrasound beam has a shorter wavelength than a lower frequency beam and therefore more cycles per second. The piezoelectric crystals generate a specific frequency determined by their size and shape and are housed in a transducer. Transducers are identified based on the frequency they produce; thus a 7.5 MHz transducer will transmit 7.5 million cycles per second. A 2 MHz probe will produce 2 million cycles per second.

In an ultrasound, depth into the patient is a function of time. The velocity of the sound wave is not affected by frequency. The speed that sound waves move through tissue is determined by the density of the tissue. Air has a very low density and ultrasound moves through it slowly; bone is very dense and sound waves move very fast. The soft tissues have different densities, ranging from 1440 to 1570 m/s [1, pp. 3–35]. The average velocity of ultrasound traveling through soft tissue is 1540 m/s, which is used to calibrate the device. By knowing the speed of sound through the body, the computer can determine the depth of a target by analyzing the time it took for the signal to return. The time for sound to travel 1 cm is 6.5> μs one way, 13 μs roundtrip. There is always a slight delay in generation of the image. This delay is generally unnoticeable to the operator.

Sound waves are also impeded on their course through the body. A high density tissue like bone may allow for rapid transmission of ultrasound waves, but the increased density also makes it difficult for the waves to move through them. Bone is said to have high *acoustical impedance*. In contrast, air has very low acoustical impedance, but because of its low density transmits ultrasound very poorly.

It has already been mentioned that when the ultrasound waves strike an object, some of those sounds waves are reflected back to the transducer. The best image quality is obtained when the target is perpendicular to the ultrasound beam. If the target is parallel to the ultrasound beam, less of the ultrasonic waves are reflected. Additionally, some waves are *refracted*, meaning they bounce off the object at an angle away from the transducer and may return from a different direction creating an artifact. When the ultrasound beam meets tissue, not all the sound waves are reflected. Some penetrate through into deeper tissue. The intensity of the ultrasound beam will weaken as it travels through the body until eventually no sounds waves can be echoed.

A term often used in diagnostic ultrasound is *echogenicity*. Echogenicity refers to how tissue reflects sound. Tissues that reflect a lot of sound are referred to as *hyperechoic* and produce a bright image. *Hypoechoic* tissues do not reflect much sound and produce a darker image. If something is referred to as anechoic then no sound is reflected and the image appears black, such as fluid-filled spaces.

Resolution is the ability to distinguish between two small separate objects. There are three types of resolution: axial, lateral, and temporal. *Axial resolution* is the ability to differentiate between two structures along the length of the ultrasound beam. A small axial resolution means a shorter wavelength leading to a better image, since the shorter wavelength will impact more objects. In contrast the lower frequency probe has a larger axial resolution because of the longer wavelength "passing over" small objects. *Lateral resolution* refers to being able to differentiate between two objects that are perpendicular to the sound wave [1, pp. 3–35]. Near field images and smaller sector width, or beam width allow for clearer images.

Temporal resolution refers to precise capture of real-time images, or how precise cardiac events are displayed in time. Temporal resolution depends on frame rate, which is the number of real-time images produced each minute. To achieve high frame rates, a higher pulse repetition frequency (PRF) is needed. The ultrasound probes will transmit a packet of ultrasound waves (at the frequency of that probe), then stop transmitting to receive the returning echoed sound waves, then transmit again. The number of times the probe can do this per second is the PRF. The PRF is related to the depth of the target and the width of the sector on the screen. To establish diagnostic quality images of fast-moving objects, a higher frame rate is needed otherwise poor-quality images will result.

The piezoelectric crystals are housed in a transducer probe which generates a specific frequency. Modern transducers are capable of generating a range of frequencies. Several types of transducers are available for diagnostic imaging including linear array probes, convex array probes and phased array probes. Linear array probes are designed for low frame rates, and a very broad gray scale. They are best suited for imaging the abdomen. Convex array and phased array probes both have a less broad gray scale, but produce very fast frame rates (Figure 6.4).

Selecting a transducer is dictated by the size of the patient. A low-frequency ultrasound wave will have a longer wavelength, having a better ability to penetrate deep tissue, but less detailed image quality. Low-frequency transducers (2–5 MHz) are good for reaching deep tissue. A high-frequency transducer (7.5–10 MHz) will not penetrate as deeply due to the shorter wavelength; yet the high-frequency transducer will have better image resolution. High-frequency transducers have better resolution of the near field producing better quality images.

Cats typically image best with a 7.5–10 MHz probe and small dogs less than 50 pounds image well with a 5–7 MHz probe. Low-frequency probes in the 3–5 MHz range are reserved for large, deep-chest breeds.

It is ideal to start the echocardiogram with a higher frequency transducer allowing for better resolution and image quality but still allowing enough depth penetration to complete the examination. It is not uncommon to need to use more than one transducer of different frequency levels to complete the study.

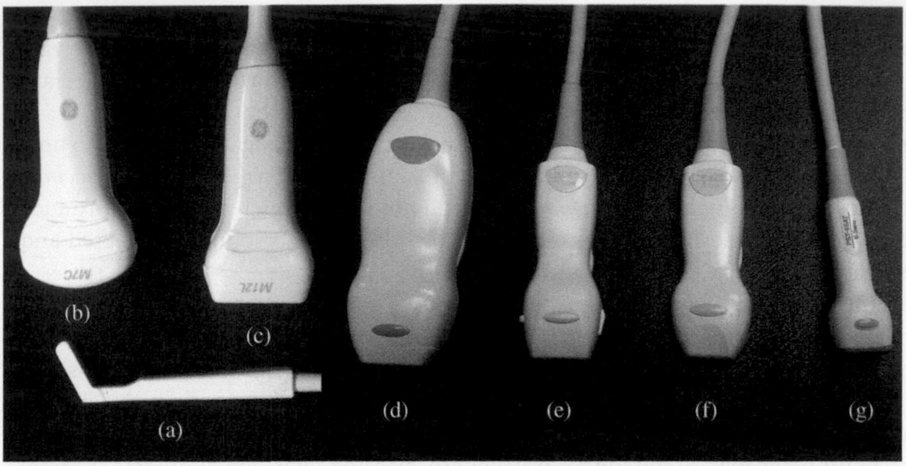

Figure 6.4 Different types of ultrasound probes. (a) 13.5 MHz small linear probe, aka, "hockey stick" commonly used for superficial small anatomy ultrasound. (b) 7 MHz convex array probe used in abdominal ultrasound. (c) 12 MHZ linear probe used for abdominal ultrasound. (d) 2.5 MHz 3-dimensional (3-D) volume probe. The newest 3-D probes will display a real time 3-D image or what is called "4-D" echocardiography. (e) 2 MHz phased array probe for echocardiography. The frequency is useful for large animal patients and larger dogs. Probes of this type typically produce 2-D images, M-mode images, and color flow Mapping and spectral Doppler modalities. (f) 5 MHz phased array probe which is similar to example (e), but this model is best suited for small to medium dogs. (g) 6.5 MHz phased array probe best suited for tiny dogs and cats.

Ultrasound Machine Controls

Each ultrasound machine has a different control layout but all machines have the same general functions. Highly sophisticated ultrasound machine often have many functions and controls for those functions. The terminology for each function may also be different, so it is incumbent on the operator to learn how their ultrasound machine operates. Common controls include: probe selection, depth, sector width, gain, freeze, time gain compensation, cine loop play, and function selections such as M-mode, continuous wave Doppler, pulse wave Doppler, and color flow Doppler.

As discussed above, multiple transducer probes are necessary for examination of different size patients. Generally, the transducers are continually attached to the machine. Each machine allows for the operator to select the correct one by simply depressing a button. This will initialize the probe and start it operating to pre-programed settings. The operator can then make various adjustments to fine-tune the image.

The operator can adjust the *depth* setting to change the amount of image in line with the ultrasound beam displayed on the monitor. A deep setting will show anatomy further away from the probe in the far field. The depth is adjusted such that the whole heart is visualized in the window without excess depth being displayed. Too much depth may show a mirror image artifact which is created by sound waves *reverberating* or passing through the heart a second time after reflecting off a bright reflector beyond the heart. The transducer perceives these ultrasound waves as taking twice as long to return to the heart and displays another image of the heart beyond the first. Correct adjustment of the depth will eliminate this artifact.

Gain refers to signal strength. It is analogous to the volume on a stereo. Increases in gain will increase the amount of gray scale pixel "fill in" on the monitor. By increasing gain, the operator makes the entire image brighter. If the image appears too bright or too dark, adjusting the gain will change the appearance of tissue echogenicity. When the operator increases the gain, they increase not just the myocardium, but the entire image so artifacts will also become more obvious. The gain should be adjusted to the point that the lumens of the cardiac chambers are fully black, but the cardiac walls are clearly visible.

Time gain compensation (TGC) controls are small slide levers on the console face. These controls allow the operator to adjust the gain at changing specific depths in the image. The slides at the bottom of the stack change the gain in the far field at the bottom of the image; the top ones control the near field (Figure 6.5).

Sector or sector width adjusts the width of the field of view. A smaller sector width will improve the resolution and frame rate, by reducing the amount of data the computer must process. Sometimes a large sector width is needed if the sonographer wants to show the relationship of chest mass/chest fluid to the heart. Generally, the sector width should be no wider than the heart itself.

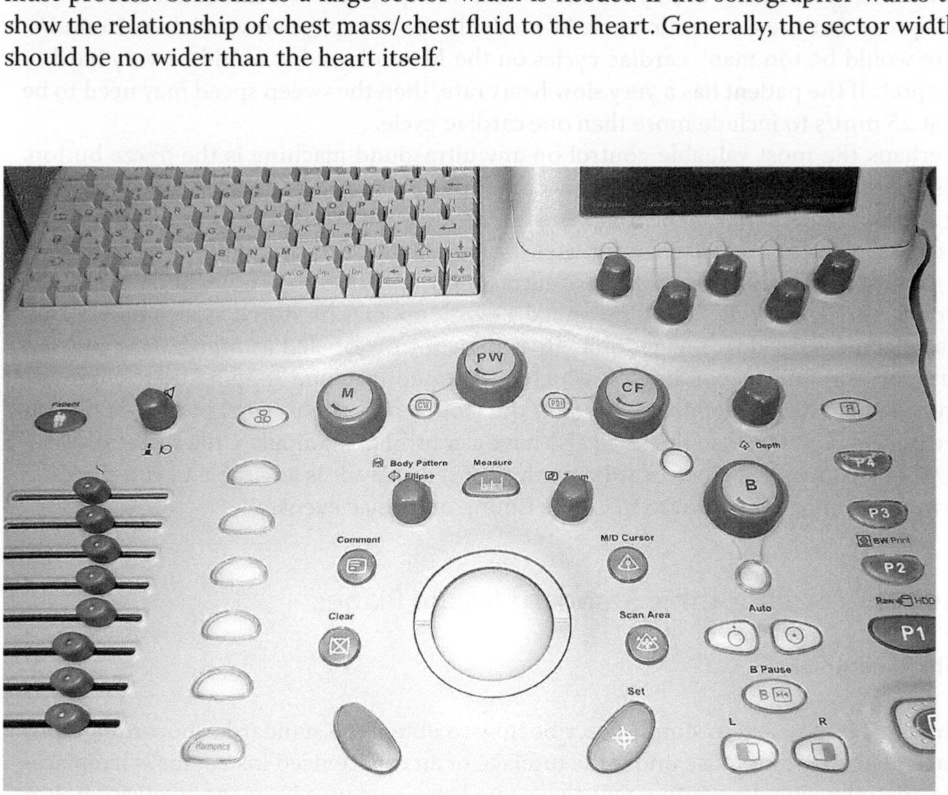

Figure 6.5 Typical echocardiograph console. The slide buttons on the left are the time gain compensation controls. The upper slides control the image gain in the near field. The lower slides control the image gain in the far field. Large knobs labeled M, PW, CF and B, control the M-mode, pulsed-wave Doppler, color-flow Doppler, and standard two-dimensional image, called B-mode, respectively. A small button labeled CW activates the continuous wave Doppler. The track ball in the lower center allows the operator to move a cursor on the screen to make selections that are then activated by the "set" button at the lower right of the track ball. Other controls seen are individual to this console, but similar functions are available on almost every echocardiograph.

All modern cardiac ultrasound machines will come equipped with an M-mode function. A button is available to activate the M-mode function. Often there is a button that may be used to toggle between the 2-D image and the M-mode to allow correct alignment of the M-mode cursor.

Ultrasound machines equipped with Doppler will have a selection of buttons for turning on or off the desired Doppler function. The continuous wave, or the CW knob, starts and stops continuous Doppler mode. Pulse wave, or the PW control, starts and stops the pulse wave mode. The color flow Doppler control may have several names (CF, CFM, or CDI), which starts and stops the color Doppler function.

M-mode, CW and PW Doppler are all displayed on a graph that sweeps across the screen. *Sweep speed* is a function of the ultrasound machine that allows the sonographer to adjust how fast an image sweeps across the screen. Sweep speeds are set at 25, 50, and 100 mm/s. The lower the sweep speed, the more cycles are being displayed on one screen. Correctly setting the sweep will depend on the patient's heart rate. For example, a cat with a heart rate of 200 bpm will need the sweep speed set a rate of 100 mm/s. This will spread out the contractions on M-mode. If the sweep speed was left at 25 mm/s, there would be too many cardiac cycles on the M-mode and it would be very hard to interpret. If the patient has a very slow heart rate, then the sweep speed may need to be set at 25 mm/s to include more than one cardiac cycle.

Perhaps the most valuable control on any ultrasound machine is the *freeze* button. This control is valuable because in uncooperative patients, the image needed for making a measurement may be fleeting. The freeze control allows the operator to freeze the image, scroll to it and capture it for later measurement. Ultrasound machines designed for cardiac work will store a loop of ultrasound images that the operator can scroll through in freeze mode. This loop, called a *cine* loop, may be stored as a complete loop or a selected individual image frame by using controls labeled as *image store* and *clip store*, for example. Depending on which ultrasound machine is being used, there are controls that change Doppler scale, shift the Doppler baselines, label images, and measure images. Cardiac machines will also have a control to manipulate the size and sweep speed of a concurrent electrocardiograph (ECG) display. It is advisable to run the ECG during the echocardiogram to mark the timing of cardiac events.

The Echocardiographic Standard Image Planes

Right Hemithorax

While it is impossible to simply describe how to obtain the standard echocardiography image planes, and practise under the tutelage of an experienced instructor is irreplaceable, the following description will give some basic guidance in image acquisition. It is in no way intended to be exhaustive or replace qualified instruction.

Learning to perform an echocardiogram requires controlling the probe in three directions in space: angulation, rotation, and placement of the probe on the chest. Angulation is typically described as zero degrees being level with the table and 90 degrees perpendicular to the table. Rotation is simply twisting the probe on its axis. Rotation is described as clockwise or counter clockwise from the perspective of looking down your arm if you held it straight out horizontally in front of you. Placement on the chest describes where the probe is placed on the chest; it is described as cranial or caudal and ventral or dorsal. Often the sonographer must adjust one of these parameters independently of the other two.

Standard imaging planes have been identified and named based on human echocardiographic terminology. The use of standardized views allows for minimal intra- and interoperator deviation, meaning comparisons of echocardiographic information is possible between different sonographers and the same sonographer over time to track the course of disease in a patient. The views are commonly referred to by the position on the chest where the image is obtained, the anatomy visible, and the orientation of the slice taken, either long axis or short axis. The long-axis views slice the heart down the sagittal plane lengthwise from apex to base. The short-axis views the transverse plane of the heart through the width of the heart fanning from apex to base. Here the terms sagittal and transverse refer to the heart only, not the patient's body. The heart does not sit perfectly square in the chest so the sagittal and transverse planes of the body would yield an oblique slice of the heart. If we imagine the heart as a pineapple, the long-axis views slice the heart like a pineapple boat. The short-axis views slice the heart like pineapple rings.

Although no exact protocol is required, images should always be acquired in the same order by each sonographer to establish a routine. Due to cardiac anatomy, 2-D images of the ventricles and atria are best imaged from the right side. In veterinary medicine the examination generally begins on the right side of the chest. This will allows for the ultrasound beam to be perpendicular to the heart for optimal image quality. The heart is imaged in both a long and short-axis plane during the study.

The long-axis views are: right parasternal long-axis "five-chamber" view, counting the aorta as the fifth-chamber (Figure 6.7) and right parasternal long-axis four-chamber view (Figure 6.8). It is standard to orient the image so the left atrium (LA) is positioned on the right side of the screen. The right parasternal long-axis five-chamber view will image the left ventricle (LV) focusing on the left ventricular outflow tract (LVOT), aortic valve (AV) and the aorta (AO). A small portion of the LA, right ventricle (RV) and right atrium (RA) will still be visible. The right parasternal long-axis four-chamber plane will contain all for heart chambers with both tricuspid (TV) and mitral valves (MV) with no aorta visible. These two imaging planes are useful in evaluating valve morphology, interventricular septum (IVS) motion, ventricular wall thickness, presence of pericardial effusion, and provide a global view of cardiac function.

Short-axis (or transverse) views are also right parasternal views. A total of four views are commonly acquired, with a possible fifth in larger dogs or in horses, by fanning the ultrasound sector from apex to base in a transverse plane imaging the LV at various levels including the papillary muscle level, chordae tendinae level (the fifth optional view), m level, heart base with aorta, and heart base with pulmonic valve (PV) and pulmonary artery (PA) (Figure 6.6).

To obtain the long-axis five-chamber image (Figure 6.7) start by holding the transducer so the reference mark is under the forefinger. With the patient in lateral recumbency, and the patient's head to the left and feet towards the sonographer, place the transducer between the third and sixth intercostal rib space where the apex beat can be felt relatively close to the sternum. The reference mark will point towards the patient's neck, the face of the transducer is angled toward the lumbar spine, and the tail (cord) is directed to the patient's elbows keeping a 45 degree angle between the transducer and

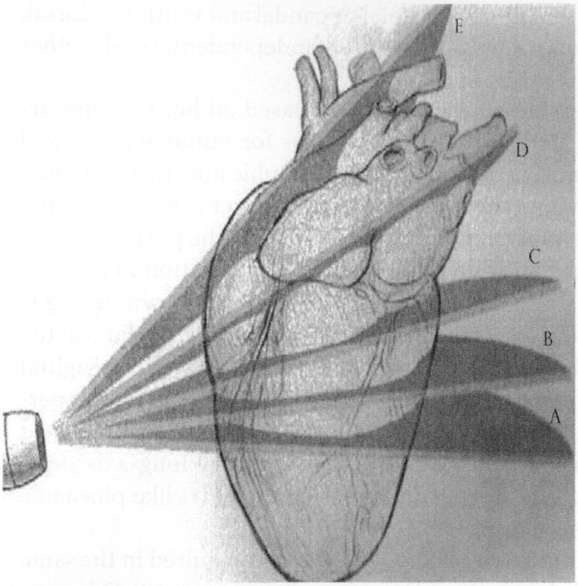

Figure 6.6 Short-axis planes bisecting the heart. The right parasternal short axis views in this drawing are shown as planes cutting through the left ventricle. Notice that the ultrasound probe is represented in one location since the images are acquired by changing the angle of the ultrasound beam in relation to the heart, not moving the probe on the chest wall. The image planes represented are right parasternal short axis views at the: A, papillary muscle level; B, chordae tendineae level; C, mitral valve level; D, aortic valve and left atrial level; E, pulmonary artery bifurcation view. Source: Data from Boon, J (2011) Veterinary Echocardiography, 2nd Edition.Wiley-Blackwell, Ames.

the imaging table. This positioning will generally provide an image of the LVOT. Rotating the reference mark counterclockwise towards the front legs will help bring more of the aorta into view and maximize the length of the LV. Slightly lifting the tail of the probe, decreasing the angle from the table, will help enhance the m and LA. Decreasing the angle too much will cause the aorta to disappear from the imaging plane.

A four-chamber image is obtained by starting with the LVOT view, then rotate the transducer counterclockwise so that the reference mark just passes the shoulders and

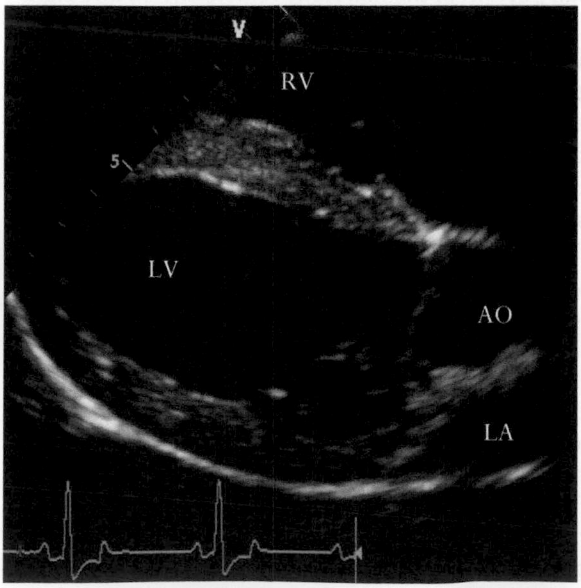

Figure 6.7 Right parasternal long-axis five-chamber view. The apex of the ventricle is to the left and the base of the heart is to the right. The cardiac chamber: LV, left ventricle; LA, left atrium; AO, aorta; RV, right ventricle. The right atrium (not labeled) is atop the aorta.

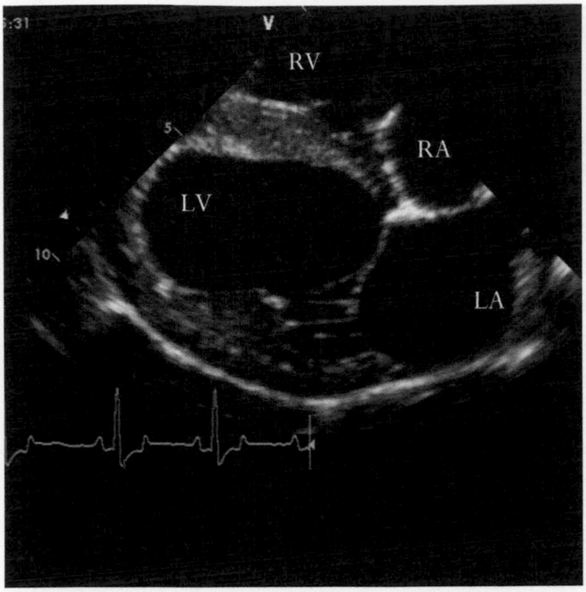

Figure 6.8 Right parasternal long-axis four-chamber view: the apex of the ventricle is to the left and the base of the heart is to the right. The chambers are identified as: LV, left ventricle; LA, left atrium; RV, right ventricle; RA, right atrium. The pericardium is the bright white line at the bottom of the LV.

the aorta is no longer in the field of view. If the image is slanted on the screen it will show the right atrium well; to maximize LV view slide the transducer dorsally up the chest wall and then angling ventral can help elongate the ventricles and improve the MV image. Lifting or dropping the tail ever so slightly may be needed to maximize the view of the LA and LV (Figure 6.8). In a four-chamber view, the heart is imaged to its fullest without any aorta or LVOT. Papillary muscles should not be visible in the LV. This view is useful for making an assessment for pericardial effusion and subjective impressions of the LV size and function. Mitral valve motion may also be assessed.

Right parasternal short-axis images are obtained by rotating the reference mark clockwise 90 degrees from the long-axis plane. The tail of the probe is dropped to about 60 degrees. The reference mark points towards the elbows and sternum. Short-axis images help evaluate overall chamber size, wall thickness and obtain M-mode images for measurement as illustrated in the next section.

To obtain the short-axis view of the LV, the reference mark points towards the elbows, the face of the probe angles toward the xiphoid. Sweep through the short-axis imaging planes starting from the apex moving up to the base of the heart. Imagine drawing a line from the xiphoid to the shoulders. Keeping the transducer in the exact same location on the chest wall, just tilt the face of the transducer along this imaginary line. Starting with the apex, image the LV in isolation with no papillary muscles or MV. From here, tilt slightly until the papillary muscles are in view, and angle more towards shoulders to image the LV at the chordae tendinae level (Figure 6.9). Ideally, this is where M-mode measurements are taken. However, in small animal medicine, this chordae tendinae level is often impossible to obtain perfectly. It is common for the M-mode of the LV to be taken at the papillary muscle level as an alternative (Figure 6.10).

Continue to angle back towards shoulders bringing in both the anterior and posterior MV (Figure 6.11). This is colloquially called the "fish mouth view" since the motion of the MV resembles the motion of a fish's mouth while feeding at the surface of the water.

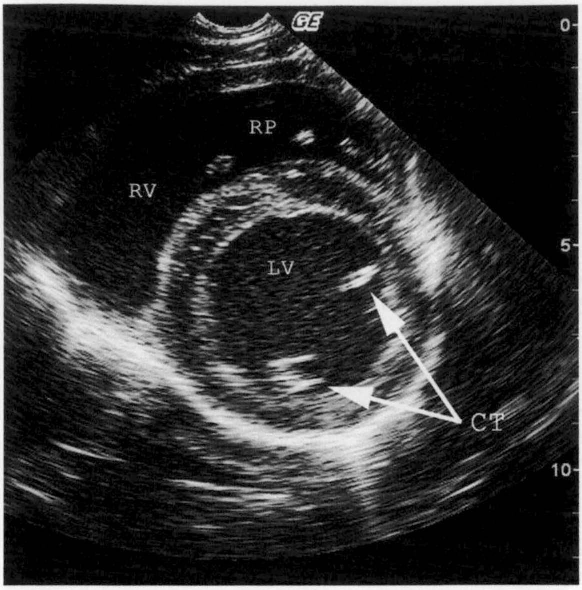

Figure 6.9 Right parasternal short-axis view at the level of the chordae tendineae (CT) in the left ventricle (LV). The papillary (RP) muscles of the right ventricle can be seen as white circular structures in the right ventricle (RV).

Another M-mode is acquired at the MV level. The angle is again adjusted closer to zero degrees by pulling the transducer tail toward the operator to image the heart base. This view will demonstrate a short-axis view of the all three AVs leaflets, and the LA, RA, and right ventricular outflow tract (RVOT) will be imaged (Figure 6.12). Often the TV can be seen in this view. Rotating the transducer slightly counterclockwise will help get the aorta evenly rounded and valves imaged properly. A final M-mode is obtained from this view.

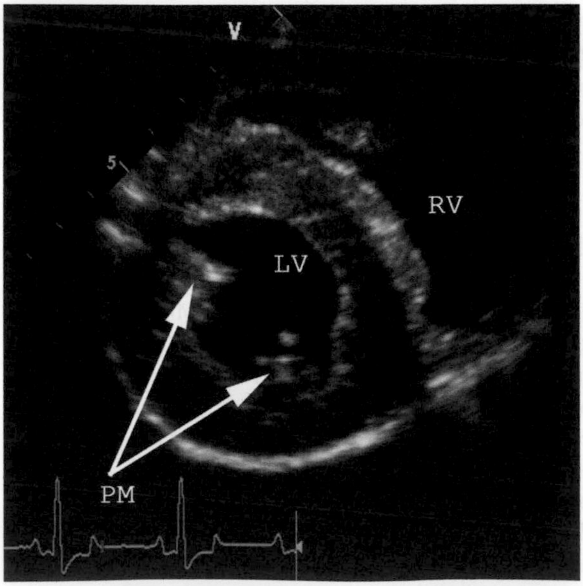

Figure 6.10 Right parasternal short-axis view at the level of the left ventricular papillary muscles (PM) in the left ventricle (LV). The right ventricle (RV) can also be seen.

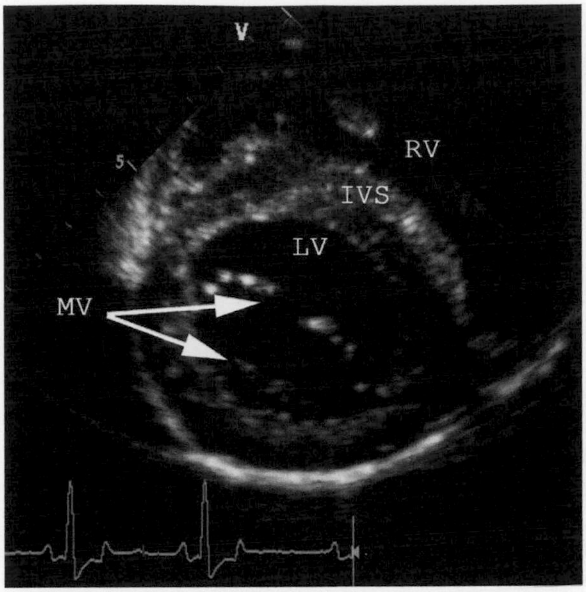

Figure 6.11 Right parasternal short-axis view at the mitral valve level. The arrows point to the cusps of the mitral valve, within the left ventricle (LV). The anterior cusp is central in the LV and closest to the interventricular septum (IVS); the posterior cusp is below that close to the LV posterior wall.

The main PA can be imaged from both the right and left parasternal chest wall. To image from the right side, start with the short-axis heart-base imaging plane. Then slightly rotate and tilt the probe towards the neck and sternum with a shallow angle almost parallel to the chest wall. The image should start with the long-axis view of the pulmonic valve to the right of the LA and angling a bit more will bring in the pulmonic bifurcation into the right and left pulmonic artery extending caudal and ventral to the LA (Figure 6.13).

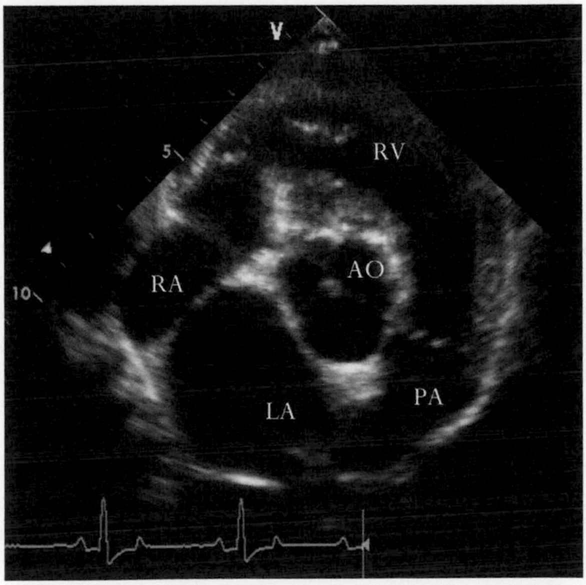

Figure 6.12 Right parasternal short-axis view at the aortic valve/left atrial level. In this view the aortic valve is seen in cross-section in a plane that allows visualization of the cusps when closed. When closed the cusps of the aortic valve form a three-pointed star shape within the circular annulus. The chambers are identified as: LA, left atrium; AO, aorta; RA, right atrium; RV, right ventricle; PA, pulmonary artery. The pulmonic valve can be seen in long axis just to the lower right of the aortic valve.

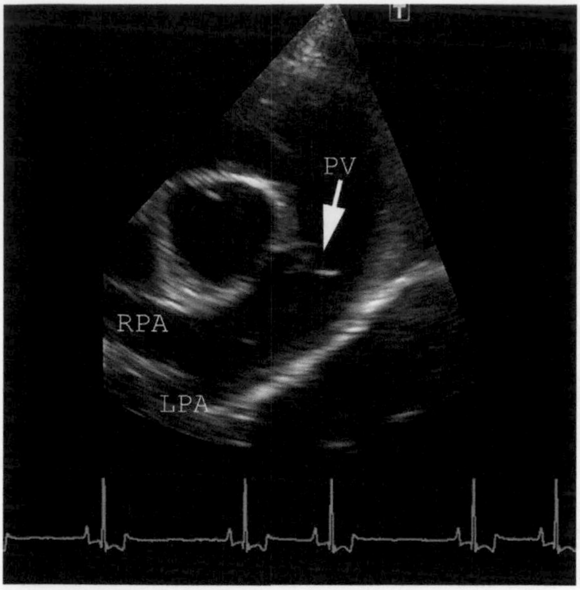

Figure 6.13 Right parasternal short-axis view: the extreme heart base dorsal to the aortic valve, showing the bifurcation of the main pulmonary artery. The pulmonic valve (PV) can be seen in long axis just to the lower right of the aortic valve. The right branch (RPA) exits to the left of the image and the left branch (LPA) exits toward the bottom of the image.

Veterinary patients have a variety of thorax conformations. When imaging cats, the heart is aligned closer to the sternum. The transducer is placed closer to the sternum, the face of the probe points towards the thoracic spine, and the tail is brought to about an angle of 10° from the table. If scanning a large or deep-chested dog, the transducer is placed about 1–3 inches (2.5–7.5 cm) dorsally up the chest wall from the sternum since their heart is more dorsally placed.

Left Hemithorax

Images taken from the left parasternal chest wall will consist of short-axis, long-axis and apical views. These left-side images are useful for evaluating valve morphology and better visualization of atrial appendages. The apical long-axis views are used for Doppler examinations.

To obtain the left apical four-chamber view, place the transducer between the fifth and seventh rib space, just cranial to the liver and close to the sternum. The reference mark is directed towards the spine, the face of the probe angles towards the patient's neck, and the tail is at an approximate 30 degree angle from the table. In this view the heart will be imaged as standing vertical, all four chambers with both MV and TV visible with the atria typically oriented at the bottom of the image (Figure 6.14). Sliding closer to the sternum, the heart becomes more vertical. Here the sonographer can access mitral and tricuspid regurgitation and obtain inflow velocities for both valves using a Doppler modality.

Starting with the four-chamber view, ever so slightly tilt the face of the transducer towards the patient's head; rotate clockwise as little as one degree to bring the aorta into view (Figure 6.15). This view can be difficult to achieve depending on the size of the patient. The sonographer may need to press firmly into the chest to get the aorta to

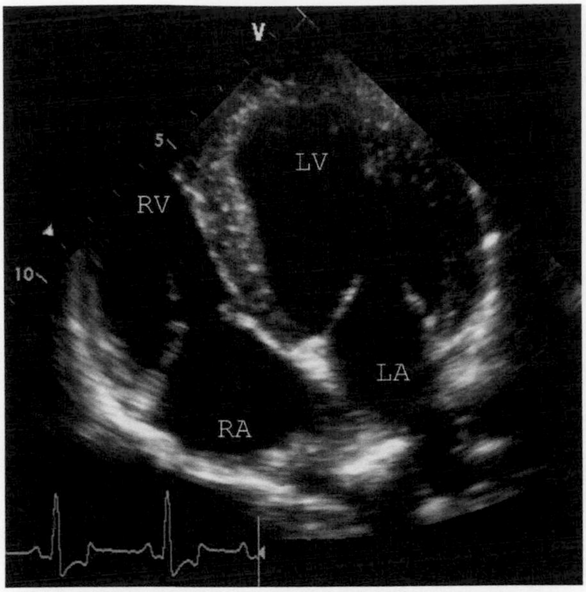

Figure 6.14 Left parasternal apical four-chamber view: from this projection the heart is seen with the left ventricular apex at the top of the screen, and the atria at the bottom. The chambers are identified as: LV, left ventricle; LA, left atrium; RA, right atrium; RV, right ventricle.

come into view. This image will provide good alignment for evaluating aortic outflow velocities.

The RA and RV, LVOT/aorta, and PA can be imaged from a more cranial position. The transducer is placed between the third and fourth rib space. The reference mark points towards the patient's neck, the face of the probe points towards the spine. Here a long-axis aorta, AVs, and the outflow tract are imaged (Figure 6.16). This view is important for visualizing chemodectomas. Dropping the tail away from the operator will bring

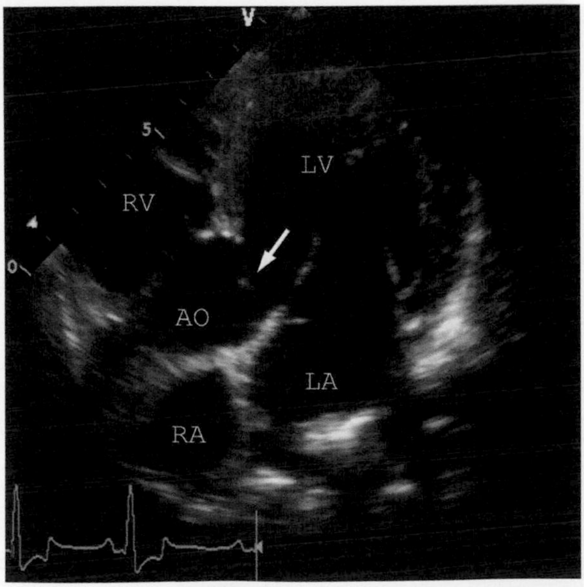

Figure 6.15 Left parasternal apical five-chamber view: the orientation of this view is the same as Figure 6.14. This image is adjusted such that the aorta is visible heading downward. The chambers are identified as: LV, left ventricle; LA, left atrium; RA, right atrium; RV, right ventricle; AO, aorta. The aortic valve is indicated by the arrow.

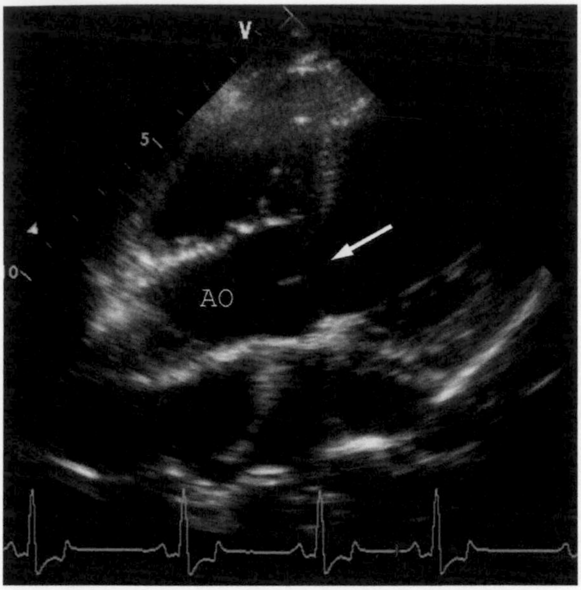

Figure 6.16 Left cranial oblique view: this image is adjusted to maximize the view of the aorta (AO) in the long axis. The heart itself is neither a long or short axis. The aorta is seen exiting the image to the left with the aortic valve (arrow) in the center.

the RV, TV, and RA into view. Better evaluation of tricuspid regurgitation and tricuspid inflow velocities are taken from this imaging plane (Figure 6.17). Dropping the tail even more will image the right atrial appendage, where hemangiosarcoma can develop. Lifting the tail past the previous aortic image to almost parallel to the chest and sliding more towards the sternum will image the PA (Figure 6.18). Sometimes this view will provide optimal alignment for Doppler evaluation of pulmonic velocities. This image plane is also useful for Doppler interrogation of patent ductus arteriosus if present.

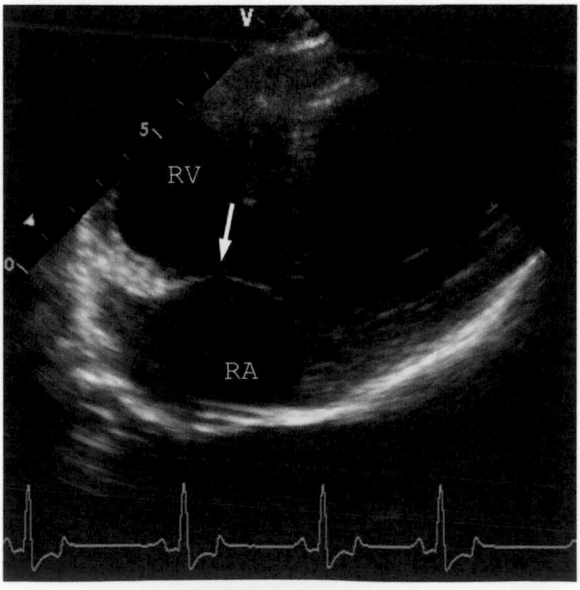

Figure 6.17 Left cranial oblique view: this image is also taken from a left cranial oblique projection with the angle adjusted to maximize visualization of the right atrium (RA) and tricuspid valve (arrow). The right ventricle (RV) is toward the top.

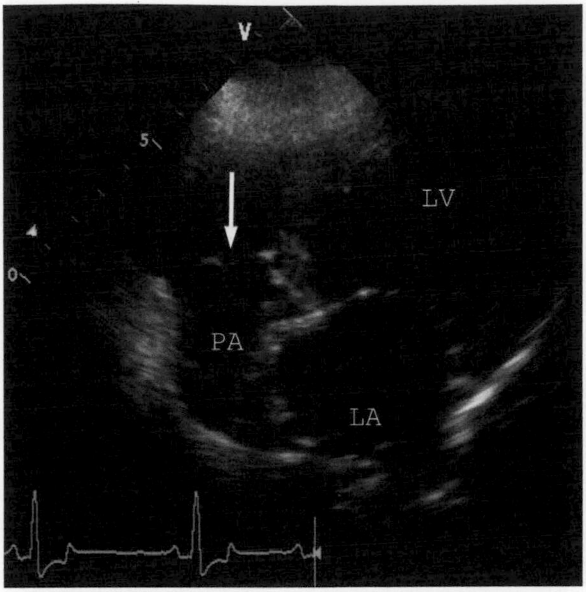

Figure 6.18 Another image from the left cranial oblique now adjusted to show the main pulmonary artery (PA) and pulmonic valve (arrow). The left atrium (LA) and left ventricle (LV) can also be identified.

The Motion Mode Images

Motion mode or M-mode is one of the earliest modes of cardiac ultrasound. M-mode is very useful in evaluating changes in wall motion, thickness, and valve motion and their relation to time. M-mode measurements are used to evaluate contractility, chamber size, and wall thickness. Diastolic measurements of the LV reflect chamber size and wall thickness. Systolic measurements assess overall contractility when compared with the diastolic measurements. M-mode uses a single ultrasound beam to provide a single line of data in the heart allowing for very precise measurements of its motion over time. Time can be matched to the electrocardiogram to make accurate assessments of the heart during specific periods of the cardiac cycle. A cursor is used to align with the cardiac anatomy on a 2-D image, and when the M-mode function is activated an image showing this area of cardiac tissue moving through diastole and systole is displayed (Figure 6.19). Still-frame images of the M-mode are then used to make measurements of wall thickness and estimate systolic cardiac function. Accuracy of M-mode measurements depends on cursor placement. If taking an M-mode measurement of the LV in a short-axis plane, it is imperative that the cursor is placed so that the LV is divided into two equal halves without papillary muscle crossing the beam. If the cursor is placed a bit more to one side than the other, papillary muscle may be included in the M-mode and give a false impression of left ventricular hypertrophy (Figure 6.20).

The most common M-mode imaging planes are from the right parasternal short axis of LV and RV (Figure 6.21), right parasternal LV at the MV level (Figure 6.22), and the short axis of aorta and LA (Figure 6.23). The difference between these planes is often very slight. A very small change of transducer angle will create dramatic differences in the image. Alternatively, M-mode views can be taken from a right parasternal long-axis four-chamber view of LV. No M-mode images are taken from the left since the anatomy is a little distorted and actual size or wall thickness may be foreshortened.

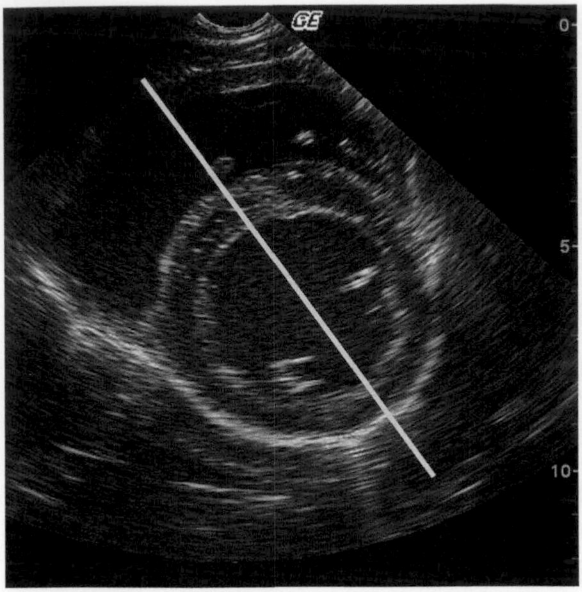

Figure 6.19 Right parasternal short-axis papillary muscle view: the correct placement of the cursor to acquire an M-mode recording of the left ventricle from the short-axis plane. The cursor is centered between the papillary muscles and bisects the interventricular septum and the left ventricular posterior wall at 90 degrees. There is sufficient inclusion of the right ventricular chamber to allow for easy determination of the endocardial borders of the interventricular septum.

Assessment of Cardiac Size and Function

A multitude of measurements may be performed on the echocardiographic images. This chapter will concentrate on those basic measurements and hemodynamic concepts required for cardiology veterinary technician specialists. A series of standard measurements are performed in virtually all echocardiograms. From these measurements information about cardiovascular status can be derived by comparing to published normal measurements (Tables 6.1–6.3). These measurements can also be compared to

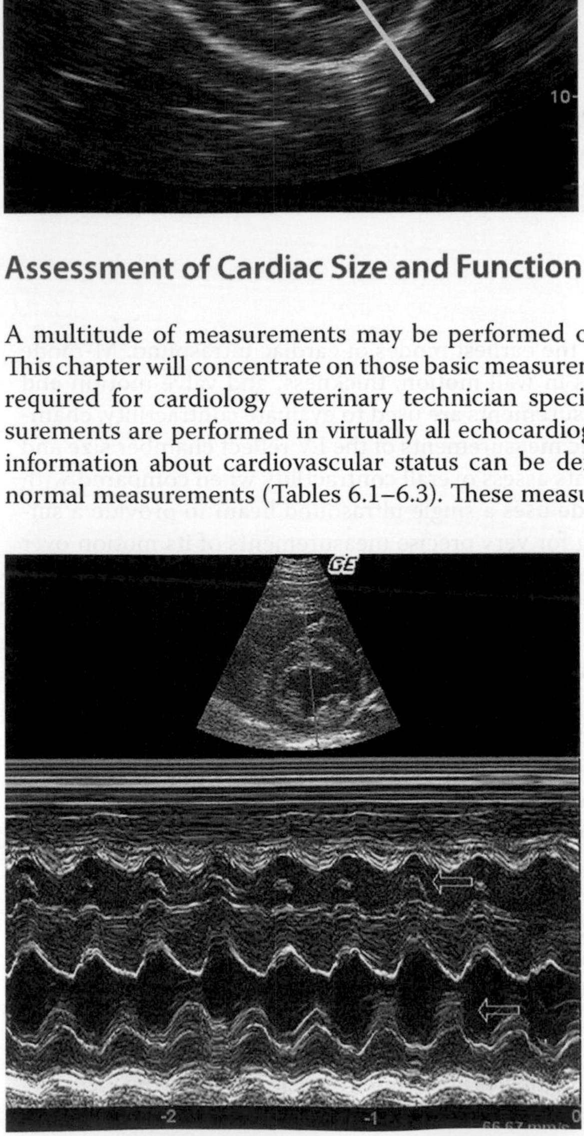

Figure 6.20 Right parasternal short-axis left ventricular M-mode. The arrows indicate the ultrasound reflection of the papillary apparatus crossing the ultrasound beam during ventricular systole. This phenomenon can be mistakenly identified as ventricular wall which could lead to erroneous measurements. The sonographer must place the guiding cursor carefully to avoid the papillary muscle; and if not possible, be aware of the artifact and exclude it from the measurement.

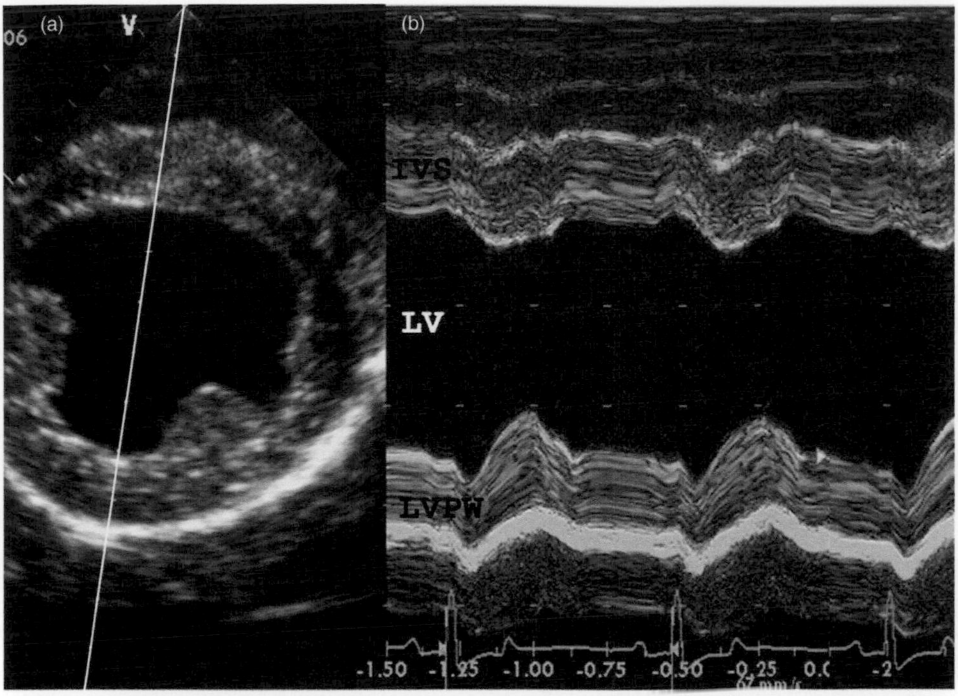

Figure 6.21 M-mode of left ventricle from the right parasternal short-axis view. (a) The left ventricle in short axis, with the M-mode cursor placed. (b) The corresponding M-mode trace. The left ventricular lumen (LV) is central between the interventricular septum (IVS) and the left ventricular posterior wall (LVPW). Above the IVS, the right ventricular lumen is seen as a hypoechoic space (black) topped by a more echogenic (greyer) section of tissue.

later measurements in the same patient to track disease progression. A simple hint for remembering what point in the cardiac cycle to take a measurement is the concept of "worst case"; this means measurements should be done when the target measure is at the point in the cardiac cycle when it should be at its biggest or smallest. For example, the diagnosis of hypertrophic cardiomyopathy (HCM) is made by an increase in the LV thickness. During systole the ventricular wall thickens normally, yet in end-diastole it will be at its thinnest; thus LV wall measurements of HCM are made at end-diastole. If the LV is thicker than normal at its thinnest then hypertrophy is present. Likewise, assessments of LA size are done at the end of systole, when the LA is at its largest.

Measurements are made on 2-D and M-mode images, and together paint a global picture of the patient's cardiac status. The most common measurements include: LA diameter, LV diameter (LVID), LV posterior wall thickness (LVPW), IVS thickness, aortic diameter, in addition to evaluation of contractility. Measurements of the right heart may be done in specialized instances. Measurements of the LV are done in systole and diastole. The measurement timing is indicated by a lower case "d" or "s". (Table 6.4) When performing cardiac measurements an average of three to five cardiac cycles is common practice. If the patient has an arrhythmia, endeavor to measure three to five sequential cycles of sinus origin. If the patient has a severe arrhythmia such as atrial fibrillation,

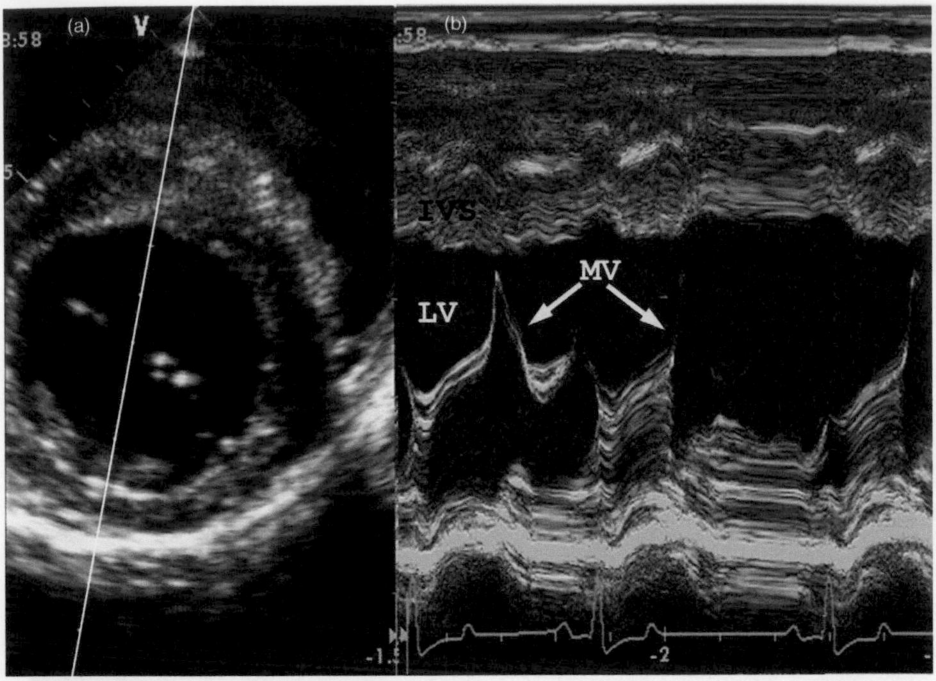

Figure 6.22 M-mode of mitral valve from the right parasternal short axis view. (a) The mitral valve in short axis, with the M-mode cursor placed. (b) The corresponding M-mode trace. The mitral valve (MV) is in the left ventricular lumen (LV) between the interventricular septum (IVS) and the left ventricular posterior wall. The two phases of mitral valve motion can be noted: the "E" wave that occurs after the T wave, and the "A" wave that is noted after the P wave on the electrocardiogram (see text and Figure 6.29 for more detail).

measure more cardiac cycles selecting those that represent an accurate picture of the patient's overall status.

When making M-mode measurements the concept of *leading edge to leading edge* is used. Leading edge measuring means the cursor to designate a measurement point is placed on the top of the margin of the section being measured (Figure 6.24). This system allows for the inclusion of one endocardial border in the measurement and is the standard system widely used in veterinary medicine. This method is used for all M-mode measurements except when measuring the *end point to septal separation (EPSS).*

Left Atrial Dimension

Assessment of LA size is very important for diagnosing and treating patients in congestive heart failure (CHF). The left atrial size will decrease with effective CHF therapy. The LA can be measured from long-axis, short-axis, and M-mode images. These data are then compared to published normal and previous echocardiographic information if available. From the right parasternal 2-D long-axis four-chamber view a measurement is made of the LA at the end of systole (Figure 6.25). This measurement is done by

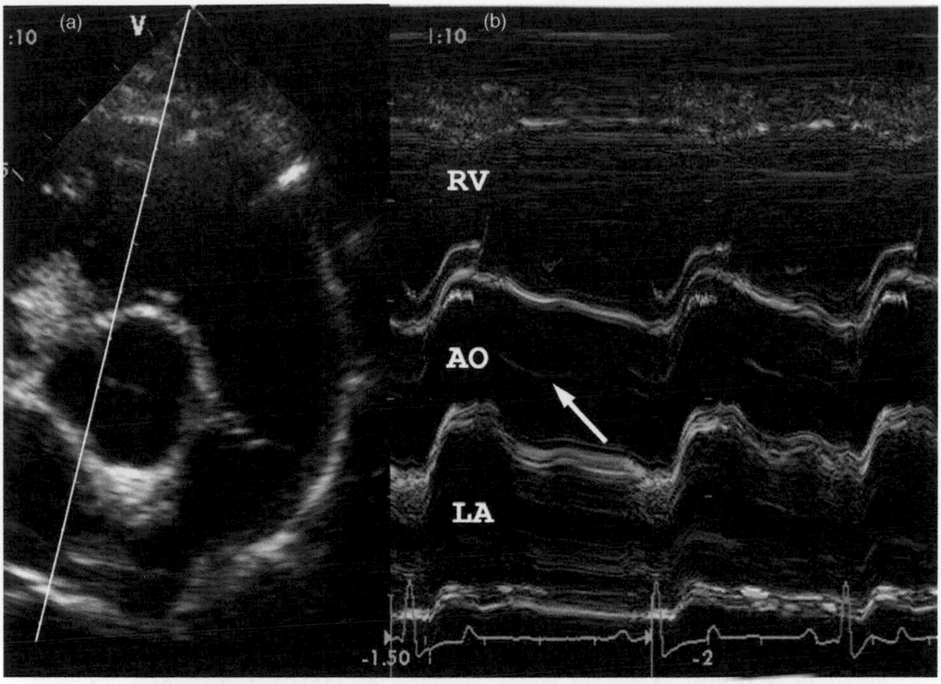

Figure 6.23 M-mode of aorta and left atrium from the right parasternal short axis view. (a) The right ventricle (RV), aorta (AO), and left atrium in short axis, with the M-mode cursor placed. (b) The corresponding M-mode trace. The RV can be seen in the near field, the middle section is the aorta, with the valve opening and closing during the cardiac cycle, and the left atrium is in the far field. The arrow indicates the aortic valve in the closed position. Just above the AO label, the aortic valve can be seen in the open position.

bisecting the LA with a line that divides it into two equal halves from atrial septum to atrial free wall parallel to the mitral annulus.

M-mode of the LA and aorta is taken from the right parasternal short-axis plane. The cursor is placed so that it falls in the middle of the aorta, catching all three aortic cusps and LA is measured as end-systole. Because of normal dog anatomy, there are instances when the cursor falls through the left auricle, not in the widest section of the atrium. This will cause the true size of the LA to be underestimated.

The LA should be measured from the M-mode taken from this same view. The aortic diameter is measured at the end of systole and the left atrial diameter is measured at the end of diastole as indicated by the end of the T wave on the ECG (Figure 6.26). In the normal patient, the LA and the aorta are approximately the same size. In normal dogs, the LA/AO ratio should be 0.83–1.13:1 and in cats 0.88–1.79:1. Horses are different in that their LA is generally smaller at 0.67–0.75:1 [1, pp. 153–266]. In patients with CHF, the LA will increase in size while the aortic size remains static. This creates a reference standard for LA size within each patient.

Left atrial size can also be measured from the 2-D right parasternal short-axis heart-base view. As mentioned earlier, the LA/AO ratio is calculated from here. This measurement takes the diameter of the aorta and the diameter of the LA and compares the

Table 6.1 Canine M-mode reference ranges (95% prediction intervals, mm).

Weight (kg)	VS d	LVID d	LVPW d	VS s	LVID s	LVPW s	AO	LA
0.5	4.44–6.78	−2.97–0.56	3.49–5.42	6.75–9.36	−4.60–2.51	6.14–8.55	8.49–11.51	8.92–12.82
0.9	4.69–6.93	3.57–5.95	3.70–5.54	7.11–9.61	−0.07–2.01	6.44–8.74	9.18–12.04	9.54–13.27
2.3	5.25–7.26	12.24–14.54	4.16–5.81	7.94–10.18	5.94–7.95	7.12–9.19	10.75–13.26	10.97–14.29
3.2	5.56–7.45	15.43–17.68	4.41–5.96	8.39–10.49	8.16–10.12	7.49–9.44	11.61–13.93	11.74–14.86
5.0	6.09–7.77	19.74–21.89	4.85–6.23	9.18–11.05	11.15–13.03	8.14–9.87	13.11–15.11	13.10–15.86
7.3	6.67–8.14	23.33–25.36	5.33–6.53	10.03–11.66	13.65–15.42	8.85–10.35	14.76–16.39	14.57–16.97
10	7.28–8.53	26.39–28.29	5.83–6.86	10.93–12.33	15.79–17.44	9.59–10.88	16.51–17.76	16.13–18.16
12.7	7.82–8.91	28.73–30.50	6.27–7.17	11.74–12.95	17.42–18.96	10.25–11.37	18.12–19.01	17.52–19.29
15	8.23–9.21	30.32–32.00	6.60–7.42	12.36–13.46	18.53–19.99	10.75–11.77	19.37–19.98	18.57–20.19
17.3	8.60–9.52	31.69–33.29	6.91–7.67	12.92–13.95	19.48–20.88	11.21–12.17	20.55–20.91	19.55–21.07
20	9.00–9.89	33.11–34.63	7.24–7.98	13.55–14.54	20.48–21.80	11.71–12.65	21.81–22.07	20.62–22.13
22.7	9.36–10.27	34.34–35.80	7.53–8.30	14.11–15.13	21.33–22.61	12.17–13.13	22.82–23.37	21.60–23.18
25	9.64–10.60	35.25–36.68	7.75–8.57	14.55–15.62	21.97–23.22	12.52–13.54	23.63–24.41	22.36–24.05
27.3	9.89–10.92	36.08–37.50	7.96–8.84	14.96–16.11	22.54–23.78	12.84–13.94	24.42–25.42	23.07–24.92
30	10.17–11.31	36.97–38.40	8.19–9.16	15.43–16.70	23 16–24.41	13.21–14.42	25.34–26.60	23.89–25.94
32.7	10.44–11.70	37.77–39.24	8.41–9.48	15.87–17.27	23.71–24.99	13.56–14.90	26.23–27.74	24.67–26.95
35	10.65–12.02	38.38–39.90	8.58–9.74	16.22–17.75	24.12–25.45	13.83–15.29	26.95–28.67	25.30–27.78
37.3	10.85–12.33	38.94–40.52	8.75–10.00	16.57–18.22	24.51–25.89	14.10–15.67	27.66–29.57	25.91–28.59
40	11.09–12.70	39.55–41.24	8.94–10.31	16.96–18.77	24.92–26.40	14.41–16.13	28.49–30.64	26.62–29.55
42.7	11.31–13.07	40.12–41.92	9.13–10.62	17.35–19.31	25.31–26.88	14.71–16.58	29.30–31.68	27.31–30.49
45	11.50–13.38	40.55–42.46	9.28–10.87	17.66–19.76	25.60–27.26	14.96–16.95	29.96–32.53	27.87–31.26
47.7	11.71–13.73	41.04–43.08	9.45–11.16	18.03–20.28	25.92–27.70	15.25–17.38	30.74–33.53	28.53–32.17
50	11.89–14.03	41.42–43.58	9.60–11.40	18.33–20.72	26.17–28.06	15.48–17.74	31.38–34.35	29.07–32.92
52.7	12.09–14.37	41.84–44.15	9.76–11.69	18.69–21.23	26.45–28.47	15.76–18.17	32.13–35.32	29.70–33.80
55	12.26–14.66	42.17–44.61	9.90–11.93	18.98–21.65	26.67–28.80	15.98–18.51	32.75–36.12	30.22–34.52
57.3	12.43–14.94	42.49–45.06	10.04–12.16	19.26–22.06	26.88–29.13	16.20–18.86	33.36–36.90	30.73–35.24
60	12.62–15.28	42.84–45.58	10.20–12.43	19.60–22.55	27.11–29.50	16.46–19.26	34.09–37.83	31.33–36.09
62.7	12.81–15.61	43.17–46.09	10.36–12.71	19.93–23.04	27.32–29.87	16.72–19.66	34.80–38.74	31.93–36.92
65	12.97–15.88	43.44–46.49	10.48–12.93	20.20–23.44	27.49–30.16	16.93–19.99	35.38 39.49	32.42–37.61
67.3	13.13–16.15	43.69–46.89	10.61–13.15	20.47–23.83	27.65–30.45	17.14–20.32	35.96–40.23	32.90–38.29
70	13.31–16.46	43.97–47.35	10.76–13.41	20.78–24.30	27.84–30.79	17.39–20.71	36.64–41.11	33.47–39.09
72.7	13.49–16.78	44.24–47.80	10.91–13.67	21.10–24.76	28.01–31.11	17.63–21.09	37.32–41.98	34.03–39.89
75	13.64–17.04	44.46–48.17	11.03–13.89	21.35–25.14	28.14–31.38	17.83–21.41	37.88–42.69	34.50–40.55
80	13.96–17.60	44.90–48.94	11.30–14.35	21.91–25.96	28.42–31.95	18.27–22.09	39.08–44.24	35.50–41.97

VS d, ventricular septum, diastole; LVID d, left ventricular diameter, diastole; LVPW d, left ventricular posterior wall, diastole; VS s, ventricular septum, systole; LVID s, left ventricular diameter, systole; LVPW s, left ventricular posterior wall, systole; AO, aorta; LA, left atrium.

Source: Data from Boon, J. (2011) *Veterinary Echocardiography*, 2nd Edition. Wiley-Blackwell, Ames.

Table 6.2 Breed-specific M-mode reference ranges.

Parameter	Cocker Spaniel (X ± SD)	Newfoundland (90% CI)	Great Dane (90% CI)	Spanish Mastiff (X ± SD)	Boxer (range)	Estrella Mtn Dog (range)
AO (cm)	–	2.6–3.3	2.8–3.4	2.86 ± 0.07	1.82-2.69	1.96-3.44
AOexc (cm)	–	0.5–1.3	0.6–1.3	–		
LA(cm)	–	2.4–3.3	2.8–4.6	2.85 ± 0.09	1.96–3.26	2.34–4.18
LA/AO	–	0.8–1.25	0.9–.5	0.97 ± 0.02		.81–1.65
LVd (cm)	3.38 ± 0.33	4.4–6.0	4.4–5.9	4.77 ± 0.14	2.90–4.80	3.89–5.89 F
						4.40–5.96 M
LVs (cm)	2.22 ± 0.28	2.9–4.4	3.4–4.5	2.90 ± 0.11	1.67–3.30	2.42–4.18
% FS	34.3 ± 4.5	22–37	18–36	39 ± 1.6		22.96–45.92
% ES	–	44–66	33–65	–		38.94–71.46
LVET (s)	–	0.14–0.20	0.12–0.18	–		
EDV (mL)						54.11–139.87
EDVi (mL/m^2)						46.42–121.62
ESV (mL)						17.66–70.23
ESVi (mL/m^2)						10.84–52.24
Vsf (cir/s)	–	1.1–2.5	1.0–2.3	–		
EPSS (cm)	–	0.3–1.4	0.5–1.2	–	0.09–0.72	.17–1.01
VSd (cm)	0.82 ± 0.13	0.7–1.5	1.2–1.6	0.98 ± 0.04	0.83–1.61	.90–1.40
VSs (cm)	–	1.1–2.0	1.4–1.9	1.56 ± 0.05	0.81–2.46	.86–1.86 F
						1.14–1.86 F
VS % Δ	–	0–45	6–32	61.2 ± 2.4		
Vsexc (cm)	–	0.4–1.0	0.2–0.8	–		
LVWd (cm)	0.79 ± 0.11	0.8–1.3	1.0–1.6	0.97 ± 0.04	0.90–1.55	.80–1.44
LVWs (cm)	–	1.1–1.6	1.1–1.9	1.52 ± 0.04	1.22–2.16	1.07–1.91
LVW % Δ	–	11–40	9–29	56.8 ± 2.5		
LVWexc (cm)	–	0.8–1.7	0.9–1.5	–		
HR	–	70–120	100–130	107 ± 5		57–143 M
						68–160 F
Age (year)					2.1–11.0	18–123 mon
kg	12.2 ± 2.3	47–70	52–75	52.4 ± 3.3	18.9–40.5	30–75
n	12	27	15	12	81	74

AO, aorta; LA, left atrium; d, diastole; s, systole; LV, left ventricle; FS, fractional shortening; EF, ejection fraction; LVET, left ventricular ejection time; EDV, end diastolic volume; EDVi, end diastolic volume index; ESV, left ventricular volume; ESVi, end systolic volume index; Vcf, velocity of circumferential shortening; circ, circumference; EPSS, E point to septal separation; VS, ventricular septum; LVW, left ventricular wall; exc, excursion; kg, kilogram; N, number; HR, heart rate; X, mean; Δ, change; SEM, standard error about the mean; mtn, mountain.
Source: Data from Boon, J (2011) Veterinary Echocardiography, 2nd Edition. Wiley-Blackwell, Ames.

two. This can be done in both the 2-D and the M-mode images. From the 2-D image a line is drawn across the diameter of the LA in line with the commissure of the left and noncoronary cusps of the AV. This diameter can also be compared with the AV measured along the commissure of the right coronary valve leaflet and the left coronary

Table 6.3 Nonanesthetized cats: M-mode refereence ranges.

Parameter	Jacobs (range)	Pipers (range)	Sisson (range)	Moise (X ± SD)	Lister non-obese cats (X ± SD)	Lister obese cats (X ± SD)	Chetboul generic (X ± SD)	Chetboul generic (min–max)	Chetboul DSH (X ± SD)	Chetboul DSH (min–max)	Schober generic (min–max)
RVd (mm)	0.0–7.0	–	0.0–8.3	–	3.9 ± 1.0	3.8 ± 0.9	3.0 ± 1.4	0.5–6.7	3.5 ± 1.5	0.9–6.7	
RVs (mm)	2.7–9.4	–	–	–							
RVWs (mm)	2.3–4.3	–	–	–			2.7 ± 0.8	1.2–4.9	2.7 ± 0.6	1.3–3.7	
RVWd (mm)					2.2 ± 0.5	3.4 ± 0.5					
LVd (mm)	12.0-19.8	11.2–21.8	10.8–21.4	15.1 ± 2.1	13.2 ± 2.3	14.7 ± 1.8	15.9 ± 2.3	9.7–21.2	14.2 ± 2.1	9.7–19.4	11.5–17.8
LVs	5.2–10.8	6.4–16.8	4.0–11.2	6.9 ± 2.2	5.2 ± 1.2	5.3 ± 1.0	8.1 ± 1.8	4.1–12.7	7.2 ± 1.8	4.5–11.2	2.6–10.9
% FS	39.0–61.0	23–56	40.0–66.7	55 ± 10.2	59.8 ± 11.6	62.9 ± 9.9	49 ± 7	33–66	49 ± 10	33–66	36–83
LVET (s)	0.10–0.18	0.11–0.19	–	–							
Vcf (cm/s)	2.35–4.95	1.27–4.55	–	–							
VSd (mm)	2.2–4.4	2.8–6.0	3.0–6.0	5.0 ± .7	4.4 ± 0.6	4.9 ± 0.6	4.6 ± 0.6	2.9–5.9	4.5 ± 0.6	3.2–5.3	3.4–5.9
VSs (mm)	4.7–7.0	–	4.0–9.0	7.6 ± 1.2			7.4 ± 1.3	4.6–12.1	6.9 ± 1.0	4.6–8.7	4.4–10.1
VS % Δ	–	–	–	33.5 ± 8.2							
LVWd (mm)	2.2–4.4	3.2–5.6	2.5–6.0	4.6 ± .5	4.2 ± .4	4.8 ± 1.0	4.3 ± 0.7	2.4–5.8	4.5 ± 0.6	3.2–5.3	3.1–5.9
LVWs (mm)	5.4–8.1	–	4.3–9.8	7.8 ± 1.0			7.5 ± 1.1	4.2–10.3	7.1 ± 1.0	5.2–9.0	5.6–9.5
LVW % Δ	–	–	–	39.5 ± 7.6							

AO (mm)	7.2–11.9	4.0–11.8	6.0–12.1	9.5 ± 1.5							
LA (mm)	9.3–15.1	4.5–11.2	7.0–17.0	12.1 ± 1.8	12.2 ± 1.9	12.8 ± 1.7					
LA/AO	0.95–1.65	–	0.88–1.79	1.29 ± 0.23	1.3 ± 0.2	1.3 ± 0.2	0.9 ± 0.1	0.5–1.2	0.9 ± 0.1	0.7–1.2	
EPSS (mm)	0.0–2.1	–	0.0–2.0	0.4 ± .7							
MAM											3.0–6.9
HR	147–242	120–240	120–240	182 ± 22	–	–	184 ± 33	100–261	187 ± 30	100–243	145–267
kg	1.96–6.26	2.3–6.8	2.7–8.2	4.3 ± 0.50	4.1 ± 0.9	7.7 ± 1.2	4.6 ± 1.2		4.0 ± 1.2		3.2–7.2
n	30	25	64–79	11	10	10	100	100	31	31	47

X, mean; SD, standard deviation; d, diastole; s, systole; mm, millimeter; RV, right ventricle; RVW, right ventricular wall; LV, left ventricle; FS, fractional shortening; LVET, left ventricular ejection time; Vcf, velocity of circumferential fiber shortening; VS, ventricular septum; LVW, left ventricular wall; AO, aorta; LA, left atrium; EPSS, E point to septal separation; MAM, M-mode mitral annular septal wall motion; HR, heart rate; kg, kilogram; N, number.
Source: Data from Boon, J. (2011) Veterinary Echocardiography, 2nd Edition. Wiley-Blackwell, Ames.

Table 6.4 Common abbreviations used in echocardiography measurement.

Measurement	Abbreviation
Interventricular septum in diastole	IVSd
Interventricular septum in systole	IVSs
Left ventricular internal diameter in diastole	LVIDd
Left ventricular internal diameter in systole	LVIDs
Left ventricular posterior wall in diastole	LVPWd
Left ventricular posterior wall in systole	LVPWs

valve leaflet (Figure 6.27). The ratio of these two measurements should be less than 1.6:1 [2]. Measuring the aorta and LA from a 2-D image is not a replacement for M-mode, but another method for evaluating the left atrial size. The aorta is measured when AVs are closed (diastole) and the LA is measured at its widest section.

Left Ventricular Dimension

Assessment of the LV is arguably the most important reason for performing an echocardiogram. Evaluation of the LV consists of chamber dimension, IVS thickness, LVPW thickness and estimates of contractility. Measurements of the LV are taken from the right parasternal 2-D long-axis, right parasternal 2-D short-axis and M-mode views acquired at the papillary or chordae tendinae level. M-mode measurements are taken from the right parasternal short-axis imaging planes. The cursor is placed so that it falls right in the middle of the LV bisecting it in two equal halves. The M-mode will display an image

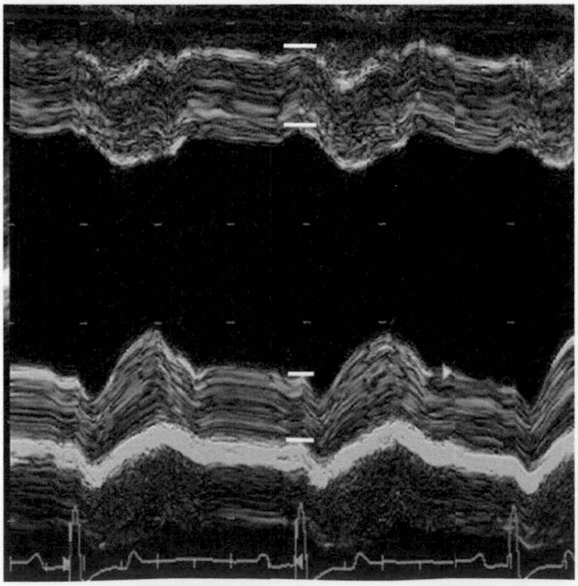

Figure 6.24 Left ventricular M-mode: the bright white lines on this image indicate the leading edges of the endocardial borders. It is at the leading edge of the endocardium that the measurement points are placed during the measuring process. The leading edge is defined as the edge closest to the top of the screen.

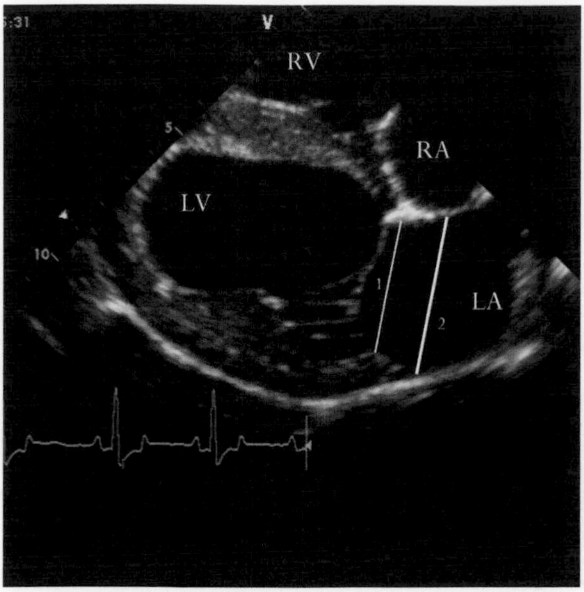

Figure 6.25 Measuring the left atrium (LA) in the right parasternal long-axis four-chamber view. Line 1 indicates the mitral annulus. Line 2 is a measurement across the body of the LA, parallel to line 1. This measurement is made at the end of systole, when the left atrium in fullest. The cardiac chambers are labeled: LV, left ventricle; LA, left atrium; RA, right atrium; RV, right ventricle.

of the left and RV as it moves throughout diastole and systole (Figure 6.21). In this view measurements are made of the IVS thickness, LV lumen dimension, and LVPW thickness all in systole and diastole. Diastolic wall thicknesses in cats are used to diagnose hypertrophic cardiomyopathy.

Modern ultrasound machines that are designed for cardiac ultrasonography will generally have a calculation package built into them. The calculation package will simplify the LV measurement process. Some ultrasound systems will automatically allow for

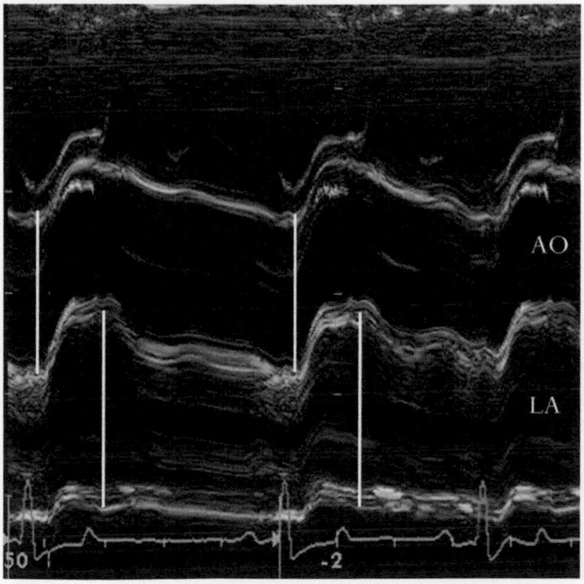

Figure 6.26 Measurement of the left atrium (LA) and the aorta (Ao) from the M-mode trace. The aorta is measured from the leading edge across the width of the aorta at the end of diastole. The end of diastole is determined by the either the ECG, or the opening of the aortic valve as seen in the image. The left atrium is measured from the leading edge across LA width at the end of systole, and indicated by the end of the T wave on the ECG. The ratio of the two measurements is calculated as the AO/LA ratio.

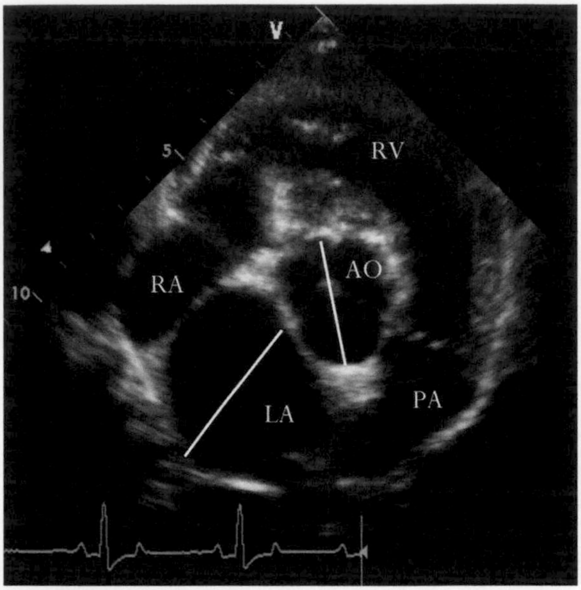

Figure 6.27 Measurement of the left atrium (LA) and the aorta (AO) in the right parasternal short-axis aortic/left atrial level 2-dimensional view. The measurement is taken at the end of systole, when the aortic valve is closed, and before the mitral valve opens. The aorta is measured parallel to the commissure of the right and left aortic valve cusps across the diameter of the aortic annulus. The LA is measured with a line parallel to the commissure of the left and septal cusps of the aortic valve, across the body of the LA. The cardiac chambers are labeled: AO, aorta; LA, left atrium; RA, right atrium; RV, right ventricle; PA, pulmonary artery.

measurement of the RV free wall. If this is the case the measurements will begin on the outside of the RV free wall and continue through the levels of the M-mode. Most often the RV measurement is not necessary and measuring begins with the IVS.

To perform measurements of the LV M-mode, start by placing the cursor on the RV side of the IVS at end-diastole, which corresponds with the onset of the Q wave, then the RV, continue with IVS, the LV, and lastly measure the left ventricular posterior wall. Then in the same order, measure the same structures in end-systole (Figure 6.28). Once the

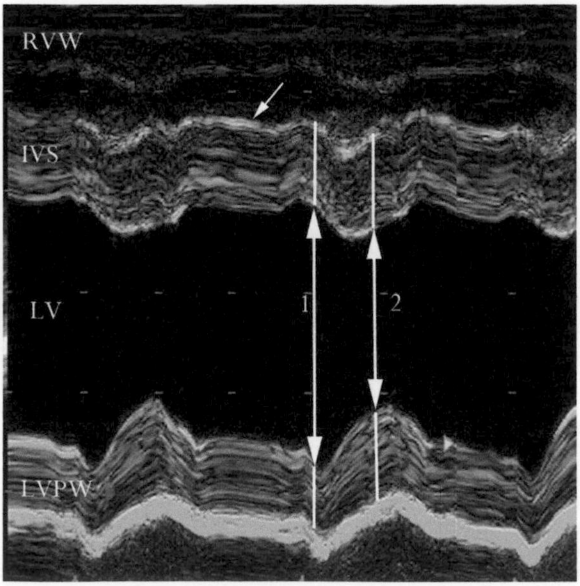

Figure 6.28 Measurement of the left ventricle from the M-mode image: the left ventricle is measured from the leading edge (small arrow) of the interventricular septum (IVS) to the endocardial border of the IVS to yield the IVS thickness (upper lines). The next measurement is from the leading edge of the endocardial border of the IVS to the leading edge of the left ventricular posterior wall (LVPW) to show the LV lumen diameter (arrowhead lines). The last measurement is the thickness of the LVPW from the leading edge of the LVPW endocardial border to the leading edge of the pericardium (lower lines). The measurements are taken in diastole and systole. The percent change in the LV lumen between diastole and systole is the percent fractional shortening (%FS).

measurements are complete, the LV internal dimensions are used to calculate fractional shortening (FS%). Often the ultrasound machine will automatically calculate FS% as an estimate of cardiac function (see Indices of Systolic Function later)

Valves of the Left Ventricle

Measurement of the MV is performed from an M-mode view. M-mode of the MV can be taken from either the right parasternal short-axis or long-axis imaging plane for LV. In a short axis, place the cursor through the LV at the level of the MV so that the cursor transects both the anterior and posterior valve equally. From the long-axis plane, the cursor is placed perpendicularly to the IVS and falls at the tips of both valve leaflets. The motion of the MV in the M-mode has the appearance of the letter "M". The first peak of the "M" is referred to as the "E" wave. The "E" wave represents the motion of the MV in *early* ventricular diastole. The valves come to a nearly closed position when pressure equalizes between the ventricle and atria. The second peak to the "M" is labeled the "A" wave and occurs after the ECG P wave, but before the QRS complex. The "A" wave represents the *atrial* contraction component of ventricular diastole. An animal in atrial fibrillation will have no "A" wave since there are no true atrial contractions.

Only one measurement is taken from the MV M-mode. Measuring the distance between the E wave and the IVS is referred to as EPSS (E point to septal separation). A large EPSS may indicate increased left ventricular pressure due to volume overload or significant aortic insufficiency. A normal canine EPSS is measured <7.7 mm and normal feline EPSS is <4 mm [3].

The EPSS measures the distance from the tip of the MV at its first opening after the T wave on the electrocardiogram to the IVS. This distance is known to increase when systolic dysfunction is present. It indicates how much the ventricle emptied its volume during the previous systole. In a normally contracting ventricle approximately 50% of the blood volume is ejected. During the next early diastolic phase, the MV will open widely nearly touching the IVS. A poorly contracting heart will not eject as much volume and the residual volume keeps the IVS further away from the IVS. This measurement is specific but may not be sensitive, and be affected by ventricular hypertrophy and preload (Figure 6.29).

Another measurement commonly taken is from the 2-D long-axis five-chamber view. The aortic diameter is measured from this image often at several places. The value of the aortic diameter can be used in conjunction with Doppler evaluation of transaortic flow to calculate cardiac output. The aortic diameter is measured at: (1) the hinge point of the AV leaflets, (2) the widest part of the sinus of Valsalva, and (3) in the tubular aorta half the distance of the sinus of Valsalva measurement away from where the sinus of Valsalva measurement was made (Figure 6.30). This should approximate the sino-tubular junction.

Indices of Systolic Function

Often the determination of cardiac function is the main indication for performing an echocardiogram. Contractility or systolic function is an assessment of how well the LV empties after filling in diastole. It is noteworthy that these indices give no information about forward flow, only how much the ventricle emptied. In the presence of valvular

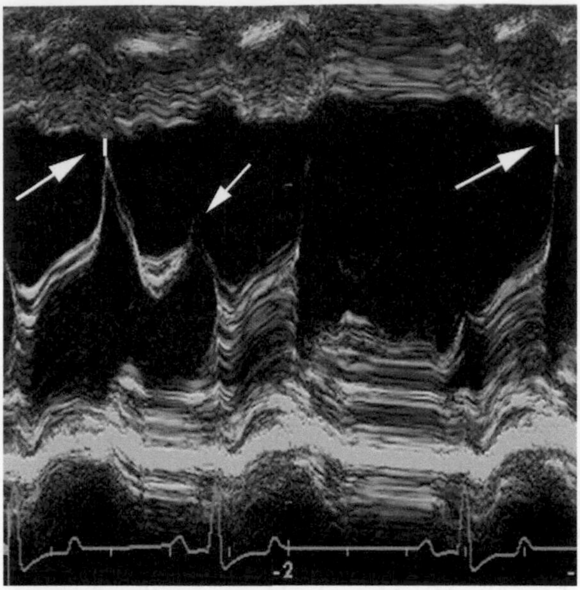

Figure 6.29 Measurement of the end point to septal separation (EPSS) in the M-mode: this M-mode image demonstrates the measurement of the mitral valve at its closest point to the interventricular septum during early diastole. The upward pointing arrows indicate the mitral valve excursion during early diastole, the "E" wave. The downward pointing arrow indicates the mitral excursion following the atrial contraction, the "A" wave. The small white lines mark the actual location of the measurement. For this measurement, the leading edge rule does not apply. Only the distance from the top of the valve leaflet to the bottom of the septum need be included.

regurgitation or a shunt, ventricular blood is leaving the ventricle, but not necessarily going forward into the aorta. In reality systolic function is a complicated process, affected by many factors such as vascular volume (preload), the pressure the ventricle is pushing against (afterload), sympathetic nervous tone, and elasticity of the myocardium. Using echocardiography there are several ways to attempt to quantify contractility. The most commonly done measurements look at the percent change in diastolic dimensions and systolic dimensions. This can be done by looking at a linear change in LV dimensions (*fractional shortening*), the area change of the LV (*shortening area*) or, a volume change

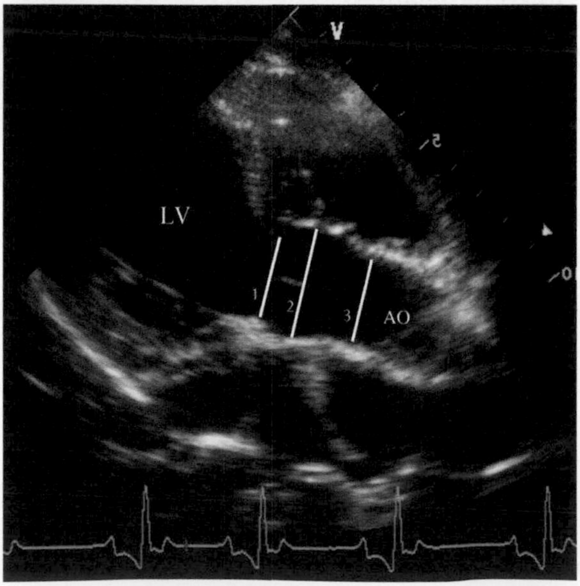

Figure 6.30 Three different methods of aortic root measurement: measurement from the right parasternal long-axis five-chamber view. Line 1 is placed across aortic valve hinge points; line 2 is placed across widest portion of the sinus of Valsalva; line 3 is placed across the sinotubular junction at half the distance of the sinus of Valsalva measurement away from the sinus of Valsalva measurement. (Line 3 placed half the distance of line 2 FROM line 2.)

of the LV (*ejection fraction*). The ejection fraction has the added advantage of calculating the LV stroke volume from which cardiac output can be derived (providing no shunt or valve regurgitation is present). One "truth" of systolic function measurement is that easy to do measurements make more mathematical assumptions, and more complicated measurements assume fewer, but are harder and more time consuming to obtain. All of these measurements are calculated from essentially the same formula (Equation 6.1) and are expressed as a percentage. The same equation can be used for the linear dimension, the area, or the volume.

$$\text{LVIMd} - \text{LVIMs}/\text{LVIMd} \times 100 = \%\,\text{CHANGE} \tag{6.1}$$

where LVIM is LVID, LVIA, or LVIV (LVID, left ventricular internal dimension; LVIA, left ventricular internal area; LVIV, left ventricular internal volume).

The determination of systole and diastole are typically made from the electrocardiogram. The measurements made for all indices of systolic function are made at the onset of the Q wave to mark end-diastole, and the end of the T wave as end-systole. Alternatively the largest diastolic frame and the smallest systolic frame can be used.

Fractional shortening (FS) is a common calculation that measures cardiac systolic function. Fractional shortening is calculated LV dimension as measured from the right parasternal short or long-axis M-mode at the chordae tendinae level (Figure 6.28). Normal fractional shortening for cats ranges from 30 to 55% and for dogs from 25 to 45% [1, pp. 153–266]. Fractional shortening measures the distance between one point on the IVS and the LVPW and how much that distance changes between diastole and systole. Additional calculations from these measurements using the Teichholz method can yield LV volumes which appear to be accurate in the normal heart but not in the failing heart [1, pp. 153–266].

Shortening area (SA) is measured from the short-axis right parasternal view at the chordae tendineae or papillary muscle level. To measure the shortening area, the operator uses the scroll function of the echocardiograph to locate a frame of the LV at end-diastole. Using the area measurement tool of the system, the internal area of the LV is traced (Figure 6.31). The operator then scrolls to an end-systolic frame and repeats the area trace. The resulting areas are then used to calculate the percent change in the LV area (Equation 6.1). A normal shortening area is between 45 and 55%. Shortening area is not commonly performed, since an ejection fraction can be carried out with less effort.

The ejection fraction (EF) is perhaps the best method of making an echocardiographic assessment of systolic function. The heart is a three-dimensional (3-D) structure that moves in all three directions simultaneously. Because FS and shortening area only change in the dimension of the LV they may not give a true representation of systolic function. Assessments of LV volume are challenging due to the geometry of the LV; it is not a simple shape such as a cylinder or a cone. There are many formulas that have been derived to attempt to calculate LV volume [4]. All of these formulas rely on some calculation of the area and length, and the ratio of area to length. The method that is most commonly employed in veterinary medicine is the Simpson's rule, also known as the summation of disks formula. For Simpson's rule, the area and length of the LV are traced by the operator. The computer then fills the traced area with a series of equally spaced disks. The sum of the area of all the disks is equated to ventricular volume (Figure 6.32). By comparing the diastolic volume with the systolic volume the ejection fraction is calculated (Equation 6.1). Simpson's rule can be applied to a single plane view

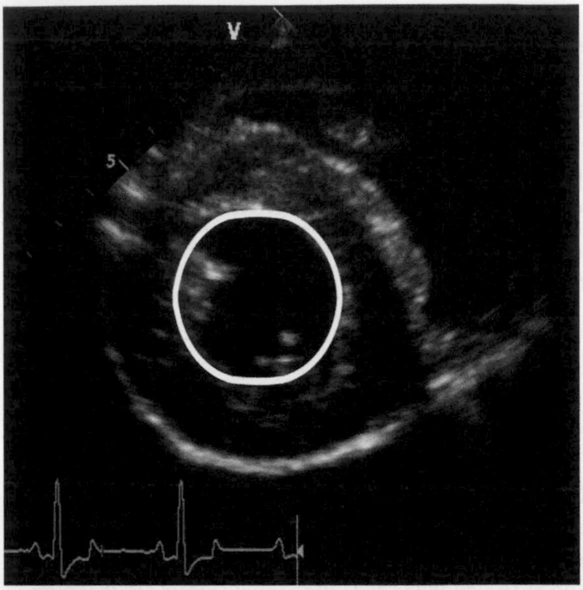

Figure 6.31 Left ventricular area measurement from the right parasternal short-axis left ventricular view: the circle placed on the ultrasound image indicates an example of the trace placed to calculate the area of the left ventricle. The measurement is taken at the end of diastole and the end of systole then the percent change calculated. For simplicity, the papillary muscles are ignored, as illustrated, while doing the trace. Including or excluding the papillary muscles are both acceptable, providing the measurement is done the same every time. The percent change in the area of the left ventricle is known as the shortening area (SA).

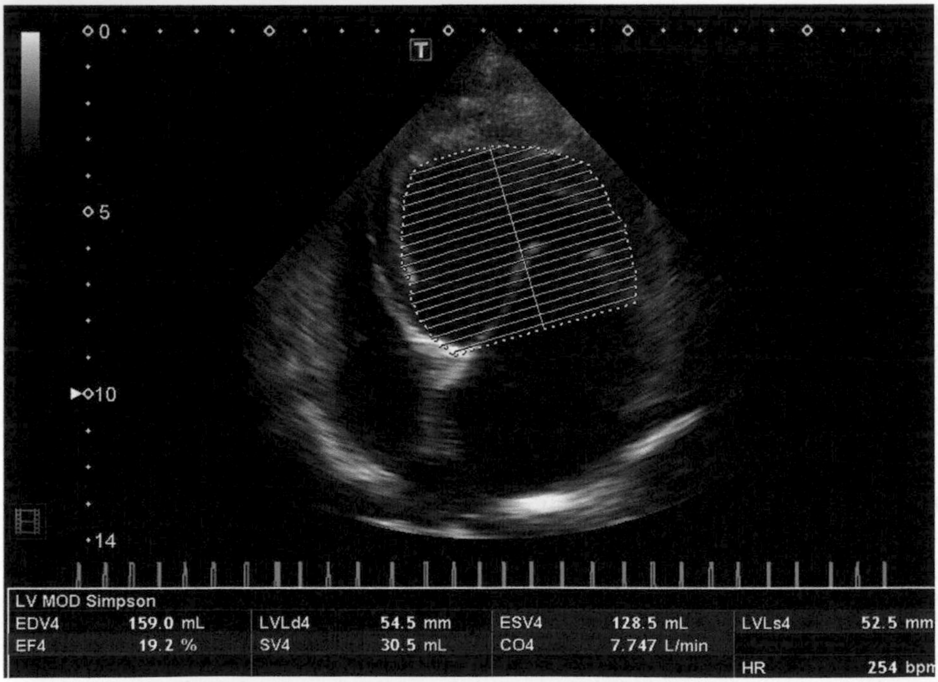

Figure 6.32 Measurement for left ventricular volume from the left apical long-axis four-chamber view: the image depicts the summation of disks method of calculating left ventricular volumes. The lines across the left ventricle represent the disks the computer places in the left ventricle after the operator has traced the area and the length of the ventricle. From this information the computer will add the disks, and then sum the area of the disks to calculate the ventricular volume. This is repeated at end systole and end diastole. The two volumes are then compared to calculate the ejection fraction (EF), which is the percent change of the ventricular volume during the cardiac cycle.

of the LV or biplane acquisition of area. All the ejection fraction formulas rely on an image plane that fully encompasses the LV. Foreshortening or off angle views of the LV will result in errors. In human medicine ejection fraction is typically calculated from the left apical four-chamber and the left apical two-chamber views to achieve bi-plane data. It is difficult in dogs to achieve left apical views that do not foreshorten the LV. Ejection fraction in veterinary medicine is performed from the right parasternal long-axis four-chamber view. This view allows for complete viewing of the LV, but limits the operator to making the assessment in a single plane.

Once the LV volume is determined the systolic and diastolic index can be calculated by dividing the volumes by the body surface area. The systolic and diastolic indexes of Simpson's formula are approximately 30 mL/m^2 and 70 mL/m^2 respectively in normal dogs [5]. Based on these numbers a normal ejection fraction for dogs is at least 42%.

The normal ranges for all the described methods reflect the many factors that change contractility. For example, a patient with mitral insufficiency will have an exaggerated FS due to increased volume available to the LV as blood moves back and forth between the LA and LV. The increase volume indices increase stretch in the LV wall which causes it to bound back vigorously making it *hypercontractile*. The greater the myocardial stretch, the greater the contraction. Added to this is the ability of the LV to pump into the low pressure LA, effectively reducing LV afterload.

In dogs that are volume depleted or dehydrated, FS, shortening area, and ejection fraction will be decreased due to a lack of preload. During diastole the LV is not filling normally, and less blood volume is available for ejection. If the diastolic dimension is lower than normal, but the systolic dimension is still normal, then the difference will be less than normal. This is a common finding in dogs with lymphoma [6].

Other Echocardiography Modalities

Transesophageal Echocardiography

Transesophageal echocardiography (TEE) is a modality that places the piezoelectric crystals of the ultrasound probe in the end of a long steerable device similar to an endoscope which allows placement down the esophagus (Figure 6.33). With TEE, different image planes can be achieved allowing for additional information about the heart to be observed. To perform TEE general anesthesia is required. It is most often used as an adjunct to fluoroscopy during cardiac catheterization of congenital heart disease. In some instances, TEE alone can be used to visualize a patent ductus arteriosus for interventional closure, or pulmonic valves for balloon valvuloplasty. During anesthesia TEE allows for direct visualization of the heart in the event of arrest or pericardial effusion.

Three-Dimensional Echocardiography

The most advanced ultrasound machines are equipped with probes that allow the sonographer to image the heart in a 3-D plane (Figure 6.34). So called "four-dimensional" echocardiography is a 3-D image moving in real time. The 3-D probe projects essentially a cone of ultrasound to acquire what is called a 3-D volume. The saved 3-D volume can then be manipulated. It can be turned and cropped. By removing some of the 3-D volume in one plane, internal cardiac structures can be seen.

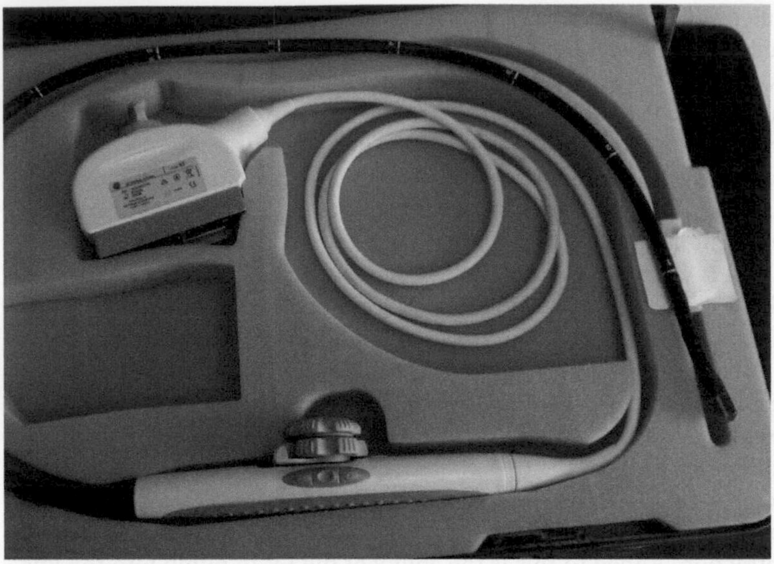

Figure 6.33 A typical transesophageal echocardiographic probe: the transesophageal probe is placed near the heart via the mouth down the esophagus. General anesthesia is required for the procedure. The depicted probe is ~1 m in length and 1 cm in diameter. The control handle allows the operator to bend the tip of the probe in up-down and right-left planes, and rotate the ultrasound crystal head within the tip.

In theory, measurements of ventricular volume are possible. This has not become widely practiced for a number of reasons. First machines that can acquire 3-D images are very expensive and usually only available at teaching institutions. Gathering of the 3-D volume is time consuming and subject to error if the sonographer is not experienced. An incomplete volume data set would create measurement errors. If a complete data set is acquired, it must be cropped properly and then the LV volume traced by hand. As technology advances automatic edge detection may speed up the process.

Contrast Echocardiography

Contrast echocardiography refers to using a highly echogenic solution injection into the blood stream to enhance imaging. Commonly referred to as a "bubble study", a gas is used as a contrast medium for the ultrasound beams. Albumin microencapsulated nitrogen gas is available as a retail product, but is rarely used in veterinary medicine due to cost and rarity of need. More commonly, simple agitated saline is injected onto a peripheral vein for the same effect (Figure 6.35).

A mixture of a small amount of the patient's blood and saline, agitated to create microscopic bubbles, is quickly injected via an intravenous catheter. The microbubbles are highly reflective of ultrasound and allow for excellent visualization of blood flow. Because the air bubbles are microscopic, the patient is not at significant risk from embolus. The majority are filtered out by the pulmonary capillaries. Contrast echocardiography is particularly useful in diagnosing right to left-shunting congenital defects

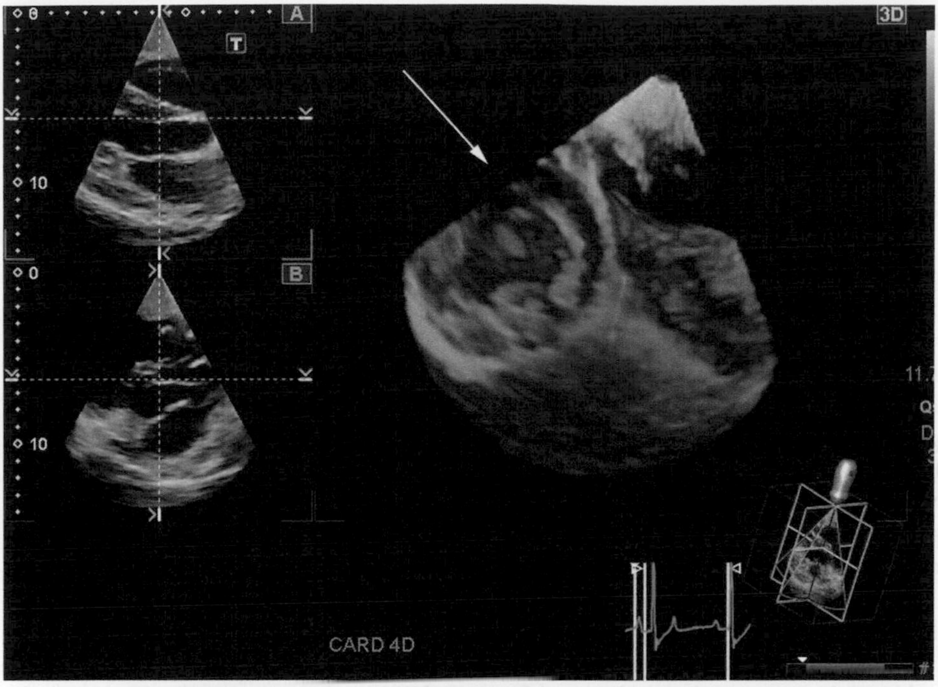

Figure 6.34 A 3-dimensional (3-D) cardiac ultrasound still image of the left ventricle. The typical short-axis left ventricular view can be seen as indicated by the arrow. The left side of the image shows the two guiding beams that the operator uses to align the ultrasound volume. The lower right corner shows an image of orientation of how the operator has rotated the image volume to see the desired structure. The main image (under the arrow) shows the left ventricle and right ventricle. The right ventricle is the open space to the right of the left ventricle.

Figure 6.35 Right parasternal long-axis four-chamber image showing an air contrast echocardiogram. An injection of agitated saline was made into a peripheral vein. The microscopic bubbles can be seen entering the right atrium (RA, arrow 1) and in this example crossing through a patent foramen ovale defect to the left atrium (LA, arrow 2). Note the right ventricular hypertrophy consistent with a pulmonic stenosis.

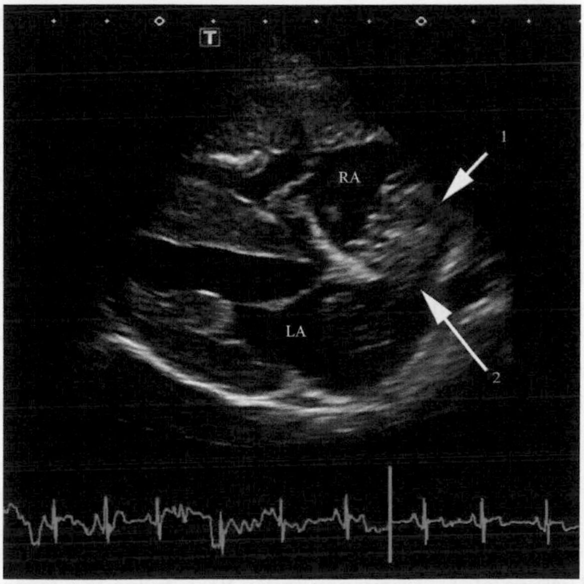

(see Chapter 10) such as Eisenmenger's syndrome, patent foramen ovale, and right to left patent ductus arteriosus.

The Doppler Study

Introduction

Doppler echocardiography is a nonimaging modality of cardiac ultrasound that is used to measure the velocity of blood flow through the heart. Doppler studies may be performed in any vessels of the body, but for the purposes of this chapter the topic will be limited to the heart and great vessels. Doppler echocardiography is another application of ultrasound technology and is typically performed in conjunction with an echocardiogram. Where the echocardiogram creates an image of the heart and provides information about the morphology and systolic function of the heart, the Doppler portion provides hemodynamic information and allows assessment of diastolic function. The Doppler study gives the cardiologist information about the direction and velocity of blood flow. It can also be used to indicate turbulent flow in the heart.

Basic Technology

Doppler studies are simply an advanced form of ultrasound that is specifically designed for blood velocity measurements. Blood is moved through the circulatory system fundamentally by pushing it from a place of high pressure to one of lower pressure. There is a predictable relationship between the pressure and the velocity of blood. By measuring the velocity, the cardiologist can make some conclusions about physiology and prognosis.

Doppler echocardiography makes use of the Doppler shift principle first described by Johann Christian Doppler in 1864. According to the Doppler principle, a sound wave emanating from a moving object as it moves toward a stationary observer will become compressed and apparently increase in frequency; conversely if the object is moving away from an observer the sound waves become rarefied or stretched out and decrease in frequency. This is a phenomenon we all have witnessed when a car passes by our standing position. The degree of frequency shift is directly related to how fast the object is moving. For a Doppler echocardiogram, the sonographer use this principle in the same way a bat uses sonar to hunt for food. An ultrasonic signal is transmitted at a known frequency from the ultrasound probe. When the signal reflects off an object it returns at a different frequency depending on which direction it is moving in relation to the probe; increased if moving toward the probe, decreased if moving away. By calculating the degree of frequency shift the ultrasound computer can measure the speed and direction of blood movement. The following formula is used by the computer to make the calculation:

$$V = \frac{C \times f_d}{2(f_o) \times \cos(\theta)} \tag{6.2}$$

where V, velocity in m/s; C, the average speed of ultrasound waves in soft tissue (1540 m/s); f_d, frequency shift; $2(f_o)$, twice the transmitted velocity; and cos (θ), the

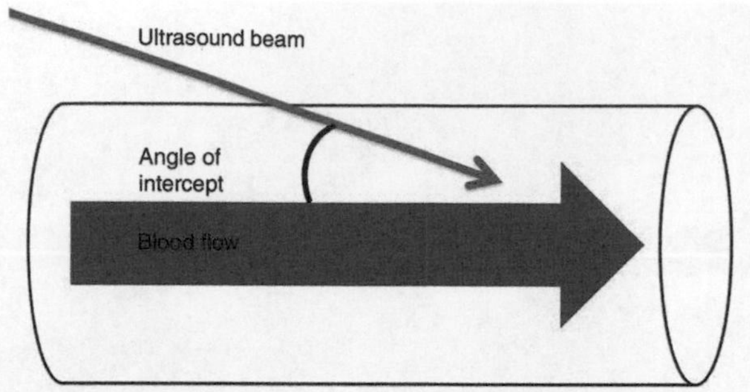

Figure 6.36 Depiction of the angle of intercept concept demonstrating the relationship between the angles of the ultrasound beam in relation to the angle of blood flow through the vessel. The closer the angle of intercept is to 0 degrees or 180 degrees, the more accurate the calculation of blood velocity will be using the Doppler equation. This is sometimes referred to as the "interrogation angle".

cosine of the angle of interrogation, also called intercept angle. The frequency shift is the difference between the transmitted frequency and the reflected frequency.

All the variables in the equation are controlled by the ultrasound machine except for the cos θ. It is the angle that the ultrasound beam strikes its target, in this case the blood pool (Figure 6.36). The most accurate calculations are made when the beam strikes the target at perfect parallel (zero or 180 degrees), and the cosine is equal to 1 or −1. As the intercept angle increases the cosine moves away from 1 and the accuracy of the calculation decreases [1, pp. 3–35]. Once the frequency is programmed into the machine, the angle of interrogation is the only variable in the equation that the operator has any control over. It is critical that the angle closest to parallel be achieved for the most accurate velocity. The operator cannot overestimate a true velocity, but can underestimate one with misalignment outside of pure parallel. Generally, angles of intercept greater than 15–20 degrees are considered unacceptable [1, pp. 3–35]. To facilitate alignment the Doppler study is performed on the left-apical four- or five-chamber view from the left hemithorax (Figure 6.14 and 6.15). This orientation allows for alignment of the Doppler cursor with blood flow heading straight up toward the transducer from the atria and straight down out of the aorta. The PA can be interrogated from a right parasternal short-axis basilar view or the cranial left basilar view (Figure 6.13 and 6.18).

Modalities

Three modalities are commonly used for cardiac Doppler measurements. Spectral Doppler includes pulsed-wave Doppler (PW) and continuous-wave Doppler (CW). Color-flow Doppler uses the same principles but the information gained is displayed as a color signal superimposed atop a 2-D echocardiographic map.

During spectral Doppler interrogation the information generated is displayed on a graph with time along the X axis and velocity on the Y axis. In the center of the graph is a baseline indicating zero flow. Returning ultrasound signals of flow toward the transducer are displayed above the baseline, and signals moving away from the transducer are displayed below the baseline. The baseline can be shifted up or down to create more graph above or below depending on the predominant direction of blood flow being recorded at the time (Figure 6.37). To use Spectral Doppler a cursor is turned on over the 2-D echocardiographic image and aligned with the blood flow to be interrogated and the Doppler of choice activated.

Pulsed wave Doppler is a modality that allows for velocity measurements at a specific location in the heart. A sample volume or "gate" is positioned along the cursor line over

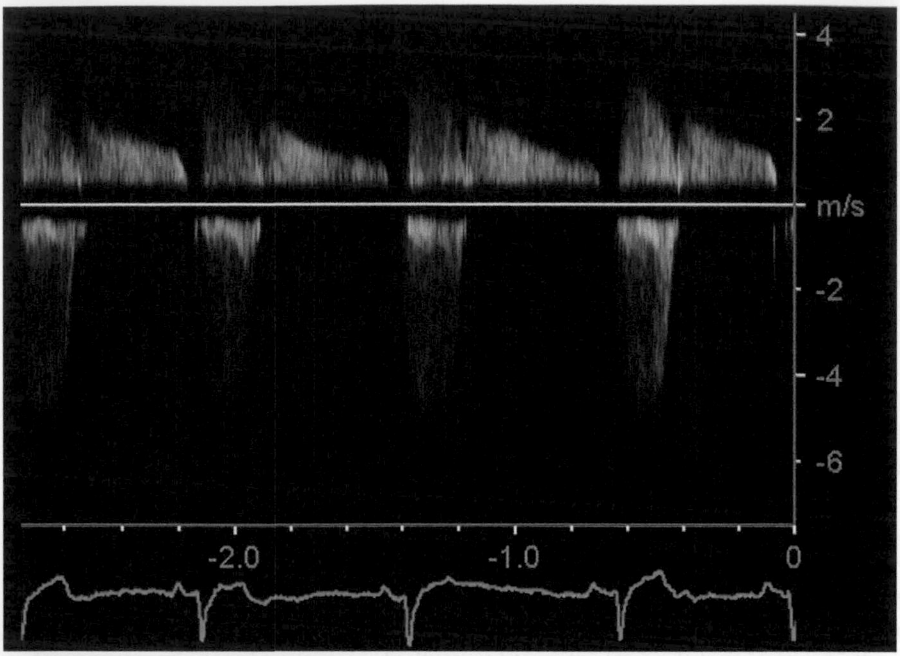

Figure 6.37 Spectral Doppler display: a continuous wave Doppler trace shows the flow toward the transducer above the baseline, and flow away from the transducer below. The X axis of the graph is marked in time with an ECG, and the Y axis is marked in velocity as m/s. The baseline has been shifted toward the top of the screen to allow for inclusion of the complete flow signal below the baseline. The velocity scale has been adjusted to an appropriate velocity scale for the flow represented. The ECG is used to mark the difference between systole and diastole.

the area for velocity measurement. The sample volume is typically reprinted by two lines crossing the cursor line and can be moved up and down the cursor to change the sample depth. The advantage of PW is the ability to record velocities at the specific depth (range specificity), but it can detect only a limited velocity range (Figure 6.38). When the PW Doppler is turned on, a piezoelectric crystal transmits a short pulse of ultrasound waves that travel to the depth designated by the sample volume while the transducer waits, and the reflected data is received by another crystal. This pattern is repeated many thousands of times a second. The number of times the crystal can transmit, shut off, wait for the returning signal and then transmit again is the PRF and represents how many times it can sample per second. The PRF is important because the faster the PRF, the faster a velocity that can be recorded. The time between pulses must be twice the sampling depth. If the returning signal has a frequency shift greater than the PRF, ambiguous information is returned to the computer. There is an inverse relationship of depth to PRF. The farther the sample gate is from the transducer, the lower the PRF due to distance and the slower a velocity can unambiguously be recorded. In essence, the returning signal is faster than the transducers ability to sample, and "*aliasing*" occurs. A similar phenomenon occurs when watching a carriage with spoke wheels move. When the carriage is moving slowly, the spokes turn at a rate slower than the human eyes ability to see them move, but as the carriage speeds up the spokes begin to appear to move backwards. Our minds know the

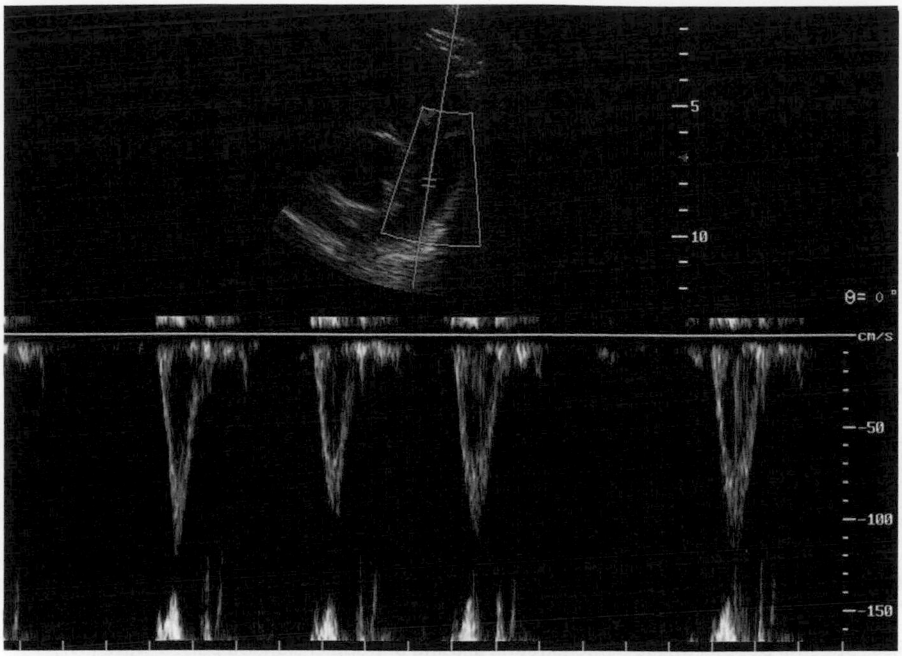

Figure 6.38 A typical spectral pulsed-wave (PW) Doppler flow signal or *envelope*. This example is from blood flow leaving the right ventricle through the pulmonic valve. The envelope is dark in the center indicating laminar flow. If the flow was to be turbulent, the centers of the envelopes would be filled in with reflected signal, indicating blood flow at multiple velocities. In this example, because all the blood accelerates together and decelerates together the signal is intense at the edges, but with very few returning soundwaves in the middle range. A smaller 2-D image is shown above for reference.

carriage is moving forward, yet because our eyes can only sample images at set speed, the spokes appear to move backwards. This known as the *Nyquist limit* and is defined as half of the PRF.

When the Nyquist limit is exceeded with PW Doppler the returning signal is displayed "wrapped around" into the opposite side of the spectral graph (Figure 6.39). The velocity at which aliasing occurs is variable due to probe frequency and depth [1, pp. 3–35]. In the small animal veterinary patient the practical average is 1.5 m/s; with small patients potentially allowing up to 1.7 m/s, and giant-breed dogs limited to about 1.0 m/s.

Continuous wave Doppler allows for measurement of very fast velocities by continuously transmitting and receiving, and is displayed the same as PW Doppler (Figure 6.40). Unlike PW Doppler, that records velocities in one site, the CW Doppler records velocities all along the length of the ultrasound beam. It is impossible for the frequency shift to be greater than the sample rate, which is continuous. This allows for extremely fast velocities to be measured and therefore provides a method of measuring the high velocity blood flow. However, the point along the ultrasound beam where the highest velocity occurs is unknown or "range ambiguous". Continuous wave Doppler is particularly useful in congenital heart disease where flow velocities can easily exceed 2.0 m/s. High velocity jets can be located with the PW Doppler and then accurately quantified by the

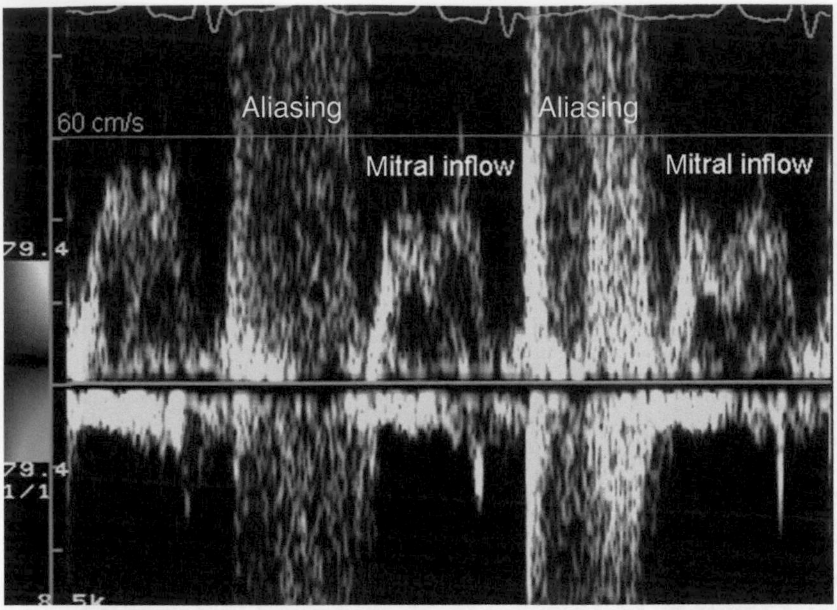

Figure 6.39 Spectral Doppler image demonstrating aliasing of Doppler signal: a pulsed-wave (PW) Doppler recording of mitral regurgitation. The transmitral ventricular filling (mitral inflow) is noted above the baseline in diastole. The "band" of Doppler signal during systole (note ECG at top) is high velocity (4 m/s) and due to the pulse repetition frequency of PW Doppler, the velocity of blood is faster than the echocardiograph's ability to record. The high velocity information gets "wrapped" from the bottom around to the top of the screen and filled in, creating the band of Doppler data. Image courtesy of John Bonagura, DVM, DACVIM.

CW Doppler. Continuous wave Doppler must still be aligned perpendicular to the direction of blood flow for the most accurate calculations. Although CW Doppler does not have a sample volume, a single line crossing the cursor is noted on most ultrasound machines. The line allows the two crystals in use to be focused at a particular region of interest.

Color-flow Doppler also known as color-flow mapping (CFM), is an advanced form of PW, but rather than the returning signal being displayed on a graph, the information is color coded and displayed atop the 2-D image. In CF Doppler there are a series of PW sample gates alongside each arranged on a plane (Figure 6.41). The ultrasound machine detects the velocity in all the sample volumes in rapid succession along with the 2-D images returning to the machine. Obviously this takes an enormous amount of computing power. Color flow Doppler can be enhanced by using the most narrow 2-D sector and smallest CFM window possible.

When the CFM feature is initiated a box appears over the 2-D echocardiographic image. This box can be moved over the region of interest and size adjusted. The colors of red and blue are traditionally used to display directions of blood flow. These colors are easily visible over the black blood pool aiding interpretation [7]. The conventional coding is: blue for away from the transducer and red for toward the transducer (Figure 6.42). The acronym BART (Blue Away; Red Toward) is often used. It is thought that this standard comes from the early use of CFM for investigating carotid blood flow in

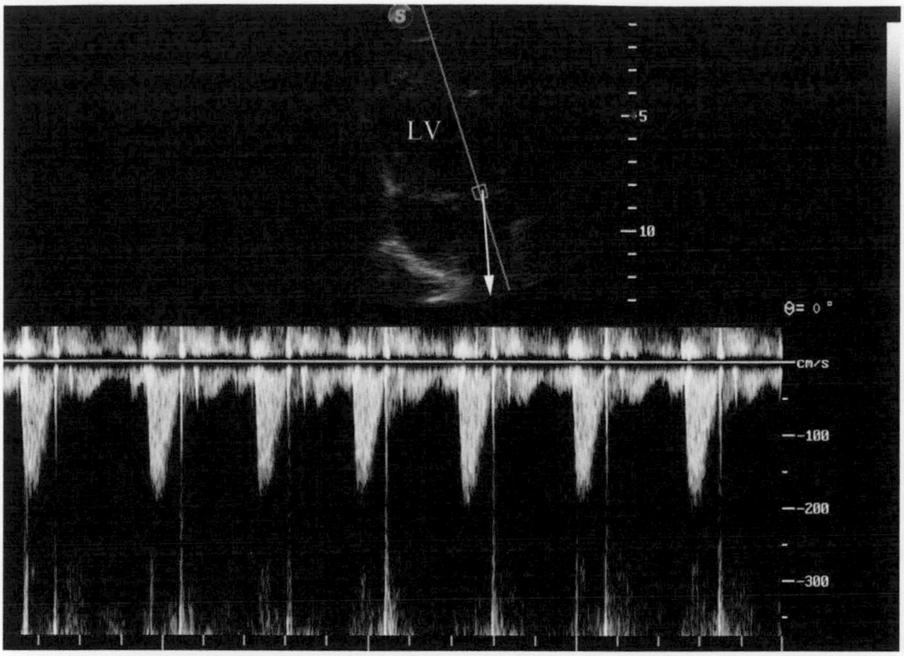

Figure 6.40 Spectral continuous wave (CW) Doppler: the measurement of aortic flow from the left apical long-axis five-chamber view. The green line indicates the path of the Doppler ultrasound beam. The white arrow shows the path of blood flow out of the aorta. The angle between the two is the angle of intercept. The yellow Doppler envelopes are projected down from the baseline indicating flow away from the probe. Because CW Doppler records all velocities down the sampling path, the low velocity are displayed with the other signal-making the envelopes uniformly filled in (compare with Figure 6.38).

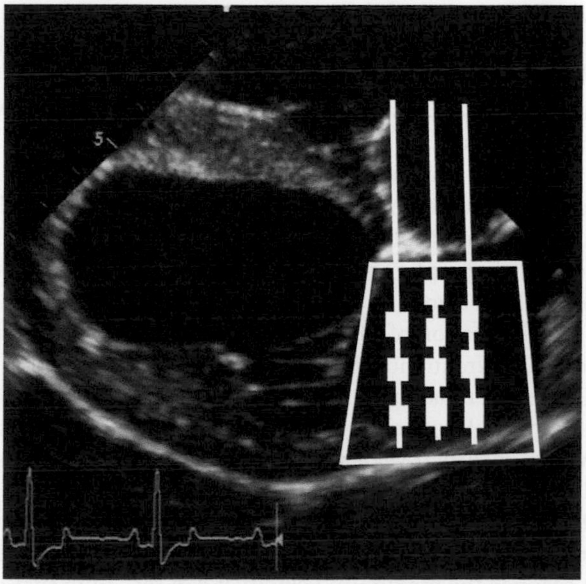

Figure 6.41 Pulsed wave sample volumes for color-flow Doppler: the white boxes and lines are an illustration of how the pulsed wave (PW) Doppler technology is used for color-flow mapping. This representation shows the concept only. The actual number of PW sample volumes is in the hundreds to thousands within the region of interest. Each sample volume is color-coded individually to display blood direction and velocity.

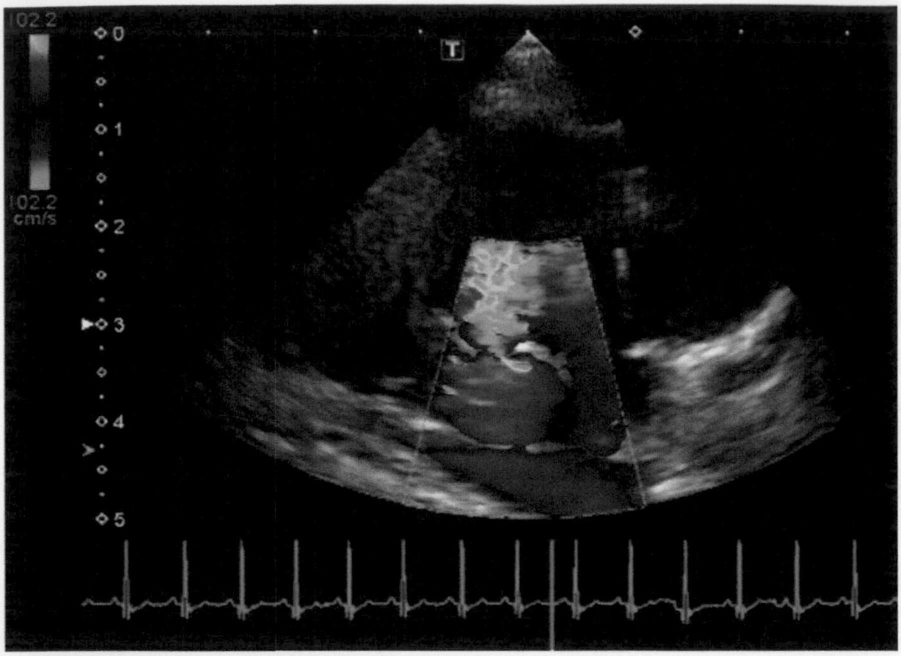

Figure 6.42 Color-flow mapping (CFM) Doppler. This example is from a patient with patent ductus arteriosus (PDA). The red signal marks blood flow toward the transducer from the aorta through the PDA. The blue signal indicates blood flow away from the transducer in the main pulmonary artery. The yellow–green mosaic represents turbulent blood flow of the high velocity transductal flow mixing with the pulmonary outflow. A small region of color aliasing can be seen just above the red section and below the turbulent flow, where the flow signal wraps from red to blue on the color wheel.

which flow toward the transducer was in the carotid artery and flow away was in the jugular vein [8]. Color flow Doppler allows the speedy identification of both normal and abnormal flow. It aids in the alignment of the PW or CW Doppler cursor for velocity measurements. It also helps locate and estimate the severity of valvular regurgitation or cardiac shunts.

An added feature of CF Doppler is variance (Figure 6.42). Variance is the term used for turbulent blood flow, which is normally laminar in the heart. Turbulence is simply blood moving in multiple directions at multiple velocities. To demonstrate turbulence most echocardiographs add a yellow–green mosaic color map interspersed with the standard red or blue signal.

The limitation of CF Doppler is that it is also subject to aliasing. As with PW when the returning frequency shift is greater than twice the PRF, then the signal gets "wrapped". In CF Doppler that means a change in color. The colors selected by the computer occur on a color wheel, with shades of blue on one half and shades of red on the other (Figure 6.43). As the recorded velocity increases in CFM, the intensity of the color increases in that direction or color. If the recorded velocity exceeds the PRF then the computer will take the next color on the color wheel. For example, if the CF signal is looking at flow away from the transducer, it will code the returning signal in blue of intensifying color until it reaches the maximum velocity it can record in that direction (the Nyquist limit) then it will use the next color in the wheel which will be a shade of red. Adjustments to the

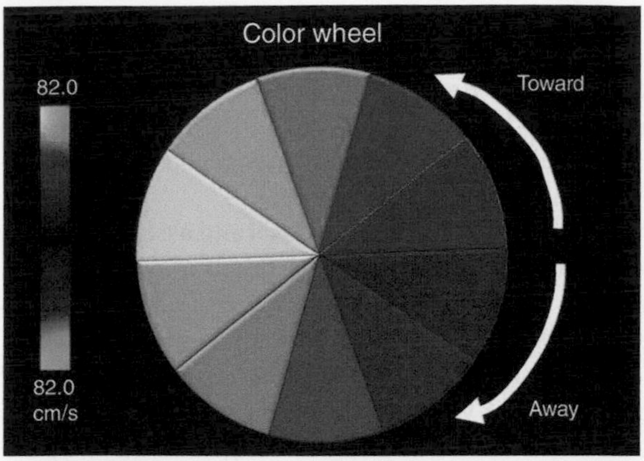

Figure 6.43 The color wheel for color-flow mapping including the color bar on the left along with the velocity scale (82 cm/s). The colors on the wheel correspond with a particular flow velocity. The arrows indicate the "zero" flow side. As blood velocity recording moves up the scale, the color that corresponds to the particular velocity will be shown on the screen. If the velocity is greater than the scale in that direction, the computer takes the next color crossing over to the colors in the opposite direction. For example if a velocity recorded is 100 cm/s toward the transducer, the computer will bypass all the red colors around the top of the wheel, and end up with the first blue color to the far left of the wheel. The recorded velocity is just over the velocity scale of 82 cm/s, thus there are not enough red colors available, and the computer will wrap all the way around to the blue shades. The crossover to the next color is *aliasing*. Source: Weyman (1994). Adapted with permission of Lippincott Williams and Wilkins.

depth of the color box, shifting the CFM baseline, or some changes in PRF may correct this problem, but only to a point. The operator will need to understand that aliasing is occurring, and not wrongly interpret the information.

Interpretation of Doppler-Derived Velocities

The practical use of Doppler echocardiography is for the determination of blood velocity from one chamber of the heart to the next. The velocity can then be used to calculate a pressure gradient (PG or ΔP). As stated earlier, blood movement within the body is based on pushing blood from a chamber of higher pressure to one of lower pressure. In the peripheral arteriole the pressure is slightly higher than the pressure in the venules driving blood through the capillaries. Pressures in the chambers of the heart change during the cardiac cycle, but the pressure of the chamber that blood is moving from will always be greater than the chamber blood is moving to. The ventricles are the driving force for the pressures in their respective systems. For example, the LV generates a pressure greater than is in the aorta during diastole to open the AV and move blood into the aorta. The velocity of blood moving from one chamber to the next is directly related to the pressure gradient by the modified Bernoulli equation:

$$PG = 4 \times V^2$$

where V is velocity in metres per second. The pressure gradient is expressed in millimetres of mercury (mmHg). The operator must understand normal cardiac physiology, especially normal cardiac chamber pressures (see Chapter 8, Table 8.3) to interpret the findings. For example, it is known that a normal velocity out of the aorta in dogs is 1.0–2.3 m/s [1, pp. 531–557]Using the Bernoulli equation indicates peak PG from the LV to the aorta is approximately 4–12 mmHg. Assuming the aortic systolic pressure is approximately 120 mmHg at peak systole, then the LV is generating a peak pressure of 124–132 mmHg. This is a normal workload for the LV.

Doppler-derived velocities have three main uses: (1) the diagnosis and assignment of severity of a stenosis of the ventricular outflow valves; (2) the estimation of chamber pressure in shunts; and (3) the noninvasive estimation of pulmonary arterial pressures.

If velocity is significantly increased via PW or CW Doppler as blood crosses the AV then subaortic stenosis is present (see Chapter 10). The velocity and calculated PG are then used to assign severity. For example, if the velocity recorded by CW Doppler is 5 m/s then using the modified Bernoulli equation a PG of 100 mmHg exists ($[5 \times 5] \times 4 = 100$). A 100 mmHg PG means the LV must then generate an extra 100 mmHg of pressure to move blood past the aortic obstruction. This represents a twofold increase in the workload of the ventricle indicating a subaortic stenosis (the normal 125 mmHg + the 100 mmHg of the stenosis). The same function is used for the pulmonic valve to diagnose and assign severity to pulmonic stenosis.

Another application of Doppler-derived pressure gradients is the estimation of normal or abnormal chamber pressures. In the case of a ventricular septal defect, Doppler can be used to detect pressure equilibration in the ventricles. An understanding of normal physiology is critical. In the normal heart, the LV systolic pressure is approximately 120–125 mmHg, and the right ventricular systolic pressure is approximately 25 mmHg. Using the Bernoulli equation to work out the velocity, with the known pressure difference between the two ventricles being approximately 100 mmHg, the operator will record a velocity at or close to 5 m/s if the ventricles still have their normal pressure (100 mmHg $/4 = 25 \rightarrow \sqrt{25} = 5$ m/s). This implies a patient whose heart is still compensating for the shunt. If the velocity recorded is significantly below 5 m/s, then decompensation may be occurring. Likewise, with mitral regurgitation (MR), the velocity of the MR jet should be 5 m/s or above since the LA pressure should be 5–10 mmHg during ventricular systole, and the LV pressure should be 125 mmHg. If the LV to LA pressure gradient is significantly below 5 m/sec, then the LV is not able to generate its normal pressure.

In cases of patent ductus arteriosus (PDA), both CW and CFM Doppler are of great benefit. In patients with PDA, blood is continuously flowing from the aorta into the main PA. By placing a CFM Doppler box over the main PA a continuous turbulent color signal will be seen and is diagnostic for PDA. The CW cursor can then be placed in the PDA aperture and a velocity through the PDA measured. The normal aortic pressure is 120–125/80 mmHg and the normal PA pressure is 20–25/10 mmHg. If the patient is well compensated, then this PG should be close to 100 mmHg. If the patient is decompensating then the trans-PDA velocity will be below 5 m/s typically indicating lower than normal aortic pressure and a failing LV.

A third application for Doppler is estimation of chamber pressures "downstream" of two adjacent chambers. This feature is used by interrogating the tricuspid regurgitation (TR) velocity to obtain a PG that can be used to estimate PA pressure. Pulmonary arterial pressures can otherwise only be determined by the invasive means of direct catheterization. First, the operator must determine the PG between the RV and the PA. If no pulmonic stenosis is present, then the peak PG from the RV to the PA would be approximately 4 mmHg. With a RV to PA pressure gradient of 4 mmHg the operator can stipulate that the RV pressure and the PA pressure are the essentially same (RV mmHg = PA mmHg). This is a commonly accepted rule of physiology as seen in published normal cardiac chamber pressures [9, 10]. The operator uses CFM to locate TR and if present measures its velocity using PW or CW Doppler. If no TR is present then this application of Doppler is unavailable.

The PG of the TR indicates the pressure difference between the RV and the RA. It was stipulated earlier that peak RV pressure is equal to peak PA pressure during systole. Therefore the PG between the RV and the RA is equal to the PG between the PA and the RA. The average normal pressure of the RA is about 5 mmHg. For blood to move through the TV it must overcome the existing 5 mmHg in the RA. The resulting TR pressure gradient added to the right atrial 5 mmHg will equal the estimated PA pressure.

An example would be a TR velocity of 4 m/s. The PG between the RV and the RA would be calculated as 64 mmHg using the modified Bernoulli equation. The 64 mmHg pressure gradient is added to the estimated RA pressure of 4–5 mmHg making a total RV pressure of 68–69 mmHg. As stipulated earlier the RV peak pressure is equal to the PA peak pressure. The conclusion is the PA pressure is also approximately 68–69 mmHg. Normal pulmonary arterial pressure in systole is reported to be 20–25 mmHg [9], therefore a pressure of 64 mmHg is indicative of pulmonary hypertension.

In addition to these uses of Doppler echocardiography, assessments of diastolic function can be made. By looking at filling patterns of the LV, and flow through the pulmonary veins as they enter the LA, the veterinary cardiologist can make some observations about relaxation of the ventricle. Doppler modalities can also be used to look at the isovolumic relaxation time; the time between the closing of the AV and the opening of the MV as a measure of cardiac relaxation. In advanced cardiac disease the isovolumic relaxation time will increase in length with decreased relaxation of the ventricle. For the interested sonographer, there are many other methods of assessing diastolic function that are beyond the scope of this text.

References

1 Boon, J.A. (2011) *Veterinary Echocardiography*, 2nd Edition. Wiley-Blackwell, Oxford.

2 Rishniw, M. and Erb, H.N. (2000) Evaluation of four 2-dimensional echocardiographic methods of assessing left atrial size in dogs. *Journal of Veterinary Internal Medicine*, **14**, 429–435.

3 Jacobs, G.J. and Knight, D.H. (1985) M-mode echocardiographic measurements in non-anesthetized cats: effects of body weight, heart rate, and other variables. *American Journal of Veterinary Research*, **46**, 1705–1711.

4 Otto, C.M. (2004) Left and Right Ventricular Systolic Function, in *Textbook of Clinical Echocardiography*. Elsevier Saunders, Philadelphia. pp. 131–165.

5 Serres, F., Chetboul, V., Tissier, R. *et al.* (2008) comparison of 3 ultrasound methods for quantifying left ventricular systolic function: correlation with diseases severity and prognostic value in dogs with mitral valve disease. *Journal of Veterinary Internal Medicine*, **22**, 566–577.

6 Fine, D.M., Selting, K., Backus, R.C. *et al.* (2014) Hemodynamic and biochemical alterations in dogs with lymphoma after induction of chemotherapy. *Journal of Veterinary Internal Medicine*, **28**, 887–893.

7 Weyman, A.E. (1994) Principle of color flow mapping, in *Principles and Practices of Echocardiography.* Lippincott Williams & Wilkins, Philadelphia. pp. 218–255.

8 Abramovich, G.N. (1963) *The Theory of Turbulent Jets.* Massachusetts Institute of Technology Press, Cambridge.

9 Moscovitz, H.L. and Wilder, R.J. (1956) Pressure events of the cardiac cycle in the dog: normal left and right heart. *Circulation Research*, **4**, 574–578.

10 Guyton, A.C. and Hall, J.E. (1996) Overview of the circulation; medical physics of pressure, flow and resistance, in *The Textbook of Medical Physiology*, 9th Edition. W.B. Saunders, Philadelphia. pp. 161–169.

7

Blood Pressure Measurement and Systemic Hypertension

H. Edward Durham, Jr.

Introduction

Systemic hypertension is defined as a sustained, abnormally elevated arterial or systemic blood pressure (ABP). This is different than pulmonary hypertension, which is not discussed in this chapter. This chapter will focus on systemic hypertension in small animal medicine. Systemic hypertension is a condition that has been reported in 30% of people [1] as well as in dogs, cats, cattle, horses, and other animal species [2, 3]. Unlike high blood pressure in humans, which is commonly a primary condition (or essential hypertension), hypertension in veterinary medicine is typically caused by other systemic diseases. Known as *secondary hypertension,* it is thought to occur in approximately 20% of the cat population [4], but is less prevalent in dogs [5].

The prevalence of hypertension tends to be much higher in cats with certain diseases. According to published research, 60–65% of cats with chronic renal failure have been reported to have hypertension [6, 7]. Hypertension is most prevalent in cats over the age of 10 years [8, 9] which may be due in part to a loss of elasticity of the vasculature in older cats [10], and to the increased incidence of renal failure in this age group. There is no gender or breed predilection for feline hypertension [5, 8].

Obesity has been associated with hypertension in dogs [11]. Variation of ABP due to the breed in dogs has also been reported [5,12]. Sight hounds may have a slightly higher ABP and small breed dogs slightly lower than reported normal values. Variations due to age, gender, and breeding status may also be present [13].

Hypertension is known as a "silent" condition because clinical signs are not apparent, and serious organ damage may occur before any clinical signs become obvious. Untreated systemic hypertension can lead to serious and irreversible damage to a number of major organ systems. This so-called *end-organ* damage most often affects the brain, eyes, heart, and kidneys [14].

Measurement of ABP has become more common since the advent of accurate non-invasive instruments. The equipment required to measure ABP is affordable and easy to operate. Blood pressure measurement can easily be obtained by a trained veterinary technician. Blood pressure should be measured in patients that are: syncopal, geriatric, have renal insufficiency, receiving diuretics or other cardiac medication, and any patient whose clinical presentation is suggestive of systemic hypertension (e.g. vision loss).

Cardiology for Veterinary Technicians and Nurses, First Edition. Edited by H. Edward Durham, Jr.

Arterial Pressure and Regulation

The exact definition of "normal" blood pressure is somewhat variable. In reality, every heartbeat generates a slightly different blood pressure. When we discuss ABP, we are really referring to the average of many beats over time. The underlying concern is to understand what the *mean arterial pressure* (MAP) is over time. Blood pressure is discussed in terms of the cardiac cycle; systolic and diastolic. During cardiac systole, the ABP is at its instantaneous peak. During diastole the closed aortic valve keeps the ABP from dropping. This ensures that the ABP will always be sufficient to provide forward flow through the capillaries for perfusion.

The MAP is roughly the average pressure in the arterial system during one cardiac cycle. It is the product of cardiac output (CO) and systemic vascular resistance (SVR). Cardiac output is the volume of blood the heart pumps in one minute; and is the product of heart rate (HR) and stroke volume (SV). Stroke volume is the amount of blood ejected during one cardiac cycle. If either HR or SV increases, more blood volume is pumped into the arteries, which in turns causes ABP to increase (Figure 7.1). Systemic vascular resistance is determined by the arterial system, and can be controlled by vasoconstriction or vasodilatation of the arterioles. As the arterioles constrict, resistance increases, increasing the pressure in the arterial system. In contrast, arteriolar dilation decreases resistance, lowering the overall pressure. Therefore, changes in either CO (determined by HR and SV) or SVR can affect blood pressure.

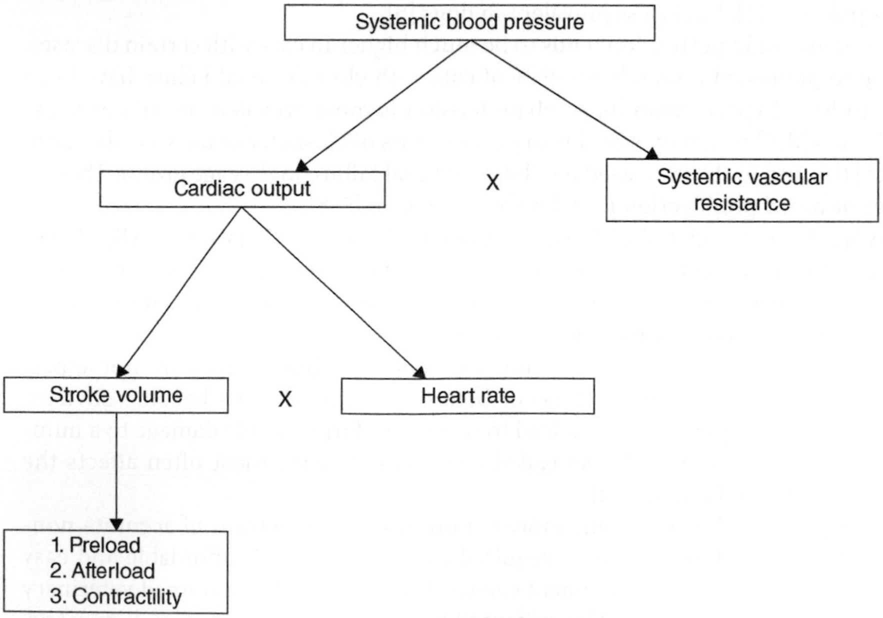

Figure 7.1 The determinants of arterial blood pressure. Blood pressure is the product of cardiac output multiplied by systemic vascular resistance. Cardiac output is the product of stroke volume multiplied by heart rate. Stroke volume is determined by the cardiac preload, the cardiac afterload and ventricular contractility.

Measuring CO in everyday practice is not practical in every patient. Estimates of MAP can be done by measuring systolic arterial pressure (SAP) and the diastolic arterial pressure (DAP) then calculating the "mean". This can be done simply using the formula:

$$\text{MAP} \approx (\text{SAP} - \text{DAP})/3 + \text{DAP} \quad (7.1)$$

However, this is not the mathematical average of the SAP and DAP. During one cardiac cycle, the pressure spends more time closer to the diastolic pressure than the SAP [15]. The calculation is taken from "area under the curve" of a direct arterial pressure trace. As HR goes up and the curve trace narrows, the MAP becomes closer to the arithmetical average.

Regulation of Arterial Pressure

Regulation of systemic blood pressure is critical to maintaining homeostasis. Disruptions in systemic blood pressure, such as hypotension and hypertension, can result in detrimental health outcomes. Hypotension decreases tissue perfusion, delivery of oxygen and nutrients, and delay the removal of metabolic waste. Hypertension can damage the organs as noted above. Mechanisms controlling blood pressure can be divided into two categories: a rapid responding short duration system, and a slower responding, yet longer in duration system. Both systems utilize manipulation of one or more components discussed previously.

The rapidly responding, shorter duration mechanism is mediated predominantly through changes in HR and SVR. The slower response, longer duration mechanism acts primarily via changes in SV by increasing total vascular volume and vasoconstriction or dilation.

Heart rate and SVR can be changed rapidly by the influence of the sympathetic nervous system (SNS). Baroreceptors, located primarily in the aorta and carotid arteries, sense changes in tension of the arterial walls, which is associated with changes in ABP. As pressure changes, the baroreceptors directly stimulate or inhibit the vasomotor center of the brain through the SNS, which causes vasoconstriction of the arterioles; thus increasing SVR. Stimulation of the SNS will also directly increase HR leading to increased CO and subsequently ABP.

An alternative method of ABP regulation is performed by chemoreceptors. Chemoreceptors are located in the proximal aorta and the carotid arteries in clusters of cells known as *aortic* and *carotid bodies*, respectively. These nerve terminals are sensitive to hypoxia, acidosis, hyperkalemia, and hypercapnia in the blood [16]. When specific chemical changes are detected, generally due to a drop in ABP, chemoreceptors can directly stimulate the vasomotor center of the brain to re-establish normal ABP.

The relatively slower responding, yet long-lasting effects of the renin-angiotensin-aldosterone system (RAAS), is regulated by the kidneys. This complex system of hormones allows the kidney to regulate vascular volume and electrolytes to aid in control of blood pressure. In addition, RAAS also impacts vascular and sympathetic neurologic tone, and can influence blood pressure via both CO and SVR. The RAAS is activated by decreases in renal perfusion and sympathetic stimulation from the baroreceptors. These stimuli cause the release of hormones in a cascade-like fashion (Figure 7.2). When the kidneys detect a decrease in their perfusion, renin is released. Renin is then combined with a plasma protein to form angiotensin-I, which is converted

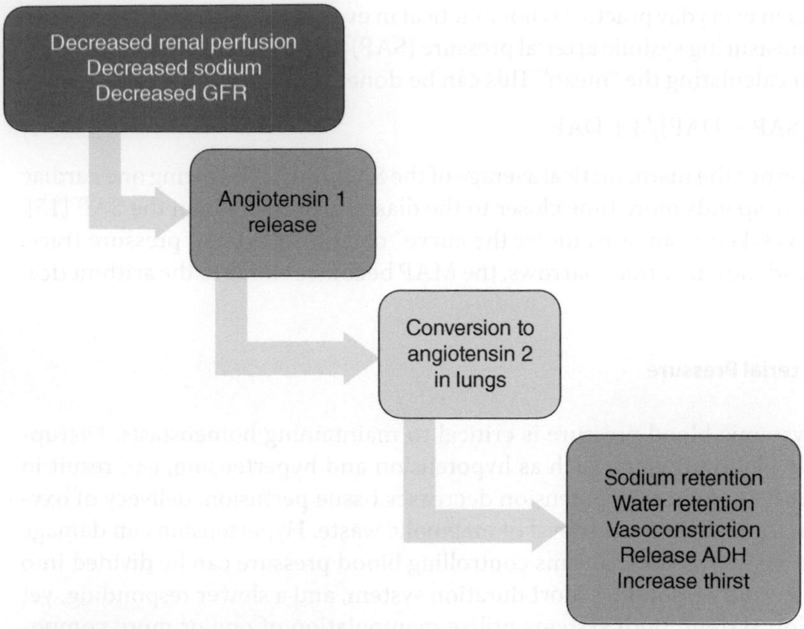

Figure 7.2 Cascade of events in the renin–angiotensin–aldosterone system (RAAS). Decreased glomerular filtration, decreased renal perfusion, and decreased sodium detection in the kidneys will incite the release of renin. Renin in turn stimulates the release of angiotensin-I. Angiotensin-I is converted to angiotensin-II in the lungs. Angiotensin-II is a potent vasoconstrictor, directly stimulates the sympathetic nervous system, stimulates the thirst center of the brain, releases antidiuretic hormone (ADH), and aldosterone. Antidiuretic hormone blocks the removal of water by the kidneys, and aldosterone retains sodium and water to increase vascular volume.

in the lungs to angiotensin-II. Angiotensin-II causes peripheral arterial vasoconstriction, increased heart rate through SNS stimulation, sodium and water retention to retain circulating volume, and stimulates thirst. Angiotensin-II causes the release of aldosterone from the adrenal glands, which further conserves sodium contributing to fluid retention. Activation of RAAS increases both blood volume (increasing SV) and vascular tone (SVR) to increase blood pressure. It generally takes RAAS about 24 hours to exert its full effect [17]. If the RAAS is suppressed, decreased blood volume and vasodilation will occur (see Chapter 15).

A simplified example of how both blood pressure regulation systems work would be a patient with acute blood loss. The sudden loss of blood volume causes the blood pressure to decrease. The baroreceptors, stimulated by the drop in ABP, increases heart rate almost immediately. The RAAS is triggered by the baroreceptors and by the direct effects of hypotension on the kidneys. Activation of RAAS results in profound vasoconstriction, water and sodium retention by the kidneys, and increased thirst. The net result of these responses is an expansion of the blood volume to maintain blood pressure.

Measurement of Blood Pressure

Measurement of ABP in animals was first performed in 1733 by Stephan Hales in a horse by directly catheterizing the mare's arterial system. Since that time, AP measurement techniques have improved in both sophistication and ease. Arterial blood pressure is usually expressed SAP over DAP; and when appropriate, MAP is included. Arterial blood pressure is expressed in millimeters of mercury (mmHg).

Although palpation of arterial pulses is an important part of the physical examination, blood pressure cannot reliably be estimated by feeling pulses. Hypotension can sometimes be indicated by "weak" pulses, but hypertension is not detectable. Pulse palpation (PP) reflects the pulse pressure, or the difference between the systolic and diastolic pressure (SAP – DAP = PP). Pulse pressure is not the same as blood pressure [17]. Patients can be hypotensive or hypertensive and have normal feeling pulses, provided the difference between the systolic and diastolic pressures is normal. To determine ABP, it must be measured.

Measuring ABP may be done directly (*invasively*) or indirectly (*non-invasively*). Invasive ABP measurement involves placing a needle, or catheter, into an artery. This catheter is then connected via saline-filled line to a pressure transducer (see Chapter 8). The pressure transducer converts the mechanical fluctuations in the fluid into an electrical signal that can be displayed on a physiological monitor with an oscilloscope or charted on a paper trace (Figure 7.3). This method is considered the "gold standard" of blood pressure measurement. This method requires sedation or general anesthesia for

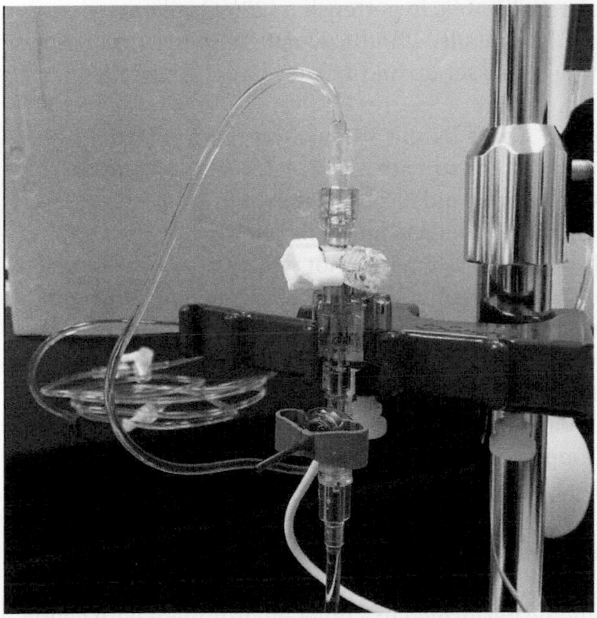

Figure 7.3 Physiological monitoring pressure transducer. The pressure transducer in this picture has a flush line that enters from the bottom, and a patient line that exits from the top from a four-way stopcock. Between the purple flush wings and the white turn valve is the chamber with the transducer membrane enclosed. One side of the membrane receives fluid oscillations from the arterial catheter. The opposite side of the membrane interfaces with the electronics that convert the motion and force of the arterial pulse into an electrical signal that can be displayed on a monitor. The cable to the monitor is seen as the white line below the transducer behind the flush valve. The monitor will generally display systolic, diastolic and mean arterial pressure with a pressure wave form. Most modern monitors capable of direct arterial measurement will also calculate the patient's pulse rate.

catheter placement. It is very useful for intra-operative monitoring and critical patients in the intensive care unit. Complications include: infection from the catheter, thromboembolism, or serious hemorrhage should the catheter become dislodged. The complications and need for substantial equipment render direct ABP measurement unsuitable for routine or outpatient use.

Indirect methods rely on some system to detect blood flow under or past a pressurized cuff. The three most popular systems are the Doppler flow detector sphygmomanometery method, oscillometric systems, and, the photoplethysmographic method. Doppler flow detected sphygmomanometery and the photoplethysmographic methods both rely on the Riva-Rocci principle [5] of detecting flow past a pressurized cuff attached to an aneroid, or mercury manometer, to estimate ABP. The oscillometric method records the motion (oscillations) of the artery under a pressurized cuff to measure blood pressure.

All three systems tend to slightly underestimate ABP when compared with invasive recordings, yet are considered clinically reliable since they are consistent over a wide range of pressures [18]. Each system has advantages and limitations. The Doppler method is very quick to perform, but is a poor estimator of diastolic pressures [18, 19]; however, SAP readings below 100 mmHg correlate well with MAP in cats [20]. Using the systolic pressure alone to manage clinical cases is acceptable since it has been reported that hypertension in cats is usually systolic alone, or systolic and diastolic but is rarely diastolic alone [7, 21]. Additionally, human medicine reports no increased risk of morbidity or mortality in the face of isolated diastolic hypertension [22]. Oscillometric systems measure the systolic and diastolic pressures, and calculates the mean pressure. Oscillometric systems are "hands free" once set up and will display the heart rate, but take more time to perform [23].

The photoplethysmographic method works by the attenuation of an infrared beam directed at the artery and a pressurized cuff to estimate ABP [24,25]. This system has the advantage of giving a continuous ABP reading and has been shown to be quite accurate in recording "beat to beat" variation [24]. Although at least one photoplethysmographic system has been validated in cats [18], these systems are not widely used in veterinary medicine. The cuffs for the photoplethysmographic system are designed for the human finger. Consequently, the size of the patient is limited to those under 10 pounds, and the cuffs don't always fit appropriately [26]. The device requires up to a minute to obtain a signal, making it less than ideal for awake patients [24]. There are also reports of difficulty obtaining readings in cats with darkly pigmented skin [5, 19]. A practical approach for device selection is to use the Doppler flow method for conscious patients and the oscillometric method for anesthetized patients.

Technique of Recording Arterial Blood Pressure

Recording ABP by any method should be performed in a quiet environment with gentle handling to minimize patient stress. Dimming the lighting, relocating to a quiet section of the veterinary hospital, and limiting unnecessary conversation enhances the procedure. The pressure cuff should be placed on a relatively cylindrical portion of the patient's extremities. Optimal sites for cuff placement include: the forelimb just proximal to the carpal joint, the rear limb either just proximal or just distal to the tibiotalar joint (hock), or the proximal tail [27]. Measurements of ABP should be done with the limb, cuff, and flow detector/device at the same level as the heart. Gravity does have an effect on ABP

Table 7.1 Common errors in measuring blood pressure.

Technical error	Consequence
Cuff overly wide	Falsely low reading
Cuff overly small or narrow	Falsely high reading
Cuff not placed snugly	Falsely elevates reading
Cuff placed over a joint	Less likely to compresses artery
Hole in cuff	Pressure leaks too fast to reliably record
Cardiac arrhythmias	Erratic readings

if the limb is below or above the heart. It is recommended that patients be in lateral or sternal recumbency, as standing encourages the patient to move about more. However, if the patient must stand to obtain an ABP measurement, it is recommended that the tail be used, as measurements on any other extremity require that limb to be lifted to the level of the heart.

Cuff selection is paramount to good technique in any system. A cuff that is too large will give erratic readings that tend to underestimate ABP, and a cuff that is too narrow will lead to falsely high readings [27,28]. Correct cuff size is related to the circumference of the limb on which the ABP is being measured. For dogs, cuff width should be 40% of the limb circumference [19,29]. For cats, a cuff width of 30% of limb circumference may be more appropriate [30]. Estimating limb circumference should be avoided. The circumference of the limb should be measured in centimeters with a soft, pliable measuring tape. The most common errors in measuring blood pressure are related to cuff selection [31]. Other factors leading to erroneous results are summarized in Table 7.1. When the objective measurement dictates a cuff size between two available cuffs, the wider of the two should be selected. The degree of error created by the cuff being slightly oversized is less than the degree of error created by an undersized cuff [29].

Doppler Flow Detected Sphygmomanometery

The Doppler flow detection method has been shown to be effective at measuring systolic ABP in cats and dogs using an inflatable human pediatric-infant cuff [19,28,32]. The Doppler flow detector utilizes an ultrasound crystal to detect the Doppler shift of blood moving through the artery (see Chapter 6 for a more detailed explanation of the Doppler shift). This method is very similar to the method used in human medicine. The technique uses the Riva–Rocci principle by having the nurse listen for the sound of blood flow (known as Korotkoff sounds) with a stethoscope past the cuff as the pressure is slowly released. The cuff is attached to an aneroid manometer, or mercury sphygmomanometer, to display the pressure. The cuff on the patient arm is inflated until no Korotkoff sounds are audible. As pressure is released from the cuff, the Korotkoff sounds become audible indicating the systolic pressure, and vanish again when the diastolic pressure is reached. In veterinary patients, Korotkoff sounds are inaudible and the Doppler crystal is employed to detect flow instead of a stethoscope. Ultrasound coupling gel is placed on the contact surface of the Doppler crystal, which is then placed distal to the cuff over the artery (Figure 7.4). The characteristic pulsatile flow signal should be audible. As the cuff

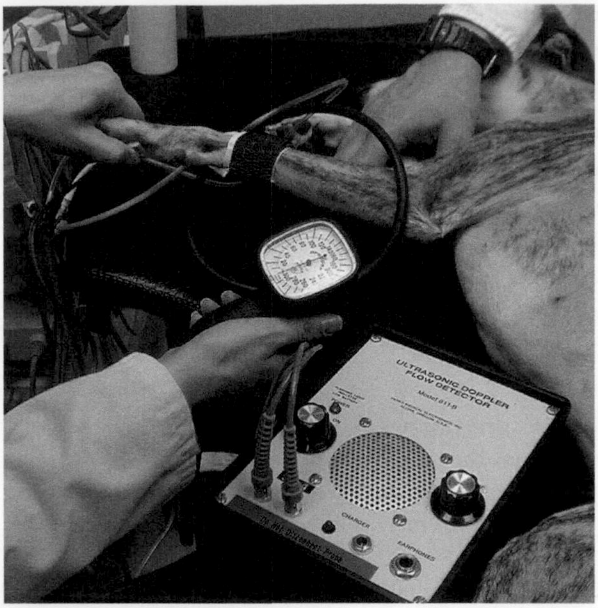

Figure 7.4 A Doppler sphygmomanometer. The operator pictured here is holding the Doppler probe on a superficial artery distal on the chosen limb to the occlusion cuff. The appropriate cuff is placed on a cylindrical anatomical site and secured if desired. The cuff is attached to an aneroid sphygmomanometer. The Doppler crystal is used to locate a pulse; then the cuff is inflated with the manometer until the Doppler pulse sound becomes inaudible. The pressure in the cuff is gradually released by a control valve on the manometer, until the first Doppler pulse sound is heard. The return of flow at the pressure in the cuff indicated by the sphygmomanometer corresponds with the systolic arterial blood pressure. See text for greater detail. (Ultrasonic Doppler Flow Detector, Model 811, Parks Medical Electronics Inc., Aloha, OR, USA. http://www.parksmed.com/.)

is inflated to a pressure greater than that of the ABP, the flow signal is lost. As the pressure in the cuff is slowly released, the flow signal will return. The first audible instance of the flow signal returning corresponds with the systolic blood pressure [33].

The equipment for the Doppler flow detected sphygmomanometery is inexpensive and easy to use, but operator technique is crucial. Cuff selection, cuff placement, and interpretation of results should all be performed carefully. A fundamental principle of all noninvasive ABP measurement is that the pressure recorded is inside the cuff when blood flow is detected, not in the vessel itself. This pressure is used to approximate ABP. The cuff should be placed snugly on the limb. Failure to do so will require extra cuff pressure to occlude flow through the artery creating a falsely high reading. If the cuff is placed over a joint, the artery may not be compressed, preventing disappearance of the Doppler flow signal. This may be misinterpreted as an ABP greater than 280 or 300 mmHg (pressures of this magnitude are rarely seen in animals).

Technical difficulties can arise in attempting to locate the flow signal with the Doppler crystal. Weak audible signal can often be attributed to insufficient coupling gel, hair interfering with the signal, or the crystal not being optimally placed over the artery. Signal is improved by clipping the site where the Doppler crystal is placed and using liberal amounts of coupling gel. Once the signal has been located, gentle manipulations of the crystal can be used to optimize the signal.

Heart rate variability and arrhythmias can add to the difficulty in interpreting the readings. As previously mentioned, every heartbeat generates its own pressure in the arterial system. When ABP is reported as "120 over 80 mmHg", it is assumed that this is an average of many heartbeats. The presence of an arrhythmia will affect the ABP of individual heartbeats. In dogs with sinus arrhythmia, the ABP of heartbeats after the longer R to R intervals will be higher than the ABP of the more rapid beats. This is a result of the longer diastolic period of the slower HR. In the event of a premature ventricular complex, little or no blood is ejected from the left ventricle. The following heartbeat will have a much higher ABP once again due to extra volume available for that heartbeat. This is known as *postextrasystolic potentiation* [34]. This effect is exaggerated with arrhythmias, such as atrial fibrillation or ventricular tachycardia. These rapid rhythms do not allow for normal filling of the ventricle during diastole, and consequently, causes widely varied stroke volumes of individual beats. Some beats will be transmitted at significantly higher pressures than others and be detected earlier as cuff pressure is released (Figure 7.5). These so-called "breakthrough" beats can be as much as 40–60 mmHg greater than other impulses. In patients with significant arrhythmias, breakthrough beats should not be used as the sole determinate of ABP. Since the majority of beats are at a lower pressure, it is reasonable to make clinical decisions based on the pressure at which the majority of heartbeats are heard most consistently.

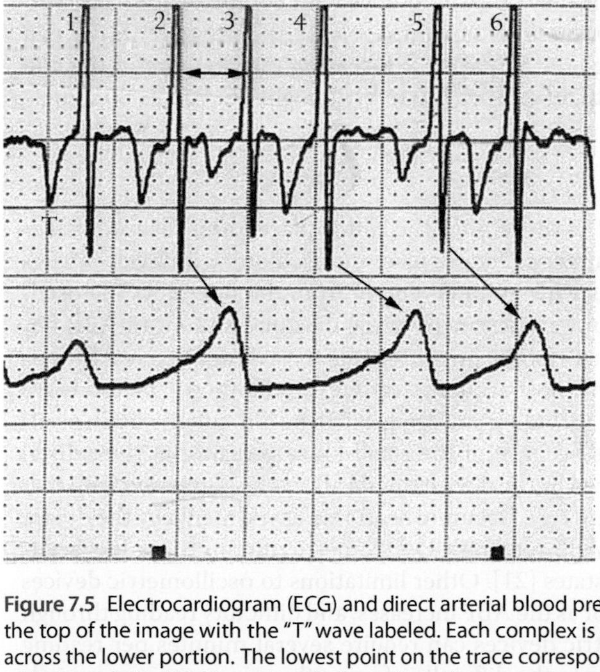

Figure 7.5 Electrocardiogram (ECG) and direct arterial blood pressure (ABP) trace. The ECG is seen at the top of the image with the "T" wave labeled. Each complex is also labeled 1 to 6. The ABP trace is across the lower portion. The lowest point on the trace corresponds to the diastolic ABP, and the peak with the systolic ABP. The arrows indicate the pulse trace generated by individual complexes. The pulse wave directly under complex 1 was generated by the previous QRS not shown, and no pulse was generated by complex 1. Due to the long diastolic period created by no ventricular outflow on complex 1, complex 2 shows a higher peak systolic pressure. Notice the short R to R interval between complex 2 and 3 (double ended arrow). Likewise complex 3 does not generate a pulse thus the output of complex 4 also shows a high peak systolic pressure. Complex 5 comes after the ventricle has had time to fill and a pulse is generated but at a less amplitude than the previous complexes. The pulse signal for complex 6 is not shown.

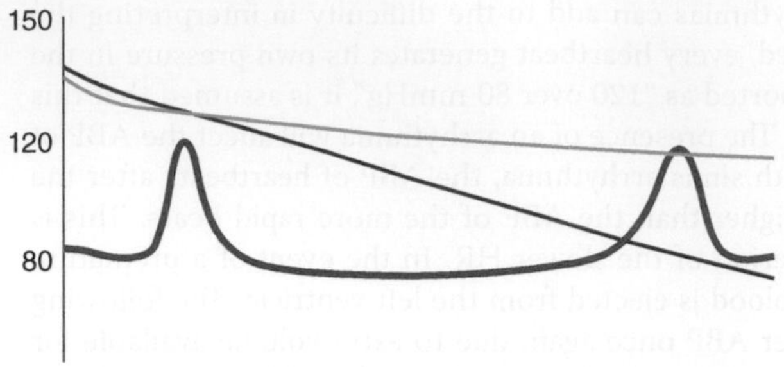

Figure 7.6 Rapid cuff deflation effect. During Doppler flow-detected sphygmomanometery the patient's heart rate dictates the speed of cuff deflation. In bradycardic animals, the cuff must have a very gradual drop in pressure to avoid "overshooting" the true arterial blood pressure (ABP). The red line in this diagram indicates the direct ABP trace. The blue line represents the cuff pressure released too rapidly in a bradycardic patient. The green line shows a more gradual cuff pressure release. Notice the blue line is at ~80 mmHg when the first pulse is detected. This indicates the blood flow is occurring, but because the pressure in the cuff is well below the true ABP, an underestimation occurs. By utilizing a flatter release slope (green line), when the first pulse appears, the pressure on the cuff will be closer to the peak systolic pressure.

Patients with profound bradycardia may present a unique problem to the Doppler method of ABP measurement. This may be seen in dogs with complete atrioventricular block. Since the HR is so slow, the operator must release the pressure in the cuff very slowly to avoid "overshooting" the actual ABP. Releasing the pressure in the cuff too quickly, can result in a dog with an ABP of 120 mmHg might be read as 80 mmHg (Figure 7.6).

Oscillometry Blood Pressure Measurement

The convenience of the "hands off" feature once the cuff is placed and secured makes oscillometry a convenient tool in surgery. Once in place the oscillometric device inflates the cuff and performs the readings with no intervention from the operator. The oscillometric method provides an accurate assessment of the diastolic and mean ABP, but somewhat underestimates the actual systolic pressure [18]. The average of five ABP values determines oscillometrically the most accurate reading. Oscillometric methods are very susceptible to motion artifact, including shivering. It can be difficult to obtain oscillometric readings in cats, perhaps because of the small pulse pressure in their distal arteries [18]. The heart rate measured by the device should always be compared with that of the patient by auscultation (Figure 7.7). Accurate heart rate assessments by the device correlate with the most accurate ABP readings. Oscillometric methods are less accurate than Doppler in hypotensive states [21]. Other limitations to oscillometric devices include an increased margin of error as the ABP increases, and difficulty reading through profound arrhythmias. Oscillometric devices can require several minutes per reading to acquire the measurement adding to the difficulty of using them in conscious animals [20].

High-Definition Oscillometry

High-definition oscillometry (HDO) blood pressure devices hold promise for eliminating some of the problems encountered with traditional oscillometric devices [5]. The

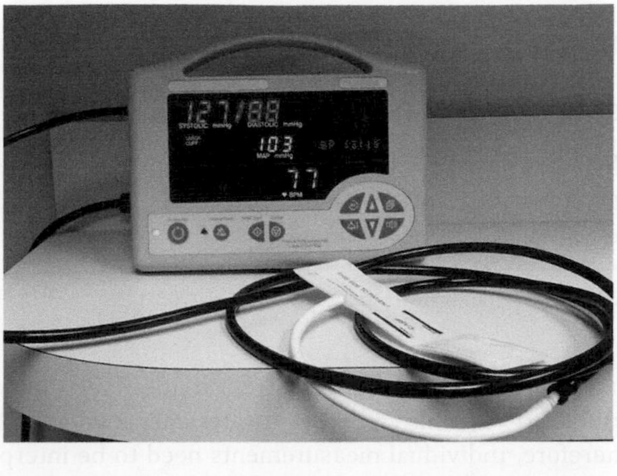

Figure 7.7 An oscillometric blood pressure device showing the systolic/diastolic ABP, the mean ABP, and the pulse rate. The patient cable and cuff can be seen in the foreground. (Cardell 9401 Veterinary Blood Pressure Monitor, CAS Medical Systems, 44 East Industrial Road, Branford, CT 06405, USA. http://www.casmed.com/.)

classic oscillometric device was taken from human medicine and repackaged for the veterinary market. The HDO was developed specifically to address the need for ABP assessment in small animals (Figure 7.8). This device has been validated when compared with invasive ABP measurement in accordance with the American College of Veterinary Internal Medicine (ACVIM) consensus panel validation criteria [35]. It currently is the only noninvasive device to meet the validation criteria.

One unique feature of the HDO is the ability to connect it to a computer and using the provided software, see a graph of the oscillations recorded by the device. If a characteristic bell-shaped curve of data is recorded, the ABP measurement is valid. This helps quickly eliminate reading that are contaminated by movement artifact.

Normal Blood Pressure

The definition of "normal" blood pressure in dogs and cats is not exact. Blood pressure is variable from moment to moment and should be viewed within a range. The methods of ABP measurement (direct vs indirect), temperament and age of the patient, intra-

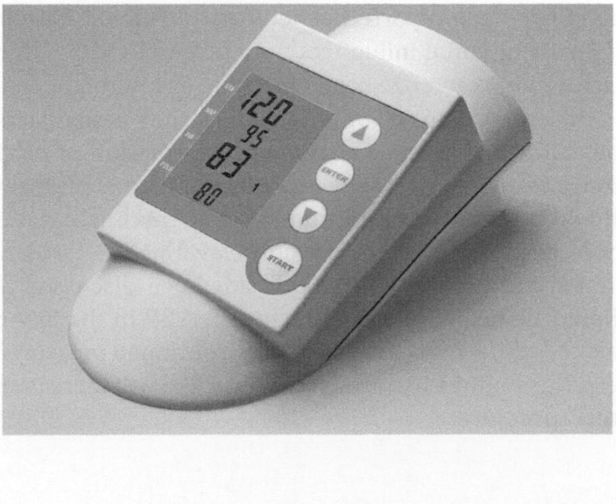

Figure 7.8 The HDO high definition oscillometric blood pressure device. The device was specifically designed for small animal veterinary medicine, and is the only non-invasive ABP measurement system that has been validated as accurate in small animal medicine (see text) (HDO Vet BP Monitor, DVM Solutions 16201 San Pedro Avenue, Suite 200 San Antonio, TX 78232, USA. http://dvmsolutions.com/memodiagnostic.htm.)

Table 7.2 General guidelines for classifying hypertension in animals.

Stage of hypertension	Measured value (mmHg)
Mild hypertension	>150/95
Moderate hypertension	>160/100
Severe hypertension	>180/120

Source: data from Brown, Atkins, Bagley *et al.* (2007) [39].

and interpatient variation, setting variation, sedation, and concurrent diseases all contribute to variability in ABP in veterinary medicine. Many factors influence ABP and therefore, individual measurements need to be interpreted in the proper clinical context. It has been purposed that an average normal for canine is ~133 mmHg systolic over ~75 mmHg diastolic; and for felines, ~124 mmHg over ~84 mmHg [33]. Sight hounds exemplify the breed variation seen in dogs with an average ABP of 149 mmHg over 87 mmHg [5]. Small breed dogs usually have normal ABP slightly above large breed dogs.

The ABP of cats in the veterinary clinic ranges from 120 to 140 systolic and 70 to 90 diastolic, with a mean of about 110 mmHg [36, 37]. Several studies have investigated the effects of hypertension and its links with systemic disease. An average value that each researcher used as the definition of hypertension is 165 mmHg [38]. Systemic hypertension has been defined as systolic pressures from 140 to 185 mmHg or above, with 160 to 180 mmHg most often defining the lower limits of hypertension. One epidemiological study of blood pressure in 203 cats showed ocular changes due to hypertension occur at a systolic pressure of 177.3 ± 28.7 mmHg [8]. In 2002, the Veterinary Blood Pressure Society announced some general guidelines for classifying hypertension in animals into mild, moderate, and severe categories (Table 7.2). These guidelines were later adopted by the American College of Veterinary Internal Medicine in 2007 [39]. One must keep in mind that these are guidelines and that patients in the mild, or even moderate, categories may only need treatment of the underlying disease. Patients in the severe category require prompt antihypertensive therapy to prevent or treat end-organ damage [5].

A phenomenon known as "white-coat" hypertension has been reported in people in whom the patient's blood pressure is elevated simply due to having it measured. This effect has been reported in veterinary patients as well [11, 39, 40]. Given the spectrum of environmental influences on a given blood pressure measurement, it may be more useful to characterize blood pressure as low, high, or "reasonable".

After recording an abnormal ABP in any patient, a determination must be made as to the validity of that measurement. Affirmation of proper technique should be verified. Improper cuff placement or technical errors can provide false data. The patient's HR should be assessed for rate and cardiac rhythm. A patient that is tachycardic suggests an increased level of stress, possibly elevating ABP, which may not be abnormal. The effect of arrhythmias on ABP has already been discussed. A series of five or more readings should be taken. A steady decline in ABP in the first one or two values can be suggestive of "white-coat" hypertension. Continued measurement until three to five repeatable readings (within 10 mmHg) are obtained will increase the likelihood for determining the "real" pressure.

When elevated ABP measurements are obtained, it is appropriate to repeat the measurement on another limb or the tail. If both readings are reasonably close, then the ABP recorded is probably real. If the readings are widely different, 40–60 mmHg, then it is likely that an error was made in one of the recordings. In true systemic hypertension, the elevated ABP should be repeatable over time. A single recording of an elevated ABP is not necessarily suggestive of hypertension. A diurnal effect has been reported [41] and immediate stress can greatly increase ABP. Ultimately, the diagnosis of hypertension relies on an elevated systemic ABP that can be reproduced and fits the clinical setting (e.g. retinal detachment or renal failure).

Pathophysiology

Systemic hypertension is most often secondary to other systemic diseases. Primary hypertension may exist, but is rare, and its diagnosis depends on excluding all other known causes of hypertension. Disease conditions which change the heart rate, vascular resistance, or blood volume affect ABP and could cause systemic hypertension (Table 7.3).

Sympathetic nervous activity from hyperadrenocorticism or hyperthyroidism increases heart rate leading to increased CO, which can cause systemic hypertension. Chronic renal failure is the most common cause of hypertension, especially in cats. Renal failure can cause systolic pressures to exceed 200–210 mmHg [7, 19]. Diabetes mellitus causes hypertension in people, but diabetic hypertension may be much less common in cats [42]. Some causes of hypertension in people, such as obesity, have been reported in dogs [11], and chronic anemia in cats. Hyperaldosteronism increases vascular volume through the effects of aldosterone on sodium and water retention.

Systemic Effects on Target Organs

There are four major organ systems that are adversely affected by systemic hypertension: the kidneys, brain, eyes, and heart. The kidneys are important because not only can renal

Table 7.3 Diseases associated with hypertension.

Disease or condition	Mechanism of action
Renal disease	Volume expansion sodium retention and/or activation of the RAAS (↑ stroke volume)
Hyperthyroidism	Increase heart rate via increased sympathetic nervous activity (↑ heart rate)
Pheochromocytoma	Increased cardiac output via increased catecholamine production (↑heart rate and stroke volume)
High-salt diet	Volume expansion via sodium retention (↑stroke volume)
Diabetes mellitus	Volume expansion via increased glucose (↑stroke volume)
Hyperaldosteronism	Volume expansion from increased aldosterone (↑stroke volume)

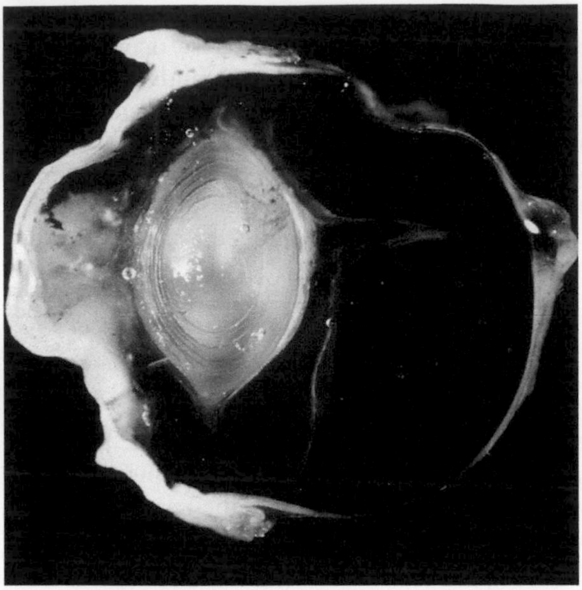

Figure 7.9 An eyeball showing a detached retina. The lens is toward the left and the retina can be seen billowing behind it to the right. Image courtesy of Elizabeth A. Giuliano, DVM, DACVO.

failure cause systemic hypertension, but the chronic hypertension leads to glomerulosclerosis. This leads to a decrease in the glomerular filtration rate causing activation of the RAAS. The sodium and water retention following RAAS activation increases the ABP creating a pathologic loop, which further damages the kidneys. It is recommended that ABP be measured regularly in any patient with chronic renal disease.

In people, hypertension is a cause of cerebral vascular accidents (CVA), more commonly known as "stroke". Signs of CVA include: seizures, ataxia, disorientation or abnormal mentation, tremors, nystagmus, head tilt, and paraparesis. Such signs have been documented in some hypertensive cats [43, 44]. In one description of systemic hypertension in cats, multifocal arteriosclerosis and focal hemorrhage consistent with CVA in the brain of two cats was described at necropsy [45]. In another study, of three cats with neurologic signs and hypertension, computed axial tomography scan results were normal but signs abated after treatment for hypertension [46].

At systolic blood pressures in excess of 200 mmHg, loss of vision may occur [6,43,47]. Cats are often presented to the veterinarian for running into furniture, or wandering aimlessly through the house. The elevated ABP can cause dilation and leakage of the arterioles of the retina [34]. Physical examination of the eyes may reveal retinal or vitreal hemorrhage, hyphema, tortuous vessels in the retina, or partial or completely retinal detachment (Figure 7.9). Although the degree of hypertension necessary to cause hypertensive retinopathy is unknown, ocular changes can be seen with sustained systolic pressures as little as 160 mmHg [46]. Arterial blood pressures should be measured in every cat with retinal detachment or sudden vision loss. Adequate control of hypertension may or may not result in regained vision. The sooner therapy can be initiated after retinal detachment, the better the outcome.

High blood pressure increases the afterload on the left ventricle, increasing the pressure generated. This increase in work causes the left ventricular wall and intraventricular septum to hypertrophy. The hypertrophy causes thickening toward the inside of the heart (concentric hypertrophy), reducing the ability of the heart to fill appropriately during diastole. To maintain a normal CO, the heart rate increases adding more work to the left ventricle, but typically does not lead to congestive heart failure [33]. Abnormal heart sounds, such as a gallop, may be ausculted, but do not appear to correlate with the degree of hypertrophy [5]. During a routine physical examination, the gallop may be the first indication of systemic hypertension. Blood pressure measurement for patients with cardiac gallops is recommended, especially cats. Hypertrophic cardiomyopathy or any other heart disease does not cause hypertension, but systemic hypertension can cause heart disease, which can alert the clinician to the condition.

Treatment

Management of systemic hypertension in veterinary medicine focuses on treating the underlying illness. In some cases, medical therapy to control ABP is necessary while the initiating disease is being investigated to prevent end-organ damage. The goal of treating systemic hypertension is to decrease the magnitude of the hypertension and the risk of end-organ damage (Table 7.2). The specific treatment will need to be tailored to the individual patient due to their specific underlying disease. Sodium restriction is not generally recommended [33]. Severe salt restriction will activate the RAAS, encouraging conservation of sodium and water that can increase ABP. Patients who have high salt diets may benefit from transition to a moderate salt diet. Certain medication may be better suited for specific conditions, such as beta-blockers for patients with hyperthyroidism. Aldosterone receptor blockers (ARB) are best suited for treating hyperaldosteroneism. Surgery is indicated for pheochromocytoma. Treatment to manage systemic hypertension specifically may possibly be withdrawn once the causative condition is controlled. Future monitoring of ABP is always recommended.

The pharmaceuticals available to treat hypertension are directed at reduction of CO or SVR. The most widely used drugs for treatment of hypertension in cats is the calcium channel blocker, amlodipine besylate [41, 47, 48]. Amlodipine is an arteriodilator that has little effect on heart rate or blood volume. Rapid in onset of action, amlodipine selectively affects the calcium channels of the arteries, but not the heart itself, minimizing adverse effects. Even though amlodipine is effective at controlling ABP in cats, it has not been shown to increase survival [49]. Amlodipine therapy may also activate the RAAS, and co-therapy with angiotensin-converting enzyme inhibitors (ACEI) in cats with renal failure is an option [33].

Angiotensin-converting enzyme inhibitors are widely selected for treatment of hypertension in dogs. This class of drug has renal and cardiac protective properties against the effect of angiotensin II and aldosterone, which slightly lowers ABP. These pharmaceuticals also reduce proteinuria, which has been associated with better outcomes [33]. Beta-blockers and diuretics are widely used in human medicine to treat hypertension. They are not typically first-choice therapy in veterinary medicine, but have use for specific cases. Diuretics are particularly useful in cases of volume overload (as seen with edema) that causes systemic hypertension. The treatment of hypertensive retinopathy with furosemide alone is not effective, and may actually be detrimental [50].

Overdose of the aforementioned drugs can cause hypotension, so monitoring of ABP in patients receiving these drugs is critical. The American College of Veterinary Internal

Medicine (ACVIM) consensus panel on systemic hypertension recommends follow-up monitoring within 1–3 days for patients at high risk of end-organ damage [33,39]. Blood pressure should be checked about 1–2 weeks after starting therapy until normal ABP is established, and then every 1–4 months as dictated by the needs of the patient. It generally is not necessary to institute emergency therapy since hypertension occurs on a spectrum. Simply reducing the risk of end-organ damage is sufficient in most cases. Only patients with rapid onset of progressive organ damage, such as encephalopathy, need aggressive emergency therapy.

Client education is a substantial part of therapy. Making sure that clients understand what systemic hypertension is, what to watch for (e.g. blindness), and the goal of therapy are important for positive outcomes. They should be instructed how to watch for the signs of hypotension, which include lethargy, exercise intolerance or weakness, and possibly anorexia related to prescribed medications. If these signs are observed, veterinary care should be sought as soon as possible.

References

1 Hajjar, I. and Kotchen, T.A. (2003) Trends in prevalence, awareness, treatment, and control of hypertension in the United States, 1988–2000. *Journal of the American Medical Association*, **290**, 199–206.

2 Giddens, W.E., Combs, C.A., Smith, O.A. and Klein, E.C. (1987) Spontaneous hypertension and its sequelae in woolly monkeys (Lagothrix Lagotricha) (Abstract). *Laboratory Animal Science*, **37**, 750–756.

3 LeBlanc, P.H., Eicker, S.W., Curtis, M. and Beehler, B. (1987) Hypertension following etorphine anesthesia in a rhinoceros (Diceros Simus) (Abstract). *Journal of Zoo Animal Medicine*, **18**, 141–143.

4 Syme, H.M., Barber, P.J., Markwell, P.J. and Elliott, J. (2002) Prevalence of systolic hypertension in cats with chronic renal failure at initial evaluation. *Journal of the American Veterinary Medical Association*, **220**, 1799–1804.

5 Egner, B., Carr, A.J. and Brown, S. (eds) (2003) *Essential Facts of Blood Pressure in Dogs and Cats*. BE Vet Verlag, Berlin.

6 Stiles, J., Polzin, D.J. and Bistner, S.I. (1994) The prevalence of retinopathy in cats with systemic hypertension and chronic renal failure or hyperthyroidism. *Journal of the American Animal Hospital Association*, **30**, 564–572.

7 Kobayashi, D.L., Peterson, M.E., Graves, T.K. *et al.* (1990) Hypertension in cats with chronic renal failure or hyperthyroidism. *Journal of Veterinary Internal Medicine*, **4**, 58–62.

8 Bodey, A. and Sansom, J. (1998) Epidemiological study of blood pressure in domestic cats. *Journal of Small Animal Practice*, **39**, 567–573.

9 Henik, R.A. (1997) Diagnosis and treatment of feline hypertension. *Compendium*, **19**, 163–179.

10 Bonagura, J.D. and Stepien, R.L. (2000) Vascular diseases, in *Saunders Manual of Small Animal Practice*, 2nd Edition (eds S.J. Birchard and R.G. Sherding). W.B. Saunders, Philadelphia. pp. 568–576.

11 Bodey, A.R. and Michell, A.R. (1996) Epidemiological study of blood pressure in domestic dogs. *Journal of Small Animal Practice*, **37**, 116–125.

12 Bright, J.M. and Dentine, M. (2002) Indirect arterial blood pressure measurement in nonsedated Irish wolfhounds. *Journal of the American Animal Hospital Association*, **38**, 521–526.
13 Meurs, K.M., Miller, M.W., Slater, M.R. *et al.* (2000) Arterial blood pressure measurement in a population of healthy geriatric dogs. *Journal of the American Animal Hospital Association*, **36**, 497–500.
14 Ware, W.A. (2000) Systemic arterial hypertension, in *Small Animal Internal Medicine*. (eds R.W. Nelson and C.G. Couto). Mosby, St Louis. pp. 193–203.
15 Levick, J.R. (2000) Haemodynamics: pressure, flow and resistance, in *An Introduction to Cardiovascular Physiology*. Arnold Publishing, London. pp. 118–147, 329–352.
16 Guyton, A.C. and Hall, J.E. (1996) Role of the kidneys in long-term regulation of arterial pressure and in hypertension: the integrated system for pressure control, in *The Textbook of Medical Physiology*, 9th Edition. W.B. Saunders, Philadelphia. pp. 221–237.
17 Wagner, A.E., Wright, B.D. and Hellyer, P.W. (2003) Myths and misconceptions in small animal anesthesia. *Journal of the American Veterinary Medical Association*, **223**, 1426–1432.
18 Binns, S., Sisson, D., Buoscio, D.A. and Scheffer, D.J. (1995) Doppler ultrasonographic, oscillometric sphygmomanometric, and photoplethysographic techniques for noninvasive blood pressure measurement in anesthetized cats. *Journal of Veterinary Internal Medicine*, **9**, 405–414.
19 Henrik, R.A. (1997) Systemic hypertension and its management. *Veterinary Clinics of North America: Small Animal Clinic*, **27**, 1355–1372.
20 Caulkett, N.A., Cantwell, S.L. and Houston, D.M. (1998) A comparison of indirect blood pressure monitoring techniques in the anesthetized cat. *Veterinary Anesthesia*, **27**, 370–377.
21 Lesser, M., Fox, P.R. and Bond, B. (2000) Non-invasive blood pressure evaluation in cats with left ventricular hypertrophic diseases. *Journal of Veterinary Internal Medicine*, **4**, 117.
22 Strandberg, T.E., Salomaa, V.V., Vanhanen, H.T. *et al.* (2002) Isolated diastolic hypertension, pulse pressure, and mean arterial pressure as predictors of mortality during a follow-up of up to 32 years. *Journal of Hypertension*, **20**, 399–404.
23 Jepson, R.E., Hartley, V., Mendl, M. *et al.* (2005) A comparison of CAT Doppler and oscillometric Memoprint machines for non-invasive blood pressure measurement in conscious cats. *Journal of Feline Medicine and Surgery*, **7**, 147–152.
24 Stokes, D.N., Clutton-Brock, T., Patil, C. *et al.* (1991) Comparison of invasive and non-invasive measurement of continuous arterial pressure using the Finapres. *British Journal of Anaesthesia*, **67**, 26–35.
25 Yamakoshi, K., Rolfe, P. and Murphy, C. (1988) Current developments in non-invasive measurement of arterial blood pressure. *Journal of Biomedical Engineering*, **10**, 130–137.
26 Tabaru, H., Watanabe, H., Tanaka, H. and Nakama, S. (1990) Non-invasive measurement of systemic arterial pressure by Finapres in anesthetized dogs. *Japanese Journal of Veterinary Science*, **52**, 427–430.
27 Carr, A.J. (1994) Blood pressure measurement in small animal practice. *Veterinary Technician*, **15**, 163–167.
28 McLeish, I. (1977) Doppler ultrasonic arterial pressure measurement in the cat. *Veterinary Record*, **100**, 290–291.

29 Valtonen, M.H. and Eriksson, L.M. (1970) The effect of cuff width on accuracy of indirect measurement of blood pressure in dogs. *Research in Veterinary Science*, **11**, 358–362.

30 Grandy, J.L., Dunlop, C.I., Hodgson, D.S. *et al.* (1992) Evaluation of the Doppler ultrasonic method of measuring systolic arterial blood pressure in cats. *American Journal of Veterinary Research*, **53**, 1166–1169.

31 Ng, K.G. and Small, C.F. (1993) Changes in oscillometric pulse amplitude envelope with cuff size: implications for blood pressure measurement criteria and cuff size. *Journal of Biomedical Engineering*, **15**, 279–282.

32 Chalifoux, A., Dallaire, A., Blais, D. *et al.* (1985) Evaluation of the arterial blood pressure of dogs by two noninvasive methods. *Canadian Journal of Comparative Medicine*, **49**, 419–423.

33 Ware, W.A. (2007) Systemic hypertension, in *Cardiovascular Disease in Small Animal Medicine* (ed. W.A. Ware). Manson, London. pp. 372–384.

34 Cooper, M. and Wayne, M.D. (1993) Postextrasystolic potentiation: do we really know what it means and how to use it? *Circulation*, **88**, 2962–2971.

35 Martel, E., Egner, B., Brown, S.A. *et al.* (2013) Comparison of high-definition oscillometry – a non-invasive technology for arterial blood pressure measurement – with a direct invasive method using radio-telemetry in awake healthy cats. *Journal of Feline Medicine and Surgery*, **15**, 1104–1113.

36 Pedersen, K.M., Butler, M.A., Ersbøll, A.K. and Pedersen, H.D. (2002) Evaluation of an oscillometric blood pressure monitor for use in anesthetized cats. *Journal of the American Veterinary Medical Association*, **221**, 646–650.

37 Detweiler, D.K. (1993) Control mechanisms of the circulatory system, in *Duke's Physiology of Domestic Animals*, 11 Edition (eds M.J. Swenson and W.O. Reece). Cornell University Press, Ithica. pp. 184–226.

38 Durham, H.E. (2005) Arterial blood pressure measurement. *Veterinary Technician*, **26**, 324–339.

39 Brown, S.A., Atkins, C., Bagley, R., *et al.* (2007) Guidelines for the identification, evaluation, and management of systemic hypertension in dogs and cats. *Journal of Veterinary Internal Medicine*, **21**, 542–558.

40 Belew, A.M., Barlett, T. and Brown, S.A. (1999) Evaluation of the white-coat effect in cats. *Journal of Veterinary Internal Medicine*, **13**, 134–142.

41 Brown, S.A., Langford, K. and Tarver, S. (1997) Effects of certain vasoactive agents on the long term pattern of blood pressure, heart rate, and motor activity in cats. *American Journal of Veterinary Research*, **58**, 647–652.

42 Sennello, K.A., Schulman, R.L., Prosek, R. and Siegel, A.M. (2003) Systolic blood pressure in cats with diabetes mellitus. *Journal of the American Veterinary Medical Association*, **233**, 198–201.

43 Maggi, F., DeFrancesco, T.C., Atkins, C.E. *et al.* (2000) Ocular lesions associated with systemic hypertension in cats: 69 cases (1985–1998). *Journal of the American Veterinary Medical Association*, **217**, 695–702.

44 Kyles, A.E., Gregory, C.R., Wooldridge, J.D. *et al.* (1999) Management of hypertension controls postoperative neurologic disorders after renal tranplantation in cats (abstract). *Veterinary Surgery*, **28**, 436–441.

45 Littman, M.P. (1994) Spontaneous systemic hypertension in 24 cats. *Journal of Veterinary Internal Medicine*, **8**, 79–86.

46 Morgan, R.V. (1986) Systemic hypertension in four cats: ocular and medical findings. *Journal of the American Animal Hospital Association*, **22**, 615–621.
47 Mathur, S., Syme, H.M., Brown, C.A. *et al.* (2002) Effects of the calcium channel antagonist amlidopine in cats with surgically induced hypertensive renal insufficiency. *American Journal of Veterinary Research*, **63**, 833–839.
48 Snyder, P.S. (1998) Amlodipine: a randomized, blinded clinical trial in 9 cats with systemic hypertension. *Journal of Veterinary Internal Medicine*, **12**, 157–162.
49 Elliott, J., Barber, P.J., Syme, H.M., *et al.* (2001) Feline hypertension: clinical finding and response to antihypertensive treatment in 30 cases. *Journal of Small Animal Practice*, **42**, 122–129.
50 Tsuboi, S. (1990) Fluid movement across the blood–retinal barrier: a review of studies by vitreous fluorophotometry. *Japanese Journal of Ophthalmology*, **43**, 133–141.

8

Angiography

Barbara P. Brewer

Introduction

Angiography is a medical imaging technique whereby a radiopaque contrast media is injected into the lumen of the vasculature for radiographic observation. It is used to visualize and evaluate blood-filled structures, including arteries, veins, and heart chambers. Angiocardiography refers to contrast injection directly into selected cardiac chambers or great vessels of the heart, to allow for visualization of chamber dimensions, function and communication between chambers of the heart or vessels.

The name "angiogram" originates from the Greek words "angeion", meaning "vessel", and "graphien", meaning "write or record". The radiographic film or image of the vascular or cardiac structure is called the angiograph or more commonly the angiogram. The Portuguese physician and neurologist, Egas Moniz, first developed the technique of contrasted X-ray cerebral angiography in 1927, for the purpose of diagnosing nervous system diseases such as tumors and arteriovenous malformations. Following the introduction of easier vascular access methods (e.g. the Seldinger technique) in 1953, the use of angiography and cardiac catheterization procedures became safer and more widely practiced.

Indications

Prior to the advent of echocardiography, angiography was the gold standard procedure for diagnosing cardiac disease. Today echocardiography with Doppler modality has become the gold standard technique for the diagnosis of both congenital and acquired heart disease. However, angiocardiography remains the most common and vital imaging modality performed during cardiac catheterization. These catheterization procedures are minimally invasive surgeries performed for the purpose of identifying and/or correcting congenital and acquired cardiac or vascular defects, including (but not limited to) patent ductus arteriosus (PDA), atrial septal defect (ASD), ventricular septal defect (VSD), pulmonic stenosis (PS), aortic or subaortic stenosis (AS or SAS), intrahepatic portosystemic shunt (PSS), pulmonary thromboembolism (PTE), and arterial thromboembolism (ATE).

Cardiology for Veterinary Technicians and Nurses, First Edition. Edited by H. Edward Durham, Jr.

During angiography, a radiopaque substance or contrast agent or dye, which absorbs X-rays, is injected into a blood vessel or cardiac chamber. During and immediately following injection of the contrast agent, the injected structures opacify, aka "highlight" or "light up" and are visualized via fluoroscopic radiation (moving X-ray). Subsequently, cardiac and vascular anomalies can be seen and definitively diagnosed, measured, and accurately assessed, usually for the purpose of correction as part of a minimally invasive cardiac catheterization surgery. A "negative" contrast study involves injecting contrast into a chamber that is believed to be receiving an abnormal shunt, such as the right atrium if an ASD is present. When the contrast is injected to fill the right atrial chamber, the shunt volume will displace the contrast. Since this "new" blood has no contrast mixed in, it does not appear in the angiogram. The absence of contrast becomes a positive finding for a left-to-right shunting ASD. This technique can prevent the need to catheterize the systemic circulation reducing the risk to the patient.

Contraindications

Angiography is not recommended in animals that have had known adverse reactions to iodinated contrast media in the past. Patients at increased risk for angiographic procedures include those with severe cardiac disease, heart failure, or pre-existing renal failure. Angiographic studies are not recommended in severely disabled animals or in cats with reduced left ventricular systolic function.

Equipment

Radiographic Equipment

Angiography ideally requires fluoroscopic capability with image intensification to reduce radiation exposure to the operator and assistants. Fluoroscopy is an examination by means of a fluoroscope, which is an instrument that allows visual observation of the form and motion of deep tissue structures of the body, by means of X-ray; it is literally a moving X-ray image, that is viewed in real time on a separate television monitor. A movable radiographic table is desirable to allow for patient positioning under the X-ray beam, without actually moving the animal itself, so that patient position will remain constant throughout the procedure. A means to record, save and play back studies is also necessary. Typically, angiographic studies are recorded either on videotape, 35 mm cinematic film or digitally. The C-arm is one type of fluoroscope that allows for multiple imaging planes without the need to reposition the patient (Figure 8.1).

Iodinated Contrast Agents

Radiopaque contrast material is an essential requirement for the performance of angiograms. All current contrast media that is used for angiography contain iodine as the X-ray absorbing element. These iodinated contrast media are divided into two categories: ionic agents and non-ionic agents.

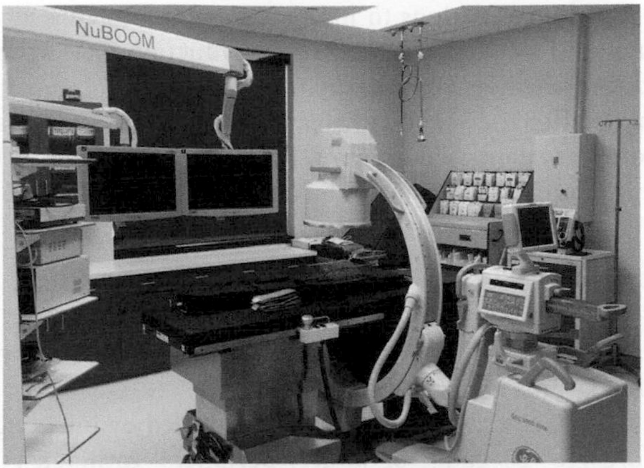

Figure 8.1 Typical fluoroscopy suite. Moving images are displayed on the television monitor and are saved digitally, for playback at regular or slow motion speed. The table is movable in four directions, to allow for constancy of patient position. The unit is operated via a foot pedal.

The older ionic contrast agents are made up of and dissociate into two ions: a negatively charged iodinated anion (e.g. diatrizoate, iodamide, iothalamate, or metrizoate) and a positively charged cation (e.g. sodium or meglumine). Sodium chloride is an example of a common ionic compound, which completely dissociates in water, with each molecule becoming two ions, one sodium and one chloride. The osmotic pressure exerted by a substance is determined by the number of particles in solution. Ionic contrast media like sodium chloride, which dissociate into two separate ions, have a greater osmolarity than that of non-ionic contrast media in which ions do not dissociate in solution. Since ionic contrast media have higher osmolarity, these agents are also hypertonic and tend to draw more solute into the plasma. For this reason, ionic agents present a higher risk, particularly in patients with heart disease, as they have the potential to increase volume overload and induce congestive signs.

Some examples of the older ionic contrast agents include: Renograffin (E.R. Squibb & Sons, Inc., New Brunswick, NJ, USA), Hypaque (Sanofi Winthrop Pharmaceuticals, New York, NY, USA) and Angiovist (Berlex Laboratories, Wayne, NJ, USA).

The newer non-ionic contrast agents do not dissociate into separate ions in solution and therefore have a lower osmolarity. These agents consist of non-ionic dimers such as iodixanol and iotrolan, which have the highest iodine to particle ratio; in the 300–400 mgI/mL range, these agents are close to being iso-osmolar with plasma, and therefore safer to use in cardiac patients. In addition, fewer allergic reactions have been reported with non-ionic contrast agents. Their disadvantages include higher cost and greater viscosity (which can be reduced by warming to 37 °C). Examples of non-ionic contrast agents include: iohexol (Omnipaque, Sinofi Winthrop Pharmaceuticals, New York, NY, USA), iopamidol (Isovue, E.R. Squibb & Sons, Inc., New Brunswick, NJ, USA), metrizamide (Amipaque, Sinofi Winthrop Pharmaceuticals, New York, NY, USA), and ioversol (Optiray, Mallinckrodt, Inc., St Louis, MO, USA).

Recommended dosage of iodinated contrast medium is 400–440 mgI/kg of contrast per injection (or 1.3–1.5 mL/kg Omnipaque 300), injected over 1–2 s using the smallest appropriate syringe [1] Large dogs are optimally injected using an automated power injector. The maximum total dosage of contrast media per study should not exceed 1000–1200 mg iodine/kg (or 3.3–4 ml/kg Omnipaque 300).

Negative reactions to iodinated contrast media include vasodilation (hypotension), arrhythmias, depressed contractile function, exacerbation of existing pulmonary edema (due to the hyperosmolarity of contrast media), renal failure and in rare cases anaphylaxis (after the second exposure to an agent). In human medicine adverse reactions to contrast agents have been reported in fewer than 0.05% of cases, and this number is thought to be even lower in veterinary angiography [1].

Catheters

There are two types of angiograms performed in veterinary medicine: nonselective angiograms and selective angiograms.

A nonselective angiogram is performed by injecting contrast media through a large bore (18–20 gauge or larger) peripheral catheter. For cardiac procedures, a jugular catheter is preferred. Following intravenous injection through the peripheral catheter, the contrast media successively opacifies the vena cava, right atrium, right ventricle, pulmonary arteries, capillaries and veins, left atrium, left ventricle, and aorta. Though the technique is simple, its disadvantages include overlap of opacified structures, making interpretation of individual structures difficult, as well as dilution of contrast as it progresses through cardiac circulation, resulting in poorer opacification of left-sided structures of the heart.

Selective angiography refers to contrast injection at specific sites in which opacification of structures demonstrates flow abnormalities in the region of the injection. In attempting to delineate cardiac abnormalities clearly, the injection of contrast material should be made as close to the abnormality as possible. With the prevalence of echocardiography in veterinary practice today, acquired and congenital cardiac defects typically are diagnosed via echocardiographic examinations. Therefore, selective angiograms are usually performed with prior knowledge of the structures that need to be identified, and into which specific chambers the injection needs to be made. Typically, the injection of contrast media is made into the upstream or preceding chamber or vessel from the defect. Some examples of common locations where angiographic injections are made to highlight the congenital defect are listed in Table 8.1.

Selective angiography or angiocardiography requires specifically designed catheters which depend upon the structures to be catheterized and the purpose of the study. Catheters used for selective angiography should be radiopaque for easy visualization, nonthrombogenic, smooth enough to slide easily through the vessel, flexible enough to bend without causing perforation and stiff enough for control of the tip by manipulation of the proximal end. The most common materials used are Dacron, polyurethane, Teflon, nylon, and polyethylene.

Sizing of Catheters

Catheters and catheter introducers are typically sized using French (F) sizing. The French sizing of catheters refers to the outer diameter of the catheter. One French is equal to 0.33 mm. For cats, most common catheter sizes are 3F to 4F; small dogs generally require 4F to 5F catheters, while for medium and large dogs 5F to 8F or larger catheters are used.

Table 8.1 Examples of angiographic injection locations.

Congenital defect	Structure into which angiographic injection is made
PS	RV
AS	LV
PDA	Thoracic aorta
ASD	LA (in a left to right shunting ASD)
	RA (in a right to left shunting ASD)
VSD	LV (in a left to right shunting VSD)
	RV (in a right to left shunting VSD)
PSS	Caudal vena cava

AS, aortic stenosis. ASD, atrial septal defect. PDA, patent ductus arteriosus. PS, pulmonic stenosis. PSS, portosystemic shunt. VSD, ventricular septal defect. LV, left ventricle. RV, right ventricle. LA, left atrium. RA, right atrium.

Types of Catheters

The type of catheter that is selected depends upon the type of study to be done, as well as the operator's personal experience and preference. Some common catheters used in cardiac catheterization/angiographic procedures include:

1) NIH catheters (with several side holes and a blunt closed tip), Lehman catheters (tapered flexible tip with two side holes proximal to the taper), Berman angiographic catheters (balloon tipped with side holes and no end hole), and the pigtail catheter (multiple side holes proximal to a curled tip with an end hole). These catheters are used for rapid angiographic contrast injections and left ventricular pressure measurement; they should have side holes and either no end hole or a tightly curved tip to avoid recoil and/or penetration of contrast into the endocardium or myocardium during delivery of contrast.
2) Swan–Ganz (balloon-tipped with end hole) is used to measure pulmonary capillary wedge pressure, right ventricular, right atrial and pulmonary artery pressures, cardiac output measurement and blood sampling.
3) Balloon-tipped end and side-hole wedge catheter is used for pulmonary artery injections; this type of catheter can be used to measure pulmonary artery, right ventricular and right atrial pressures, as well as for blood sampling studies (Figure. 8.2).
4) Pigtail catheters should always be used for transversing the aortic valve during angiography and for measurement of pressures primarily in the left ventricle.
5) The Cournand catheter is a flexible catheter with an end hole only; the Goodale–Lubin catheter is a flexible catheter with an open tip and two side holes close to the tip; both of these catheters are used for pressure measurement primarily in the left ventricle and aorta, and for blood sampling.
6) Many multipurpose catheters with various end configurations are available for use, depending on the structure or vessel to be assessed (Figure 8.3).

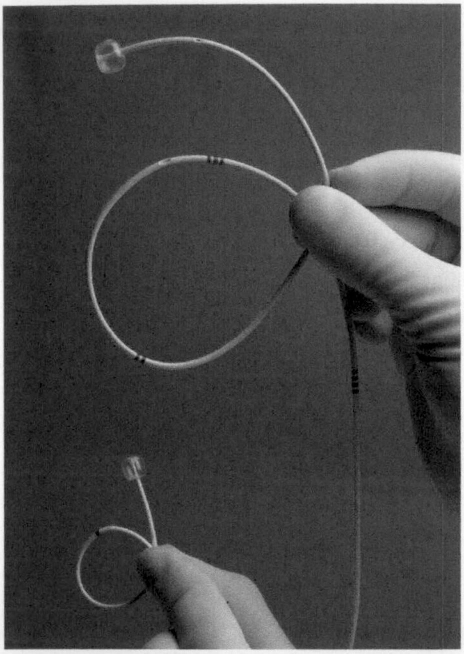

Figure 8.2 Swan–Ganz type pulmonary catheters with balloon tip inflated: 5F (left) and 7F (right). These catheters have an end hole as well as proximal and distal side holes, and are used primarily for right-sided catheterization and pulmonary arterial wedge pressure measurement.

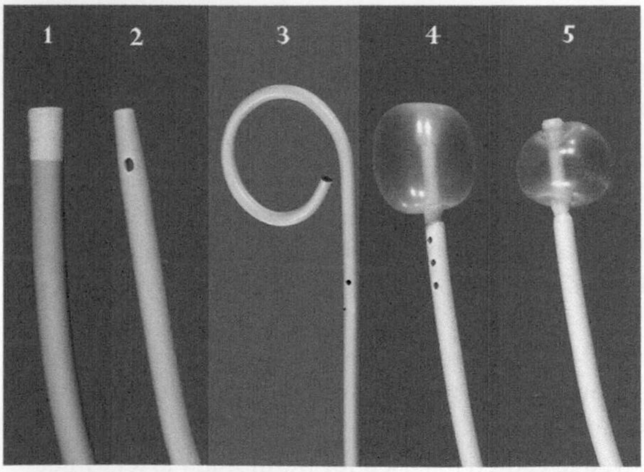

Figure 8.3 An array of catheter tips from catheters commonly used in cardiac catheterization and angiographic studies. 1, 4F multipurpose A1-type small curve angiographic catheter with an end hole and no side holes (Cordis, Inc., Milpitas, CA 95035, USA. https://www.cordis.com/en_us.html). 2, 6F multipurpose A2-type angiographic catheter with an end hole and two side holes (Cordis, Inc.) 3, 5F pigtail catheter with an end hole, multiple side holes and a tightly curved tip (Cordis, Inc.). 4, 5F Berman angiographic balloon catheter with balloon inflated; this catheter has no end hole and multiple side holes and is used in angiographic studies to avoid catheter recoil and/or penetration of contrast into the endocardium or myocardium during delivery of contrast (Arrow International/Teleflex, Research Triangle Park, NC, USA. http://www.arrowintl.com/). 5, 5F Wedge pressure catheter with balloon inflated, with an end hole and no side holes; this catheter is used primarily for right heart catheterization (Arrow, Inc.).

Vascular Access

The site of vascular access is dependent on the type and location of the abnormality to be visualized and the correction of the malformation that is planned. For example, for PDA visualization and correction, vascular access is typically via the femoral artery, as this approach allows the catheter a fairly straight path to the aorta and ductal anatomy. For balloon valvuloplasty to correct a severe pulmonic stenosis, either the jugular vein or (less commonly) the femoral vein is used. Veterinary patients are typically under general anesthesia for angiography and the vascular access procedure.

Two main types of vascular access are employed in veterinary cardiac catheterization: the Seldinger technique and vascular cut-down procedure.

The Seldinger Technique

The Seldinger technique, first described in 1953 by Sven Ivar Seldinger, is a method of obtaining vascular access via placement of a percutaneous sheath introducer (Figure 8.4) without a direct cut down to the vessel. It is performed mostly for right-sided catheterization, in medium- to large-sized dogs.

The sequential steps of the Seldinger technique are:

1) A wide area around the puncture site is clipped, sterilely prepared and draped.
2) The vessel is located by digital palpation.
3) A small puncture incision with a #11 surgical blade can be made to facilitate catheter or sheath passage through the skin.
4) A vascular cannula with stylet or an 18 gauge vascular needle is inserted into the vessel; venous access can be confirmed by a slow, continuous flow of dark blood, whereas arterial access produces strong pulsatile bright red blood flow.
5) If present, the stylet is removed, and a flexible guidewire is inserted through the needle or cannula into the vessel.
6) The needle is then removed, leaving the guidewire in place.
7) A dilator sheath combination, usually with a hemostasis port to prevent backflow of blood, is threaded over the guidewire into the vessel; the purpose of the dilator is to ease entry of the sheath introducer into the vessel.
8) The dilator is removed and the sheath introducer is sutured in place and flushed with heparinized saline; catheters can then be easily introduced and exchanged through the sheath introducer, with minimal vascular trauma at the entry site.
9) Upon removal of the sheath introducer at the end of the procedure, continuous direct vascular pressure should be applied until hemostasis is achieved (up to 20–30 min if an arterial puncture was performed) (Figure 8.5).

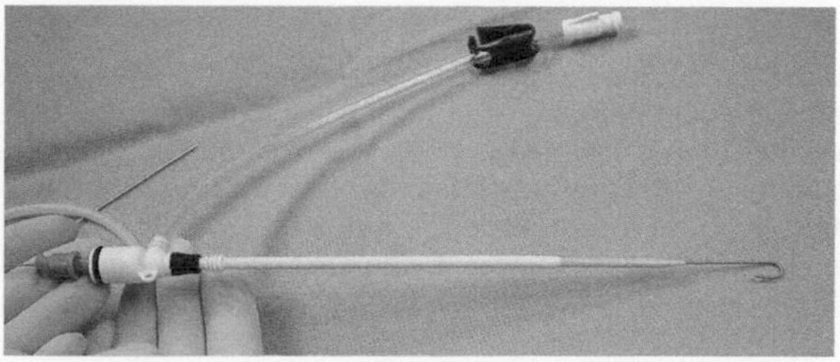

Figure 8.4 Sheath introducer with guidewire and hemostasis port; sheath is usually placed via the Seldinger technique, for the purpose of catheter introduction and exchange, and has the advantage of reducing vessel trauma and blood loss.

(a)

(b)

(c)

(d)

(e)

(f)

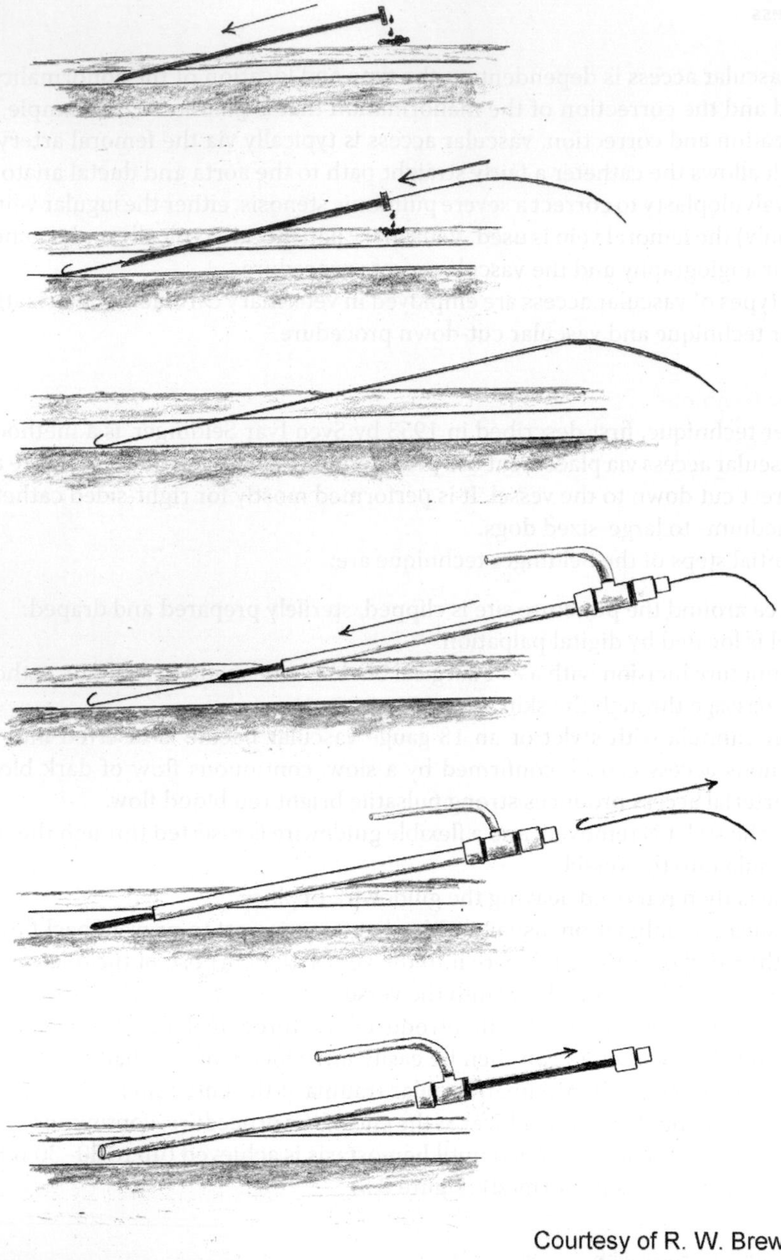

Courtesy of R. W. Brewer

Figure 8.5 The steps of the Seldinger technique to place a percutaneous sheath introducer. (a) The vessel is digitally palpated and an 18 gauge thin-walled needle is inserted into the vessel; placement into the vessel is confirmed by backflow of blood through the needle. (b) A flexible J-tip guidewire is threaded through the needle into the vessel. (c) The needle is removed leaving the guidewire in place. (d) An end hole sheath introducer with vascular dilator is threaded over the guidewire into the vessel. (e) The guidewire is removed. (f) The vascular dilator is removed, sheath introducer is flushed, and sutured in place. The sheath is now ready to accommodate passage of catheters through the vessel.

Cut-Down Procedure

The most direct and rapid access into the vessel lumen is to surgically expose the vessel in a cut-down procedure. The most common vessels accessed in this fashion are the external jugular vein, carotid artery, femoral vein, or femoral artery. The steps typically involved in a surgical cut-down vascular access procedure are:

1) A wide area around the site is clipped, sterilely prepared and draped.
2) A 1–1.5 inch incision is made over the vessel, taking care not to lacerate the vessel by pulling the skin slightly away while the skin is incised.
3) Blunt dissection is performed using either forceps or scissors to expose the desired vessel; in cats and small dogs lidocaine without epinephrine can be drizzled over the exposed vessel to prevent vasospasm/vasoconstriction.
4) Once the vessel is exposed, it is secured proximally and distally to the puncture site by means of a nonabrasive suture (e.g. 2-0 silk), umbilical tape or rubber bands.
5) A small incision is made into the vessel using vascular scissors or a #11 surgical blade; if an artery is being accessed mild tension should be applied to the proximal ligature to decrease the amount of bleeding.
6) The catheter is introduced into the vessel and the occluding ligatures are tightened, with the proximal ligature loose enough to allow for passage and manipulation of the catheter, but tight enough around the catheter and vessel to prevent bleeding.
7) Once the catheter is in the blood vessel, it is flushed initially and periodically thereafter with heparinized saline (1–2 IU/mL).

Guidewires

Guidewires are used with vascular access catheters to facilitate the placement, manipulation, and exchange of the catheters. Most guidewires are made of a stainless steel coil that surrounds an inner core that runs the entire length of the wire for additional strength. The sizing of guidewires can be somewhat confusing. In North America, the diameter of the wire is measured in inches (a measurement held over from the guitar string days) and the length is expressed in centimeters. Most common guidewires range in diameter from 0.001 inch to 0.052 inch, with 0.035 to 0.038 inch being the most frequently used. Typical guidewire length ranges from 125 to 260 cm. At one end, the guidewire tip lacks a central core, making it more flexible, and this tip may be straight or "J" in shape, to further decrease the risk of vascular or endocardial perforation (Figure 8.6). Some guidewires have a movable core allowing the operator to adjust the amount of the tip that becomes flexible. By pulling the movable core back, more of the tip becomes floppy; pushing the core out decreases the amount of wire that is flexible.

Some uses for guidewires include:

1) To decrease the likelihood of circulatory perforation and to protect the endothelium of vessels and chambers from catheter induced trauma.
2) As a preplacement guide for insertion of catheters into specific sites (especially stiff or balloon dilatation catheters); in this case the flexible tip of the guidewire is inserted into the vessel and maneuvered to the desired location; the catheter is then inserted over the guidewire to the region of interest.
3) For maintaining vessel access during exchange of catheters.

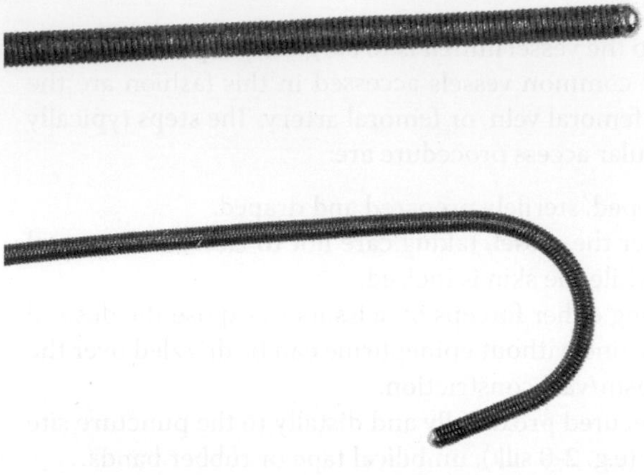

Figure 8.6 Flexible tip guidewires used for catheter exchange and manipulation during cardiac catheterization. Straight tip (top) and J-tip (bottom) (which is less traumatic to the intima of the vessel).

4) For straightening of a curved catheter (e.g. a pigtail catheter) for the purpose of maneuvering it to the desired location.
5) To add core strength to a softer more flexible catheter, in order that it may be maneuvered into the desired location.

Interventional Devices

One of the major indications for use of angiography in veterinary medicine today is to delineate cardiac malformations immediately prior to and as part of the interventional procedure to correct the defect. The major malformations that are corrected with minimally invasive interventional cardiac catheterizations at the time of writing are shunt lesions such as PDA, PSS, VSD, ASD and stenotic or dysplastic valves such as in PS, mitral stenosis or mitral dysplasia and less commonly AS or SAS.

For correction of PDA and PSS via catheterization techniques, embolization coils, Amplatz canine ductal occluders® (Infiniti Medical Supply, Menlo Park, CA, USA, http://infinitimedical.com/index.html) and caval stents are currently being employed.

Gianturco helical coils (Cook Medical Bloomington, IL, USA, http://www.cookmedical.com/) are made of stainless steel wire coated with Dacron fibers, which are thrombogenic (Figure. 8.7). Each coil is packaged individually in a thin straight metal sheath, that allows it to be pushed via a guidewire, into a catheter. Following angiographic identification of ductal anatomy, the catheter is advanced into the ductus and the soft end of a guidewire is used to advance the coil out of the catheter into the ductus, under fluoroscopic guidance. Once deployed, clot formation on the Dacron fibers of the coil occurs within about 10–15 min, essentially closing the ductus. Recommended coil size is about twice the width of the minimal ductal diameter. The coil embolization procedure is appropriate only in those PDAs that have a tapered morphology, in order that the coils will "get stuck" and become well seated in the narrow end of the taper. Following deployment of each coil, an angiogram is performed, with the catheter tip in the descending aorta just distal to the ductal opening, to assess whether any ductal patency remains; this is determined by the presence of contrast appearing in the main pulmonary artery. Multiple coils can be placed until no further evidence of shunting is seen on the angiogram (Figure. 8.8).

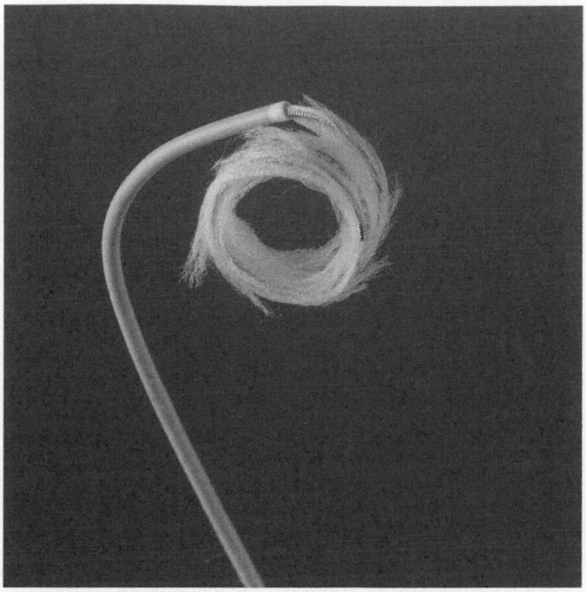

Figure 8.7 4F catheter with an embolization coil partially extruded; coils are made of steel embedded with Dacron fibers, which promote thrombus formation and subsequent patent ductus arteriosus occlusion.

The Amplatz Canine Ductal Occluder® (Infiniti Medical Supply, Menlo Park, CA, USA, http://infinitimedical.com/index.html) (Figure 8.9) is the newest device currently used for PDA closure, replacing embolization coils in all but the smallest animals (see Chapter 16) This device is also deployed using a catheter and cable, so that an initial disk made of wire mesh is seated through the ductal aperture on the pulmonary artery side, and the remaining larger aortic disk is deployed into the ampulla of the PDA. Complete occlusion via thrombosis around the device is usually achieved in 10–15 min, and only one device is sufficient for closure of the ductus. An angiogram is repeated after about 10–15 min to assure ductal occlusion.

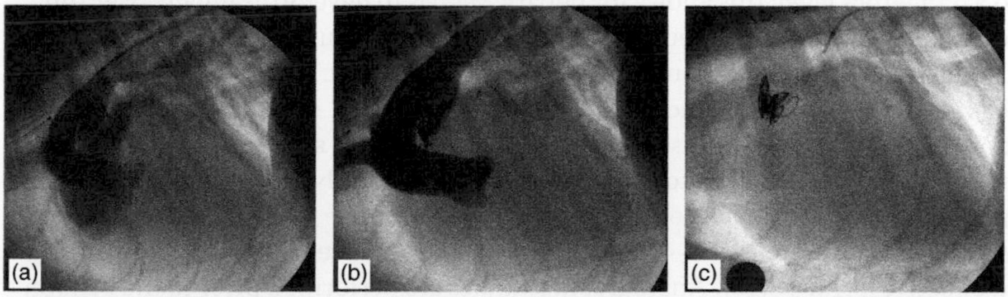

Figure 8.8 Images taken during a patent ductus arteriosus (PDA) coil occlusion procedure. (a) Angiogram from a dog with a large PDA; with the dog in lateral recumbency, a catheter has been inserted into the femoral artery and advanced into the aorta to the level of the PDA. The aortic root fills with contrast and the PDA is visualized, documenting communication between aorta and main pulmonary artery. Note that the main pulmonary artery also fills well with contrast. (b) Angiogram of a dog with several coils occluding a PDA; repeat angiogram of the dog in (a), following placement of a number of thrombogenic coils within the PDA. Note the lack of contrast in the main pulmonary artery, indicating successful closure of the PDA using the coil embolization technique. (c) Radiographic view obtained following deployment of several embolization coils within the PDA of the dog in (a) and (b).

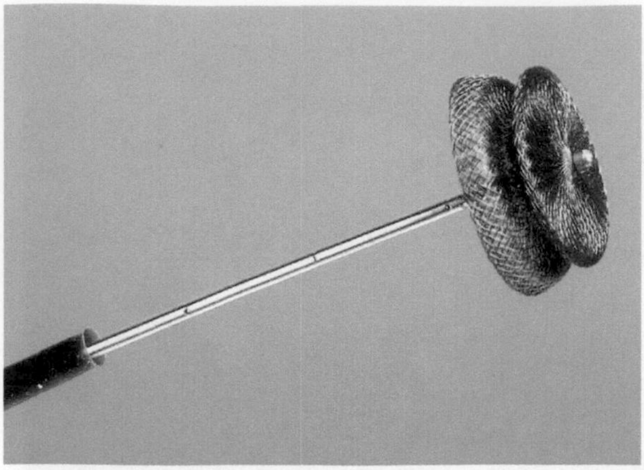

Figure 8.9 Amplatz Canine Ductal Occluder® (Infiniti Medical Supply, Menlo Park, CA, USA, http://infinitimedical.com/index.html) fully deployed and still attached to the delivery cable with guiding catheter visible. The detachable nitinol mesh device has a short waist in the middle that separates a flat distal disk (which is deployed across the pulmonary arterial ostium of the ductus) from a cupped proximal disk (which is deployed into the ampulla of the patent ductus arteriosus).

Intrahepatic PSS are difficult, invasive surgical cases, since a gradual closure of the shunt is desired in order to promote neovascularization of hepatic circulation while at the same time avoiding the development of portal hypertension, which can result following abrupt shunt closure. Embolization coils together with caval stents are being deployed successfully through minimally invasive catheterization procedures to gradually and partially occlude these shunting vessels, and thus allow for hepatic neovascularization. Angiograms are performed to delineate shunt morphology. Caval stents are then deployed in the caudal vena cava, covering the area where the shunt empties into the vena cava. Coils are then deployed via catheter inserted through the holes of the stent, into the shunting vessel; the stent serves the purpose of preventing coils from dislodging and flowing out into the vena cava. Angiograms are performed following the deployment of each coil, to assess for optimal attenuation of flow, ideally allowing some of the shunting flow to continue but to a lesser degree. Portal pressure, measured via pressure transducer and portal vein catheter, also helps to determine at which point to cease deploying coils. Optimally, shunting is attenuated while portal vein pressure is not elevated to a dangerous level; this allows for hepatic vessels to develop gradually over time.

Balloon valvuloplasty is another minimally invasive procedure that is performed via cardiac catheterization, for the purpose of alleviating stenotic valvular malformations (see Chapter 16). Pulmonic stenosis is the congenital lesion that best lends itself to correction via balloon valvuloplasty. In balloon valvuloplasty, a large diameter balloon catheter is fed over a guidewire to the area of the stenotic valve, and inflated to dilate or open the valve by fracturing or stretching the obstructive tissue. Low profile balloon catheters with diameter 1.2–1.5 times the valvular orifice have been shown to be safe and effective (Figure 8.10). Angiographic studies are performed prior to the balloon dilation, to delineate the stenotic region and to rule out the presence of an anomalous left coronary artery (coronary artery which encircles the pulmonary artery and is at risk of rupture during balloon dilatation; balloon valvuloplasty is contraindicated in these cases). Pressure gradients in the right ventricle are measured before and after each balloon dilatation to assess postprocedural improvement. During the procedure, the balloon is inflated one to three times using a 5:1 solution of saline and contrast. Using fluoroscopy, a "waist" is initially seen in the balloon, demarcating the region of stenosis, which disappears as the balloon is dilated further and the obstructive lesion is partially torn open by the pressure of the fully inflated balloon (Figure 8.11).

Figure 8.10 Catheters used for balloon valvuloplasty. Two catheters used for balloon dilation of congenital defects such as pulmonic or aortic stenosis. The balloon catheter on the left is an older more rigid type, while the balloon catheter on the right is a newer low-profile balloon catheter.

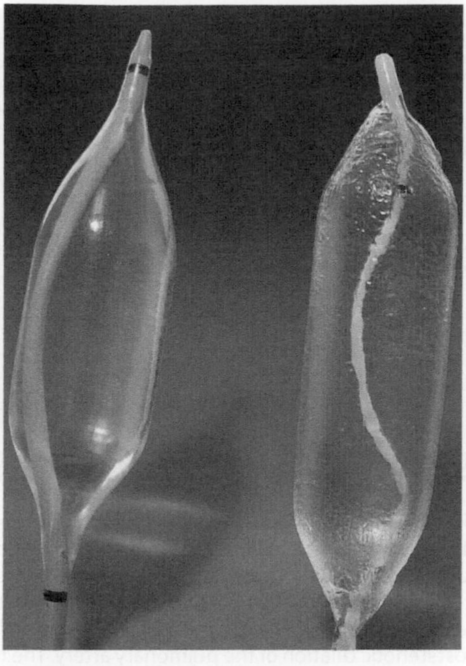

Balloon dilatation may also be helpful in alleviating conditions of mitral stenosis, tricuspid stenosis, subaortic stenosis, and cor triatriatum dexter or sinister. Amplatzer septal occluders are newer devices that are in the early stages of being used to correct ASD and VSD cases.

Additional Equipment

A Luer-lock syringe or automated power injector is required for making the injection of contrast media into the desired location. For small animals, injections may be made by hand, using a Luer-lock syringe. Specially designed Luer-lock syringes are available with finger rings for added high pressure control. A large bolus of contrast should be rapidly injected over 1–2 s under fluoroscopic visualization. It is of utmost importance that all air be removed from the syringe, the connection with the catheter and from any catheter or tubing between syringe and patient, and that no air be injected, especially into the left side of the heart, where one small bubble could occlude a coronary or cerebral artery and lead to acute myocardial infarction or stroke.

Power injectors have the capability to deliver an adequate volume of contrast rapidly, while allowing for calibration of pressure and rate of injection delivery, facilitating successful angiographic studies in larger animals. As is true with hand-operated syringe injections, appropriate precautions should be taken to ensure that all air is removed from the power injection syringe and tubing to prevent air embolism.

A multichannel physiologic recorder is often used as adjunct equipment during an angiographic procedure, particularly if therapeutic correction of a cardiac malformation is to be performed. Examples of these types of procedures include balloon valvuloplasties and PDA occlusions. The physiologic recorder is used to record intracardiac pressure, and must be calibrated to zero as well as to an appropriate range of pressure

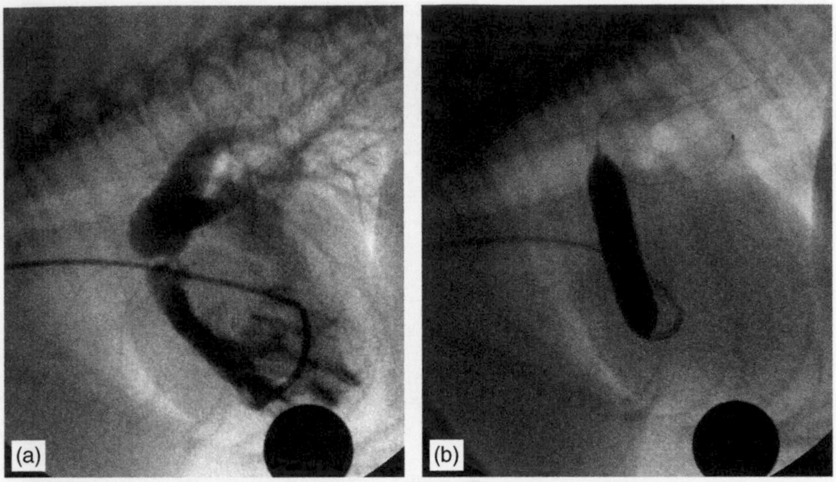

Figure 8.11 Images taken during a pulmonic stenosis balloon valvuloplasty procedure. (a) Angiogram of a dog with severe pulmonic stenosis. With the dog in lateral recumbency, a catheter has been advanced through the jugular vein into the right ventricle of a dog with severe valvular pulmonic stenosis, and contrast was injected into the right ventricle and pulmonary artery. Note the filling defect at the level of the pulmonic valve, resulting from valve thickening and dysplasia, as well as the poststenotic dilation of the pulmonary artery. The right ventricular wall is also thickened. (b) Angiogram showing a balloon dilatation catheter inflated over the stenotic region of the dog in (a). The catheter has been inserted into the jugular vein and advanced into the right ventricle, across the pulmonic valve and into the pulmonary artery, with the balloon placed at the stenotic region of the valve. The balloon has been fully inflated, to dilate the narrowed pulmonic valve.

according to the procedure to be performed and the severity of the animal's condition. For example, during a balloon valvuloplasty in a patient with a pressure gradient of 200 mmHg across the pulmonic valve, right ventricular pressures will need to be recorded as high as 200 mmHg, and the pressure channel for the right ventricle will need to be calibrated to measure pressures this high. Pressure calibrations are performed through the use of pressure transducers, which are connected between both physiologic recorder and specialized pressure tubing and the catheter being used. Three way stopcocks are placed at all catheter and tubing connections. Aside from cardiac pressures, the physiologic recorder also has the capability to continuously display an ECG and other monitoring variables.

Other ancillary necessities include anesthetic and monitoring equipment to maintain a safe level of patient restraint. A direct current defibrillator should be available, as well as cardiac emergency drugs, in the event of a serious rhythm abnormality or cardiopulmonary arrest.

Angiographic Technique

Angiography is considered a surgical procedure with regard to sepsis and due all the standard sterile surgery precautions, including full cap, mask and gown with sterile gloving. A sterile field should be maintained at all times.

Selective Angiography

1) Pre-anesthesia sedation and general anesthesia with endotracheal intubation are accomplished, and a light plane of inhalation anesthesia is maintained, with continuous anesthetic monitoring.
2) The area of catheter insertion is clipped, sterilely prepared and draped.
3) Vascular access is accomplished via either a percutaneous sheath introducer or surgical cut-down procedure.
4) All catheters and introducer sheaths are flushed with sterile heparinized saline (1500–3000 IU/L).
5) A cardiac catheter with multiple side holes is recommended to prevent recoil, and/or penetration of contrast into the endocardium or myocardium during contrast injection.
6) Catheter is guided via fluoroscopy to the desired vessel or cardiac chamber; common locations for angiographic injection include:
   - midcavity of the right ventricle or right ventricular outflow tract for PS procedures.
   - main pulmonary artery or its branches to detect PTE.
   - midcavity of the left ventricle or left ventricular outflow tract for AS/SAS.
   - root of aorta to diagnose the severity of aortic insufficiency.
   - aortic arch or thoracic aorta to assess and measure PDA morphology.
   - distal aorta to diagnose aortic/systemic thromboembolism.
7) A small volume test injection, using a 50:50 dilution of contrast and sterile saline, can be given to assure optimal catheter placement.
8) A large bolus of undiluted radiographic iodinated contrast is rapidly injected with fluoroscopic observation and recording; the angiogram is saved and can then be replayed (ideally in slow motion) for identification of morphology and cardiac function.
9) Angiocardiography/ventriculography dosage is 400–440 mgI/kg or 1.3–1.5 mL/kg Omnipaque 300 per injection, injected over 1–2 s, using the smallest appropriate syringe [1].
10) As previously emphasized, care must be taken not to inject air, especially in systemic circulation injections.
11) Catheters should be frequently flushed to prevent thrombus formation.
12) Postprocedurally following catheter removal, if the cut-down procedure was performed, vessels are repaired or ligated. If a percutaneous approach was used, continuous pressure is applied for several minutes over a venotomy site, or for 20–30 min over an arterotomy site, to assure hemostasis. Bandaging is applied as necessary and normal postanesthetic parameters are monitored.

Nonselective Angiography

1) A large bore (18–20 gauge or larger) intravenous catheter is placed, preferably in the jugular vein.
2) A large bolus of contrast is rapidly injected intravenously over 1–2 s.
3) Dose of contrast is typically 0.75–1.5 mL/kg of Omnipaque 300, or maximally 400–440 mgI/kg per injection [1].

Table 8.2 Suggested times for radiographic exposures postcontrast injection into a jugular venous catheter.

RA	0.5–1 seconds
RA, RV, PA	1–2.5 seconds
PV, LA, LV	3–5 seconds
LV, Ao with CHF	8–12 seconds

LV, left ventricle; RV, right ventricle; LA, left atrium; RA, right atrium; PA, pulmonary artery; PV, pulmonary vasculature; Ao, aorta; CHF, congestive heart failure.

4) Radiographic exposures are obtained 0.5–15 s postinjection; shorter times are needed for evaluation of the right heart and pulmonary arteries, while longer times are required for left-heart evaluation, in larger animals and in animals with heart failure or slow circulation times. Some suggested times for radiographic exposures postcontrast injection into a jugular venous catheter are see in Table 8.2.

In general, contrast delineation of abnormalities may be satisfactory using nonselective angiography, but optimal opacification typically requires injection as close to the abnormality as possible.

Contrast/Hemodynamic Studies

In animals with normal anatomy, contrast studies would follow the normal path of blood flow through the heart and vasculature.

Right-Heart Catheterization

Right-heart catheterizations are typically accomplished either via an external jugular vein or femoral vein. An external jugular venous approach generally allows for easier passage of the catheter into the right ventricle or pulmonary artery than does a femoral venous approach. Right-heart catheterization with semirigid catheters is risky due to the potential for cardiac puncture by the catheter tip. Therefore, guidewires and flow-directed balloon-tipped catheters, such as the Berman angiographic catheter (Arrow International/Teleflex, Research Triangle Park, NC, USA. http://www.arrowintl.com/), balloon wedge pressure catheter or the Swan–Ganz thermodilution catheter, are recommended. These catheters have a balloon at their tips, that when inflated protects the catheter tip from damaging the endocardial/myocardial surface. The inflated balloon also tends to be swept with the direction of blood flow, aiding in catheter placement into the desired chamber or vessel (Figure 8.12).

Once access is established either via sheath introducer or cut-down procedure, the catheter is threaded down the jugular vein and into the cranial vena cava and right atrium under fluoroscopic guidance. Occasionally the catheter will enter the azygous vein or caudal vena cava, rather than the right ventricle, especially if the catheter is very straight. Working a slight curve into the catheter tip can facilitate maneuvering of the

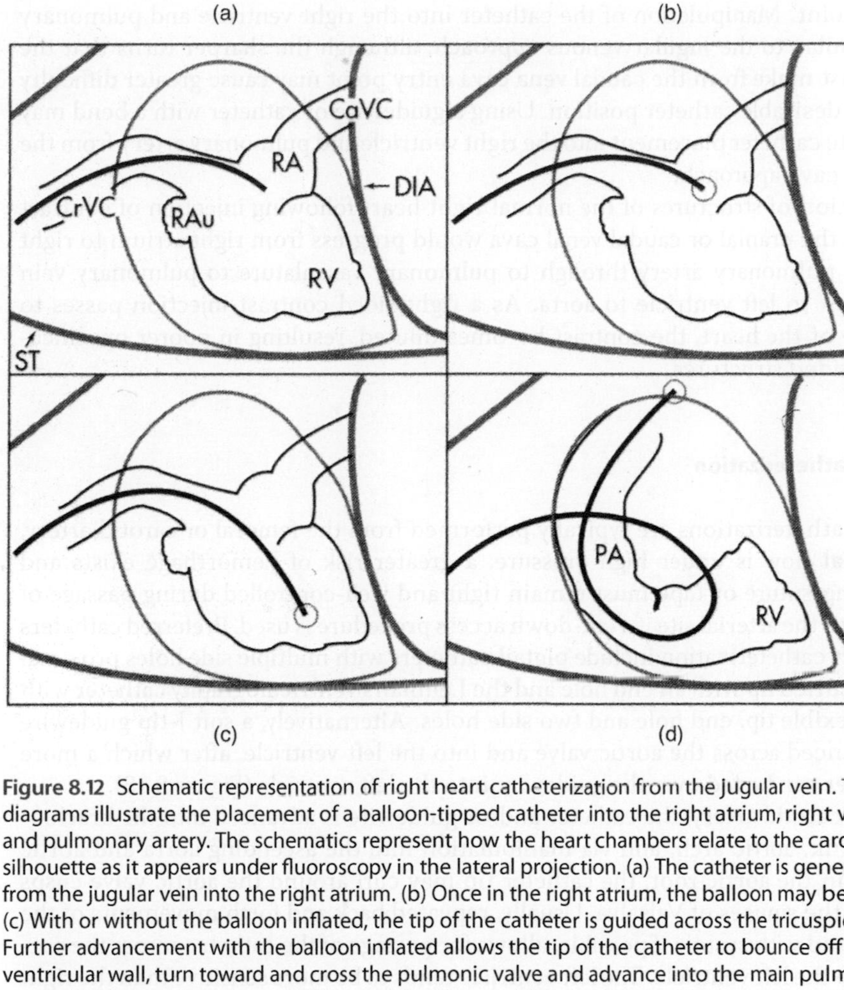

Figure 8.12 Schematic representation of right heart catheterization from the jugular vein. The diagrams illustrate the placement of a balloon-tipped catheter into the right atrium, right ventricle, and pulmonary artery. The schematics represent how the heart chambers relate to the cardiac silhouette as it appears under fluoroscopy in the lateral projection. (a) The catheter is generally placed from the jugular vein into the right atrium. (b) Once in the right atrium, the balloon may be inflated. (c) With or without the balloon inflated, the tip of the catheter is guided across the tricuspid valve. (d) Further advancement with the balloon inflated allows the tip of the catheter to bounce off the right ventricular wall, turn toward and cross the pulmonic valve and advance into the main pulmonary artery. CrVC, cranial vena cava; CaVC, caudal vena cava; DIA, diaphragm; RA, right atrium; Rau, right auricle; RV, right ventricle; PA, pulmonary artery; ST, sternum.

catheter into the right atrium. The balloon tip is inflated once the catheter has entered the right atrium, the catheter is angled ventrally and slightly caudally, and passed across the tricuspid valve into the right ventricle. Once in the right ventricle, with the balloon still inflated, the catheter is manipulated around the right ventricular apex into the right ventricular outflow tract. This is facilitated by the "flow-directed" quality of the balloon-tipped catheter. Once the catheter is directed toward the right ventricular outflow tract, it is advanced into the pulmonary artery; at this point, the balloon is deflated to prevent occlusion of the pulmonary vasculature.

From a femoral vein approach, the catheter would be advanced through the caudal vena cava into the right atrium. The multiple branches of vessels that come off the caudal vena cava may make it difficult for the flexible catheter to pass; the insertion of a guidewire into the catheter, with slow and careful catheter advancement under fluoroscopic guidance can facilitate the passage of the catheter into the right atrium from this entry point. Manipulation of the catheter into the right ventricle and pulmonary artery is similar to the jugular venous approach, although the sharper turns that the catheter must make from the caudal vena cava entry point may cause greater difficulty in attaining desirable catheter position. Using a guidewire or catheter with a bend may help facilitate catheter placement into the right ventricle and pulmonary artery from the caudal vena cava approach.

Opacification of structures of the normal right heart following injection of contrast media from the cranial or caudal venal cava would progress from right atrium to right ventricle to pulmonary artery through to pulmonary vasculature to pulmonary vein to left atrium to left ventricle to aorta. As a right-sided contrast injection passes to the left side of the heart, the contrast becomes diluted, resulting in poorer opacification of left-sided structures.

Left-Heart Catheterization

Left-heart catheterizations are typically performed from the femoral or carotid artery. Since arterial flow is under high pressure, a greater risk of hemorrhage exists and the occluding suture or tape must remain tight and well-controlled during passage of catheters into the arterial site if a cut-down access procedure is used. Preferred catheters for left-heart catheterization include pigtail catheters with multiple side holes proximal to a tightly curled tip with an end hole and the Lehman's ventriculography catheter with a tapered flexible tip, end hole and two side holes. Alternatively, a soft J-tip guidewire can be advanced across the aortic valve and into the left ventricle, after which a more rigid catheter can be fed over the guidewire into the left ventricle (Figure 8.13).

From the carotid artery, the catheter and/or guidewire is advanced into the brachiocephalic trunk, aortic arch, and via manipulation into the ascending aorta and aortic root. Once in the aortic root, the catheter tip may curl around the aortic valve cusps and snag in the sinuses of Valsalva. Usually, repeated back and forth movements of the catheter, timed with systole if possible, allows for passage of the catheter across the aortic valve into the left ventricle. The left ventricle tends to be more sensitive than the right ventricle, and ventricular arrhythmias can be induced by stimulation from the catheter tip. In this case, the catheter tip needs to be moved to a less arrhythmogenic location. The ECG should be continuously monitored. Because of the tight curve that a catheter must make to proceed from the left ventricle across the mitral valve to the left atrium, and also because of the greater arrhythmogenicity of the left ventricle, left atrial catheterizations are not routinely performed. Left-atrial catheterization can be performed using a curved flexible catheter or via a transeptal approach from the right atrium, but this procedure is technically more difficult and requires an experienced operator.

From the femoral artery, the catheter is guided through the abdominal and descending aorta to the aortic arch and aortic root. The curvature of the aortic arch makes left-heart catheterization from the femoral artery more difficult, as the catheter tip is a greater distance from the point of entry/operator control, and more difficult to maneuver. The catheter may tend to pass into the straight path of the left subclavian artery or brachiocephalic trunk. Use of a catheter with a curved tip or a flexible guidewire may help facilitate left-heart catheterization from this location.

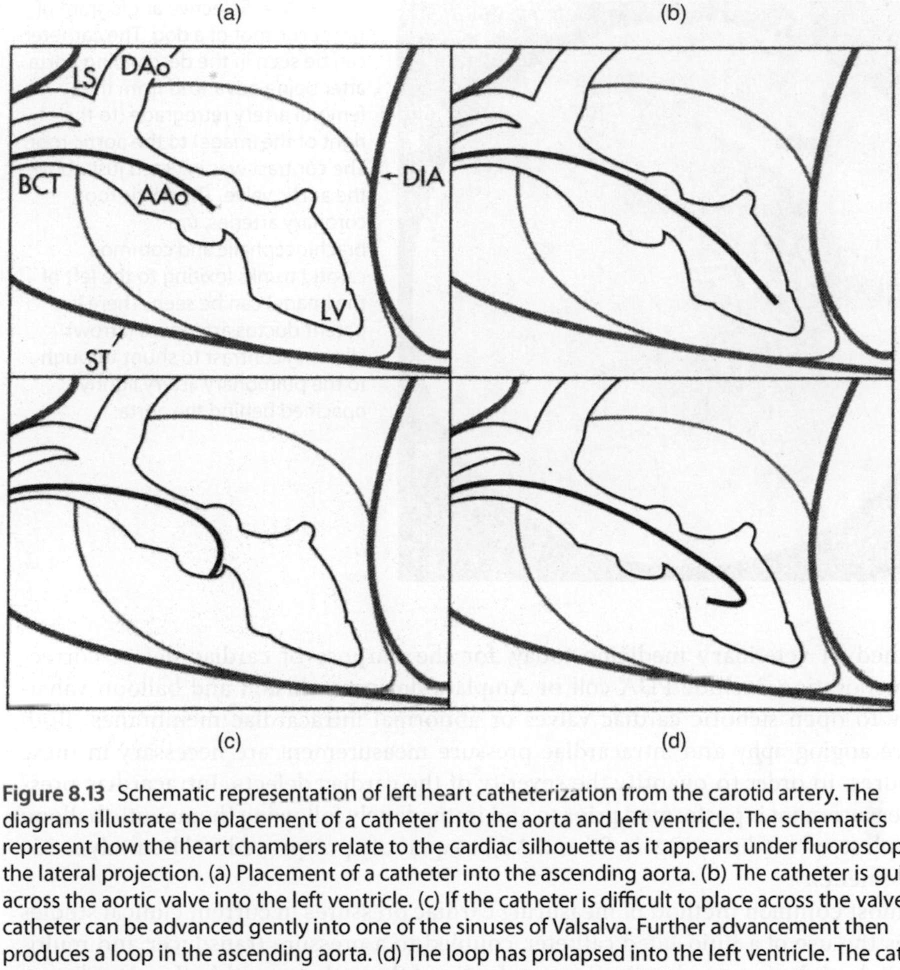

Figure 8.13 Schematic representation of left heart catheterization from the carotid artery. The diagrams illustrate the placement of a catheter into the aorta and left ventricle. The schematics represent how the heart chambers relate to the cardiac silhouette as it appears under fluoroscopy in the lateral projection. (a) Placement of a catheter into the ascending aorta. (b) The catheter is guided across the aortic valve into the left ventricle. (c) If the catheter is difficult to place across the valve, the catheter can be advanced gently into one of the sinuses of Valsalva. Further advancement then produces a loop in the ascending aorta. (d) The loop has prolapsed into the left ventricle. The catheter is then withdrawn to eliminate the loop (b). AAo, ascending aorta; BCT, brachiocephalic trunk; DAo, descending aorta; DIA, diaphragm; LS, left subclavian artery; LV, left ventricle; ST, sternum.

Opacification of structures of the normal left-heart following contrast injection from the left ventricle would outline the aorta, coronary arteries, aortic arch, and its branches (Figure 8.14).

Cardiac Pressures

Normal Cardiac Pressures and Waveforms

Intracardiac pressure measurement is an important and crucial hemodynamic measurement that is often an integral component of cardiac catheterization/angiographic procedures. The most common cardiac catheterization and angiographic procedures

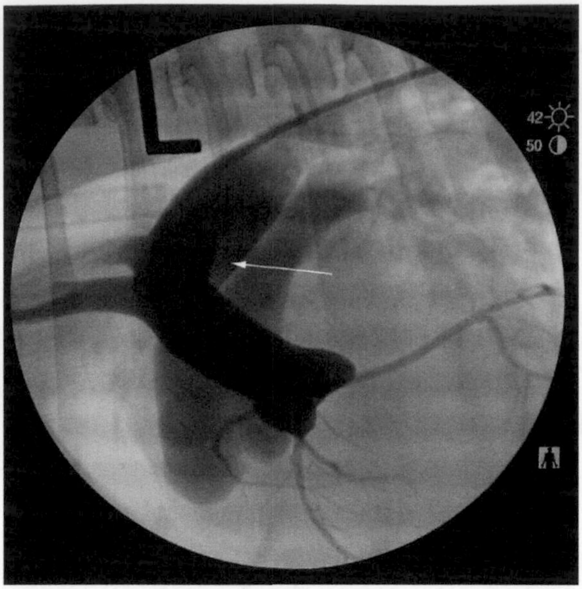

Figure 8.14 Selective angiogram of the aortic root of a dog. The catheter can be seen in the descending aorta after being advanced from the femoral artery retrograde (to the right of the image) to the aortic root. The contrast was injected just above the aortic valve. The aortic root, coronary arteries, the brachiocephalic and common carotid trunks (exiting to the left of the image) can be seen. There is a patent ductus arteriosus (arrow) allowing contrast to shunt through to the pulmonary artery lightly opacified behind the aorta.

performed in veterinary medicine today, for the purpose of cardiac defect correction/amelioration, include PDA coil or Amplatz device occlusion and balloon valvuloplasty to open stenotic cardiac valves or abnormal intracardiac membranes. Both selective angiography and intracardiac pressure measurement are necessary in these procedures, in order to quantify the severity of the cardiac defects. Intracardiac pressure measurement is performed prior to and immediately following therapeutic balloon valvuloplasty procedures (e.g. in PS and AS), to quantify postprocedural hemodynamic improvements.

The most common method of measuring cardiac pressures in current clinical studies involves the use of a fluid-filled catheter, coupled to a pressure transducer and multichannel physiologic recorder. Pressure at the tip of the catheter within the chamber or vessel to be measured is transmitted by small fluid movements through the catheter to the transducer. The pressure is then converted into voltage and then amplified and displayed on the physiologic recorder, in oscilloscopic form.

In order for pressure to be accurately recorded, the following criteria must be met:

1) The transducer must be calibrated to 0 mmHg and 100 mmHg, and confirmed via a mercury manometer.
2) The catheter tip and transducer must be at the same vertical level, which is typically standardized at the midsternal location for a laterally recumbent animal.
3) Air bubbles, small thrombi, fluid leaks, kinked catheters, overly long or very narrow catheters should be avoided, due to their hindrance to free fluid movement within the catheter–transducer system; such hindrances cause "over-damping" of the pressure signal.
4) The catheter is flushed prior to pressure measurement and the catheter tip should be free in the lumen of the chamber or vessel to be measured, except when measuring pulmonary wedge pressure.

Table 8.3 Normal intracardiac pressures.

	Systole (mmHg)	Diastole (mmHg)
Right atrium	4–6	0–4
Right ventricle	15–30	0–5
Pulmonary artery	15–30	5–15
Pulmonary wedge	6–12	4–8
Left atrium	5–12	<8
Left ventricle	95–150	<10
Aorta	95–150	70–100

Normal pulmonary wedge pressure is obtained by "wedging" the end hole of the catheter into a small pulmonary vessel in a right-heart catheterization, thereby occluding forward flow and thus measuring "back pressure" from the pulmonary capillaries, veins, and left atrium. The pulmonary wedge pressure tracing reflects left atrial pressure, and is slightly less than pulmonary artery pressure.

Upon withdrawal from the "wedged" location, the catheter then can be used to measure pressures in the pulmonary artery, right ventricle and right atrium successively. The right ventricular outflow tract is commonly a sensitive region of the heart that is prone to ventricular extrasystoles as the catheter tip traverses this area. Should this occur, the catheter tip should be pulled back to a region that is less sensitive to arrhythmia.

In left-heart catheterizations, pressure is measured during withdrawal of the catheter tip from the left ventricle into the aorta. Normal cardiac pressures are listed in Table 8.3.

Normal arterial pressure tracings have a peak systolic pressure, a dicrotic notch (associated with semilunar valve closure), and a diastolic pressure. In the normal ventricle, systolic pressure should be the same as the corresponding artery pressure; diastolic pressure is close to atrial pressure and near zero. End diastolic pressure is measured after atrial contraction (a-wave) and before the rapid early systolic upstroke. Pulmonary artery diastolic pressure should be close to left ventricular end diastolic pressure and left atrial pressure in the normal animal.

Abnormal Pressures

Abnormal intracardiac pressures tend to occur as a consequence of resistance or obstruction to blood flow. Flow obstructions are characterized by a pressure gradient (difference) across the obstruction, between the proximal and distal sides of the obstruction. For example, valvular stenoses cause an abnormal pressure gradient or difference between the pressure in the chamber proximal to the stenosis and the chamber distal to it. Valvular stenoses can be located at the valvular level, in the subvalvular region or the supravalvular area.

Common valvular stenotic lesions include pulmonic stenosis, aortic or subaortic stenosis, mitral stenosis, tricuspid stenosis, and double-chambered right ventricle (akin to a subvalvular pulmonic stenosis). Other cardiac malformations or conditions leading to abnormally elevated cardiac pressures include cor triatriatum dexter, cor triatriatum sinister, pulmonary hypertension or systemic hypertension.

Some abnormal pressure measurements and their grade of severity in various cardiac congenital malformations are detailed below:

1) In pulmonic stenosis, there is an abnormal pressure gradient between the right ventricle and pulmonary artery during systole, which is caused by the obstruction to flow created by the narrowed pulmonic valve. Mild conditions of pulmonic stenosis typically have a pressure gradient of 20–50 mmHg across the pulmonic valve during systole; the pressure gradient in cases of moderate pulmonic stenosis is 50 to 80–100 mmHg, and pressure gradients above 80–100 mmHg are classified as severe (see Figure 8.15).
2) In aortic or subaortic stenosis, there is an abnormal pressure gradient between the left ventricle and aorta during systole, which is caused by the obstruction to flow created by the narrowed aortic valve or subvalvular region. Mild conditions of aortic/subaortic stenosis typically have a pressure gradient of 20–50 mmHg across the aortic valve during systole; the pressure gradient in cases of moderate aortic/subaortic stenosis is 50–100 mmHg, and pressure gradients above 100 mmHg are classified as severe (see Figure 8.16).

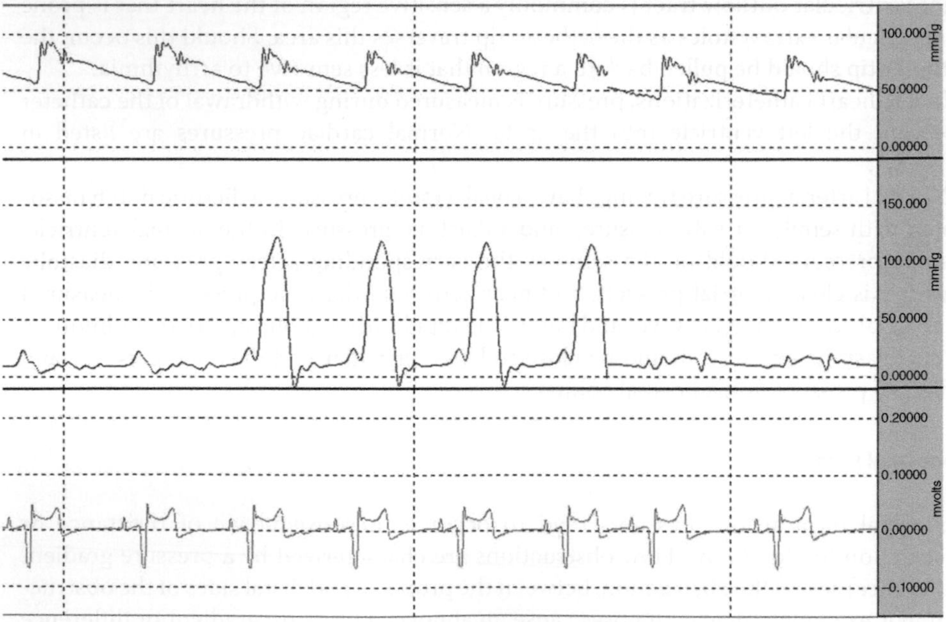

Figure 8.15 Pressure tracings and ECG recording of an anesthetized dog with pulmonic stenosis and tricuspid regurgitation. The top tracing reflects aortic pressure (~88/50 mmHg), obtained from a catheter in the aorta. The middle graph reflects serial pressures recorded from the right atrium (~20/4 mmHg; left side of graph), right ventricle (~121/12 mmHg; middle of graph), and pulmonary artery (~20/8 mmHg; right side of graph), as the catheter was advanced from the right atrium to right ventricle and then into the pulmonary artery. High right ventricular systolic pressure is secondary to pulmonic stenosis and there is a gradient of approximately 100 mmHg across the stenotic pulmonic valve. The high right atrial pressure is likely due to right heart failure and tricuspid regurgitation.

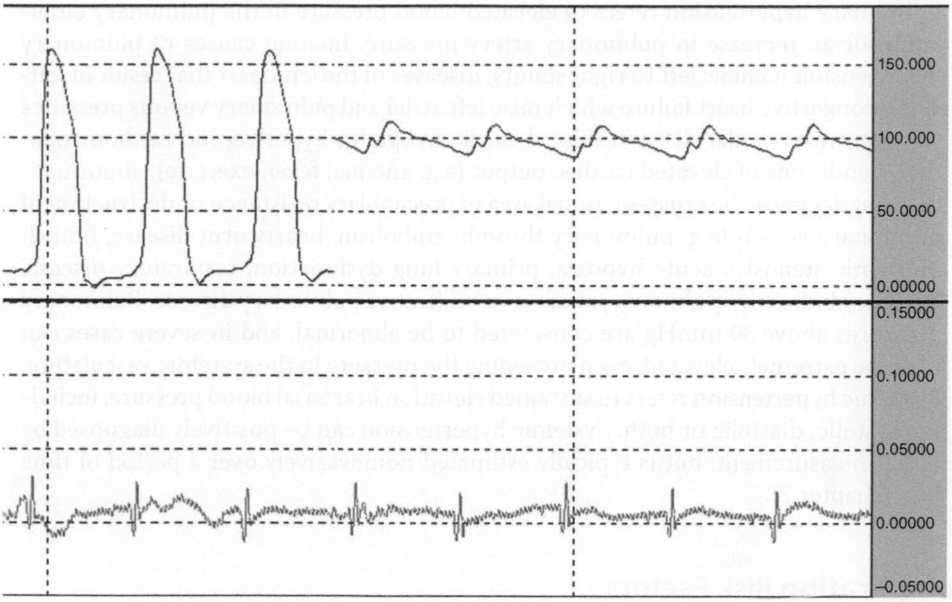

Figure 8.16 Pressure and ECG recordings of an anesthetized dog with subaortic stenosis (SAS). The upper graph shows a recording of left ventricular pressure (159/10 mmHg; left side of graph) and aortic pressure (~114/90 mmHg; right side of graph), as a catheter was pulled from the left ventricle into the aorta. The higher systolic pressure in the left ventricle is secondary to SAS, with an estimated peak pressure gradient of nearly 50 mmHg. Note the narrowed arterial pulse pressure difference of less than 30 mmHg, which is the graphical manifestation of the weak arterial pulses typically present in dogs with subaortic stenosis. The lower graph shows a simultaneous ECG recording.

3) In mitral stenosis, direct pressure measurements are difficult to obtain as previously described. Echocardiography is the less technically challenging method of evaluating left atrial to left ventricular pressure gradients. Mitral inflow velocities via Doppler echocardiography range from 1.4 to 2.5 m/s with pressure gradients of 8–25 mmHg across the mitral valve, indicating that left atrial pressure is from 8–25 mmHg higher than left ventricular pressure in diastole [2].
4) Tricuspid stenosis is rarely seen in veterinary medicine. However, tricuspid dysplasia is occasionally seen and can result in both a stenotic and an incompetent valve. In tricuspid dysplasia, pressure gradients across the tricuspid valve range from 9 to 36 mmHg, resulting in markedly elevated right atrial pressures (e.g. in the 15–45 mmHg range) [2].
5) Cor triatriatum dexter and cor triatriatum sinister are congenital defects in which an embryonic membrane divides the right (dexter) or left (sinister) atria into two right or left atrial chambers. The small communication or hole in the membrane dividing the atrium causes resistance to flow and an effective stenosis between the cranial (closer to the AV valve) and caudal (closer to the vena cava or pulmonary veins) atrial chamber. This results in increased pressure in the caudal chamber, which is transmitted back to the upstream veins and capillaries. Pressure measurements of cor triatriatum sinister again are difficult to obtain; however, cor triatriatum dexter pressure gradients can often be measured by direct catheterization as described above for right-heart pressure measurements.

6) Pulmonary hypertension refers to elevated blood pressure in the pulmonary circulation or an increase in pulmonary artery pressure. Inciting causes of pulmonary hypertension include: left to right shunts, diseases of the left heart that result in left-sided congestive heart failure which raise left atrial and pulmonary venous pressures (e.g. chronic valvular disease, dilated cardiomyopathy, hypertrophic cardiomyopathy), conditions of elevated cardiac output (e.g. anemia, fever, exercise), abnormalities that decrease the cross-sectional area of precapillary resistance or destruction of pulmonary vessels (e.g. pulmonary thromboembolism, heartworm disease, branch pulmonic stenosis), acute hypoxia, primary lung dysfunction, respiratory disease, chronic obstructive pulmonary disease or infiltrative pulmonary disease. Pulmonary pressures above 30 mmHg are considered to be abnormal, and in severe cases can become extremely elevated, even exceeding the pressure in the systemic vasculature.
7) Systemic hypertension refers to sustained elevation in arterial blood pressure, including systolic, diastolic or both. Systemic hypertension can be positively diagnosed by direct measurement, but is typically estimated noninvasively over a period of time (see Chapter 7).

Complicating Risk Factors

As with any invasive procedures, there are a few inherent risks associated with angiographic procedures.

Arrhythmias may occur secondary to catheter-induced ventricular irritability. When these occur the catheter should be promptly repositioned to a less irritable location. The right ventricular outflow tract is particularly sensitive to catheter manipulation, and right bundle branch block is a frequent transient or permanent sequela of right-heart catheterization, particularly postballoon valvuloplasty procedures. Emergency drugs and a direct current defibrillator should *always* be ready for immediate use.

Cardiac tamponade may result from ventricular or valvular rupture secondary to vigorous catheter manipulation. Careful gentle manipulation as well as proper selection of catheters and guidewires should always be maintained.

Catheter breakage/foreign body embolization can occur, especially secondary to resterilization and re-use in veterinary medicine, making catheters more prone to splitting and cracking, especially near the tip. If catheter breakage occurs, the embolus must be promptly retrieved, either via long endomyocardial forceps or surgical procedure.

A rare but potentially disastrous complication is perforation of a cardiac chamber by a cardiac catheter or guidewire. Perforations of the atria are most common due to their thin walls, but often will not lead to serious adverse events (Figure 8.17) Perforation of a ventricle is less common but potentially more dangerous. Due to their relative high pressure as compared to the atria, hemorrhage is more likely and ventricular arrhythmias are possible.

Hemorrhage, hematoma formation or blood clots may occur at the incision site or around the catheter tip. Catheters should be frequently flushed, routinely aspirating blood back prior to each flush to assure that no blood clots have formed. Incision sites should be properly closed with control of dead space, vessels ligated or repaired, and adequate bandaging or proper use of direct pressure should be assured to minimize these complications.

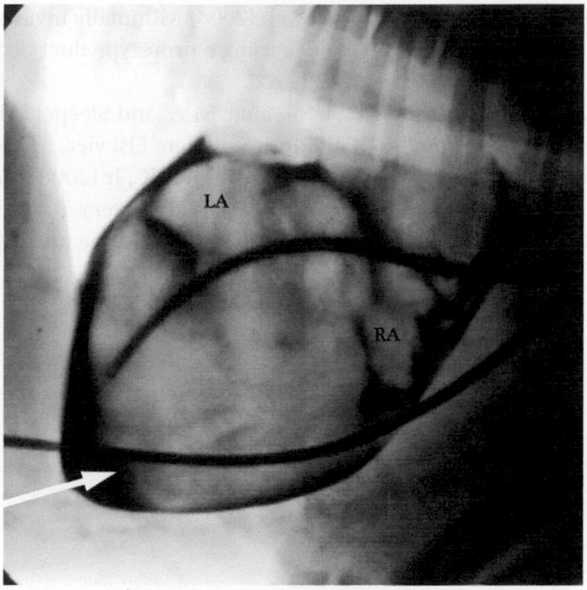

Figure 8.17 Contrast pericardiogram: in this fluoroscopy image a catheter (upper dark line superimposed over heart) has been inadvertently advanced through the right atrial wall into the pericardial space. A low volume hand injection of contrast was made into the pericardial space. The outer structures of the heart are visible. The paraconal interventricular grove (arrow) can be appreciated at the apex, and the atria (RA, right atrium; LA, left atrium) are outlined near the base of the heart. The lower dark line is an ECG monitoring cable in the image.

Conclusion

Angiography and angiocardiography are good and relatively safe, minimally invasive techniques for evaluating cardiac lesions and other vascular anomalies. Nonselective angiography is most useful in identifying abnormalities of large veins, right-heart structures, right-to-left shunts and to confirm venous thromboembolism. Selective angiography/angiocardiography is a necessary step during therapeutic catheterization procedures for the correction of defects such as pulmonic stenosis, aortic stenosis, patent ductus arteriosus, and portosystemic shunts. Improvements in occlusion and therapeutic devices is ongoing and will likely increase the frequency of successful minimally invasive procedures in the future, during which angiography will continue to play a vital role.

References

1 Wallack, S.T. (2003) *The Handbook of Veterinary Contrast Radiography*. San Diego Veterinary Imaging, Inc., Solana Beach.
2 Kittleson, M.D. and Kienle, R.D. (1998) *Small Animal Cardiovascular Medicine*. Mosby, St Louis.

Further Reading

Abbott, J.A. (2000) *Small Animal Cardiology Secrets*. Hanley & Belfus, Philadelphia.
Baim, D.S. (2006) *Grossman's Cardiac Catheterization, Angiography and Intervention*, 7th Edition. Lippincott Williams & Wilkins, Philadelphia.
Fox, P.R., Sisson D. and Moise, N.S. (1999) *Textbook of Canine and Feline Cardiology*, 2nd Edition. W.B. Saunders, Philadelphia.

Nguyenba, T.P. and Tobias, A.H. (2008) Minimally invasive per-catheter patent ductus arteriosus occlusion in dogs using a prototype duct occluder. *Journal of Veterinary Internal Medicine*, **22**, 129–134.

Tilley, L.P., Smith F.W.K., Jr, Oyama, M.A. and Sleeper, M.M. (2008) *Manual of Canine and Feline Cardiology*, 4th Edition. Saunders Elsevier, St Louis.

Vaden, S., Knoll, J., Tilley, L.P., Smith, F.W.K., Jr (2008) *Blackwell's Five-Minute Veterinary Consult: Diagnostic Procedures and Laboratory Tests.* Blackwell Publishing, Ames.

Wise, M. (1982) Non-selective angiography in the normal dog and cat. *Veterinary Radiology*, **23**, 144–151.

9

Cardiac Biomarkers

Kristin Hohnadel

Introduction

Detection of cardiac disease in veterinary patients is typically by thoracic radiography, electrocardiography, echocardiography, and most importantly, physical examination. However, these tests can occasionally provide ambiguous results or fail to detect disease that is not structural. Patients can also have more than one disease contributing to their clinical signs. In these cases, biochemical assays can be very useful. Specific cardiac biomarkers have become the standard of care in human medicine, and they are gaining in usefulness in veterinary medicine. They are of use in many applications, including detection, monitoring, and screening for cardiac disease. There are still limitations, however. Veterinary patients who would benefit from these diagnostic tests tend to be very ill, but these tests are not typically available as point of care tests, which would allow for expeditious diagnoses. Also, very few tests have been evaluated for any other species but canines.

Leakage Markers

Creatine Kinase

Creatine kinase (CK) is a component of skeletal and cardiac muscle. With muscular damage, this enzyme is released and can be detected with specific assays. Creatine kinase muscle/brain (CK-MB) is the gold standard for detection of acute myocardial infarction in humans. However, CK-MB is found in very low quantities in dogs and horses. It is also not cardiac specific in animals: in equine athletes and large breed dogs, this level can increase with skeletal muscle damage [1]. Additionally, acute myocardial damage is not commonly a part of cardiac disease in veterinary patients.

Some types of acute muscular damage are associated with cardiac disease. Specifically, arterial thromboembolism (ATE) can be associated with severe disease, typically cardiac, in felines. When other diagnostics are not available, ambiguous, or the patient is too critical, CK is useful in screening patients in whom an ATE is suspected. While other types of muscular damage such as trauma, restraint, or even intramuscular

Cardiology for Veterinary Technicians and Nurses, First Edition. Edited by H. Edward Durham, Jr.

injections can increase CK, the typical result with an ATE is ten- to even a hundredfold over normal in the author's personal experience. Though rare, thromboembolic disease is also reported in canines generally with diseases that cause coagulopathy, e.g. immune-mediated hemolytic anemia, protein-losing nephropathy, and hyperadrenocorticism. CK could be useful in evaluating a patient that presents with lameness due to suspected thromboembolism that may not be due to cardiac disease.

Troponin

Troponins are a part of the normal troponin–tropomyosin complex in skeletal and cardiac muscle. It contains three types of troponin: C, T and I. These biomarkers can be detected in the blood with muscle damage. Cardiac troponin I (cTnI) is found in cardiac muscle and therefore assays that can effectively reflect the levels in blood have the most potential to be useful in detecting disease. In humans, the degree of elevation has been correlated with severity of myocardial damage. It is nearly undetectable in healthy animals with current assays [2].

Theoretically, any condition that can cause myocardial damage can cause elevated levels of cTnI. Elevated levels have been detected in a variety of diseases, not necessarily specific to cardiac disease, including renal disease, gastric dilatation volvulus, and blunt chest trauma [3]. Specific cardiac conditions are also associated with elevated levels of cardiac cTnI. Pericardial effusion can cause an increase in cTnI, and measuring levels may be helpful in distinguishing whether the effusion is secondary to a right atrial hemangiosarcoma or idiopathic disease. However, more investigation is necessary to evaluate for heart base tumors [4]. CTnI levels have also been evaluated to determine if these assays can be useful in determining cardiac-associated dyspnea from noncardiac dyspnea. This does not seem to be the case [5]. At specific doses, doxorubicin chemotherapy is known to cause cardiomyopathy characterized by arrhythmias and systolic dysfunction which may lead to congestive heart failure. Elevated levels of cTnI have been reported after chemotherapy and prior to cardiac changes, but in a limited evaluation [6]. Babesiosis has also been associated with elevated troponin levels [7].

Cardiac troponin I has also been evaluated in cats with hypertrophic cardiomyopathy (HCM), and levels were elevated when compared with normal cats. Symptomatic cats with HCM had higher troponin levels than asymptomatic cats [8].

Natriuretic Peptides

Atrial Natriuretic Peptide

Atrial natriuretic peptide (ANP) is a protein that causes release of sodium (natriuresis) in response to atrial stretch or increased atrial tension [1]. In cardiac disease, this generally happens in response to increased atrial size from mitral regurgitation. ANP has a short half-life, and attempts to create a useful assay have been difficult because of its instability and necessity for specific labor-intensive processing. Plasma levels of *N*-terminal proANP (NT-proANP) are much more stable and detectable and occur in higher quantities. There is also significant homology between human and animal ANP, so tests developed for humans may be utilized for veterinary patients [9]. In humans, NT-proANP is useful in predicting left ventricular systolic dysfunction including acute myocardial infarction. However, this does not seem to be the case with veterinary patients, specifically canines. NT-proANP may be most useful for detection of atrioventricular valvular regurgitation that is nearing decompensation or has actually decompensated to congestive heart failure [9]. However, this may be confounded by increased levels due to other conditions. Exercise, increased blood volume, and renal or hepatic disease in humans have been proven to cause increased ANP levels [1].

Brain Natriuretic Peptide

Brain natriuretic peptide (BNP) is another protein responsible for natriuresis, but it is released by the body in response to ventricular stretch or distension as well as atrial. Like ANP, BNP is found in low quantities in plasma, has a short half-life, and must be treated with care to measure the assay accurately. BNP does not have the same homology with human BNP as does ANP. Therefore, specific veterinary tests must be developed [10]. However, there appear to be more applications for BNP than ANP. Increased levels of BNP are also associated with certain noncardiac diseases, including renal disease [11]. Certain medications, including diuretics, have also been reported to alter BNP levels. Breed and age variances may play a role in BNP level variability, as well [12]. Therefore, clinical evaluation must take these factors into account.

Distinguishing patients with occult dilated cardiomyopathy (DCM) has a very valuable role in veterinary medicine. Dog breeds, specifically Doberman pinschers and Great Danes, are highly predisposed to DCM. Unfortunately, the first sign of disease in these dog breeds is decompensation to congestive heart failure, syncope, and even sudden death. BNP has been evaluated in predicting occult dilated cardiomyopathy, and while it seems to have a role in predicting the myocardial disease in preclinical stages, it does not seem applicable in arrhythmogenic cardiomyopathy [13]. Similarly, golden retriever muscular dystrophy, a skeletal and cardiac muscle disease characterized by muscle necrosis and replacement with fibrous tissue and eventually left ventricular systolic dysfunction and congestive heart failure, can be predicted in more severe stages of the disease [14]. Unfortunately in these types of cases, BNP does not seem sensitive enough to indicate disease prior to significant changes. This may allow patients that are genetically predisposed to these fatal conditions to enter the gene pool before they are diagnosed.

Other studies have assessed BNP's ability to distinguish cardiac from noncardiac dyspnea. Clinical evaluation in these cases may be precluded by the severity of the patient's condition, and traditional diagnostics could have a detrimental effect on the patient's status. Venipuncture may be tolerated by a patient that would not tolerate more time-intensive and restraint-intensive tests. In these cases, a test to evaluate the cause of dyspnea quickly would be ideal. The BNP assay has been proven applicable by several studies, but unfortunately, has not yet reached this level of convenience. There has also been conflicting results generated from these studies. For instance, in one study, NT-proBNP was found to be higher in dogs [15]. The same study reported elevations in BNP with pulmonary hypertension. Pulmonary hypertension is generally a secondary condition. In veterinary patients, it often develops in response to primary lung disease and causes cardiac changes, or *cor pulmonale*, which may lead to right-sided congestive heart failure. While treatment is still warranted, the cause of pulmonary hypertension must be evaluated. Other studies have not attempted to make a distinction between causes of congestive heart failure [5]. One study did not report a difference between congestive heart failure and dilated cardiomyopathy [16]. Another limitation of these studies seems to be the lack of differentiation of BNP levels between cases that include both lung disease and cardiac disease in the same patient. Many veterinary patients have complex and confounding diseases that include more than one potential cause of dyspnea, and BNP would be most useful if it could help practitioners distinguish between them for the best treatment of the patient.

BNP in cats is reportedly sensitive to the presence of cardiac disease, but further studies seem to be appropriate to evaluate this [10].

Clinical Assays

Cardiac Troponin I Assays

A variety of assays are available and validated for use in the detection of cTnI in canines. These include the AxSYM system from Abbott, Dade Behring's Stratus CS, the Access AccuTnI from Beckman Coulter, Biosite Triage Meter and many more [2, 3, 5, 17]. Each has differing levels of sensitivity and specificity. These assays are not created equal, and they are not applicable across other species. Normal values are consistently at or below 0.03 ng/mL. However, there is no standard on which the tests are based, and there is no specific test that is considered "gold standard" [18]. Therefore, each test must be validated on its own.

ANP/NT-proANP Assays

Because of the difficulty of the assay process with ANP, the process is detailed and complex. However, due to the homology of animal ANP with human ANP, assays developed for humans can be used cross-species [10]. This is also true for NT-proANP. The radioimmunoassay is a simpler process, and NT-proANP occurs in larger, more stable amounts in plasma. It is, however, more sensitive to noncardiac effects, including azotemia.

BNP/NT-proBNP Assays

As mentioned previously, BNP does not have the same cross-species homology as ANP. This means that these tests must be developed specifically for veterinary patients. Similar to ANP, the assay for BNP is a complicated and complex process. Special care of the sample must be taken to ensure accurate results. A commercial test has become available for both canine and feline NT-proBNP by Veterinary Diagnostics Institute, who validated the tests. Recently a feline SNAP® (IDEXX Laboratories, Westbrook, ME, USA. https://www.idexx.com/corporate/home.html) has become available, and the previously utilized radioimmunoassay kits, including Biosite are still available [13].

Use of Clinical Assays

These assays, while extremely useful, work best as an adjunct to available traditional tests. Clinical judgment cannot be replaced by these tests, but they can be extremely valuable in cases where standard diagnostics are unavailable or unfeasible. To the general practitioner, they could be utilized as a screening tool after detection of an abnormality like a murmur, gallop rhythm, or arrhythmia and prior to referral to a cardiologist. To a cardiologist, these tests could help assess a critical patient not able to undergo the stress of time and restraint for traditional tests, and assist in distinguishing misleading information. None of the biomarker assays have yet been marketed as a point of care test, but because of the often critical nature of patients with cardiac disease, this would be a very practical advancement. Hopefully, these biomarker assays will also gain utility as screening tools for breeding purposes to evaluate breeding dogs for cardiac disease, along with the expertise of a genetic counselor. Reducing the number of veterinary patients with cardiac disease, or knowing how to correctly assess and treat them, is an ambitious goal for cardiac biomarkers, and while recent advancements are promising, more assessment and development is necessary.

References

1 Archer, J. (2003) Cardiac biomarkers: a review. *Compendium Clinical Pathology*, **12**, 121–128.

2 Sleeper, M.M. (2001) Cardiac troponin I in the normal dog and cat. *Journal of Veterinary Internal Medicine*, **15**, 501–503.

3 Burgener, I.A., Kovacevic, A., Mauldin, G.N. and Lombard, C.W. (2006) Cardiac troponins as indicators of acute myocardial damage in dogs. *Journal of Veterinary Internal Medicine*, **20**, 277–283.

4 Shaw, S.P., Rozanski, E.A. and Rush, J.E. (2004) Cardiac troponins I and T in dogs with pericardial effusion. *Journal of Veterinary Internal Medicine*, **18**, 322–324.

5 Prosek, R., Sisson, D.D., Oyama, M. and Solter, P. (2007) Distinguishing cardiac and noncardiac dyspnea in 48 dogs using plasma atrial natriuretic factor, B-type natriuretic factor, endothelin, and cardiac troponin-I. *Journal of Veterinary Internal Medicine*, **21**, 238–242.

6 DeFrancesco, T., Atkins, C., Keene, B. *et al.* (2002) Prospective clinical evaluation of serum cardiac troponin T in dogs admitted to a veterinary teaching hospital. *Journal of Veterinary Internal Medicine*, **16**, 553–557.

7 Lobetti, R., Dvir, E. and Pearson J. (2002) Cardiac troponins in canine babesiosis. *Journal of Veterinary Internal Medicine*, **16**, 63–68.

8 Herndon, W., Kittleson, M., Sanderson, K. *et al.* (2002) Cardiac troponin I in feline hypertrophic cardiomyopathy. *Journal of Veterinary Internal Medicine*, **16**, 558–564.

9 Haggstrom, J., Hansson, K., Kvart, C. *et al.* (2000) Relationship between different natriuretic peptides and severity of naturally acquired mitral regurgitation in dogs with chronic myxomatous valve disease. *Journal of Veterinary Cardiology*, **2**, 7–16.

10 Sisson, D.D. (2004) Neuroendocrine evaluation of cardiac disease. *Veterinary Clinics: Small Animal*, **34**, 1105–1126.

11 MacDonald, K.A., Kittelson, M., Munro, C. and Kass P. (2003) Brain natriuretic peptide concentration in dogs with heart disease and congestive heart failure. *Journal of Veterinary Internal Medicine*, **17**, 172–177.

12 Oyama, M.A., Fox, P.R., Rush, J.E. *et al.* (2008) Clinical utility of serum N-terminal pro-B-type natriuretic peptide concentration for identifying cardiac disease in dogs and

assessing disease severity. *Journal of the American Veterinary Medical Association*, **232**, 1496–1503.

13 Oyama, M.A., Sisson, D.D. and Solter, P.F. (2007) Prospective screening for occult cardiomyopathy in dogs by measurement of plasma atrial natriuretic peptide, B-type natriuretic peptide, and cardiac troponin-I concentrations. *American Journal Veterinary Research*, **68**, 42–47.

14 Chetboul, V, Tessier-Vetzel, D, Escriou, C. *et al.* (2004) Diagnostic potential of natriuretic peptides in the occult phase of golden retriever muscular dystrophy cardiomyopathy. *Journal of Veterinary Internal Medicine*, **18**, 845–850.

15 DeFrancesco, T.C., Rush, J.E., Rozanski, E.A. *et al.* (2007) Prospective clinical evaluation of an ELISA B-type natriuretic peptide assay in the diagnosis of congestive heart failure in dogs presenting with cough or dyspnea. *Journal of Veterinary Internal Medicine*, **21**, 243–250.

16 Fine, D.M., DeClue, A.E. and Reinero, C.R. (2008) Evaluation of circulating amino terminal-pro-B-type natriuretic peptide concentration in dog with respiratory distress attributable to congestive heart failure or primary pulmonary disease. *Journal of the American Veterinary Medical Association*, **232**, 1674–1679.

17 Adin, D.B., Oyama M.A., Sleeper M.M. *et al.* (2006) Comparison of canine cardiac troponin i concentrations as determined by 3 analyzers. *Journal of Veterinary Internal Medicine*, **20**, 1136–1142.

18 Wells SM and Sleeper M. (2008) Cardiac troponins. *Journal of Veterinary Emergency and Critical Care*, **18**, 235–245.

Section III

Cardiac Diseases

10

Congenital Heart Diseases

H. Edward Durham, Jr.

Introduction

Congenital disease of the heart can often be complex and confusing. Understanding normal circulation can be challenging, but when it gets deranged in development, a new level of confusion can ensue. Congenital heart disease typically changes the loading conditions in the cardiac chambers in one of two ways: by increasing the pressure load or by increasing the volume load in one or more heart chambers. Combinations of the two loads can exist. By understanding if the condition presents a volume load or a pressure load will aid in the diagnosis and therapy of patients with congenital heart disease.

The prevalence of congenital cardiac disease in dogs was reported to be approximately 0.5–0.85% in 1992 [1]. The Veterinary Medical Database (VMD) is a central storage database for diagnosis information of cases submitted by five veterinary teaching institutions. The author reviewed the VMD from 1965 to 2003 which revealed that of all dogs entered, 0.09% had a diagnosis of some type of congenital cardiac defect. The most commonly reported congenital heart defect was the patent ductus arteriosus (PDA), followed by subvalvular aortic stenosis (SAS) and pulmonic valve stenosis (PS). Some breeds of dogs are overrepresented with certain congenital defects, such as SAS in the golden retriever. Table 10.1 shows the most common congenital defects and the dog breeds in which they are most frequently seen.

Classifications of Congenital Heart Disease

A thorough knowledge of normal cardiac anatomy is essential in understanding congenital defects. Grouping cardiac congenital defects by the hemodynamic consequences they cause aids in understanding their development. Valvular dysplasias are malformations of the cardiac valve apparatus that result in either a stenosis, regurgitation, or both. Stenosis is seen in a valve orifice that is too small for the workload required of it. It is analogous to a narrowing in a river that causes the increased speed of flow and turbulence that are rapids. Dysplasias can be seen at any of the four cardiac valves and tend to create increased pressure in the cardiac chamber upstream.

Shunts are abnormal hemodynamic communications between two portions of the cardiovascular anatomy. The most commonly seen shunts are patent ductus arteriosus

Cardiology for Veterinary Technicians and Nurses, First Edition. Edited by H. Edward Durham, Jr.

Table 10.1 The commonest congenital heart defects and the most susceptible dog breeds for each disease.

Patent ductus arteriosus	
	Bichon Frise
	Chihuahua
	Cocker Spaniel
	Collie
	English Springer Spaniel
	German Shepherd
	Keeshond
	Labrador Retriever
	Maltese
	Newfoundland
	Poodle Breeds
	Pomeranian
	Shetland Sheepdog
	Yorkshire Terrier
Subaortic stenosis/aortic stenosis	
	Bouvier de Flandres
	Boxer
	Bull Terrier
	English Bulldog
	German Shepherd
	German Shorthair Pointer
	Golden Retriever
	Great Dane
	Newfoundland
	Rottweiler
	Samoyed
Pulmonic stenosis	
	Airdale Terrier
	Beagle
	Boykin Spaniel
	Boxer
	Chihuahua
	Cocker Spaniel
	English Bulldog
	Mastiff

Table 10.1 (*Continued*)

Pulmonic stenosis (*continued*)	
	Samoyed
	Schnauzer Breeds
	Terrier Breeds
	West Highland White Terrier
Ventricular septal defect	
	English Bulldog
	English Springer Spaniel
	Keeshond
	West Highland White Terrier
Tricuspid valve dysplasia	
	Boxer
	German Shepherd
	Golden Retriever
	Great Dane
	Labrador Retriever
	Old English Sheepdog
	Weimaraner

(PDA), ventricular septal defects (VSD), or atrial septal defects (ASD). Most shunts flow from the systemic circulation to the pulmonary circulation due to the greater pressure of the systemic circulation, and tend to create an increased volume load on the heart. Cyanotic heart diseases are typically shunts in which hypoxic blood from the pulmonary circulation enters the systemic circulation, leading to systemic hypoxia and cyanosis. Congenital cardiac malformations do not always present as a single defect. The term complex congenital defect simply refers to abnormalities that may include more than one of the above classifications, such as a PDA with a PS. Virtually all significant congenital cardiac defects cause a murmur that can be heard during auscultation, but exceptions do occur. Generally, the loudness of the murmur does not correlate well with the severity of the disease. Echocardiography has become the most common modality for diagnosing congenital heart defects. An algorithm has been proposed to aid is sorting out the complex cardiac abnormalities commonly seen with congenital heart disease [2].

Subaortic Stenosis

Subvalvular aortic stenosis or subaortic stenosis (SAS) is an important cardiac congenital defect seen in Newfoundlands, golden retrievers, boxers, Rottweilers and other large-breed dogs. It is notable that the defect is rarely diagnosed in Labrador retrievers. This defect is a fibromuscular ring that develops in the left ventricular outflow tract (LVOT) between the left ventricle (LV) and the valve proper. The fibrous ring creates an obstruction to blood flow from the LV through the aortic valve. The severity of SAS is determined by degree of pressure load added to the LV to eject blood. Subaortic stenosis is present at birth in affected animals, and can progress in severity up to approximately one year of age, at which time a final diagnosis of severity can be made.

The increased pressure in the LV can lead to ventricular hypertrophy, decreased coronary perfusion, myocardial ischemia, and fibrosis [3]. The amount of these changes is related to the severity of the stenosis and the amount of pressure overload it exerts on the LV. Severe obstructions lead to marked LV hypertrophy and ischemia, and mild obstructions showing little or no obvious hypertrophy.

Clinical Presentation

Often this condition has no outward clinical manifestations until the onset of heart failure, or in the cases of severe stenosis, sudden death may be the first sign. Typically, SAS is first suspected when a murmur is heard during a routine veterinary examination in breeds that are predisposed. This usually occurs during the well-puppy visit. The physical examination may reveal an audible, left basilar systolic murmur, as well as hypokinetic femoral pulses. The murmur often is a crescendo or diamond-shaped murmur, a so called "ejection" murmur. The loudness of the murmur does not always coincide with the severity of the stenosis, but generally very loud murmurs (grades 4–6/6), are often associated with severe disease, and may radiate cranially through the carotid arteries making the murmur audible on the dog's head.

Diagnostics

Radiographs typically show a normal-size cardiac silhouette in the lateral projection with occasional loss of the cranial cardiac waist. From the ventrodorsal (VD) view there is widening of the mediastinum caused by a poststenotic dilation of the aortic arch, with a bulge over the cranial heart projecting toward the patient's left side (Figure 10.1). Left ventricular and left atrial (LA) enlargement may rarely be seen with severe SAS that also affects the mitral valve as a result of mitral regurgitation.

Echocardiography is the standard of care in diagnosing and prognosticating for a SAS. Echocardiographic findings correlate with severity. Echocardiography of mild to moderate SAS typically shows that left ventricular dimensions typically remain within normal limits. In severe SAS some degree of LV hypertrophy may be appreciated and the fibrous ring that creates the obstruction of a narrowed LVOT is sometimes visible. This "imaging lesion" appears as a ridge of tissue on the septal and posterior wall on the LVOT (Figure 10.2). Some dogs will also have abnormalities in their mitral valve leading to mitral regurgitation and potentially LA enlargement.

Using Doppler echocardiography with color flow mapping, an image of the aorta will show turbulent blood flow during systole in the aorta (Figure 10.3). During diastole, aortic insufficiency is commonly seen [3, 4] (Figure 10.4).

Definitive diagnosis is acheived by measuring the velocity of blood moving across the aortic valve recorded with spectral Doppler imaging (Figure 10.5) (see Chapter 6). Doppler-derived velocities over 2.25 m/s are considered abnormal in all breeds of dog [1, 3]. The velocity is translated into a pressure gradient between the LV and the aorta

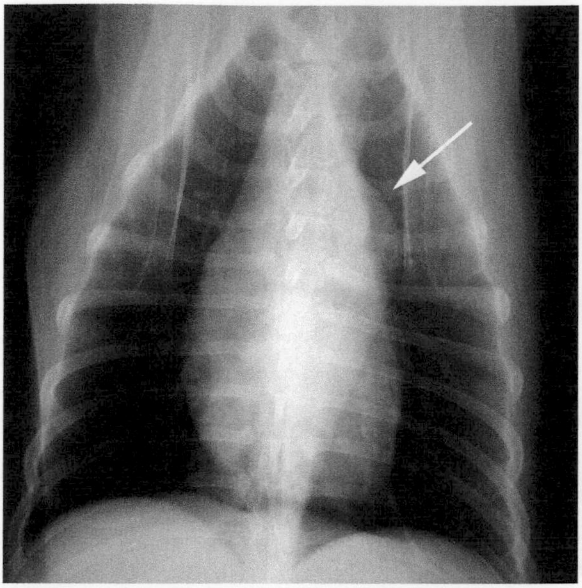

Figure 10.1 A ventrodorsal radiograph of a dog with subaortic stenosis: note the aortic bulge in the 1–2 o'clock region indicated by the arrow. This is a result of the poststenotic dilation of the aortic arch. The remaining cardiac silhouette is normal size and shape. The pulmonary parenchyma is normal, as are the other thoracic vascular structures.

by use of the modified Bernoulli equation, which states that four times the velocity squared will equal the pressure difference or *pressure gradient* (PG) between two chambers (Equation 10.1). Doppler assessment of the aortic outflow velocity is done from the left apical five-chamber view and the subcostal view. The subcostal view has been shown to provide the best alignment for measuring the PG across the aorta [5].

$$4^*V^2 = \Delta P \tag{10.1}$$

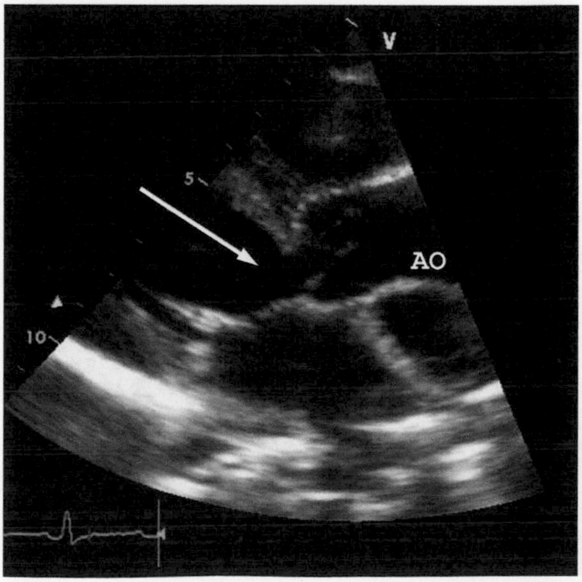

Figure 10.2 Long axis echocardiographic view of subaortic stenosis lesion: the arrow points to the narrowed left ventricular outflow tract. The fibrous obstruction protrudes downward in the image. The aortic valve cusps are seen centrally between the arrow and the aorta (AO) label. They are extending upwards and towards the right. The left atrium is in the far field, and the right atrium in the near field.

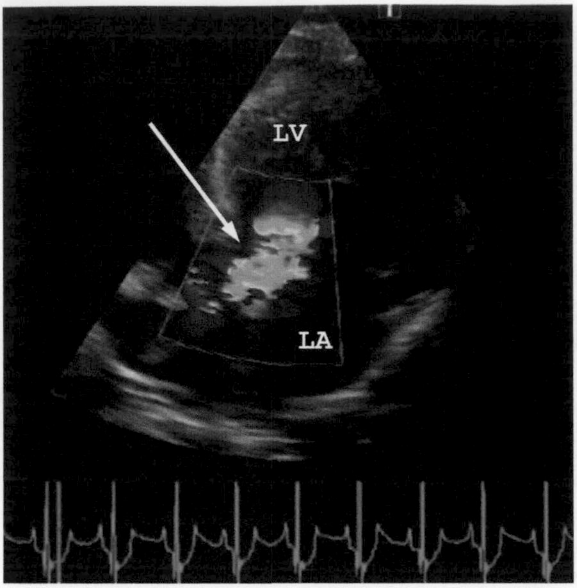

Figure 10.3 Left apical long axis view of turbulence in the aorta: the yellow–green mosaic of high velocity turbulent blood flow by color-flow Doppler in the aorta during ejection is typical for subaortic stenosis. The left atrium (LA) and left ventricle (LV) are labeled. Notable in the color mapping is the blue shell of downward flow nearest the top of the image, which as blood accelerates changes from flat blue to ice blue to high velocity variant flow.

where V = Doppler-measured blood velocity expressed in m/s and ΔP = the PG between the two cardiac chambers that the blood was moving between during the velocity measurement.

Although the exact classification of SAS severity is not uniform among veterinary cardiologists, most agree that dogs with a PG of 25–50 mmHg are classified as having mild SAS, those with 50–80 mmHg as moderate, and those with 80 mmHg or above as having severe SAS [4; 6, pp. 477–525] in nonanesthetized dogs. Some authors classify severe

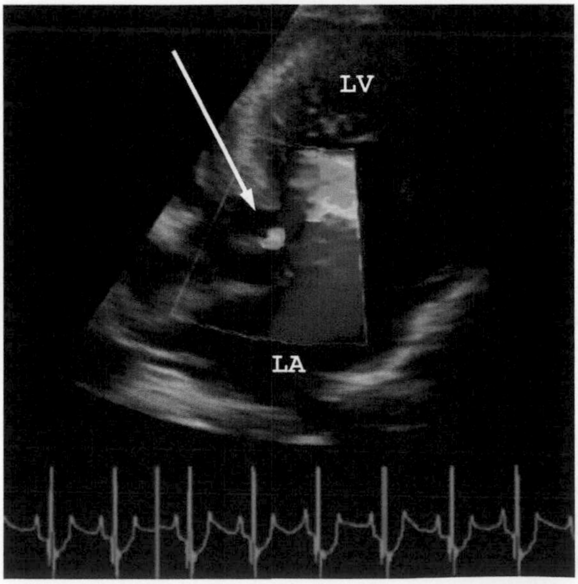

Figure 10.4 Left apical long axis view of aortic insufficiency: the arrow points to the red retrograde flow through the aortic valve during diastole of aortic insufficiency commonly seen in subaortic stenosis cases. The left atrium (LA) and left ventricle (LV) are labeled. The red Doppler signal of blood filling the LV from the LA can be seen to the right of the aortic valve.

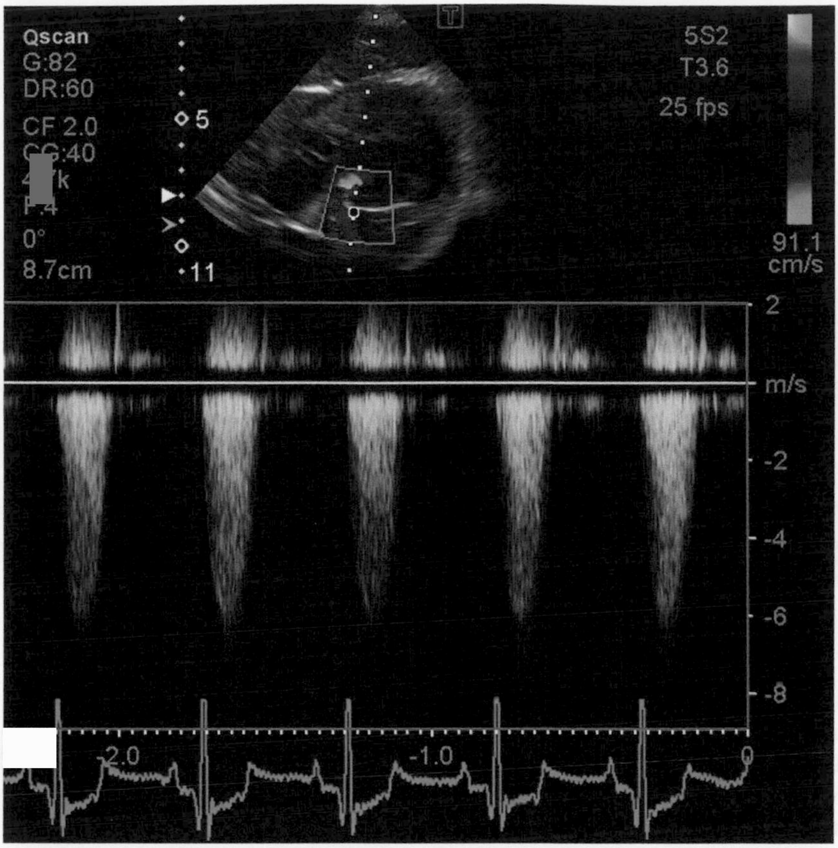

Figure 10.5 Continuous wave spectral Doppler of severe subaortic stenosis. The spectral Doppler image here shows the peak velocity across the stenotic aortic valve to be greater than 6 m/s, which corresponds with a peak pressure gradient of greater than 144 mmHg. Dogs with pressure gradients of greater than 130 mmHg have an increased risk of morbidity and mortality. The velocity scale is on the right of the spectral graph. An ECG is provided for timing of the cardiac cycle. The cursor line can be seen aligned with the color of turbulent blood flow in the reference image above.

SAS as a PG above 100 mmHg [1,3]. Research from 2014, however, demonstrated that dogs with a PG equal to or less than 133 mmHg, were at no greater risk of mortality than those with a PG between 80 and 130 mmHg, suggesting that reclassification of severe SAS is warranted [7].

It must be remembered that the transaortic velocity is dependent on many factors. Increased sympathetic tone or cardiac shunts may falsely elevate velocity, whereas negative inotropic drugs, anesthesia, and myocardial failure will decrease transaortic velocities. Normal velocities are generally considered to be less than 1.7 m/s, thus an equivocal zone exists between the normal 1.7 m/s and the clearly abnormal of 2.25 m/s [3]. Owners with breeding dogs that fall in this category must counsel with the veterinary cardiologist carefully to determine the dog's potential to pass on an inheritable heart condition to their offspring.

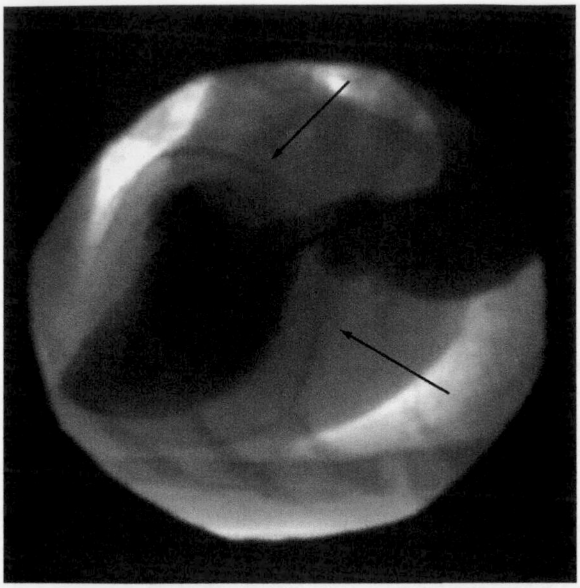

Figure 10.6 Angiogram of subaortic stenosis: the pigtail catheter is entering the image from the right side. The catheter is placed in the carotid artery and advanced through the aortic root past the aortic valve, and into the left ventricle. An injection of contrast is made into the left ventricle. This frame is taken at end diastole. The narrowing of the stenosis can be seen between the left ventricle and the aorta. The arrows point to the coronary arteries as they wrap around the ventricles. The left ventricle should have an opening into the aorta as wide as the aortic root. The poststenotic dilation can be seen to the right of the image.

Prior to the widespread use of echocardiography to diagnose SAS, many cases were diagnosed via cardiac catheterization. During cardiac catheterization a PG could be measured directly by means of intracardiac catheters and pressure transducers. Anesthesia will reduce the PG by approximately half as compared with Doppler derived PG [8]. Additionally, radiographic contrast imaging of the left ventricular outflow tract could be performed (Figure 10.6).

Therapy

Currently, there is no curative treatment for SAS. Several methods have been attempted to partially relieve the degree of obstruction for severe cases in an attempt to move dogs to the moderate category including: balloon valvuloplasty (Figure 10.7), open-heart surgical intervention [9], interventional catheters with cutting balloons [10] and medical therapy with beta-blockers. None of these treatment options have been shown to extend life better than another. At this time beta-blocker therapy is the most widely accepted treatment due to the low-risk-to-benefit ratio [3]; however, the benefits may not be as hopeful as initially thought [7]. If signs of congestive heart failure (CHF) and/or arrhythmias become present then traditional therapy with diuretics, angiotensin-converting enzyme inhibitors and anti-arrhythmic therapy is warranted (see Chapter 15).

Patients with mild stenosis generally live normal lives with no clinical signs. Dogs with moderate SAS may develop syncope, CHF and/or ventricular arrhythmias; however, they may live a full life with the disease. Dogs with severe SAS may show syncope or will often die of CHF or of ventricular arrhythmias. Any degree of SAS predisposes the patient to bacterial endocarditis. Because the obstruction is actually not the valve leaflets themselves but "below" the valve, the high velocity jet impacts the valve leaflets at the onset of systole. Over time the damage from this impact damages the valve leaflet

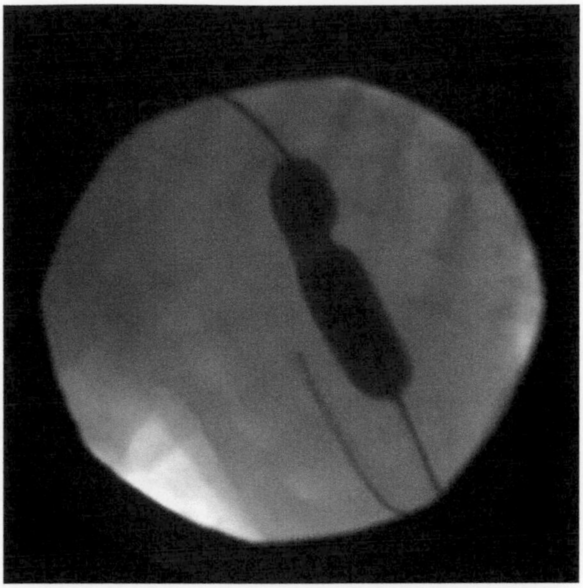

Figure 10.7 Fluoroscopic view of aortic balloon valvuloplasty: a cardiac guidewire has been passed from the carotid artery to the aorta and across the aortic valve into the left ventricle. It can be seen curling back towards the top of the heart. The interventional balloon can be seen inflated with contrast agent across the stenosis. A visible waist is noted in the balloon where the stenosis is located.

surface, roughening them which allows for adherence of bacteria present in the bloodstream from normally occurring bacteremia (see Chapter 11). The general recommendation for any dog suspected or diagnosed with subaortic stenosis undergoing surgical or invasive procedures (including dental prophylaxis, spay or neuter, endoscopy, or severe infections) is to be provided with an extended course of prophylactic antibiotics.

Pulmonic Stenosis

Pulmonic stenosis is a malformation of the pulmonic valve. Unlike subaortic stenosis, PS occurs in the valve itself. This anomaly can present in different forms. One variation is a narrowed annulus with fairly normal valve leaflets. A second version appears as a normal valve annulus with tethered and fused leaflets. Pulmonic stenosis is most often seen in terrier breeds, bulldogs, and other small breed dogs. Although PS can occur in any breed, it is not commonly seen in large-breed dogs except for the boxer and to a lesser extent, the Labrador retriever. Bulldogs and boxers present an unusual challenge for the veterinary cardiologist since they can develop a third type of pulmonic stenosis that involves the coronary arteries. In dogs, two coronary arteries typically leave the aortic root, one to the left heart and one to the right. In 1990, four variations of the origin of the right coronary artery were described, subcategorized as R1 and R2. The R1 anomaly is a single coronary artery that circumnavigates the entire heart with no major branches. The R2 anomaly is an artery of single aortic origin, but branches into right and left main branches. Three different variations have been reported: R2a, R2b, and R2c. The R2b and R2c do not cause any clinical sign, so the prevalence in the general population is hard to predict. The R2a anomaly is a cause of pulmonic stenosis (Figure 10.8). The R2a anomaly occurs mostly in bulldogs and boxers in which the right coronary artery may be absent,

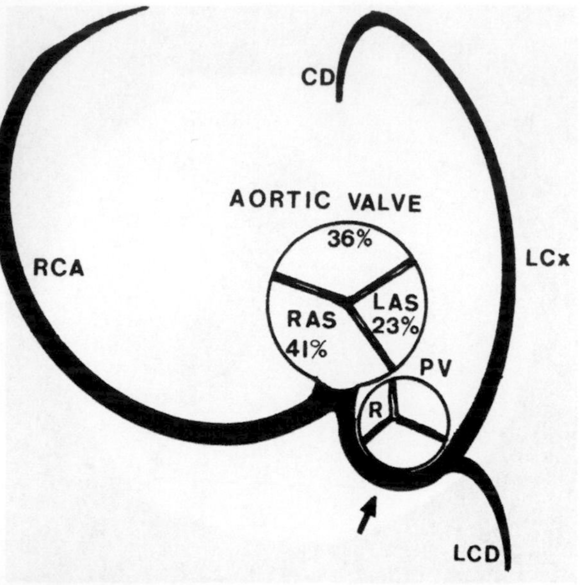

Figure 10.8 A single coronary artery arrangement in pulmonic stenosis: the single left coronary artery (arrow) exits the aorta towards the bottom of the image and courses over the pulmonic valve (PV) narrowing the orifice. The pulmonic cusps and sinuses (R) are hypoplastic. The mean portion of aortic circumference associated with each cusp for a small group of dogs are indicated by the percentages. The left aortic sinus (LAS) does not have a coronary sinus and represents only ~23% of aortic circumference. The right cusp and sinus (RAS) is nearly twice the size of the LAS. The left cranial descending coronary artery (LCD) arises from the anomalous left main coronary ostium. The right coronary artery (RCA) traverses the right ventricle. The caudal descending coronary artery (CD) is a terminal branch of the left circumflex coronary artery (LCx). Source: Buchanan (1990) [11]. Reproduced with permission of JAVMA.

causing a branch of the left coronary artery to literally wrap around the pulmonary artery creating the stenosis [11].

Clinical Presentation

Similar to SAS, PS is often suspected after routine examination when a left basilar systolic murmur is heard. The intensity of the murmur correlates somewhat with the severity of the stenosis, but loud murmurs may be present with moderate stenosis. This may be due to the relatively small size of the most common patients seen with PS vs SAS, creating loud murmurs with even moderate PG. Similar to SAS, the quality of the murmur often is an ejection quality (crescendo or diamond-shaped) murmur loudest at the left heart base. Other clinical manifestations of PS include exercise intolerance, syncope, and ascites from right ventricle (RV) failure. A palpable thrill is often felt in cases with severe PS in the left axillary region.

Diagnostics

Radiographic findings will show evidence of right ventricular and right atrial enlargement with a prominent poststenotic dilation of the main pulmonary artery visible in

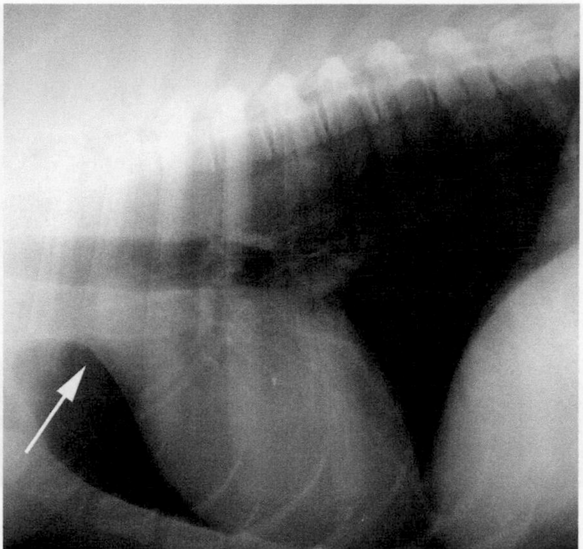

Figure 10.9 Lateral radiograph of a dog with pulmonic stenosis: the arrow in this image points to the enlarged pulmonary artery. It is noticed as a loss of the cranial waist in the cardiac silhouette. The overall cardiac silhouette is normal in shape and size. A normal reference image is available in Chapter 5.

both the lateral and VD views (Figures 10.9 and 10.10). The remaining pulmonary vascular may appear to be under circulated. If signs of right-heart failure are present then a dilated caudal vena cava may also be seen.

An electrocardiogram can be useful in distinguishing SAS from PS by calculating the mean electrical axis (MEA) (see Chapter 4). Right ventricular hypertrophy will cause the MEA to deviate toward the right axis in PS, while MEA remains normal in SAS, even

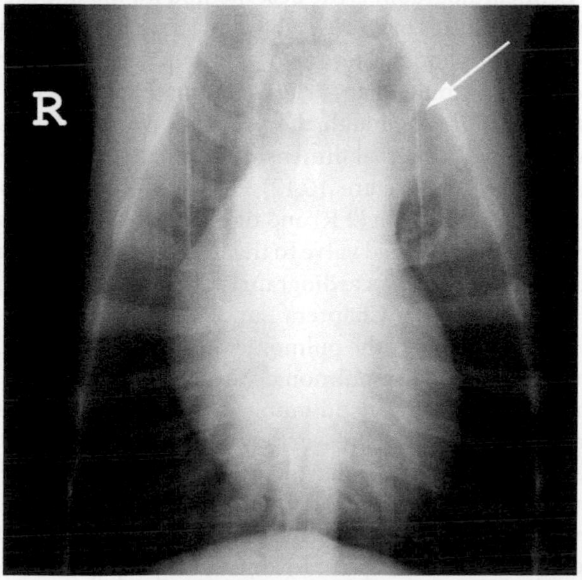

Figure 10.10 Ventrodorsal radiograph of a dog with pulmonic stenosis: the arrow in this image indicates the poststenotic dilation creating a noticeable bulge at the left cranial aspect of the cardiac silhouette. Using the clock-face analogy, the bulge is at 1 o'clock.

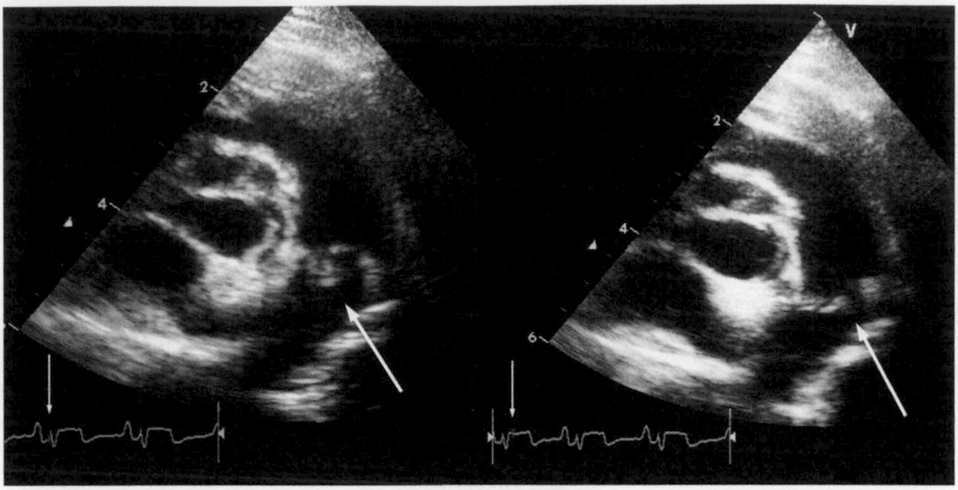

Figure 10.11 Echocardiographic view of a stenotic pulmonic valve: this short axis view of the heart base shows a stenotic pulmonic valve. The twin image shows the pulmonic valve at the start of systole. The small arrows at the bottom shows the electrocardiogram (ECG) indicating the red line in the early QRS complex. The ECG demonstrates a right axis shift in the predominantly negative QRS complex. The left image is just before the valve should open. The valve cusps (large arrows) can be seen as thickened and billowing upwards towards the right ventricle. The right image shows the cusps as they try to open. In a normal pulmonic valve, the cusps should not be visible during systole, but in this image they are prominent and thick.

in the presence of LV hypertrophy. The "P" wave amplitude can measure greater than normal ("P" pulmonale) if right atrial enlargement is present.

Echocardiography is the best method for making the definitive diagnosis. Echocardiographic features of PS are right ventricular hypertrophy, enlargement of the right atrium (RA), poorly mobile, tethered pulmonic cusps, and/or a hypoplastic valve annulus and poststenotic pulmonary artery dilation (Figure 10.11). The increase in pressure and lack of forward flow through the pulmonic valve (PV) also affects the LV. In severe PS, a decreased LV internal dimension and flattening of the interventricular septum (IVS) is usually present (Figure 10.12). Evaluation with Doppler color mapping can show tricuspid regurgitation (TR) and due to the elevated pressure in the RV being transmitted through the tricuspid valve to the RA, a patent foramen ovale (PFO) is sometimes noted. An air-contrast echocardiogram is useful in confirming the suspected diagnosis of a PFO (Figure 10.13) (see Chapters 1 and 6).

Color Doppler of the pulmonic valve will demonstrate highly turbulent blood flow and insufficiency of the pulmonic valve is also noted [1] (Figure 10.14). Spectral Doppler interrogation of transpulmonic flow reveals elevated velocities across the pulmonic valve (Figure 10.15). Pressure gradients greater than 80–100 mmHg are considered to be severe, pressures between 50–80 mmHg are moderate and less than 50 mmHg are mild pulmonic stenosis [1, 3]. However, a 2011 study suggests that dogs with a PG greater than 60 mmHg are at increased risk of cardiac mortality [12]. The transpulmonic valve velocities can be acquired from the right parasternal short axis basilar view, or from

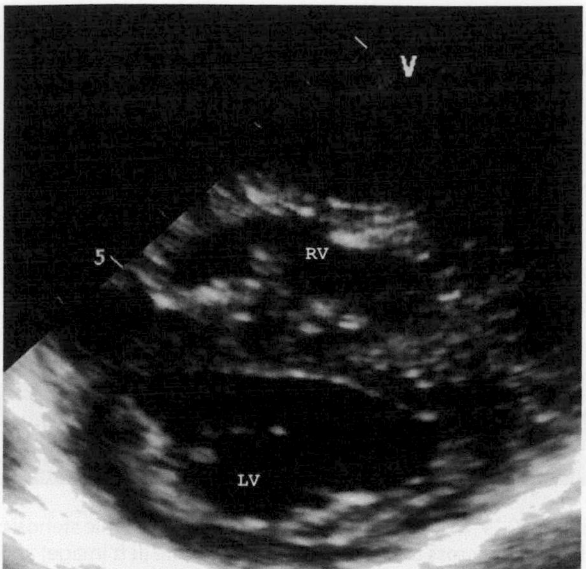

Figure 10.12 Echocardiographic short axis view of ventricles in canine pulmonic stenosis: the right ventricle (RV) at the top of the image exhibits RV hypertrophy. The RV should be approximately one-third as thick as the left ventricle (LV). The LV is approximately normal thickness, while the RV is seen as the same as the LV. The intraventricular septum is flattened rather than rounding towards the RV due to the excessive RV pressure. A normal reference image is available in Chapter 6.

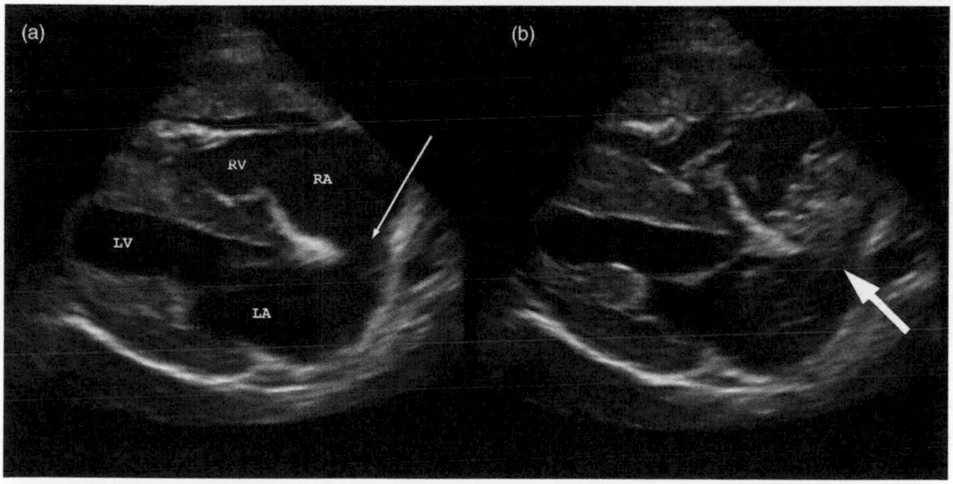

Figure 10.13 Echocardiographic image of a patent foramen ovale (PFO): this twin image shows a long axis four-chamber of a canine heart with pulmonic stenosis. The chambers are labeled as: LV, left ventricle; LA, left atrium; RA, right atrium; RV, right ventricle. (a) The heart just before a microbubble air-contrast echocardiogram. The PFO is apparent by the hypoechoic area in the interatrial septum (arrow). The right ventricle is hypertrophied in response to the increased work added to it by the stenotic valve. The left ventricle is decreased in chamber dimension due to poor cardiac output from the right ventricle. The RA appears slightly larger than the LA and the RV papillary muscle and tricuspid chordae tendineae are visible as the hyperechoic structure in the RV. (b) The microbubbles entering the RA from the right of the image during later diastole frame. An injection of agitated saline was made into a cephalic vein. As the microbubbles enter the RA, increased pressure in the RA from tricuspid regurgitation as a result of a pressure overload of the RV pushes the bubbles into the LA through the PFO (wide arrow). The microbubble air-contrast echocardiogram is diagnostic for a right-to-left shunting septal defect.

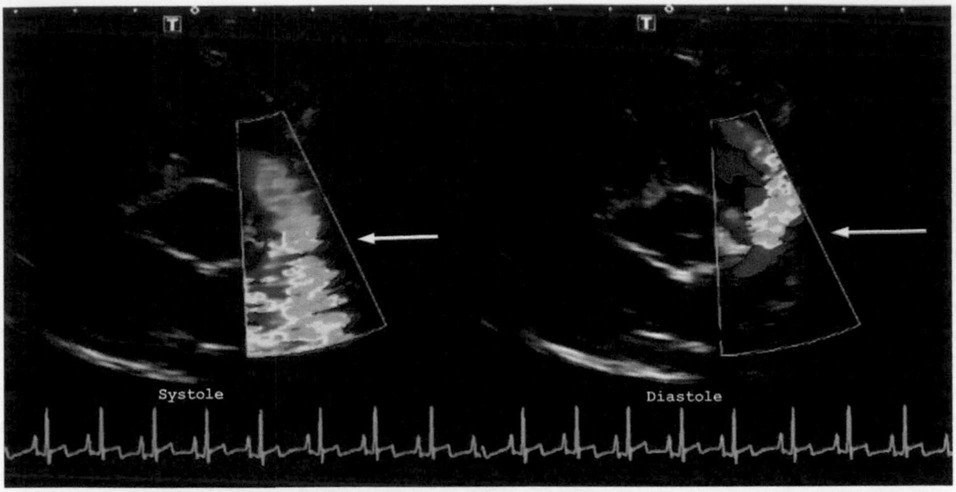

Figure 10.14 Doppler color-flow mapping of pulmonic stenosis: this twin image shows turbulent blood flow across the pulmonic valve in systole (left image) and diastole (right image). The arrows indicate the level of the valve for reference. During systole, blood moves downward in this view and is coded in blue, until it reaches the valve, where it increases in velocity and becomes turbulent. The yellow–green mosaic of color beyond the valve indicates turbulence. In diastole, the incompetent valve allows blood to flow retrograde into the right ventricle or upwards in this view and is coded as red. This pulmonic insufficiency also is somewhat turbulent.

the left cranial right ventricular outflow tract view [6, pp. 37–99] with transthoracic echocardiography.

Cardiac catheterization of the RV allows for recording of elevated RV pressure. Angiography demonstrates the narrow orifice of the pulmonic valve and the prominent poststenotic dilation (Figure 10.16).

Therapy includes medications, surgery or balloon valvuloplasty via cardiac catheterization. Cases of mild to moderate PS can often be very successfully managed with medical therapy alone or may not require any treatment. These patients may show no clinical signs other than exercise intolerance after periods of heavy activity. Patients with severe PS often benefit from an interventional procedure to reduce their PG in the mild to moderate range. Negative inotropic drugs such as beta-blockers or calcium channel blockers are used to treat PS when definitive therapy is not an option or as a bridge to intervention.

Several surgical procedures have been tried in dogs with PS, but most require extracorporeal perfusion and are not cost-effective for most clients. Surgeries to open the pulmonic orifice can be performed using a tubular graft to create a conduit around the stenosis [11] (Figure 10.17). Placement of an overlaying patch graft to create a structurally sound aneurysm around a bisected valve or similar techniques have been used [13, 14]. Valve replacement requires cardiopulmonary bypass.

Balloon valvuloplasty is a widely utilized treatment for dogs since open heart surgery is often risky and cost prohibitive. Balloon valvuloplasty is a cardiac catheterization procedure which can be performed via a transvenous catheter introducer whereby catheters are advanced into the right heart from the jugular vein following flow [15, 16]

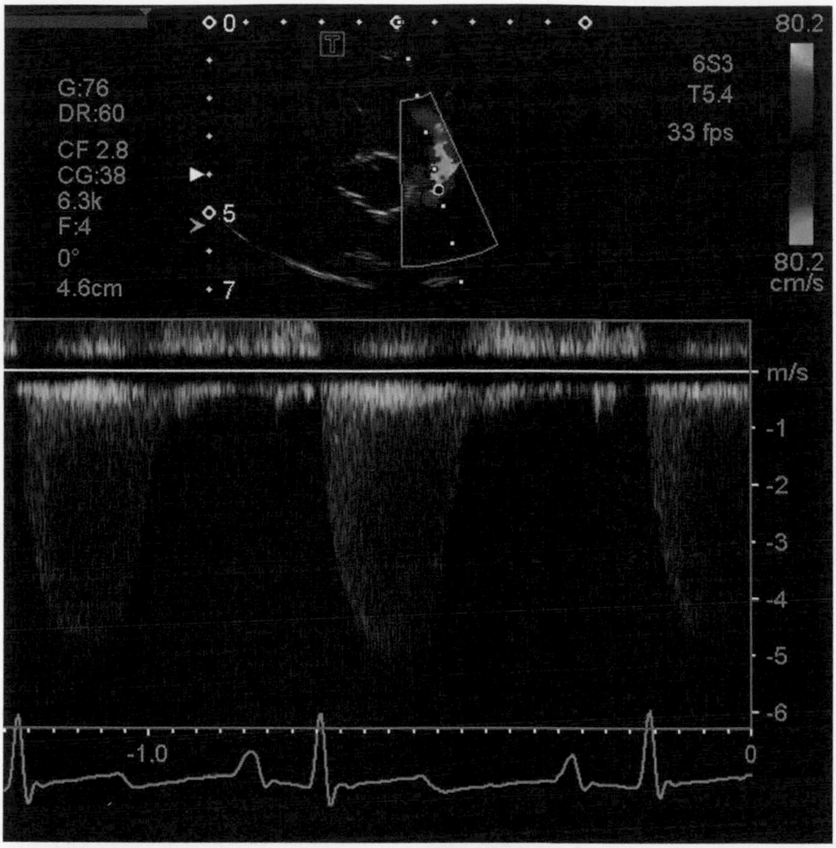

Figure 10.15 Spectral continuous wave Doppler of transpulmonic blood flow: the top portion of the image shows the reference echocardiographic image, and the Doppler cursor can be seen passing through the pulmonic valve area. The aorta is seen in cross-section in the center of the heart. The graph is a recording of the transpulmonic blood velocity. Normal blood velocity across the pulmonic valve is typically equal or less than 1.5 m/s. In this example the velocity scale on the right indicates a velocity of approximately 5 m/s which corresponds with a pressure gradient (see Chapter 6) of approximately 100 mmHg. This would equate to the right ventricle generating approximately 125 mmHg or five times greater than normal right ventricular pressure to eject blood though the stenotic valve.

(see Chapters 8 and 16). A special interventional balloon catheter is inflated across the valve to dilate it (Figure 10.18). The goal is to open the valve leaflets and subsequently reduce the transpulmonic PG. During this procedure it is possible to measure the PG directly with catheterization before and after the procedure. Balloon valvuloplasty is particularly suited to dogs with valve fusion and a normal valve annulus. Dogs with a hypoplastic valvular annulus may still benefit, but the outcome is not as positive and these dogs may see their PGs rise again over time. Evidence indicates that for dogs with high, moderate and severe PS, some intervention does improve their quality and quantity of life [17].

The R2a anomaly eliminates balloon valvuloplasty as a treatment option, as inflation of the balloon would rupture the coronary artery causing immediate death (Figure 10.19).

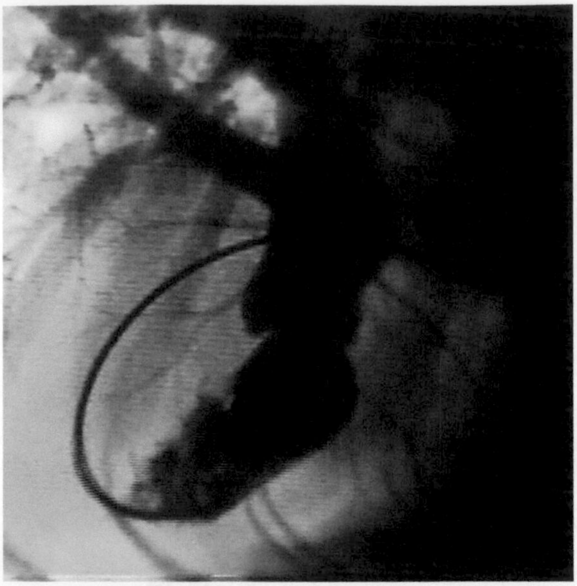

Figure 10.16 Fluoroscopic angiogram of canine pulmonic stenosis. The catheter is entering the image on the right from the cranial aspect of the patient; the spine is at the top. The catheter runs from the jugular vein, cranial vena cava, right atrium, then finally through the right ventricle and out of the pulmonic valve. A radiopaque contrast is injected into the right ventricle. A prominent narrowing separates the pulmonic root (upper) and right ventricular outflow tract (lower). In the center of the stenosis is a dark contrast jet of maximal flow. The subtle noncontrasted light lines to either side of the central jet are the restricted valvular cusps. The poststenotic dilation is above the pulmonic root. The two pulmonary arterial branches and some of the pulmonary vasculature can also be seen.

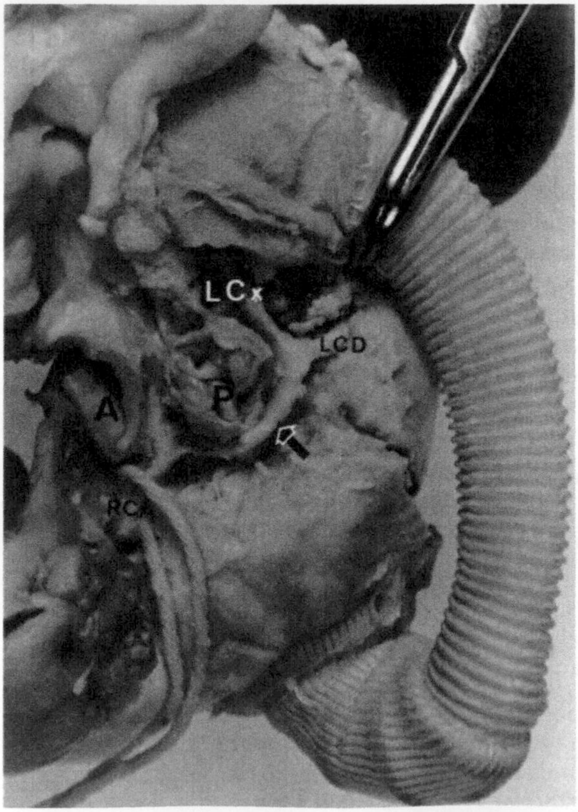

Figure 10.17 Pulmonic bridging conduit postmortem in a dog with R2a coronary artery anomaly: the anomalous left main coronary artery (arrow) runs cranial and adjacent to the constricted pulmonic valve (P) before dividing in the left circumflex (LCx) left cranial descending (LCD) coronary arteries. The right coronary artery (RCA) courses in a normal fashion after bifurcating a few millimeters away from the large right aortic sinus (A). Source: Buchanan (1990) [11]. Reproduced with permission of JAVMA.

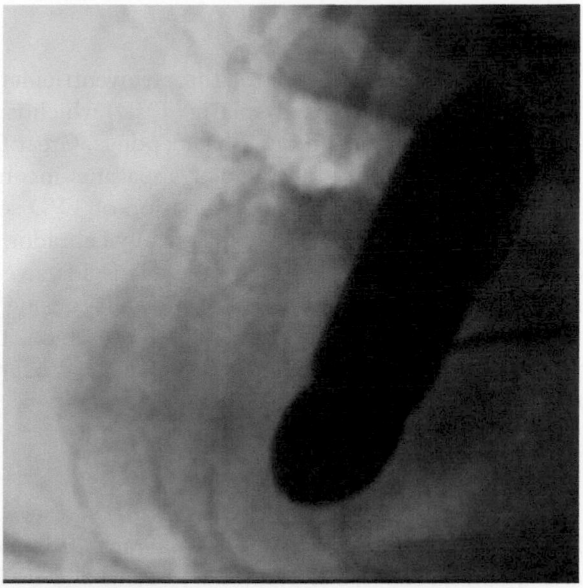

Figure 10.18 Fluoroscopic image of pulmonic balloon valvuloplasty. This image shows an interventional dilation balloon for pulmonic stenosis being inflated. The narrowed waist is at the point of the valvular stenosis. The balloon is inflated for several seconds, then deflated; this is repeated two to three times to achieve maximal effect. The catheter portion of the interventional balloon is entering the image on the right. The catheter runs from the jugular vein, cranial vena cava, right atrium, then finally through the right ventricle and out of the pulmonic valve.

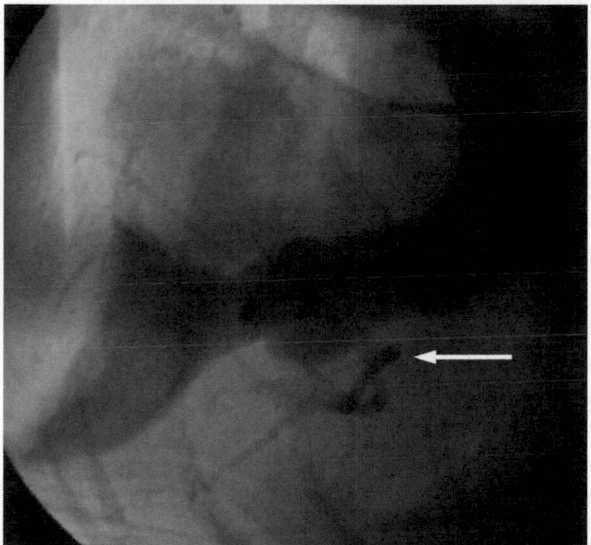

Figure 10.19 Fluoroscopic angiogram of canine single coronary aortic root: the pigtail catheter entering from the right is being advanced from the carotid artery and is positioned atop the aortic valve. A radiopaque contrast is injected to record this diastolic angiogram. The single coronary artery can be seen exiting the aorta to the lower right, and traverses over the pulmonary trunk (arrow). Smaller coronary branches may be appreciated coursing around the outer surface of the heart. There is aortic regurgitation, most likely due to the catheter deforming the aortic valve. Figure 8.14 demonstrates normal coronary arterial courses. A catheter may also be seen in the upper right quadrant of the image. The catheter is being advanced through the jugular vein, to the cranial vena cava, and sits resting in the right atrium in preparation for a right ventriculogram.

Atrioventricular Valve Dysplasia

The most common dysplasia of the atrioventricular (AV) valves seen in veterinary medicine is tricuspid valve dysplasia (TVD) which is a breed concern in the Labrador retriever. Also seen in Old English sheepdogs, Great Danes and boxers, TVD may take many shapes and leave the valvular apparatus incompetent and/or stenotic [18, 19]. Ebstein's anomaly is a particular variation of TVD seen in humans that may be analogous to forms of TVD in dogs, specifically Labrador retrievers [20]. Ebstein's anomaly is characterized by the location of the tricuspid valve leaflets below the valve annulus, and tethering of these leaflets to the RV walls causing them to have poor mobility.

Likewise mitral valve dysplasia (MVD) presents with a wide variation of deformities to the valve apparatus. Mitral valve dysplasia has been reported to occur in cats, Great Danes, German shepherds and bull terriers [1].

Clinical Signs

Clinical manifestations of MVD or TVD range from none to rapid onset of CHF. Mitral valve dysplasia can lead to pulmonary edema and TVD to ascites associated with right-heart CHF. Cases with moderately functional valves may only exhibit signs of exercise intolerance or lethargy. A murmur may not always be present on physical examination, but when noted, MVD is most often associated with a left apical systolic murmur of mitral regurgitation, and TVD with a right-sided systolic murmur. Murmur intensity can be variable, ranging from grade 2 to 5/6 and generally does not correlate well with the severity of the dysplasia. Examination of the neck in patients with TVD may reveal jugular pulses associated with tricuspid regurgitation. A positive hepato-jugular reflux test (see Chapter 3) indicates elevated RA pressures.

Diagnostics

Radiographs show enlargement of the atria if there is significant regurgitation in the corresponding AV valve of the heart. Some ventricular enlargement may also be noted for the corresponding valve. If the valves are stenotic, the engorgement of the "upstream" vessels will be seen as enlargement of the cranial or caudal vena cava in TVD, and enlargement of the pulmonary veins in MVD (Figure 10.20).

Electrocardiography in patients with AV dysplasia may show atrial arrhythmias such as atrial fibrillation, atrial flutter, or atrial premature complexes (APC). A left axis shift with LA and/or LV enlargement pattern, such as "P" mitrale, can be noted in MVD cases. In dogs with TVD, "P" pulmonale, or a deviation of the MEA toward the right, is likely. Conduction defects through the ventricle, such as right bundle branch blocks or "splintering" of the QRS complex (Figure 10.21) are common findings on an ECG. If the stage of decompensation is advanced ventricular premature complexes (VPC) are also possible.

Echocardiography is the most useful modality for diagnosing AV dysplasia. The morphology of the valve itself can be viewed for abnormal placement, abnormal movement and abnormal connection of the papillary muscles and chordae tendineae. The atria associated with the dysplastic valve are generally enlarged, and in some cases severely.

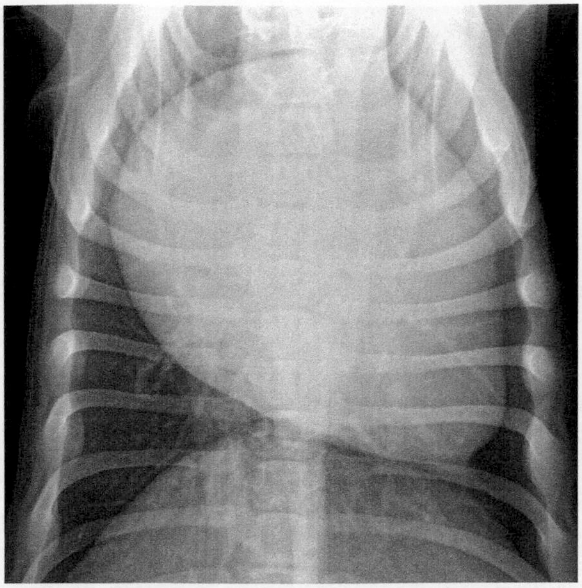

Figure 10.20 Ventrodorsal radiograph of canine tricuspid dysplasia showing marked enlargement of the cardiac silhouette. In this example it is the right ventricle and atrium that are enlarged. The dysplastic valve allows for severe tricuspid regurgitation.

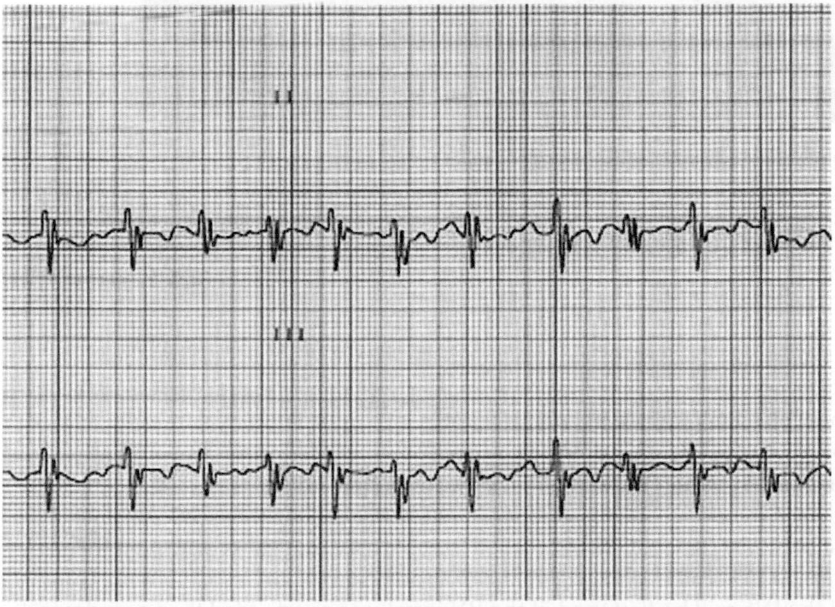

Figure 10.21 Electrocardiogram of QRS splintering recorded at 25 mm/s and standard calibration and shows leads II and III. The baseline is uneven, but clear P waves can be identified before each QRS complex. The QRS has an extra positive deflection after the S wave, but before the T wave. This "splintering" of the QRS complex is a characteristic commonly seen with tricuspid dysplasia.

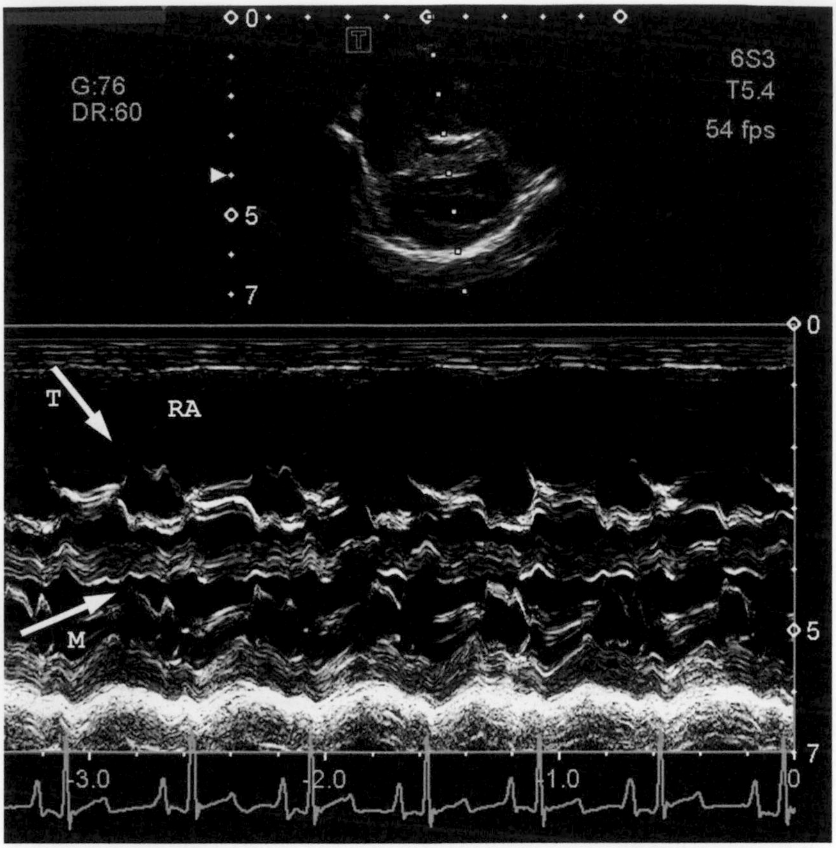

Figure 10.22 Short axis M-mode echocardiogram image of tricuspid dysplasia showing the characteristic "double fish-mouth" of right atrial enlargement (RA). This is recorded in the echocardiographic plane used to record the mitral valve motion. The upper arrow (T) points to the tricuspid valve and the lower arrow (M) points to the mitral valve. The interventricular septum is between the two valves.

Commonly, the chordae tendineae may be absent with the valve leaflet directly attached to the papillary muscle. Ventricular function and size can be abnormal, usually dilated, with poor contractility. M-mode of the valve motion may show poor movement of the leaflets in diastole, especially with MVD.

Dogs with TVD may have such severe RA dilation that a short-axis image of the tricuspid valve can be appreciated. This so called "double fish-mouth" is only seen with RA dilation (Figure 10.22). The IVS may develop an abnormal motion also. If RV pressure is very elevated the IVS will be flattened; if the RV is volume overloaded then paradoxical IVS motion may be seen in which the IVS moves away from the LV posterior wall in systole (Figure 10.23). Three-dimensional echocardiography can provide view of the valve, which allows for planemetry measurements, as well as permits visualization previously uncommon in veterinary medicine (Figure 10.24).

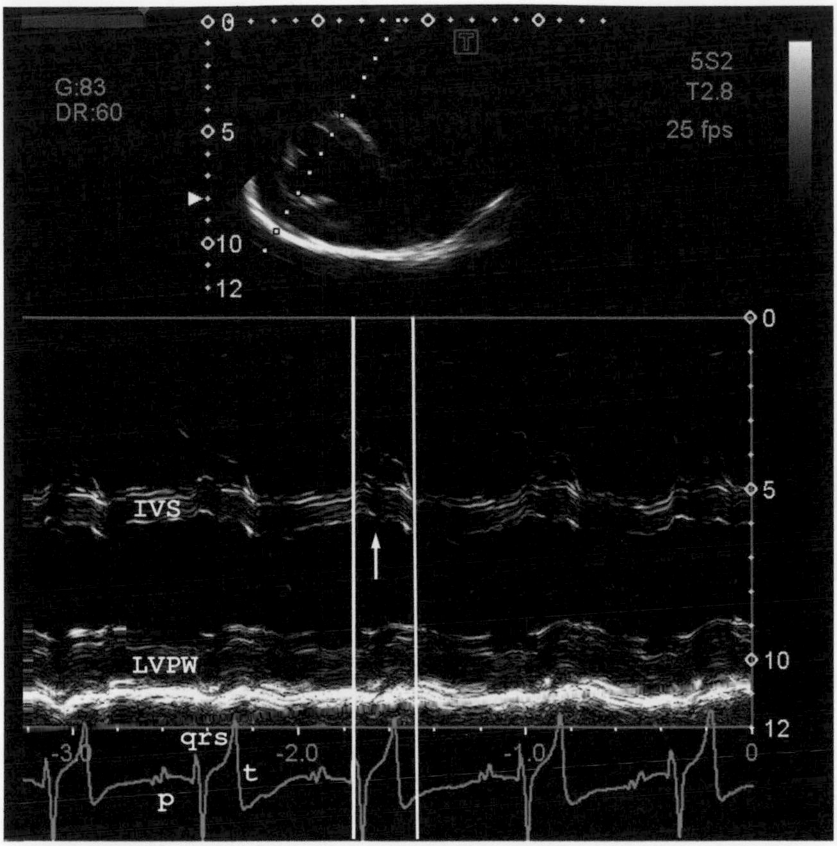

Figure 10.23 M-mode echocardiographic image of paradoxical septal motion: in the presence of right ventricular volume overload, the interventricular septum (IVS) will move away from the center of the left ventricular lumen rather than towards it as usual during systole. The parts of the electrocardiogram are labeled P (p), QRS (qrs), and T (t) along with the left ventricular posterior wall (LVPW). Note the negative QRS complex in lead II typical of a mean electrical axis shift towards the right. The vertical lines indicate the duration of systole in the third cardiac contraction shown. The IVS can be seen moving upwards (arrow) away from the left ventricle between the lines (see Chapter 6 for normal reference).

Using Doppler modalities, PGs across the valves can be estimated and regurgitation diagnosed with color flow mapping (Figures 10.25 and 10.26). An increase in velocity of blood from the atria to the ventricles is indicative of a stenotic valve.

Unfortunately, short of open heart surgery, there is little that veterinary cardiology has to offer. Valve replacement surgery is costly, and has rarely been performed in AV valve dysplasia. As the patient ages the long-term hemodynamic consequences are virtually identical to acquired valve disease. Medical management of the hemodynamic effects with standard heart failure therapy is the most common treatment. In the case of a stenotic tricuspid valve, cardiac catheter balloon valvuloplasty is possible, but more often TVD lesions are only regurgitant [18].

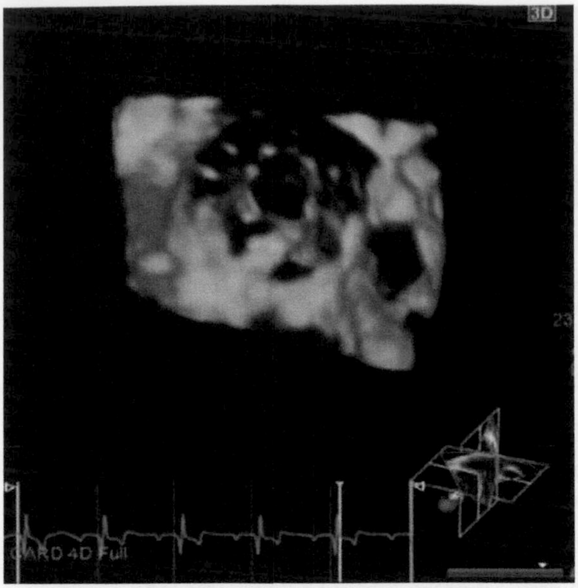

Figure 10.24 Three-dimensional echocardiographic image of a dysplastic tricuspid valve (larger dark circular shape) from the right ventricular side of the valve looking towards the right atrium. The area of the valve can be measured. There is a large hole (smaller dark circle within the larger one) in the center of the valve where the valve would be incompetent. The area of the defect could also be measured from this view.

Intercirculatory Shunts

Intercirculatory shunts are abnormal hemodynamic communications between the pulmonic and systemic circulations. They can occur at any level of the circulation; in the heart itself, in the central vasculature, or in the peripheral vessels. Shunts between the

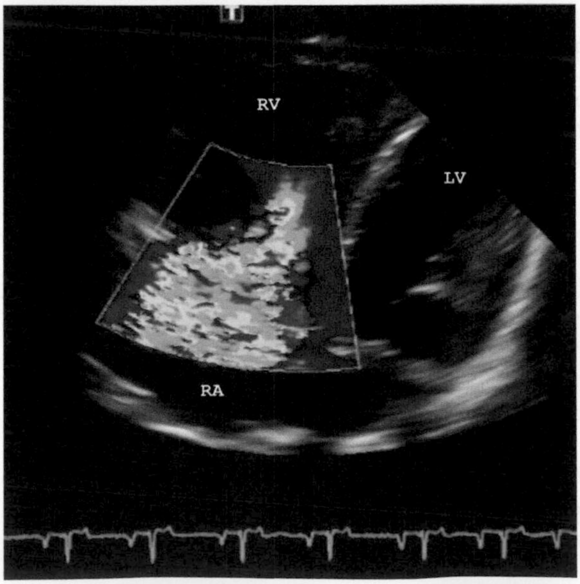

Figure 10.25 Color-flow mapping Doppler image of tricuspid regurgitation: this is a left apical four-chamber view of a canine heart with tricuspid dysplasia. The right ventricle (RV) is towards the top and the right atrium (RA) is at the bottom. The left ventricle (LV) is to the right of the image. The presence of tricuspid regurgitation is demonstrated by the large turbulent color-flow signal in this image. On the RV side of the valve, the blue color signal represents blood flow away from the transducer, or down in this example. As the blood reaches the tricuspid regurgitant orifice, it accelerates to become the high velocity turbulent color image shown. The red color on the edges of the yellow–green mosaic is aliasing of the color signal.

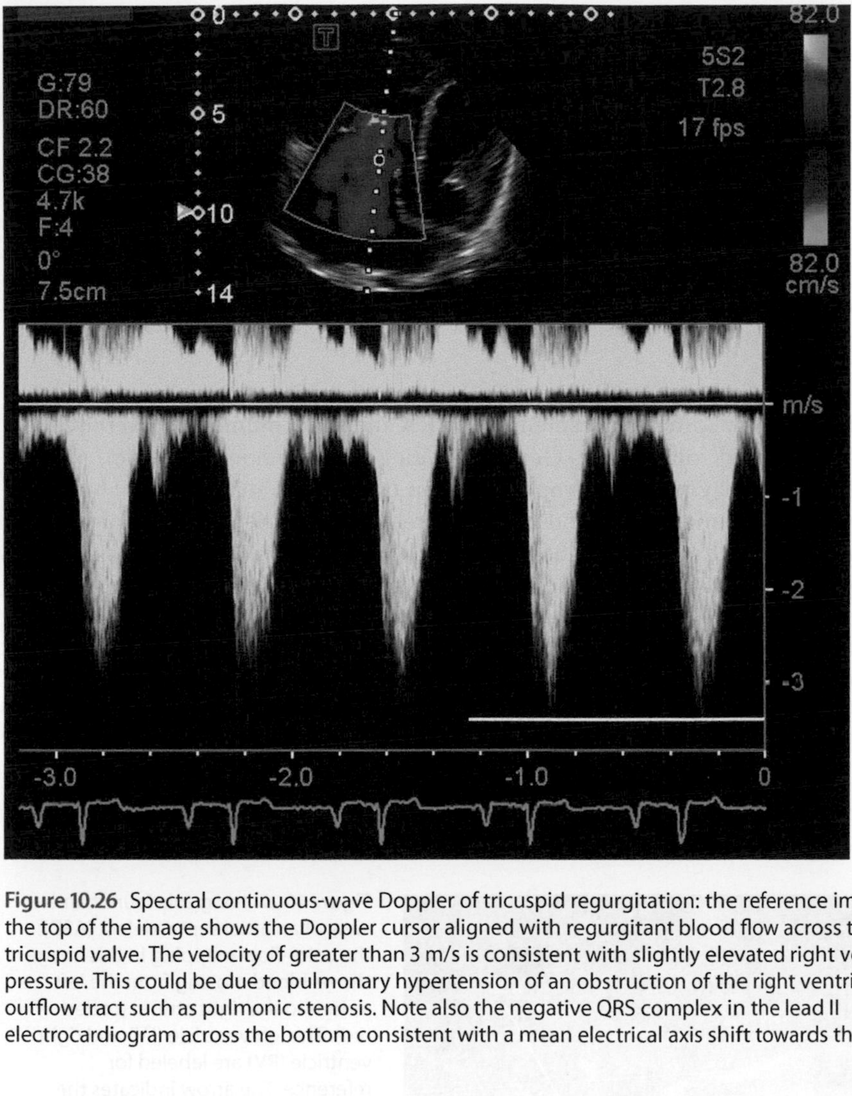

Figure 10.26 Spectral continuous-wave Doppler of tricuspid regurgitation: the reference image near the top of the image shows the Doppler cursor aligned with regurgitant blood flow across the tricuspid valve. The velocity of greater than 3 m/s is consistent with slightly elevated right ventricular pressure. This could be due to pulmonary hypertension of an obstruction of the right ventricular outflow tract such as pulmonic stenosis. Note also the negative QRS complex in the lead II electrocardiogram across the bottom consistent with a mean electrical axis shift towards the right.

cardiac chambers are termed *septal defects* and can be atrial or ventricular. Central vasculature anomalies may be persistent flow through the fetal ductus arteriosus or aortopulmonary windows [1]. Aortopulmonary windows are a failure of the spiral septum to completely develop with the *truncus arteriosus* of the embryo. They are extremely rare and create an ostium or "window" between the aorta and the main pulmonary artery. Shunts that occur out in the peripheral vasculature are termed an *arteriovenous fistula*. Shunts can flow from the arterial circulation to pulmonary (so called *left to right* shunts) or pulmonary to arterial (*right to left*). Due to the greater blood pressure in the arterial system, most shunts flow from left to right. Shunts provide an abnormal volume load to one or more parts of the circulation. The size of the defect and the load it represents determines the severity of cardiac effects.

Atrial Septal Defects

Atrial septal defects are very uncommon and often have little or no clinical significance unless the patient is an athlete, which could explain a lack of peak performance in an otherwise perfect specimen. They are often incidental findings on echocardiogram that was performed for some other reason. Unless increased RV and RA pressures are present, ASDs will shunt from the LA to the RA during diastole. ASDs rarely present with murmurs; however, when a murmur is heard, they are often soft, left basilar systolic murmurs due to relative pulmonic stenosis from increased flow through the right ventricular outflow tract [1].

Diagnostics

Radiographs may show some enlargement of the RA and some pulmonary overcirculation from the increased volume load. Generally radiographs are nondiagnostic.

Echocardiography may reveal a "drop out" lesion on the interatrial septum, but this area is fairly nonechogenic anyway and overinterpretation must be avoided. Color-flow Doppler can be used to demonstrate flow across the defect. This will be noted as a low-velocity flow generally coded in red and is best appreciated during longer diastolic periods (Figure 10.27).

Patent foramen ovale is the result of nonclosure of a fetal physiological shunt that passes blood from the placental circulation entering the RA to the LA then LV. This is not a true ASD because the atrial septum is anatomically correct. Typically after birth, a flap of tissue that was held open by the flow from the maternal circulation through the foramen ovale closes when the right atrial pressure drops (see Chapter 1). If RA pressures never drop below LA then the ovale may remain patent. When PFO is present,

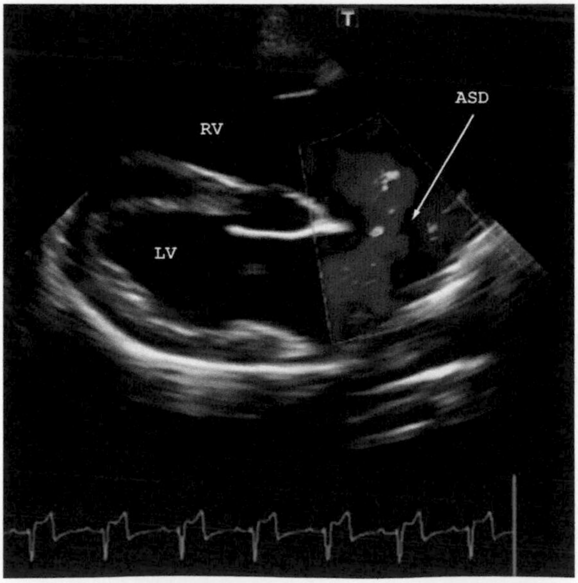

Figure 10.27 Long axis four-chamber view of an atrial septal defect (ASD): the color-flow mapping in this image shows blood moving from the left atrium to the right atrium (coded red). The left ventricle (LV) and right ventricle (RV) are labeled for reference. The arrow indicates the opening between the two atria filled with the Doppler color signal. This portion of the interatrial septum often will be seen as hypoechoic, and a false diagnosis of ASD is possible. The color-flow mapping assists in determining a true ASD from a normal interatrial septum with echo "drop-out".

PS or pulmonary hypertension and TR are almost always present as well. As previously stated, a contrast echocardiogram is very helpful in diagnosing a PFO.

Treatment

Typically, no treatment is needed for the ASD since they are small and have minimal hemodynamic consequences. In dogs with large ASDs, transcatheter placement of closure devices can be attempted [21].

Ventricular Septal Defect

Shunting resulting from a hole in the IVS is known as a VSD. These defects most often occur in membranous or perimembranous regions of the heart just below the aortic valve, tricuspid valve or pulmonic valve of the RV and near the aortic valve as viewed from the LV. In the embryological development of the heart this area is the last to be closed by union of the IVS and the spiral septum of the truncus arteriosus. The proximity of the VSD to the aortic valve may lead to prolapse of an aortic valve leaflet. Ventricular septal defects can occur in the muscular portion of the IVS in horses and cattle, but rarely occur in small animals. The size of a VSD can be quite variable ranging from 1 to 2 millimeters to several centimeters, and can affect the cardiac architecture as seen with tetralogy of Fallot.

Clinical Presentation

Patients will present with a loud right-sided basilar systolic murmur (grade 5–6/6) as juveniles. They may exhibit exercise intolerance or syncope during exercise, but are otherwise normal. If the defect is very small or *restrictive*, the patient may never develop cardiac signs. If a diastolic murmur is present, then aortic prolapse and regurgitation should be suspected.

Diagnostics

Radiographs generally show enlargement of the LA and LV with pulmonary overcirculation with enlargement of the complete pulmonary vasculature. If the shunt volume is large and cardiac output compromised, evidence of CHF may also be present.

Electrocardiography is typically within normal limits with the exception of potential LV and LA enlargement patterns. In late-stage disease, atrial or ventricular arrhythmias may be present.

Echocardiography demonstrates an enlarged LV and LA as rounded, volume-loaded chambers (Figure 10.28). Systolic function may be impaired. The defect itself may be hard to visualize unless it is large, but color-flow Doppler will reveal a high-velocity jet moving from the LV to the RV during systole near the aortic valve in the long axis five-chamber view and the short axis heart base view [6, pp. 437–475] (Figure 10.29).

Spectral Doppler interrogation of this jet indicates the PG between the LV and RV. This yields information on prognosis as an assessment of chamber pressures. Assuming the pressure in the ventricles is within normal limits, the PG should be approximately 100 mmHg at peak systole. Using the modified Bernoulli equation, the velocity measured should be near 5 m/s (Equation 10.2) (Figure 10.30).

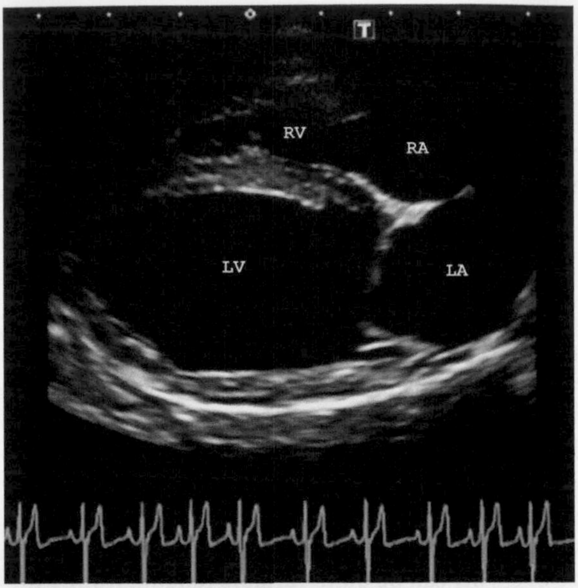

Figure 10.28 Long axis four-chamber view of a canine heart with volume overload. The chambers are labeled as: LV, left ventricle; LA, left atrium; RV, right ventricle; RA, right atrium. The LV shows an enlarged rounded shape and the LA is also enlarged. This is a typical-looking LV in dogs with ventricular septal defects due to the overcirculation of blood through the pulmonary vasculature. As blood shunts from the LV to the RV the additional volume from the LV is carried to the lung and return directly to the LV causing the pictured changes in the heart.

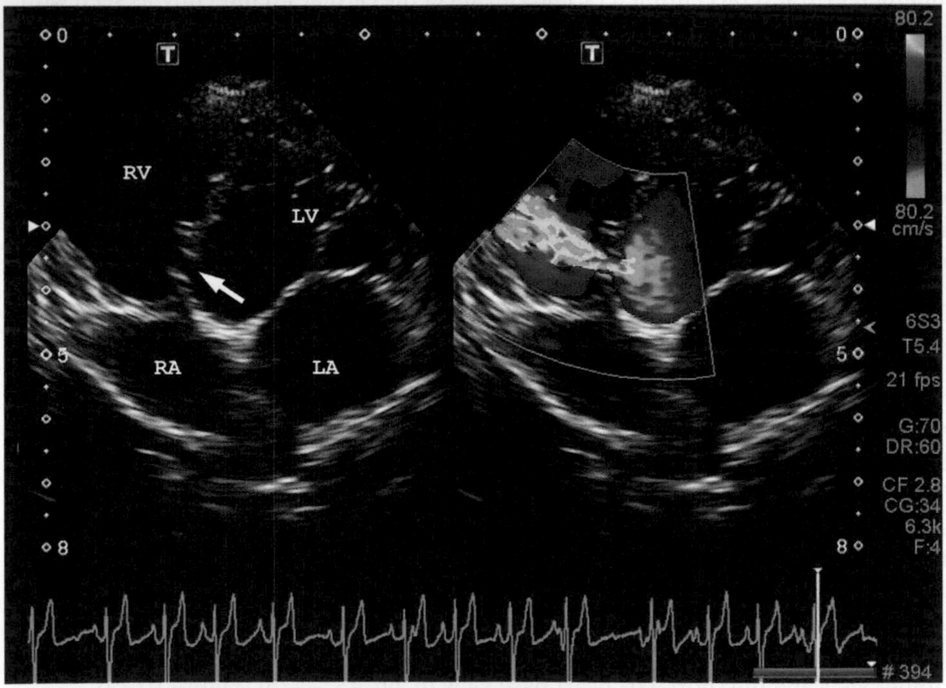

Figure 10.29 Twin image of a ventricular septal defect (VSD) with and without color-flow mapping: this image is from the left apical four-chamber projection. The left image shows the VSD (arrow) as a hypoechoic space in the interventricular septum. The chambers are labeled as: LV, left ventricle; LA, left atrium; RV, right ventricle; RA, right atrium. The right portion shows the exact same image with the Doppler color-flow mapping added, demonstrating the trans-septal flow. The large blue signal is blood being ejected from the LV as it heads out the aorta. A yellow–green mosaic high-velocity turbulent blood flow jet can be seen crossing through the VSD into the RV.

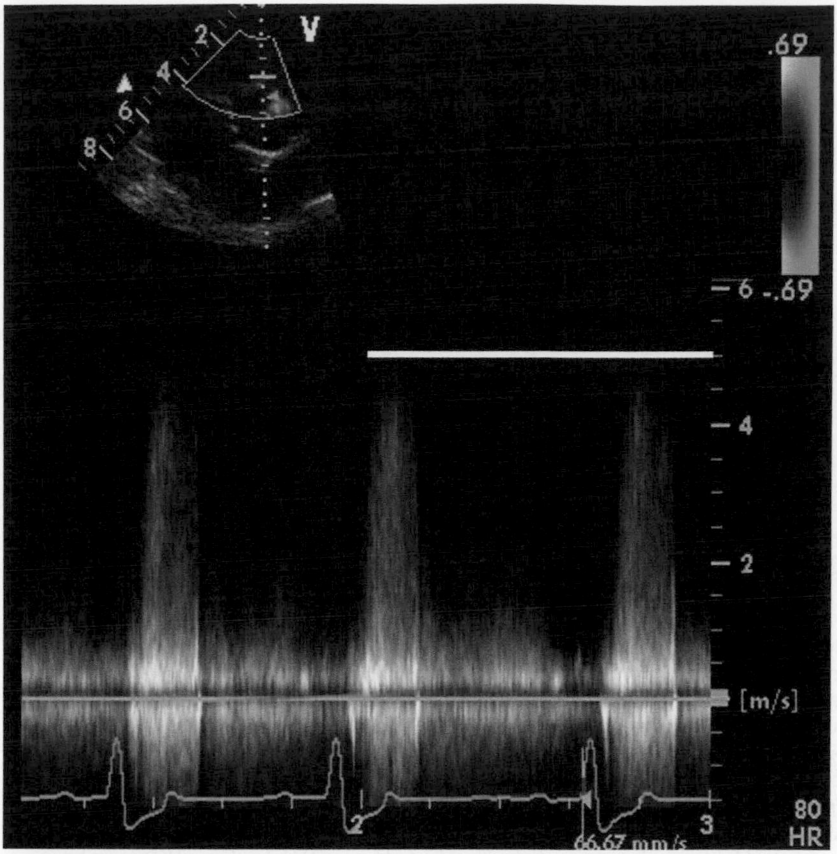

Figure 10.30 Spectral Doppler velocity image of blood flow through a ventricular septal defect: the blood flow from the left ventricle to the right ventricle recorded in this spectral Doppler image is moving towards the transducer, thus is displayed upwards from the baseline. It also is seen as the red signal within the reference image at the top. The velocity scale indicates the velocity to be approximately 5 m/s (line). Using the modified Bernoulli equation, the calculated pressure gradient would be approximately 100 mmHg between the ventricles. This implies normal ventricular chamber pressures associated with a heart in compensation for the condition.

RV peak systolic pressure = ~25 mmHg. LV peak systolic pressure = ~125 mmHg. Thus LV pressure – PV pressure = ~100 mmHg.

$$\begin{aligned} &4 * V^2 = \Delta P \\ &4 * V^2(\mathrm{m/s}) = 100\,\mathrm{mmHg}. \text{ Solve for } V^2 \\ &100\,\mathrm{mmHg}/4 = 25 \\ &\sqrt{25} = 5\,\mathrm{m/s} \end{aligned} \tag{10.2}$$

If cardiac catheterization is performed, an injection of contrast into the LV will be seen passing through the IVS into the RV outflow tract (Figure 10.31). With the advent of echocardiography, cardiac catheterization is uncommon.

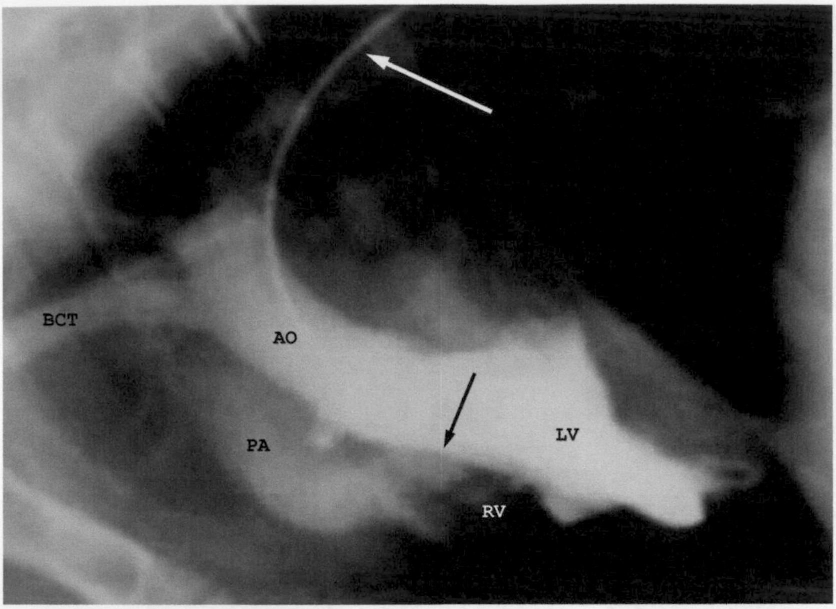

Figure 10.31 Fluoroscopic ventriculogram of a ventricular septal defect: the heart is seen here in a right lateral projection with the patient's head to the left. The major anatomical features are labeled: AO, aorta; LV, left ventricle; RV, right ventricle; PA, pulmonary artery; BCT, brachiocephalic trunk. A pigtail catheter (white arrow) has been advanced from the femoral artery retrograde through the descending aorta, around the aortic arch, through the aortic valve, then into the apex of the left ventricle. The contrast was injected into the LV, and is seen passing through a ventricular septal defect (VSD) (black arrow). The contrast is simultaneously highlighting the LV and RV outflow tracts, PA and proximal AO. Although the contrast jet of trans-VSD flow is difficult to appreciate, the reader should understand that for the highlighted structure to be illuminated from a LV injection, a VSD must be present. This image also demonstrates the VSD flow heading directly out the PA, and not filling the RV with contrast. This is typical for the VSD since the shunt occurs during systole, and the defect is located in proximity to pulmonic valve.

Treatment

The pathophysiology of the VSD generally leads to volume overload of the LA and LV. The shunt occurs during systole which protects the RV from the additional volume. The shunt volume travels from the LV directly out of the pulmonary artery in most cases, circulating through the lungs and back to the LA then LV. Added to the shunt volume is the returning volume from the body to the RA. If the shunt volume adds 2.5 times the normal volume to the LV, then LV failure is likely [1]. Most patients with large VSDs eventually succumb to left-heart CHF as the volume of the LV increases by the shunt volume returning to the left heart through the lungs. Consequently, the systolic function can be depressed and the heart goes into low output failure. As LV end-diastolic pressure rises and systolic function decreases, the PG between the LV and the RV can drop, as well as the LV to RV VSD velocity, providing a clue to the decompensation of the LV. During this time, the loudness of the systolic murmur may decrease as compared with when the diagnosis was first made. Surgical closure of VSD has been reported [22]. but because of cost, surgery is not generally practiced. Transcatheter occlusion has been performed

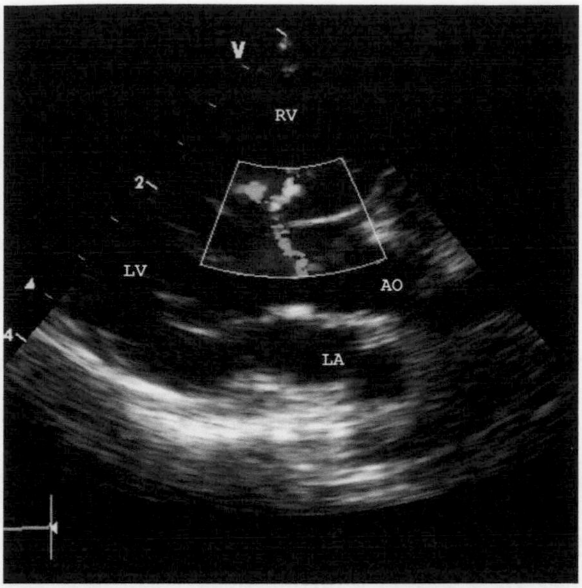

Figure 10.32 Long axis four-chamber image of a right-to-left shunting ventricular septal defect. The chambers are labeled as: LV, left ventricle; RV, right ventricle; AO, aorta; LA, left atrium. The color-flow signal in the center of the images demonstrates blood flowing from the RV to the LV, as indicated by the predominately blue color of flow away from the transducer. The yellow–green mosaic superimposed on the blue indicates turbulence as the blood crosses the defect.

with various occlusion devices [23–25]. Transcatheter occlusion for muscular VSD is more promising than for membranous and perimembranous VSD. Deployment of an occlusion device in the membranous and perimembranous regions comes with the risk of entrapping a portion of the aortic valve and inducing significant aortic insufficiency. Management of left-sided CHF is carried out with standard therapy with diuretics, ACE inhibitors, and positive inotropes.

In rare cases, the overcirculation of the pulmonary vasculature makes the vessels hyperreactive and they become stiff, leading to increased pulmonary vascular pressures. If they should rise to the point of exceeding systemic pressure, then the shunt will reverse from left to right to right to left (Figure 10.32 and 10.33). This condition, known as Eisenmenger's syndrome, leads to cyanosis and hypoxemia and is often fatal. It can also be confirmed by a contrast echocardiogram. Right-to-left shunting VSDs also show dilation of the large pulmonary arteries but undercirculation to the lung periphery, and the size of the heart generally remains normal on a radiograph [1]. Some newer drugs can be used to lower pulmonary hypertension [26] increasing blood flow to the lungs, and to combat secondary polycythemia, but a heart–lung transplant is the only curative treatment.

Patent Ductus Arteriosus

Patent ductus arteriosus is considered the most common cardiac defect in dogs, especially poodles, Shetland sheepdogs, collies and Maltese (see Table 10.1). Fortunately, it is rare in cats and may normally persist for a week in foals prior to closing. This shunt is formed by a failed closure of the ductus arteriosus (DA) of the fetal circulation which allows blood to bypass the lungs *in utero*. The DA is formed from the left sixth aortic

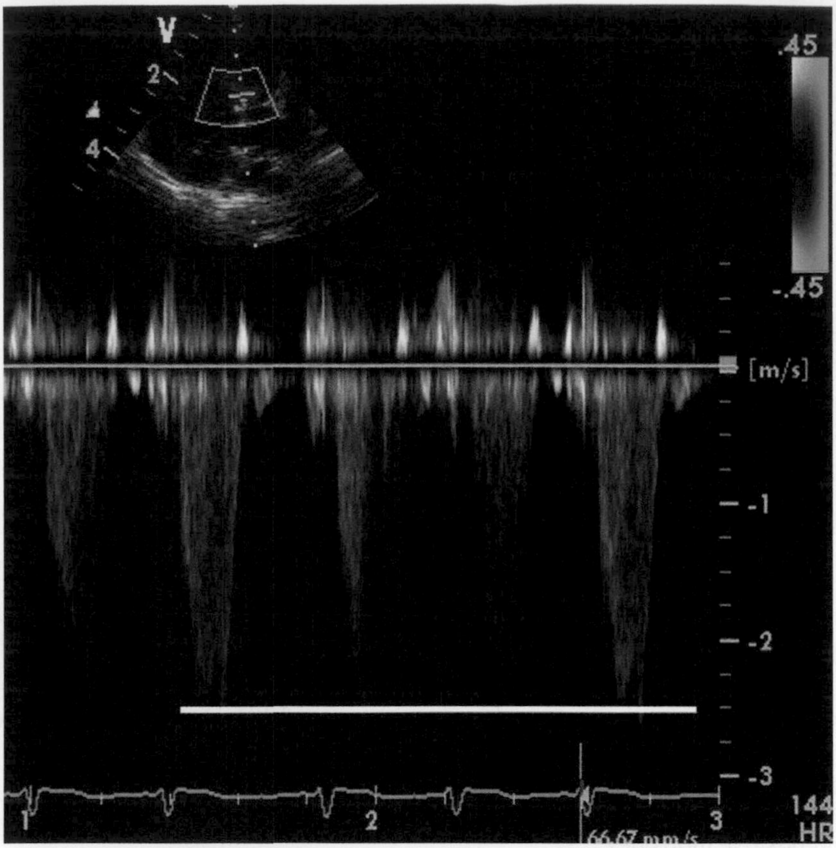

Figure 10.33 Spectral Doppler image of a right-to-left shunting ventricular septal defect: the Doppler cursor is aligned with the right-to-left shunt in the upper reference image. The velocity is recorded below the baseline as blood moves away from the transducer. The velocity seen here is approximately 2.5 m/s. Initially this velocity may seem insignificant, but when applied to the clinical context a grim picture emerges. Using the modified Bernoulli equation, this velocity represents a 25 mmHg pressure gradient (see chapter 6) between the RV and LV. Because the shunt is right to left, the RV pressure must be greater than LV pressure. If LV pressure is even approximating normal peak systole pressure of 120 mmHg, this implies the RV pressure is nearly 145 mmHg, or roughly six times normal. Unless the patient has concurrent pulmonic stenosis, this elevated pressure is due to the pulmonary hypertension of Eisenmenger's physiology.

arch in the embryo and allows blood from the RV to cross directly into the descending aorta. The DA normally closes once the pulmonary vascular resistance drops postparturition. Once the pulmonary vascular pressure dips below systemic pressure, if the DA does not close and the DA remains patent, blood flows from the descending aorta to the main pulmonary artery distal to the pulmonic valve. This arrangement keeps the right heart protected from the extra volume. Similar to the VSD, the extra blood is shunted to the main pulmonary artery then travels to the left heart through the lungs creating a volume overload of the LA and LV. Two-thirds of dogs with a PDA will develop CHF by one year of age [1].

Clinical Presentation

Puppies with a PDA are often diagnosed during the initial veterinary examination by the characteristically loud (grade 4–6/6) continuous murmur in the axillary region of the left cardiac base. The murmur is very characteristic; sometimes described as a "machinery" murmur because the sound resembles the sound of a washing machine agitating clothes. If auscultation is performed at the left apex, typically only a grade 4–6 systolic murmur is appreciated. By moving to the craniodorsal axillary region the diastolic portion of the continuous murmur becomes apparent. They may appear as "poor doers" or runts compared with littermates or are normal with only exercise intolerance noted.

During diastole the blood shunting from the aorta to the pulmonary artery lowers the diastolic arterial blood pressure. This results in a greater than normal pulse pressure (see Chapter 3) and palpation of the femoral arteries is described as *hyperkinetic,* or bounding pulses.

Diagnostics

Radiographs show LV enlargement patterns in both lateral and VD views and a multiple bulge effect at the 12–3 o'clock position on the VD view indicating dilation of the aorta, pulmonary artery, and the left auricular appendage (Figure 10.34). Pulmonary overcirculation is present. If the patient is diagnosed later in life, then signs of CHF may also be present.

Electrocardiography shows a normal MEA with dramatic enlargement of the QRS complex in lead II indicating LV enlargement (Figure 10.35). Advanced cases may have atrial fibrillation, APCs or VPCs.

Echocardiography confirms the LV and LA enlargement and allows for assessment of systolic function. Patients with PDA may have marked to severe LV and LA dilation. Systolic function may be normal, but depending on the age at diagnosis, can

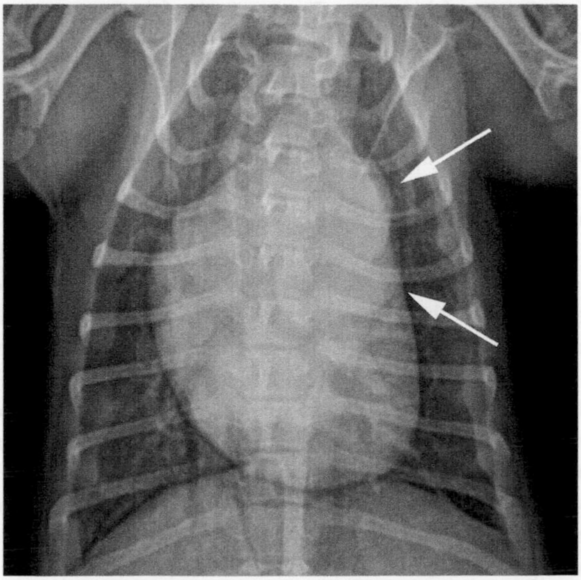

Figure 10.34 Ventrodorsal radiograph of canine patent ductus arteriosus: the upper arrow indicates the location of a bulge in the aorta. The lower arrow marks the location of a second bulge made by the pulmonary artery. The luminary vasculature is also prominent due to the additional blood flow created by the shunt.

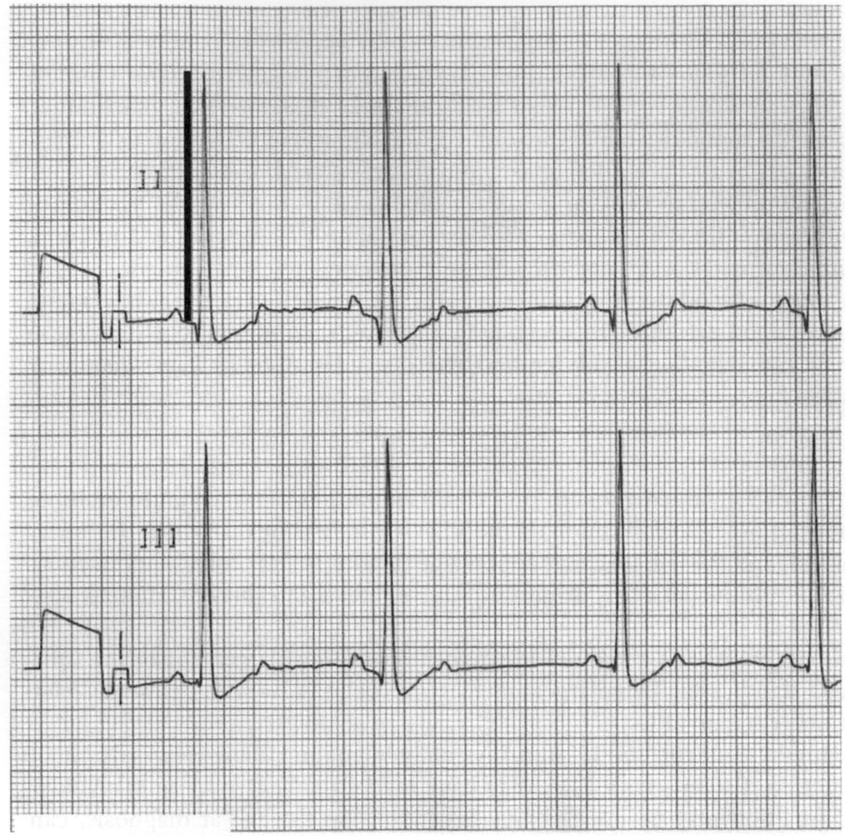

Figure 10.35 Electrocardiogram showing a left ventricular enlargement pattern: the calibration in this electrocardiogram (ECG) is 1 cm/mV, and the paper speed is 50 mm/s. The black line marks the height of the R wave of this patient. The amplitude of the R wave measures 4.1 mV. This is 1.1 mV greater than normal and is typical of dogs with patent ductus arteriosus.

be compromised. Earlier diagnosis generally provides for persevered contractility. The RV and RS are usually within normal limits. Color-flow mapping of the pulmonary artery from the right short axis heart base view shows continuous turbulent blood flow [6, pp. 437–475]. During the Doppler examination of PDA, a continuous turbulent color-flow pattern will be seen circulating in the main pulmonary artery. This color-flow pattern is virtually pathognomonic for PDA. The inflow jet of blood coursing from the aorta can often be appreciated around the 5 o'clock region of the image (Figure 10.36). Because a PDA is not in the heart itself, the actual DA can be difficult to visualize. An alternative echocardiographic view is from the left heart base view of the pulmonary artery. The PDA appears as a small tubular structure entering the distal main pulmonary artery (Figure 10.37). Spectral Doppler of the transductal flow is expected to reveal peak systolic velocities of 4–5 m/s providing pulmonary artery and aortic pressures are normal (Figure 10.38). Velocities less than 4 m/s imply poor cardiac output and a failing LV.

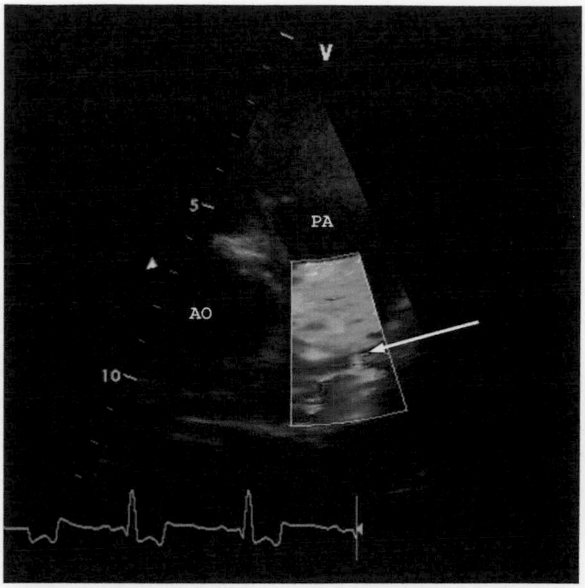

Figure 10.36 Color-flow Doppler of a patent ductus arteriosus (PDA) in the short axis heart base view: the aortic root (AO) and the main pulmonary artery (PA) are labeled. The arrow points to the narrow jet of yellow turbulent blood flow through the aperture of the PDA. The red signal below is blood flowing towards the transducer from the aorta (a section out of the view) through the PDA towards the aperture into the PA. The blue signal is pulmonic outflow moving away from the transducer. Above the arrow is the yellow–green mosaic of turbulent blood flow where the ductal flow mixes with the right ventricular outflow.

Treatment

Treatment of PDA is best accomplished by closure of the shunt. This has traditionally been accomplished with surgical ligation [27, 28] for which results have been excellent [29]. Surgical ligation is an open thoracic procedure but not open heart. Entering through a left hemithoracotomy, the surgeon isolates and then ligates the PDA, in some cases bisecting the PDA after placement of two ligatures. Bisecting the PDA eliminates

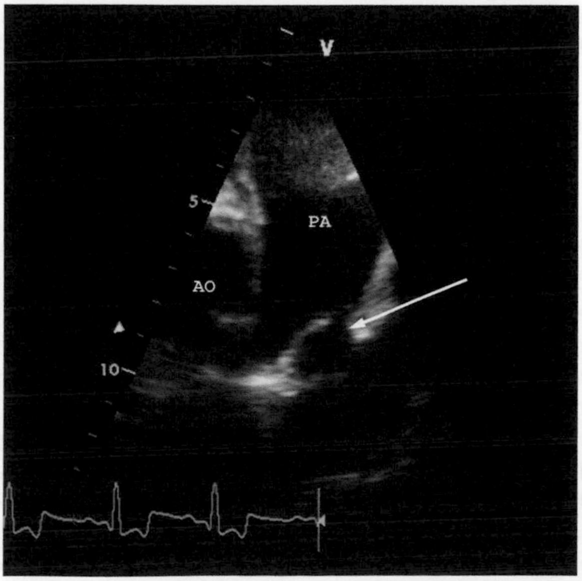

Figure 10.37 Echocardiographic short axis heart base view of a patent ductus arteriosus: this is similar to Figure 10.35 without the color Doppler added. The aorta (AO) is central, with the main pulmonary artery (PA) on the right. In the lower right quadrant of the image is the ampulla of the ductus arteriosus (arrow). The aperture of the ampulla into the PA is just at the tip of the arrow.

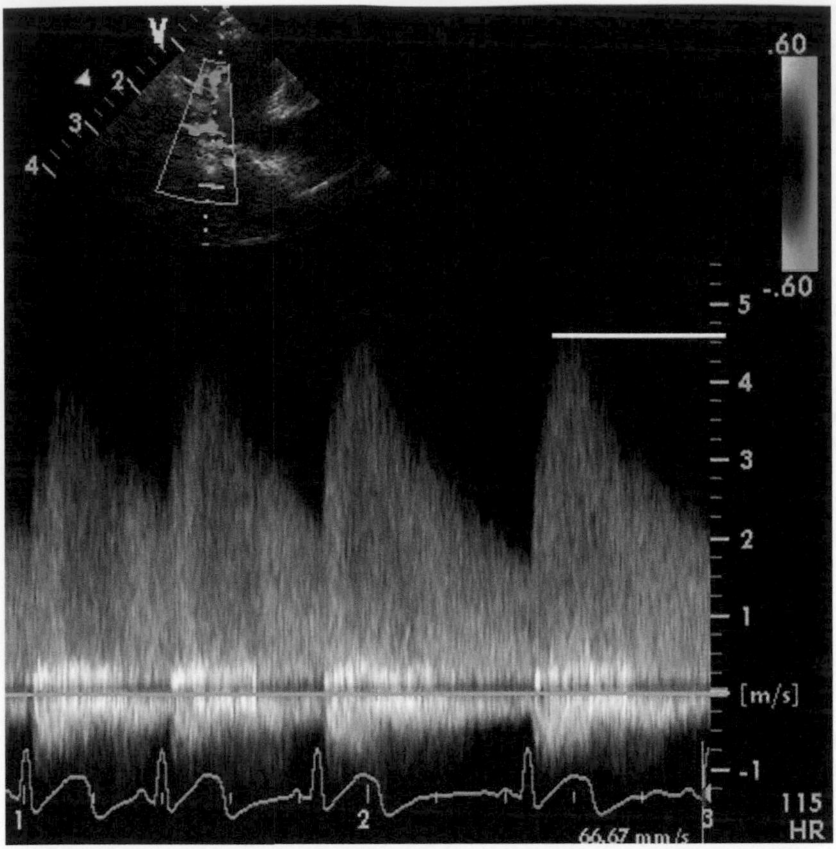

Figure 10.38 Spectral Doppler recording of transductal flow: the Doppler cursor is aligned with blood flow through the patent ductus arteriosus. The velocity trace in the lower portion demonstrates a peak velocity of approximately 4.5 m/s during systole, and velocity at end diastole of near 2.0 m/s. The exact end diastolic velocity is determined by the length of diastole. Longer diastolic periods allow for more shunting of flow out of the aorta continually lowering the pressure. The peak systolic velocity of 4.5 m/s represents a pressure gradient of 81 mmHg between the aorta and the pulmonary artery. This difference is only slightly abnormal and generally implies a heart compensating for the abnormal blood flow.

the possible complication of recanalization of the PDA, which can occur [30]. Generally, surgery should be as soon as possible once the diagnosis has been made. Delaying surgery can potentially allow time for permanent remodeling of the myocardium leading to persistent systolic dysfunction. The risk of tearing the aorta, pulmonary artery, or the PDA is always present, but more so in older dogs. Surgery should ideally be performed in dogs under the age of 2 years [1].

Transcatheter occlusion is an alternative to surgery; both treatments are curative. Transcatheter occlusion is a method of deploying a device in the PDA from inside the vasculature and occurs in the cardiac catheterization laboratory (see Chapter 16). A variety of devices have been developed including [31, 32]: embolization coils, vascular plugs, and most recently the Amplatz Canine Ductal Occluder® (Infiniti Medical Supply,

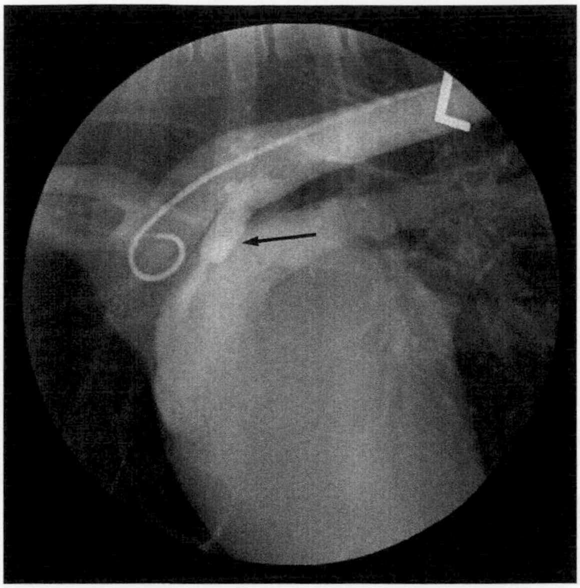

Figure 10.39 Fluoroscopic angiogram of patent ductus arteriosus (PDA) in a dog: the catheter was advanced from the femoral artery retrograde through the descending aorta to the cranial portion of the aortic arch in this right lateral view. The radiopaque contrast is injected in the proximal aorta to highlight the structure of the aortic arch. The PDA is indicated by the arrow. A small jet of contrast can be seen streaming into the main pulmonary artery through the PDA. The brachiocephalic and common carotid arteries can be seen cranial to the pigtail catheter. The arrow is sitting inside the main pulmonary artery.

Menlo Park, CA, USA, http://infinitimedical.com/index.html). These devices are introduced into the PDA through arterial vasculature usually via the femoral artery through the abdominal aorta to the descending aorta and the PDA. Occasionally this procedure is done via the pulmonary artery [32]. Initially, an angiogram of the PDA is performed (Figure 10.39) and the anatomy positively identified. A cardiac catheter is then directed through the vasculature to the PDA where the cardiologist can then place an occlusion device in the lumen of the PDA (Figure 10.40). The occlusion devices are self-expanding

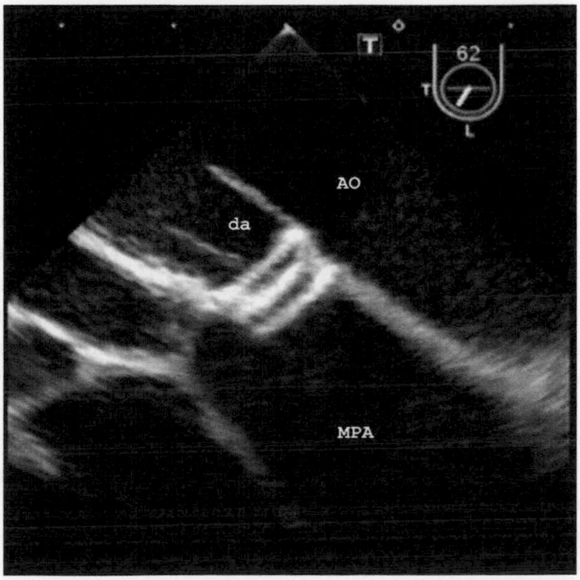

Figure 10.40 Transesophageal echocardiographic image of an Amplatz® Canine Ductal Occluder. The central three-lined hyperechoic structure is an Amplatz® Canine Ductal Occluder being positioned with the patent ductus arteriosus (da). The bright line below the "da" label is the deployment cable. AO, aorta. MPA, main pulmonary artery.

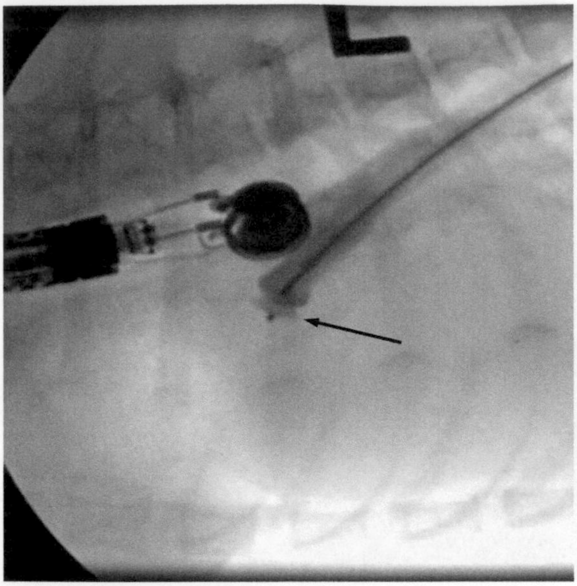

Figure 10.41 Fluoroscopic angiogram of patent ductus arteriosus in a dog after closure: the catheter was advanced from the femoral artery retrograde through the descending aorta to the cranial portion of the descending aorta in this right lateral view. The catheter contains the Amplatz® Canine Ductal Occluder (arrow) and deployment cable. The instrument above the ductus arteriosus is a transesophageal ultrasound probe. An injection of radiopaque contrast is made through the catheter directly into the ductus arteriosus. No contrast can be seen flowing past the Amplatz® Canine Ductal Occluder.

and can be collapsed to pass through the cardiac catheter. Once positioned in the PDA, the occlusion device is released from its deployment catheter. The devices are thrombogenic and usually will take 10–20 minutes to completely occlude blood flow. A second angiogram will verify complete occlusion (Figure 10.41). Surgery and transcatheter occlusion have excellent success rates and long-term outcomes [29, 31] although, rarely, complications such as embolization device dislodgement or infection do occur [33].

Cyanotic Conditions

The complex congenital and cyanotic heart conditions are extremely rare in small animal medicine. It would be beyond the scope of this text to delve too deeply into their pathophysiology. Congenital cardiac conditions that cause a mixing of blood from the pulmonary circulation into the systemic circulation can cause the patient to be cyanotic. Conditions, such as tetralogy of Fallot (TOF), Eisenmenger's syndrome, reversed PDA, right-to-left ASDs, and endocardial cushion defects can all cause deoxygenated blood from the pulmonic circulation to mix with systemic blood. However, these conditions are rare. Some patients do adapt to these conditions and can live normal lifespans; however, they rarely exercise well due to poor oxygenation. The low oxygen saturation of the blood perfusing the kidneys stimulates the release of erythropoietin, which in turn creates a secondary polycythemia.

Tetralogy of Fallot is a combination of four defects typically seen together; a large VSD, dextropositioning of the aorta, PS and RV hypertrophy (Figures 10.42 and 10.43). Tetralogy of Fallot was first described by Niels Stensen in 1672, but was named for Etienne-Louis Arthur Fallot [34] who linked the defect to "blue baby syndrome" in 1888. The

Figure 10.42 Long axis five-chamber echocardiographic view of a heart with tetralogy of Fallot. The chambers are labeled as: LV, left ventricle; RV, right ventricle; AO, aorta. A large interventricular septal defect is indicated by the arrow. The aorta has shifted over the mid-septum and receives blood flow from both ventricles. The aortic valve is just above the "AO" label. Portions of the mitral and tricuspid valves can be seen as thickened hyperechoic linear structures in their respective ventricles. Hypertrophy of the RV can be seen just above the RV label.

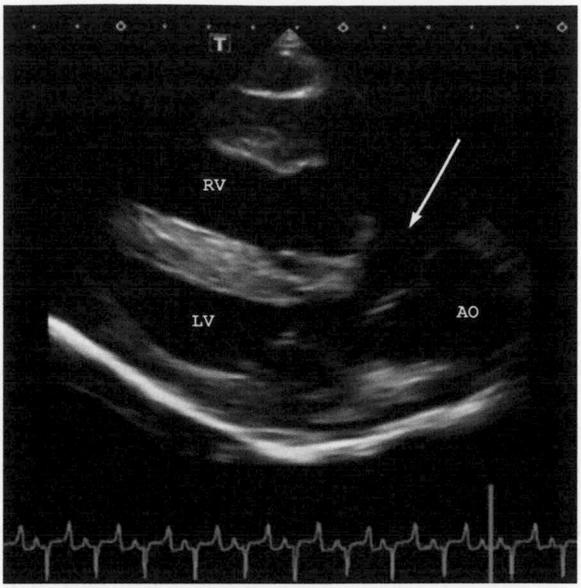

large VSD obliterates the support structure for the aorta, so it shifts to a position centered over where the IVS would be effectively pushing it toward the RV, known as dextroposition, or "overriding" aorta. Because of the PS, the blood returning to the RV is shunted into the overriding aorta mixing with the oxygenated blood returning from the lungs as it heads toward the body. Dogs with TOF may have a systolic murmur related to the PS, but often are silent.

Figure 10.43 Short axis basilar echocardiographic view of a heart with tetralogy of Fallot. The chambers are labeled as: LA, left atrium; RA, right atrium; RV, right ventricle; PA, pulmonary artery. The aorta is in the center of the image. The white arrow points to the interventricular septal (IVS) defect just under the aortic valve. The aortic valve is distorted by the lack of support from the IVS. The black arrow indicates the thickened leaflets and narrow orifice of the pulmonic valve.

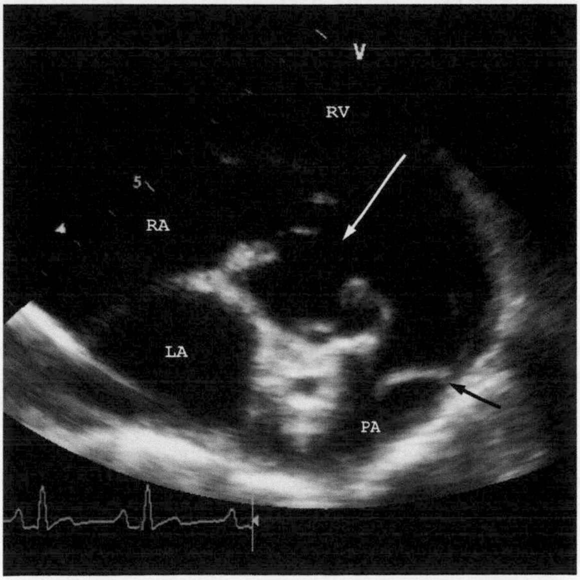

A thoracic radiograph of a dog with TOF will show a bulging aorta, enlarged right heart and pulmonary undercirculation from the PS. The mixed venous and arterial blood is then sent to the body causing peripheral cyanosis. The PS also causes the RV to hypertrophy. Surgical correction has been performed in dogs during cardiopulmonary bypass [35]. Due to cost, most patients receive medical management for blood hyperviscosity, and ultimately succumb to complications from hypoxemia, hyperviscosity and/or cardiac arrhythmia [1].

The so called "reverse" PDA or more properly *persistent fetal flow* is also extremely rare and has a similar pathophysiology to Eisenmenger's syndrome, which is a right-to-left shunting VSD due to pulmonary hypertension. In such cases, pulmonary hypertension (Eisenmenger's physiology) can also be present with a PDA causing the flow to shunt from the pulmonary artery to aorta; opposite of the common PDA. The development of pulmonary hypertension happens very early in life, perhaps even such that after parturition, the pulmonary vascular resistance does not reduce, and the fetal path of blood flow is maintained. Typical presentation is an animal showing exercise intolerance, lethargy, syncope, and/or abnormal blood work. These cases usually have a normal auscultation, but have the unique physical examination finding of *differential cyanosis.* Differential cyanosis is noted by observing pink mucus membranes cranially (e.g. the gums or eyes) and cyanotic mucus membranes caudally (e.g. vulva or prepuce). Since the

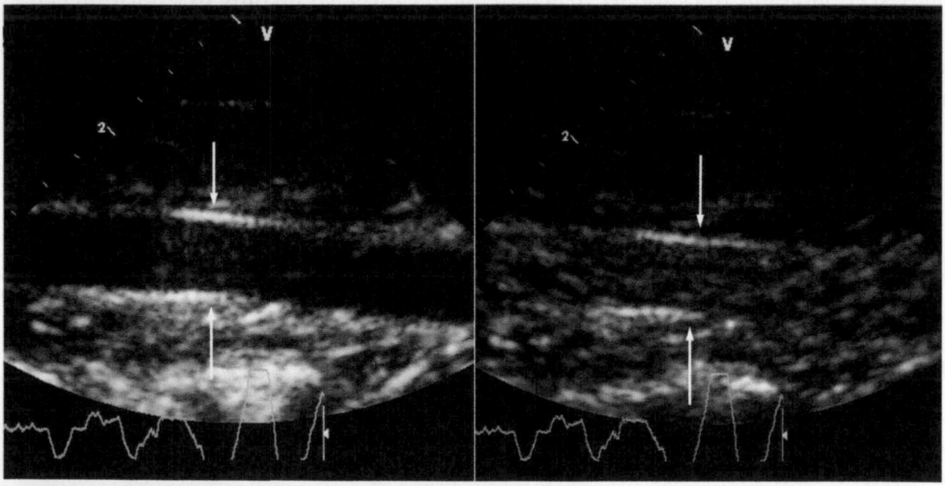

Figure 10.44 Ultrasonic view of the abdominal aorta with positive air-contrast diagnosis of right-to-left shunting patent ductus arteriosus: the left image shows the abdominal aorta before the microbubble injection. The arrows indicate the walls of the aorta seen as two bright lines. The lumen of the aorta is black. The grey area in the center of the aorta is an ultrasound artifact of the highly reflective aortic vascular walls. The right image is the aorta filled with the microbubbles coursing through. The only path for microbubbles to enter this section of the aorta is through a shunt distal to the brachiocephalic and carotid arteries. The only common communication between the pulmonary circulation and the systemic circulation is the ductus arteriosus. If the right-to-left shunting of fetal flow persists after birth, then the so-called "reverse" patent ductus arteriosus is present. Consequently, microbubbles injected into the venous system will travel to the right atrium, right ventricle, and out of the pulmonary artery. The microbubbles will then pass through the ductus arteriosus from the pulmonary artery to the descending aorta where they are visualized in the abdominal aorta.

shunt occurs in the descending aorta, distal to the brachiocephalic and common carotid arteries, only blood caudal to the shunt is mixed with hypoxic blood from the pulmonary artery.

Radiographs of a reverse PDA typically shows dilation of the main pulmonary artery, and lobar branches and a "ductal bump" can sometimes be seen in the VD projection. Echocardiography can be used to diagnose a reverse PDA. Typical findings are PV hypertrophy, dilation of the pulmonary artery, and color-flow Doppler of the main pulmonary artery demonstrates flow through the DA. An air-contrast echocardiogram of the abdominal aorta is positive if microbubbles are seen in the aorta after injection into a peripheral vein. The air contrast microbubbles travel from the venous return, to the RV, to the pulmonary artery, across the DA and into the aorta where they travel caudally (Figure 10.44).

Treatment of reverse PDA entails management of polycythemia and hyperviscosity with phlebotomy or drugs. Surgical closure in dogs with reverse PDA is not recommended. The supersystemic pulmonary vasculature pressure will overburden the RV if the shunt is closed, leading to sudden death. Medications, such as sildenifil can be used to lower pulmonary arterial pressures in other right-to-left shunts [6, pp. 437–475] but their use is still novel in reverse PDA.

Cor triatriatum dexter and sinister are a developmental defect of the atria (right=dexter, left=sinister) in which a third atria is created by an abnormal extra membrane restricting flow into the atria and on to the ventricle (Figure 10.45). Cor triatriatum dexter has been reported in dogs, but not in cats. It may cause signs of right heart failure and has been palliated with balloon dilation of the abnormal membrane [36, 37].

Cor triatriatum sinister has only been reported in cats, along with supervalvular mitral stenosis [38, 39] (Figures 10.46 and 10.47). This condition leads to left-sided CHF. In the case of cor triatriatum sinister, standard cardiac catheterization is difficult due to the anatomical arrangement preventing passage of catheters from the arterial circulation

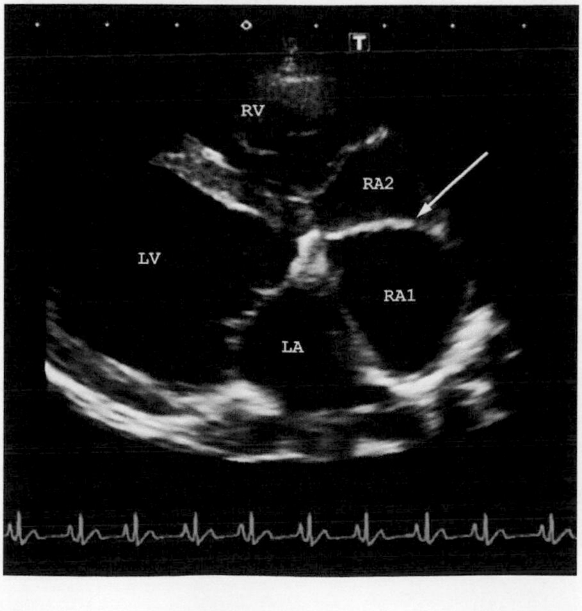

Figure 10.45 Long axis echocardiographic view of cor triatriatum dexter: the chambers are labeled as: LA, left atrium; LV, left ventricle; RA1, distal right atrial chamber; RA2, proximal right atrial chamber; RV, right ventricle. The arrow indicates the membrane separating the two portions of the right atrium. A small non-valved ostium allows blood flow to enter RA2 from RA1. The severity of disease is related to the opening; larger orifices leading to better outcomes.

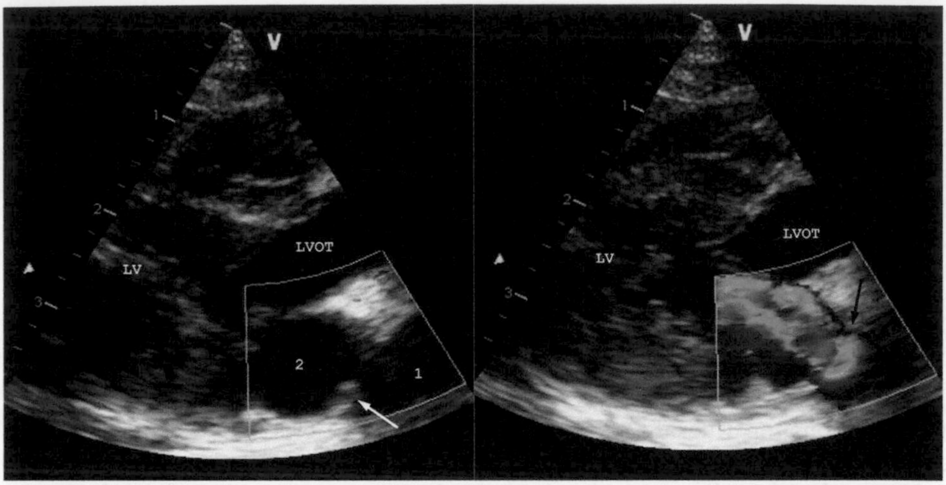

Figure 10.46 Long axis echocardiographic view of cor triatriatum sinister (CTS): this twin image shows the two chambers of the left atrium in CTS. The left image chambers are labeled as: LV, left ventricle; LVOT, left ventricular outflow tract; 1, distal left atrial chamber; 2, proximal left atrial chamber. A slight hyperechoic area (arrow) between 1 and 2 is the membrane separating the two atria. The right image is the same view with color-flow Doppler to demonstrate high-velocity blood flow. The arrow marks the location of the ostium through the membrane at the narrowing of the color Doppler signal. The dome shape color to the lower right shows the point at which blood become turbulent as it enters the opening. The blood then streams directly through the proximal chamber 2, and into the LV. The severity of disease is related to the opening; larger orifices leading to better outcomes.

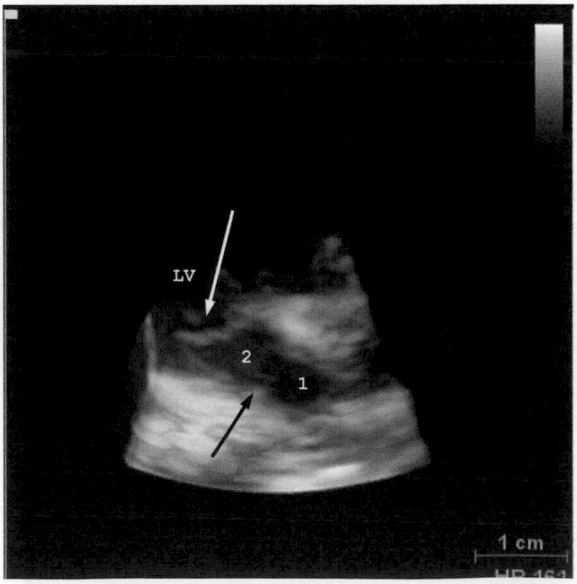

Figure 10.47 Three-dimensional image of cor triatriatum sinister. It should be viewed as one does a block suspended in space, with one corner visible. The viewer sees mostly one side (yellowish) and only a portion of a side going away on the left (blue). The distal left atrial chamber is labeled 1 and the proximal chamber labeled 2. The left ventricle (LV) is back and away from the viewer. The white arrow points to the mitral valve and the black arrow to the membrane separating 1 and 2.

retrograde to the LA. A hybrid open heart surgery and balloon dilation procedure has been reported with some success [40]. Medical management of CHF is most commonly elected by clients.

References

1 Bonagura, J.D. and Lehmkuhl, L.B. (1999) Congenital heart disease, in *Textbook of Canine and Feline Cardiology* (P.R. Fox, D.D. Sisson and N.S. Moïse, eds). WB Saunders, Philadelphia. pp. 471–535.

2 Oyama, M.A. and Sisson, D.D. (2001) Evaluation of canine congenital heart disease using an echocardiographic algorithm. *Journal of the American Animal Hospital Association*, **37**, 519–535.

3 Ware, W.A. (2007) Congenital cardiovascular diseases, in *Cardiovascular Disease in Small Animal Medicine* (W.A. Ware, ed.). Manson, London. pp. 228–262.

4 Kittleson, M.D. and Kienle, R.D. (1998) Aortic stenosis, in *Small Animal Cardiovascular Medicine* (M.D. Kittleson and R.D.Kienle, eds). Mosby, Inc., St Louis. pp. 260–272.

5 Bonagura, J.D. and Lehmkuhl, L.B. (1994) Comparison of transducer placement sites for doppler echocardiography in dogs with aortic stenosis. *American Journal of Veterinary Research*, **55**, 192–198.

6 Boon, J.A. (2011) *Veterinary Echocardiography.* Wiley–Blackwell, Oxford.

7 Eason, B.D., Fine, D.M., Leeder, D. *et al.* (2014) Influence of beta blockers on survival in dogs with severe subaortic stenosis. *Journal of Veterinary Internal Medicine*, **28**, 857–862.

8 Bonagura, J.D., Lehmkuhl, L.B. and Jones, D.E. (1995) Comparison of cardiac catheterization and doppler-derived pressure gradients in a canine model of subarotic stenosis. *Journal of the American Society of Echocardiography*, **55**, 192–198.

9 Nelson, D.A., Fossum, T.W., Gordon, S. and Miller, M.W. (2004) Surgical correction of subaortic stenosis via right ventriculotomy and septal resection in a dog. *Journal of the American Veterinary Medical Association*, **225**, 705–708, 698.

10 Kleman, M.E., Estrada, A.H., Maisenbacher H.W. *et al.* (2012) How to perform combined cutting balloon and high pressure balloon valvoloplasty for dogs with subaortic stenosis. *Journal of Veterinary Cardiology*, **14**, 351–361.

11 Buchanan, J.W. (1990) Pulmonic stenosis caused by a single coronary artery in dogs; four cases. *Journal of the American Veterinary Medical Association*, **196**, 115.

12 Francis, A.J., Johnson, M.J., Culshaw, G.C. *et al.* (2011) Outcome in 55 dogs with pulmonic stenosis that did not undergo balloon valvuloplasty or surgery. *Journal of Small Animal Practice*, **52**, 282–288.

13 Hunt, G.B., Pearson, M.R., Bellenger, C.R. and Malik, R. (1993) Use of a modified open patch-graft technique and valvulectomy for correction of severe pulmonic stenosis in dogs: eight consecutive cases. *Australian Veterinary Journal*, **70**, 244–248.

14 Orton, E.C., Bruecker, K.A. and McCracken, T.O. (1990) An open patch-graft technique for correction of pulmonic stenosis in the dog. *Veterinary Surgery*, **19**, 148–154.

15 Bright, J.M., Jennings, J., Toal, R. and Hood, M.E. (1987) Percutaneous balloon valvuloplasty for treatment of pulmonic stenosis in a dog. *Journal of the American Veterinary Medical Association*, **191**, 995–996.

16 Johnson, M.S. and Martin, M. (2004) Results of balloon valvuloplasty in 40 dogs with pulmonic stenosis. *Journal of Small Animal Practice*, **45**, 148–153.

17 Johnson, M.S., Martin, M., Edwards, D. *et al.* (2004) Pulmonic stenosis in dogs: balloon dilation improves clinical outcome. *Journal of Veterinary Internal Medicine*, **18**, 656–662.

18 Kunze, S.P., Abbott, J.A., Hamilton, S.M. and Pyle R.L. (2002) Balloon valvuloplasty for palliative treatment of tricuspid stenosis with right-to-left atrial-level shunting in a dog. *Journal of the American Veterinary Medical Association*, **220**, 464, 491–6.

19 Chetboul, V., Tran, D., Carlos, C. *et al.* (2004) Congenital malformations of the tricuspid valve in domestic carnivores: a retrospective study of 50 cases. *Schweiz Arch Tierheilkd*, **146**, 265–275. [In French]

20 Eyster, G.E., Anderson, L., Evans, A.T. *et al.* (1977) Ebstein's anomaly: a report of 3 cases in the dog. *Journal of the American Veterinary Medical Association*, **170**, 709–713.

21 Gordon, S.G., Miller, M.W., Roland, R.M. *et al.* (2009) Transcatheter atrial septal defect closure with the Amplatzer atrial septal occluder in 13 dogs: short- and mid-term outcome. *Journal of Veterinary Internal Medicine*, **23**, 995–1002.

22 Shimizu, M., Tanaka, R., Hoshi, K. *et al.* (2006) Surgical correction of ventricular septal defect with aortic regurgitation in a dog. *Australian Veterinary Journal*, **84**, 117–121.

23 Margiocco, M.L., Bulmer, B.J. and Sisson, D.D. (2008) Percutaneous occlusion of a muscular ventricular septal defect with an Amplatzer muscular VSD occluder. *Journal of Veterinary Cardiolgy*, **10**, 61–66.

24 Saunders, A.B., Carlson, J.A., Nelson, D.A. *et al.* (2013) Hybrid technique for ventricular septal defect closure in a dog using an Amplatzer® Duct Occluder II. *Journal of Veterinary Cardiolgy*, **15**, 217–224.

25 Bussadori, C., Carminati, M. and Domenech, O. (2007) Transcatheter closure of a perimembranous ventricular septal defect in a dog. *Journal of Veterinary Internal Medicine*, **21**, 1396–1400.

26 Nakamura, K., Yamasaki, M., Ohta, H. *et al.* (2011) Effects of sildenafil citrate on five dogs with Eisenmenger's syndrome. *Journal of Small Animal Practice*, **52**, 595–598.

27 Buchanan, J.W., Soma, L.R. and Patterson, D.F. (1967) Patent ductus arteriosus surgery in small dogs. *Journal of the American Veterinary Medical Association*, **151**, 701–707.

28 Breznock, E.M., Wisloh, A., Hilwig, R.W. and Hamlin, R.L. (1971) A surgical method for correction of patent ductus arteriosus in the dog. *Journal of the American Veterinary Medical Association*, **158**, 753–762.

29 Eyster, G.E., Eyster, J.T., Cords, G.B. and Johnston, J. (1976) Patent ductus arteriosus in the dog: characteristics of occurrence and results of surgery in one hundred consecutive cases. *Journal of the American Veterinary Medical Association*, **168**, 435–438.

30 Eyster, G.E., Whipple, R.D., Evans, A.T. *et al.* (1975) Recanalized patent ductus arteriosus in the dog. *Journal of Small Animal Practice*, **16**, 743–749.

31 Singh, M.K., Kittleson, M.D., Kass, P.H. and Griffiths, L.G. (2012) Occlusion devices and approaches in canine patent ductus arteriosus: comparison of outcomes. *Journal of Veterinary Internal Medicine*, **26**, 85–92.

32 Glaus, T.M., Berger, F., Ammann, F.W. *et al.* (2002) Closure of large patent ductus arteriosus with a self-expanding duct occluder in two dogs. *Journal of Small Animal Practice*, **43**, 547–550.

33 Wood, A.C., Fine, D.M., Spier, A.W. and Eyster, G.E. (2006) Septicemia in a young dog following treatment of patent ductus arteriosus via coil occlusion. *Journal of the American Veterinary Medical Association*, **228**, 1901–1904.
34 https://en.wikipedia.org/wiki/Tetralogy˙of˙Fallot#– Wikipedia page for tetralogy of Fallot.
35 Orton, E.C., Mama, K., Hellyer, P. and Hackett, T.B. (2001) Open surgical repair of tetralogy of Fallot in dogs. *Journal of the American Veterinary Medical Association*, **219**, 1089–1093.
36 Atkins, C. and DeFrancesco, T. (2000) Balloon dilation of cor triatriatum dexter in a dog. *Journal of Veterinary Internal Medicine*, **14**, 471–472.
37 Adin, D.B. and Thomas, W.P. (1999) Balloon dilation of cor triatriatum dexter in a dog. *Journal of Veterinary Internal Medicine*, **13**, 617–619.
38 Heaney, A.M. and Bulmer, B.J. (2004) Cor triatriatum sinister and persistent left cranial vena cava in a kitten. *Journal of Veterinary Internal Medicine*, **18**, 895–898.
39 Fine, D.M., Tobias, A.H. and Jacob, K.A. (2002) Supravalvular mitral stenosis in a cat. *Journal of the American Animal Hospital Association*, **38**, 403–406.
40 Stern, J.A., Tou, S.P., Barker, P.C.A. *et al.* (2013) Hybrid cutting balloon dilatation for treatment of cor triatriatum sinister in a cat. *Journal of Veterinary Cardiology*, **15**, 205–210.

11

Acquired Heart Diseases

Stacey Leach

Introduction

There are a number of acquired cardiac diseases in veterinary medicine. In humans, coronary arterial disease, cardiomyopathies, and valve degeneration are all frequently diagnosed. Animals also develop various forms of cardiomyopathy and valvular degeneration, although coronary arterial disease is extremely rare. Furthermore, the incidence of these conditions is often species or breed specific. Cats for instance, rarely develop dilated cardiomyopathy (DCM), but are known to have hypertrophic cardiomyopathy (HCM) or similar conditions like restrictive cardiomyopathy (RCM). Dogs on the other hand seem to segregate along breed size lines. Large-breed dogs more commonly develop DCM, while small-breed dogs more commonly develop chronic valvular degeneration. Some breeds, such as the cocker spaniel, have been reported to develop both. Although cardiac hypertrophy does occur with ventricular outflow tract obstructions such as pulmonic and subaortic stenosis in dogs, naturally occurring HCM is rare in dogs, and when diagnosed may be due to iatrogenic hyperthyroidism [1]. Each of these diseases will be considered individually.

Canine Cardiomyopathies

Cardiomyopathies, which are primary diseases of the cardiac muscle, include primarily arrhythmogenic right ventricular cardiomyopathy (ARVC) and DCM in dogs.

Arrhythmogenic Right Ventricular Cardiomyopathy

Arrhythmogenic right ventricular cardiomyopathy, commonly referred to as boxer cardiomyopathy, is an inherited cardiomyopathy in boxers that is characterized by fibro-fatty infiltration of the myocardium, primarily the right ventricle. A genetic mutation has recently been found to be associated with the development of ARVC in boxers and a commercial test is available [2]. ARVC can present in one of several forms: asymptomatic with a ventricular arrhythmia (occult), symptomatic with ventricular arrhythmias only, or symptomatic with systolic ventricular dysfunction and dilation.

Cardiology for Veterinary Technicians and Nurses, First Edition. Edited by H. Edward Durham, Jr.

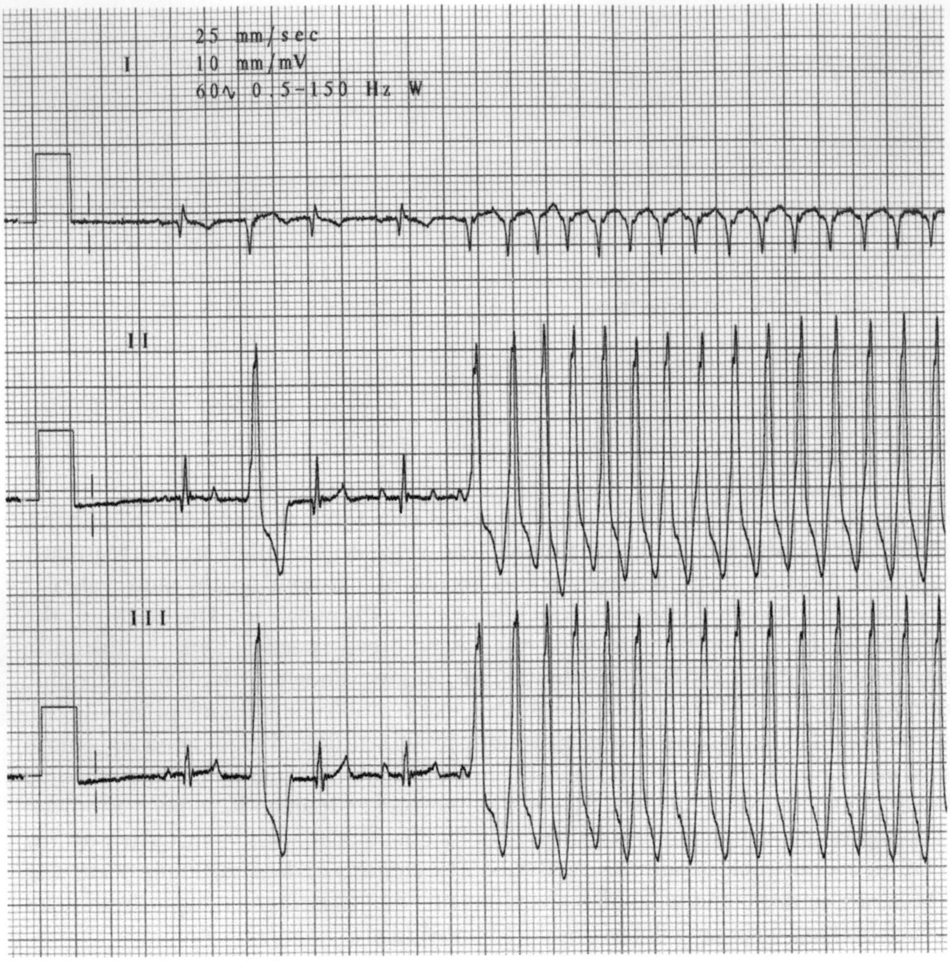

Figure 11.1 Electrocardiogram (25 mm/sec; 10 mm/mv) from a boxer with arrhythmogenic right ventricular cardiomyopathy. The first, third, and fourth complex are all sinus. The second complex is a ventricular premature complex conducted with a left bundle branch block morphology. After the fourth sinus complex a run of ventricular tachycardia occurs with a rate of 300 bpm.

The frequency of the arrhythmia is of significance, since very frequent ventricular premature complexes (VPCs) or runs of VPCs may lead to ventricular tachycardia, ventricular fibrillation, and sudden death. Clinical signs may include episodic weakness, exercise intolerance, syncope, sudden death, and less commonly congestive heart failure (CHF). The typical electrocardiographic (ECG) findings usually include predominantly upright VPCs on lead II suggesting origination within the right ventricle (left bundle branch block morphology) (Figure 11.1). Given the intermittent nature of the ventricular arrhythmias, a normal ECG does not rule out ARVC. A 24-hour ambulatory ECG (Holter monitor) may provide better insight into the complexity and frequency of the arrhythmias. Blood pressures and an echocardiogram should be evaluated in suspected cases. Echocardiography is generally unremarkable, although a small subset of boxers may have evidence of systolic dysfunction and ventricular dilation [3]. Antiarrhythmic therapy is recommended to reduce the frequency and severity of arrhythmias and clinical signs; however, there is no evidence to date that the risk of sudden death is reduced with therapy. Commonly used antiarrhythmics include mexiletine, sotalol, or a combination of mexiletine with sotalol or atenolol [4].

Dilated Cardiomyopathy

Dilated cardiomyopathy is characterized by declining myocardial contractility resulting in progressive systolic dysfunction and subsequent dilation of the cardiac chambers, most notably the left ventricle, yet both ventricles may be affected. In humans a large percentage of DCM is considered familial, the result of various genetic mutations. The overall prevalence has been reported to be approximately 0.5%; however, it is much higher in specific breeds [5]. The cause of primary canine DCM is unknown but may also be related to familial inheritance of genetic mutations, or the end result of a variety of myocardial insults. Dilated cardiomyopathy has been shown to develop secondary to drug exposure (doxorubicin), infectious agents (parvovirus, Chagas' disease), nutritional deficiency (taurine), and persistent sustained tachycardia. Breeds most commonly affected are large- and giant-breed dogs, including the Doberman pinscher, Great Dane, boxer, Newfoundland, and Irish wolfhound. A mutation in the gene encoding pyruvate dehydrogenase kinase 4, located on canine chromosome 14, has been associated with the development of DCM in some American Doberman pinschers [6] while a different study utilizing a European cohort, found a marker on canine chromosome 5 [7]. Although not considered a large-breed dog, the American cocker spaniel and standard schnauzer have also been reported to develop DCM [8, 9]. A mutation in the gene encoding RBM20, a ribonucleic acid binding protein gene, has been recently identified in standard schnauzers with DCM [10]. Although primary DCM typically has a long occult (asymptomatic) phase, it eventually progresses to the overt (symptomatic) phase. The occult phase may last up to 4 years in Doberman pinschers prior to the onset of clinical signs. There are breed variations in the clinical course of disease, as the overt phase is much more rapidly progressing in Doberman pinschers [5]. The clinical signs may range from acute CHF to sudden death. Coughing, dyspnea, and exercise intolerance may be noted with left-sided CHF, and ascites with right-sided CHF. Syncope or episodic weakness secondary to cardiac arrhythmias may also be observed. Doberman pinschers and boxers are more likely to experience syncope and sudden death than other breeds with DCM.

Physical examination may reveal a low-pitched gallop due to a dilated, noncompliant ventricle. DCM may progressively stretch the tricuspid and mitral valve annulus and allow for regurgitant blood flow. As a result, soft systolic heart murmurs may be auscultated over the regions of the mitral and tricuspid valves. Thorough auscultation may also reveal an irregular rhythm. These arrhythmias may include either VPCs, premature atrial complexes, ventricular or supraventricular tachycardia, or atrial fibrillation. Careful palpation of the arterial pulses may reveal noticeably irregular pulse rates and pulse deficits associated with premature beats or atrial fibrillation. Signs of right-sided CHF such as distended jugular veins, jugular pulsation, ascites and hepatomegaly may be detected. Pleural effusion may result in muffled heart and lung sounds. Harsh lung

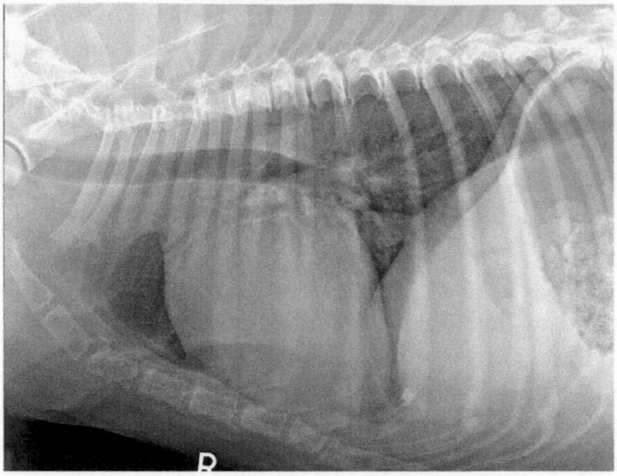

Figure 11.2 Lateral thoracic radiograph of a dog with dilated cardiomyopathy. Generalized cardiomegaly is present.

sounds and crackles may be auscultated suggestive of pulmonary edema from left-sided CHF. Cardiac cachexia may also be noted with more chronic presentations of CHF.

Initial diagnostics should include a blood chemistry panel, complete blood count (CBC), and urinalysis to identify any other comorbid conditions and to guide therapeutic decisions. Blood chemistry abnormalities are generally nonspecific and may include mild electrolyte derangements, mild increases in blood urea nitrogen, creatinine, and alkaline phosphatase. The CBC and urinalysis are typically unremarkable. Blood and plasma taurine concentrations are indicated in cocker spaniels with DCM or any atypical breed presenting with DCM. Blood pressures are warranted to identify hypotension as a result of reduced cardiac output. Serial blood gas and pulse oximetry may be useful in monitoring response to therapy for CHF.

Electrocardiographic changes may reveal underlying arrhythmias. Atrial fibrillation is commonly noted in giant-breed dogs while ventricular tachycardia and VPCs are commonly detected in Doberman pinschers and boxers. Cardiac chamber enlargement patterns such as P-mitrale and tall R waves may be seen. Given the paroxysmal nature of the arrhythmia, a 24-hour ambulatory ECG recording may help reveal the frequency and intricacy of the arrhythmia as well as response to therapy.

Thoracic radiographs should be performed to evaluate for any evidence of CHF and evaluate the cardiac silhouette. Left atrial and left ventricular enlargement may be noted in particular with Dobermans and boxers, while generalized cardiomegaly is a common finding in most large- and giant-breed dogs (Figure 11.2). Signs of CHF may be noted and include left atrial enlargement, pulmonary venous distension, and an interstitial to alveolar lung pattern in the perihilar and caudodorsal lung fields. Pleural fissure lines and blunting of the long lobes may be noted with pleural effusion and right-sided CHF. Other radiographic signs of right-sided CHF may include an enlarged caudal vena cava, hepatomegaly, and ascites.

Echocardiography is required to definitively diagnose DCM and characterize chamber enlargement and systolic function. Two-dimensional and M-mode echocardiography may detect dilated atrium and ventricles (Figures 11.3 and 11.4). The left ventricular fractional shortening, ejection fraction, and fractional shortening area may all be decreased suggestive of systolic dysfunction. The E-point septal separation is

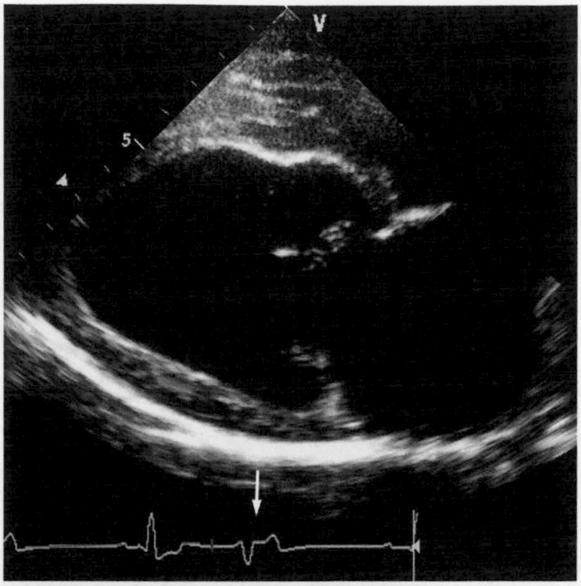

Figure 11.3 Right parasternal four-chamber view from a dog demonstrating left atrial and ventricular enlargement secondary to dilated cardiomyopathy. A ventricular premature complex (arrow) can be seen on the electrocardiogram during the echocardiographic study. Patients with dilated cardiomyopathy often have concurrent arrhythmias.

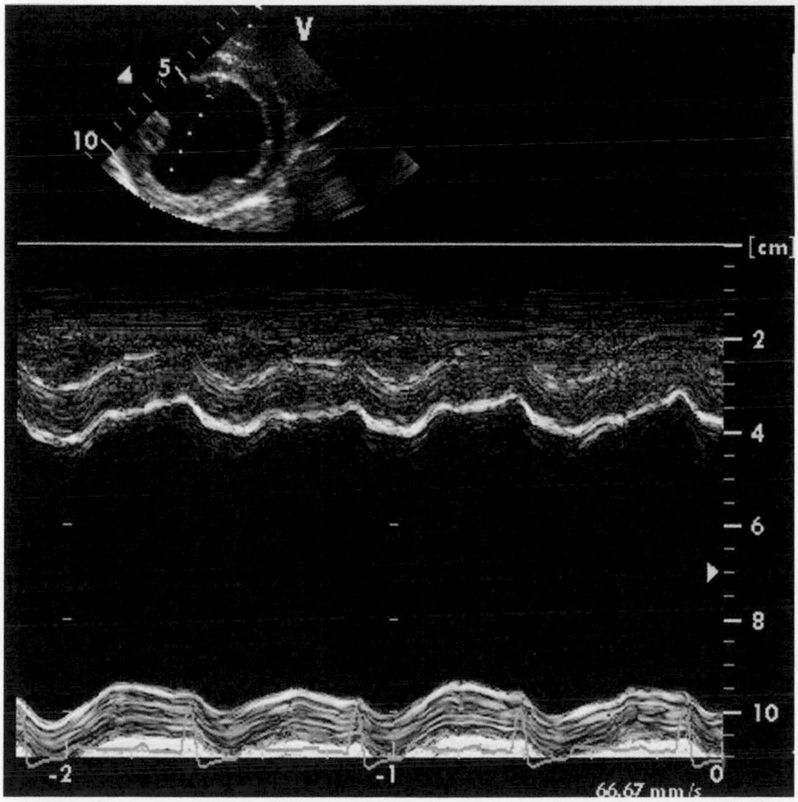

Figure 11.4 An M-mode echocardiogram recorded at the level of the left ventricle in a dog with dilated cardiomyopathy. The left ventricular end-systolic and end-diastolic diameters are increased indicating systolic dysfunction and volume overloading, respectively.

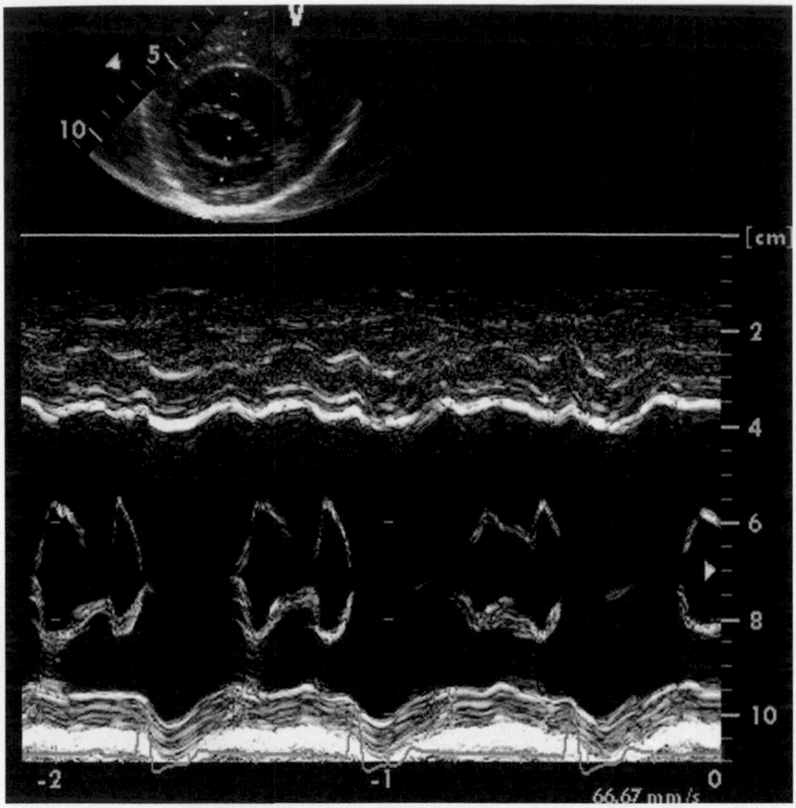

Figure 11.5 An M-mode echocardiogram recorded at the level of the mitral valve demonstrating a markedly increased E-point-to-septal separation in a dog with dilated cardiomyopathy.

also typically increased as a result of a decreased ejection fraction (Figure 11.5) and is discussed in further detail in Chapter 7. Doppler echocardiography can detect the presence and severity of valvular insufficiency (Figure 11.6).

The long-term prognosis for DCM is generally considered poor as all cases are ultimately fatal, unless potentially reversible causes such as taurine deficiency or sustained tachycardia are identified and treated. Therapy with pimobendan (Vetmedin®) and angiotensin-converting enzyme inhibitors (ACEI) have both been shown to delay the onset of CHF in Doberman pinschers with occult DCM [11, 12]. Whether these medications are beneficial to other breeds with DCM remains unknown. The presence of pulmonary edema, pleural effusion, ascites, atrial fibrillation, and a younger age of onset are all negative prognostic indicators [13–16]. With overt DCM the goal of treatment is to palliate the clinical signs and improve quality of life. Current medical management may include antiarrhythmics, positive inotropes such as pimobendan (Vetmedin®) and digoxin, ACEI, and diuretics. Acute CHF may require aggressive treatment consisting of oxygen support and intravenous diuretics and vasodilators and is discussed in further detail in Chapter 15. Periodic abdominocentesis may be useful in alleviating discomfort and respiratory distress from profound ascites. Severe hypotension as a result of myocardial failure may necessitate the use of intravenous inotropes such as dobutamine.

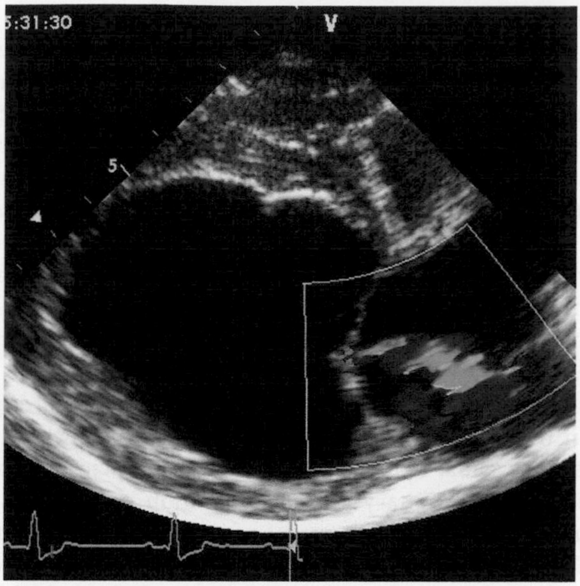

Figure 11.6 An echocardiogram with color-flow Doppler demonstrating mitral valve regurgitation in a dog with dilated cardiomyopathy. Volume overloading associated with dilated cardiomyopathy can result in distension of the annulus of the atrioventricular valves and subsequent regurgitation.

Digoxin is often used as it is both a positive inotrope and a useful antiarrhythmic for rate control of atrial fibrillation. Combination therapy with other antiarrhythmics is often necessary to achieve adequate heart rate control [17]. Ventricular arrhythmias resulting in clinical signs should also be addressed with appropriate antiarrhythmics. Chronic therapy consists of furosemide, an ACEI, as well as positive inotropes.

Acquired Valve Disease

The majority of acquired valve diseases are due to a chronic degenerative condition (endocardiosis), whereas a smaller percentage may be due to infectious inflammatory processes (endocarditis).

Endocardiosis

Endocardiosis, also known as chronic myxomatous valvular degeneration or degenerative valve disease, is the most commonly acquired cardiac disease reported in the dog, typically affecting the mitral valve [18, 19]. Both atrioventricular valves can be affected whereas isolated tricuspid valve and semilunar valve involvement is less common.

Endocardiosis commonly occurs in middle-age to older, small- to medium-sized breeds including Cavalier King Charles spaniels, dachshunds, toy poodles, Chihuahuas, and cocker spaniels. The severity and prevalence of disease increases with age although, Cavalier King Charles spaniels are noted to have a higher prevalence and earlier onset of disease. The underlying cause is unknown; however, a genetic origin is likely.

Endocardiosis is a noninflammatory, progressive, myxomatous degenerative process involving fibrosis, loss of collagen, and glycosaminoglycan accumulation within the chordae tendineae and valve leaflets. The chordae tendineae may thicken and stretch and the valve leaflets may prolapse. The leaflets also become thickened, with nodular shortened margins resulting in decreased valvular strength and valve prolapse, reduced coaptation, and regurgitation of blood. The regurgitation into the atrias increases the atrial pressures. If the mitral valve is affected, the increased left atrial pressures result in dilation of the left atrium, which can progress to increased pulmonary capillary pressures and resultant pulmonary edema. With tricuspid valve involvement, increased right atrial pressures may lead to right atrial enlargement and the development of ascites.

Dogs may be well compensated and asymptomatic for years, although the development of certain sequelae may cause acute decompensation [20]. Potential sequelae may include the development of arrhythmias, rupture of a chordae tendineae, rupture of the atrial wall, and the development of pulmonary hypertension. Rupture of a chordae tendineae can allow for a sudden increase in the amount of regurgitation and initiate sudden and fulminant CHF. Chronic mitral regurgitation can cause jet lesions on the endocardial surface of the left atrium which may eventually rupture, leading to pericardial hemorrhage and acute cardiac tamponade. Chronic mitral regurgitation and pulmonary venous congestion may increase pulmonary vascular resistance and lead to the development of pulmonary hypertension, exacerbating clinical signs. Coughing is usually the first clinical sign noted with endocardiosis and may be due to either congestive heart failure or mainstem bronchial compression from an enlarged left atrium. Increased respiratory effort, dyspnea, exercise intolerance, weakness, syncope, and weight loss are other presenting complaints. Physical examination of asymptomatic patients may reveal a systolic click or a systolic heart murmur over the regions of the mitral or tricuspid valves.

Guidelines have been established by the American College of Veterinary Internal Medicine (ACVIM) Specialty of Cardiology consensus panel for the diagnosis, staging, and treatment of endocardiosis in dogs [21]. This classification scheme describes four basic stages of heart disease. Briefly, stage A identifies dogs at a high risk for developing heart disease but without any evidence of current heart disease. Stage B identifies dogs with structural heart disease as evident by a heart murmur but no clinical signs, and is further subdivided into those with no radiographic or echocardiographic evidence of cardiac enlargement (stage B1), and those with evidence of cardiac enlargement (stage B2). Stage C refers to dogs with past or current clinical signs attributable to heart failure, and stage D denotes dogs with end-stage disease that is refractory to standard therapy. Thoracic radiographs are important in the staging and management of endocardiosis, and are required for the diagnosis of CHF. With increasing mitral regurgitation the left atrium may become enlarged. Moderate to severe left atrial enlargement may elevate and compress the left mainstem bronchus (Figure 11.7). Distended pulmonary veins and an interstitial to alveolar pattern are suggestive of left-sided CHF. Caudal vena caval distension, pleural effusion, hepatomegaly, and ascites may be noted with right-sided CHF.

A sinus rhythm or sinus tachycardia is most commonly noted on ECG; however, atrial and ventricular chamber enlargement patterns may be recognized. Various atrial and ventricular arrhythmias may be noted with advanced disease and include most commonly APCs and atrial fibrillation. Atrial fibrillation, an arrhythmia associated with chronic mitral regurgitation and left atrial enlargement, results in a loss of organized atrial contraction which decreases ventricular filling and can lead to a significant reduction in cardiac output and signs of weakness or syncope.

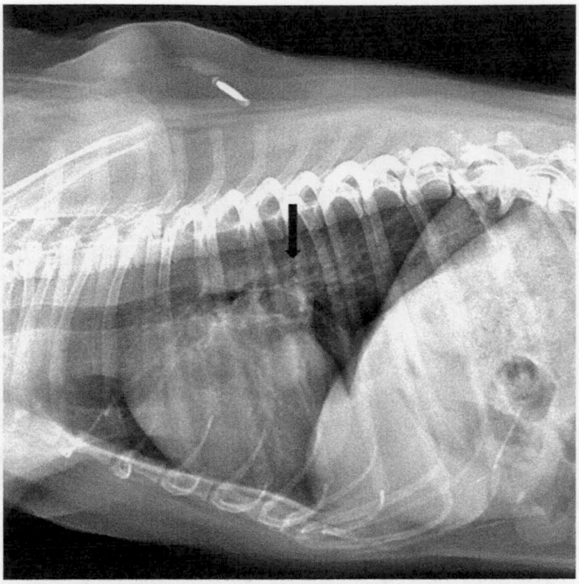

Figure 11.7 Lateral thoracic radiograph of a dog with chronic myxomatous mitral valve disease. There is loss of the caudal cardiac waist consistent with left atrial enlargement. The left mainstem bronchi (black arrow) is elevated and compressed secondary to the enlarged left atrium.

Echocardiography is useful for evaluating the degree of cardiac chamber dilation and identifying valvular regurgitation. Echocardiographic changes may include systolic prolapse of the atrioventricular valves (Figure 11.8) into the atrium and variable degrees of nodular thickening of the valve leaflets. Left atrial enlargement may also be apparent (Figure 11.9). Flail leaflets and ruptured chordae tendineae may be visualized. Indices of systolic function such as fractional shortening may be increased due to a reduced left ventricular afterload and increased preload from mitral regurgitation; however, normalized or reduced fractional shortenings may result with progressive myocardial

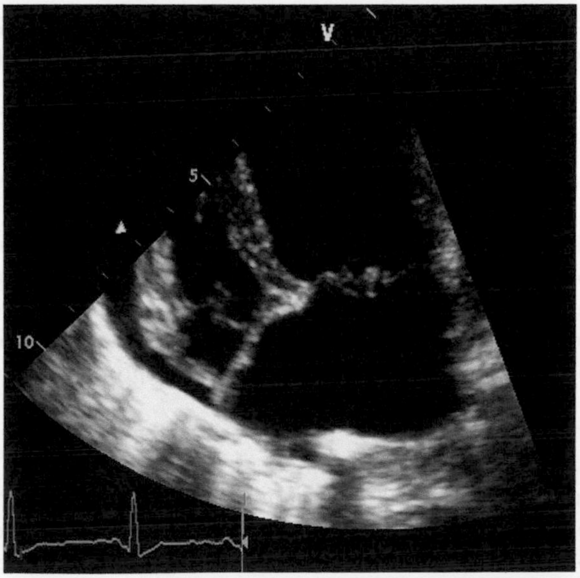

Figure 11.8 Left apical four-chamber view in a dog with chronic myxomatous valvular degeneration. There is enlargement of the left atrium and both atrioventricular valves appeared thickened with areas of prolapse.

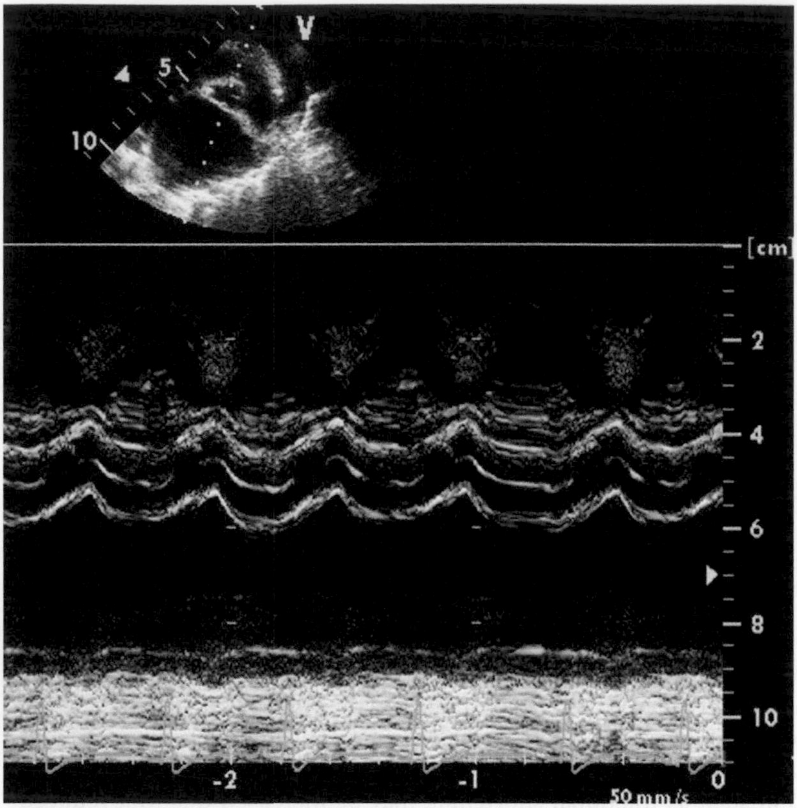

Figure 11.9 An M-mode echocardiogram recorded at the level of the heart base in a dog with chronic myxomatous mitral valve degeneration. The left atrial diameter is enlarged.

dysfunction. Color-flow Doppler and spectral Doppler interrogation can identify regurgitant blood flow through the affected valves (Figure 11.10).

Recently, the results of a large prospective multicentered clinical trial revealed that pimobendan administration to dogs with radiographic and echocardiographic cardiomegaly (i.e. stage B2) slowed the progression of disease and delayed the onset of congestive heart failure [22]. Despite the lack of compelling evidence, many cardiologists also advise the use of ACEI in dogs with stage B2 disease [21,23,24]. Once congestive heart failure has occurred (i.e. stage C), cases are managed medically with the goals of relieving pulmonary edema, enhancing cardiac output, and blunting the maladaptive neurohormonal response of the renin–angiotensin–aldosterone system. Most dogs may remain asymptomatic for years, and many dogs can survive beyond 1 year following the onset of clinical signs from CHF with appropriate medical care.

Endocarditis

Infective endocarditis is an infectious inflammatory disease of the endocardial surface or valves of the heart, and is relatively rare in the dog with a reported prevalence of 6.6% or less [25–27]. The aortic and mitral valves are the most commonly involved in

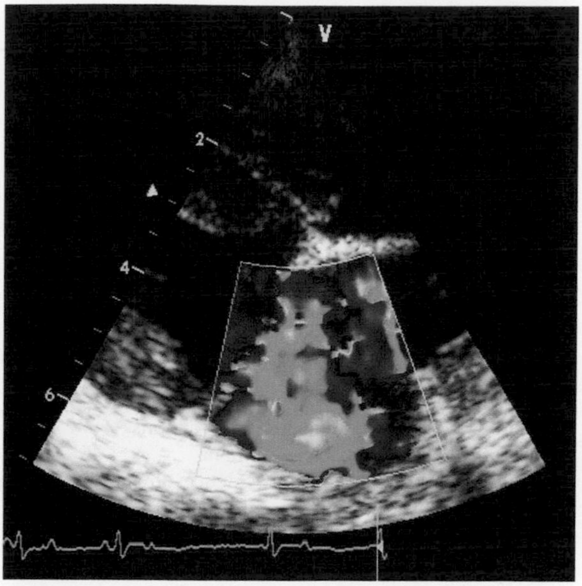

Figure 11.10 An echocardiogram with color-flow Doppler demonstrating marked mitral valve regurgitation in a dog with chronic myxomatous mitral valve degeneration.

dogs. Persistent or transient bacteremia is required to establish an infection. Endothelial damage and disturbed blood flow may allow for the formation of a thrombus at the site. This aggregate of platelets and fibrin can serve a nidus for bacterial colonization and invasion. Valvular insufficiency results as a consequence of valvular vegetations. These vegetations can be friable and embolize, shedding bacteria into systemic circulation. Subaortic stenosis is a well-recognized risk factor for infective endocarditis likely due to increased turbulence resulting in valvular endothelial damage and exposure of the underlying collagen. The most common acquired valvular disease, endocardiosis, has not been associated with an increased risk of endocarditis, nor has severe dental disease.

Clinical signs are variable and may include signs of left-sided CHF or nonspecific signs of lethargy, lack of appetite, lameness, weakness, collapse, or intermittent fever. Physical examination may reveal a heart murmur. The type of murmur depends on the valve involved. Types of murmurs include a diastolic murmur of aortic insufficiency, a systolic murmur of mitral valve regurgitation, or murmurs with both a diastolic and systolic component, also known as "to and fro" murmurs. Signs of polyarthritis such as joint swelling, lameness, and pain may be noted.

Definitive diagnosis requires the combination of clinical signs, laboratory results, and echocardiographic imaging (Table 11.1). Clinical laboratory findings may reveal evidence of inflammation or infection. Neutrophilia with a left shift and varying degrees of thrombocytopenia may be observed. Serum chemistry may reveal azotemia, increased hepatic enzyme concentrations, and hyperglobulinemia. Proteinuria, hematuria, and pyuria may be present on urinalysis. Urine cultures should also be performed to identify any causative agents. Blood cultures prior to antibiotic therapy are helpful in establishing a diagnosis of endocarditis and guiding treatment. Ideally, multiple blood samples should be taken using aseptic techniques from different venous sites at least 1 hour apart and is further described in Chapter 16 (Figure 11.11). The most common bacteria isolated from cultures are *Staphylococcal* and *Streptococcal* species or *Escherichia*

Table 11.1 Criteria for diagnosis of endocarditis.

Definitive diagnosis:
- Two major criteria
- One major and three minor criteria
- Five minor criteria

Probable endocarditis:
- One major and one minor criteria
- Three minor criteria

Unlikely endocarditis:
- Firm alternative diagnosis
- Resolution of clinical signs within 4 days of antibiotic therapy

Major criteria:
- Positive blood culture on separate occasions
- Evidence of endocardial involvement
  - Positive echocardiographic evidence: obvious oscillating mass or abscess
  - New murmur of valvular insufficiency

Minor criteria:
- Fever
- Immune-mediated condition (i.e. glomerulonephritis, polyarthropathy)
- Predisposing condition (i.e. subaortic stenosis)
- Serologic evidence of infection
- Other echocardiographic findings

Adapted from [44].

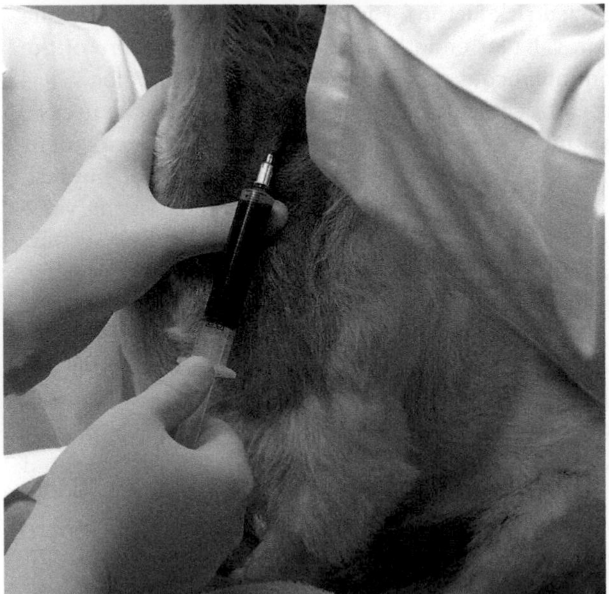

Figure 11.11 Blood culture samples require the use of sterile gloves, needles, syringes, and commercial blood culture bottles. The venipuncture sites should be clipped and thoroughly cleaned with antiseptics such as 2% chlorhexidine gluconate and 70% isopropyl alcohol.

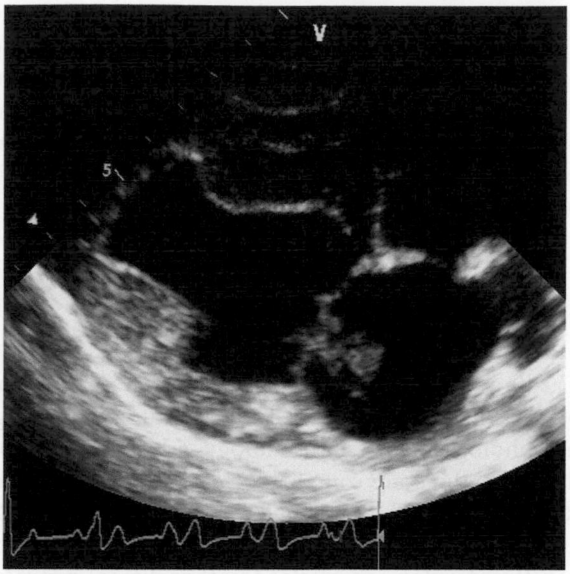

Figure 11.12 Right parasternal four-chamber view from a dog presenting with lethargy, anorexia, fever, and a recently diagnosed heart murmur. An oscillating vegetative lesion is visible on the atrial aspect of the anterior mitral valve leaflet.

coli. *Bartonella* has recently become recognized as an important cause of endocarditis [28]. Serologic testing and polymerase chain reaction for *Bartonella* may be useful, as it is difficult to successfully culture. Radiography may be unremarkable or may reveal cardiomegaly and CHF.

Echocardiography may reveal the presence of vegetative lesions on the affected valves (Figure 11.12). These may appear as valve thickening or as an oscillating hyperechoic mass associated with the valve. It may be difficult to distinguish valvular changes of endocardiosis from infective endocarditis on echocardiographic appearance alone. Color-flow and spectral Doppler should identify valvular insufficiency (Figure 11.13).

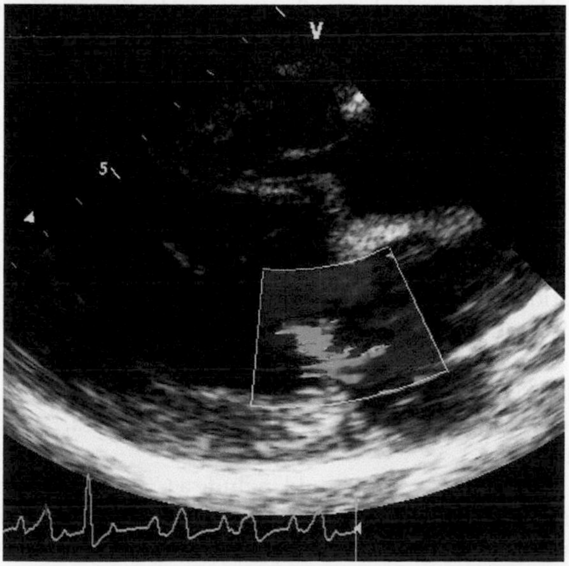

Figure 11.13 An echocardiogram with color-flow Doppler demonstrating mitral regurgitation secondary to mitral valve endocarditis.

Long-term antibiotics are the cornerstone of treatment. Antibiotic choice should ideally be based on culture and sensitivity; however, empiric therapy with broad spectrum antibiotics should be instituted while awaiting culture results. Repeat cultures are recommended both during and following antibiotic treatment. Other supportive care may be needed including the management of CHF and arrhythmias. Long-term prognosis is usually poor to guarded, as most dogs succumb to CHF, sudden death from arrhythmias, or thromboembolic disease.

Feline Cardiomyopathies

Cardiomyopathies are the most common heart diseases in cats. Cardiomyopathies can be classified by various methods including physiologic or clinical features, phenotypic morphologic expression, etiology, and type of myocardial dysfunction. Primary cardiomyopathies are considered idiopathic and include: hypertrophic cardiomyopathy, RCM, DCM, and unclassified cardiomyopathy (UCM). Secondary myocardial disorders are due to identifiable metabolic or systemic disease processes. Myocardial hypertrophy can also develop as sequelae to other disease processes including hyperthyroidism and systemic hypertension.

Hypertrophic Cardiomyopathy

Primary HCM, the most common cardiomyopathy of cats, is characterized by concentric myocardial hypertrophy, most notably in the left ventricle. The underlying cause is unknown, although a genetic basis is likely. Genetic mutations have been identified in both Maine coon and Ragdoll cats with HCM [29, 30]. Many cats with primary HCM also have a dynamic obstruction to the left ventricular outflow tract, referred to as hypertrophic obstructive cardiomyopathy (HOCM). HOCM is characterized by a narrowing of the left ventricular outflow tract (LVOT), systolic anterior motion (SAM) of the mitral valve, and increased left ventricular outflow pressure gradients. SAM is identified on echocardiogram as a portion of the septal mitral valve leaflet moving into the LVOT during systole. This may increase wall stress and myocardial oxygen demand and promote myocardial ischemia. Concentric hypertrophy and myocardial fibrosis decrease the compliance of the left ventricle contributing to diastolic dysfunction. Many cats may be asymptomatic for years or present in CHF. Other physical examination findings may include auscultation of heart murmurs, gallops, or arrhythmias. Murmurs may develop due to either left ventricular outflow tract obstruction or from mitral regurgitation. Tachypnea and dyspnea may occur secondary to pulmonary edema or pleural effusion.

Arterial thromboembolism (ATE) is important sequelae to any form of feline cardiomyopathy and may result in a sudden occlusion of blood flow to the limbs, most commonly the hind limbs, leading to weakness, lameness, and severe pain in the affected limbs.

Initial diagnostics should include a CBC, serum chemistry panel, and urinalysis. Additionally, in order to rule out reversible causes of myocardial hypertrophy, blood pressures and serum thyroid concentrations should be evaluated. ECG abnormalities may

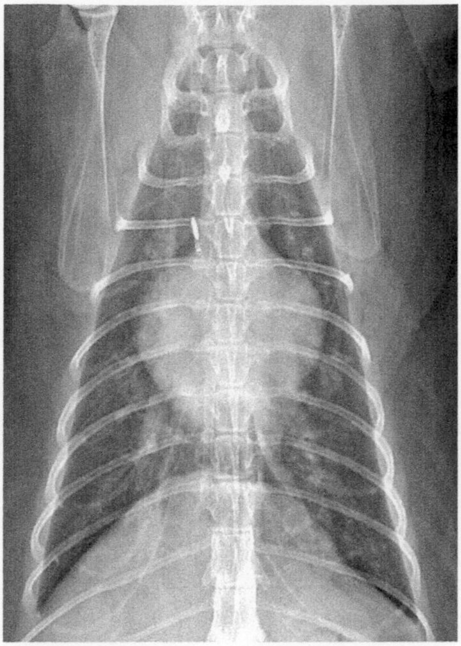

Figure 11.14 Dorsoventral radiograph of a cat with hypertrophic cardiomyopathy. There is marked left atrial enlargement giving a "shield" or "valentine" shape to the cardiac silhouette.

include ventricular, and less commonly, supraventricular tachyarrhythmias, as well as conduction disturbances such as left anterior fascicular block patterns.

Thoracic radiographs may be unremarkable or show variable degrees of left atrial and left ventricular enlargement (Figure 11.14). Symptomatic cats may also have pulmonary venous congestion, interstitial to alveolar infiltrates, and/or pleural effusion (Figure 11.15).

Echocardiography is required to diagnose and differentiate feline myocardial diseases. Diffuse or focal hypertrophy may be noted in the left ventricular free wall, septum, and papillary muscles (Figure 11.16). Left atrial enlargement is often marked (Figure 11.17). The fractional shortening is often normal or increased and there may be near complete systolic left ventricular cavity obliteration. The papillary muscles and myocardium may appear hyperechoic potentially due to ischemic injury and fibrosis. SAM is occasionally noted, causing a dynamic obstruction to the left ventricular outflow tract (Figure 11.18). Doppler interrogation of the transmitral inflow patterns may demonstrate diastolic dysfunction.

Treatment of symptomatic patients relies upon improving the clinical signs of CHF. Oxygen therapy is often warranted in cases of emergency presentation. Any stress, such as physical restraint for examination or diagnostic procedures may exacerbate dyspnea, which may lead to death. Thoracocentesis should be performed in cases suspected of having pleural effusion. Diuretics such as furosemide should be given parenterally to help resolve pulmonary edema. Furosemide should be given at regular intervals or as a constant rate infusion until the respiratory rate and character have improved. Nitroglycerin cream may be advantageous to help reduce afterload on the failing heart, although its efficacy is unknown. Long-term therapy is the same as with other forms of CHF.

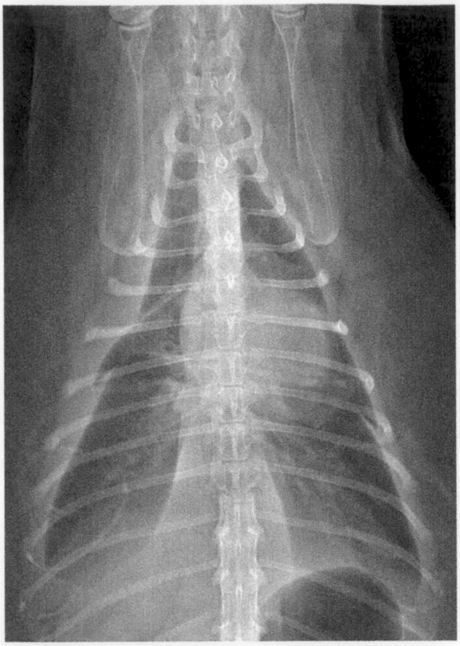

Figure 11.15 Dorsoventral radiograph of a cat with pleural effusion due to hypertrophic cardiomyopathy.

There is no consensus on the benefit of treating asymptomatic HCM. Beta-blockers and calcium channel blockers are recommended by some to slow the heart rate and thereby enhance ventricular filling, potentially reduce systolic outflow tract obstruction, and reduce myocardial oxygen consumption. However, in one study therapy with atenolol, a β_1-selective blocker, failed to show a benefit in survival times [31]. Given the potential for ATE in cats with enlarged left atriums or a previous history of ATE,

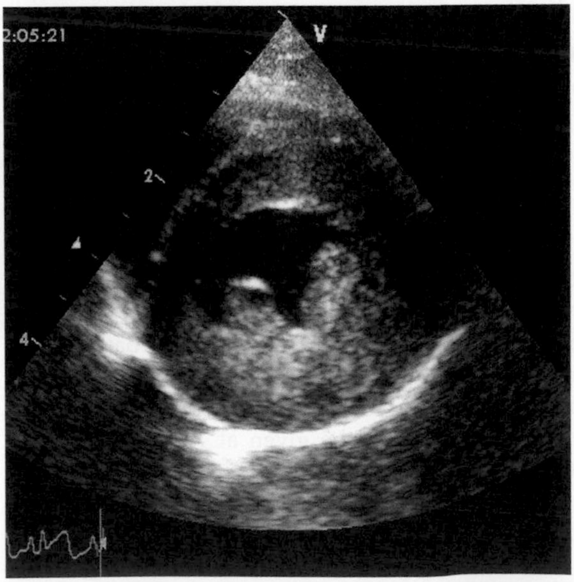

Figure 11.16 Right parasternal short-axis view at the level of the left ventricle in a cat with hypertrophic cardiomyopathy. The papillary muscles appear prominent and there is marked myocardial thickening, most notably in the left ventricular free wall.

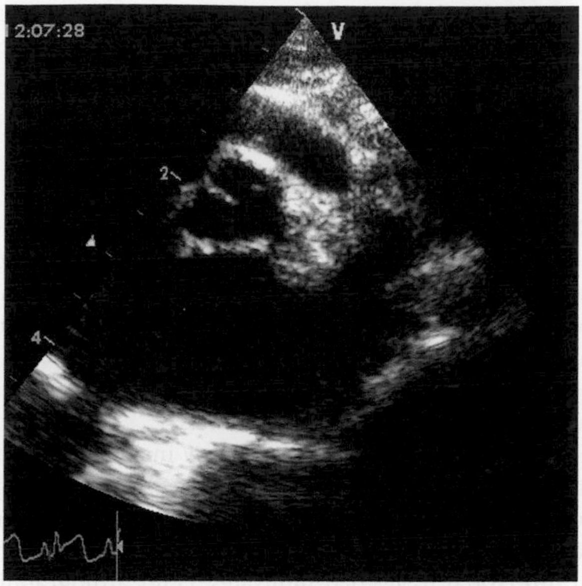

Figure 11.17 Right parasternal short-axis view at the level of the heart base in a cat with hypertrophic cardiomyopathy. Marked left atrial enlargement is evident.

prophylactic therapy with low-dose aspirin or clopidogrel (Plavix®) may be beneficial in reducing the occurrence of thromboembolic disease. Clopidogrel has recently been shown to be superior to aspirin in reducing recurrent ATE in cats [32]. If clinical signs of ATE are present, then appropriate treatment should be initiated (discussed later in the chapter). Prognosis of HCM and HOCM is quite variable as many cats with HCM remain asymptomatic for years. Some cats will progress rapidly into CHF, develop ATE,

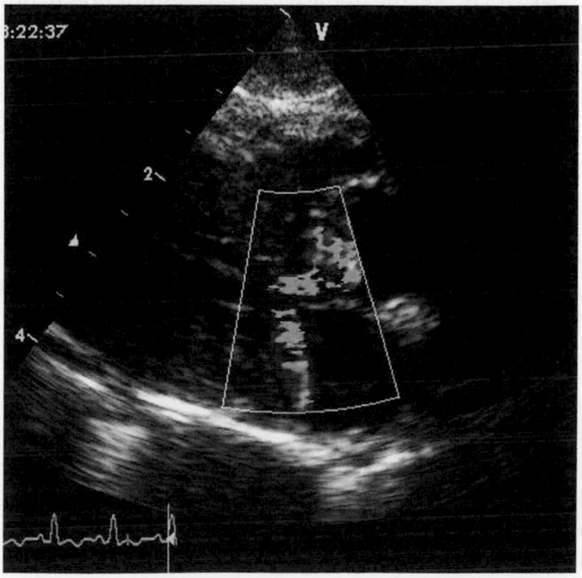

Figure 11.18 An echocardiogram with color-flow Doppler demonstrating two turbulent jets associated with systolic anterior motion of the mitral valve in a cat with hypertrophic obstructive cardiomyopathy.

or die suddenly (perhaps from a lethal tachyarrhythmia). Cats that present in CHF generally have a poor prognosis with a median survival of anywhere from 3 to 18 months [33, 34].

Restrictive Cardiomyopathy

Restrictive cardiomyopathy is uncommon and characterized by significantly reduced diastolic filling and decreased ventricular compliance with essentially normal systolic function and left ventricular wall thickness. The cause of RCM is unknown but may result from a variety of myocardial insults that lead to endocardial, subendocardial, or myocardial fibrosis. The clinical presentation of RCM is similar to those of other feline cardiomyopathies. Physical examination may reveal soft murmurs of mitral or tricuspid regurgitation, gallops, or arrhythmias.

Electrocardiographic findings may include supraventricular or ventricular arrhythmias, conduction disturbances, and/or chamber enlargement patterns. Left atrial or biatrial enlargement, as well as tortuous dilated pulmonary veins may be noted on thoracic radiography. Cats with congestive heart failure may have evidence of pleural effusion, or interstitial to alveolar infiltrates. Echocardiographic characteristics may include left atrial enlargement, a thickened hyperechoic endocardial surface, and either normal or only slightly reduced measurements of systolic function.

The prognosis of RCM is typically poor. There is an increased risk of progression to CHF, ATE, or sudden death, and treatment is mostly supportive.

Unclassified Cardiomyopathy

Unclassified cardiomyopathies (UCM) are myocardial diseases that share many characteristics of other cardiomyopathies and do not fit into distinct categories of HCM, RCM, or DCM. The underlying cause is unknown; however, in some cases it may reflect the advancement or regression of other cardiomyopathies. The clinical presentation of UCM is similar to that of other feline cardiomyopathies.

Thoracic radiography may reveal biatrial or left atrial enlargement as well as pleural effusion and interstitial to alveolar lung patterns consistent with CHF. Echocardiography typically reveals enlarged dilated atria. Mild systolic dysfunction may be noted as well, yet ventricular wall measurements may be within the normal range.

Prognosis is variable and depends on the clinical presentation. Asymptomatic cats with mild left atrial enlargement have a better prognosis. Cats with concurrent CHF tend to have a poor prognosis, although some may respond well to supportive care and standard CHF therapy.

Dilated Cardiomyopathy

The incidence of feline DCM, once the most common feline cardiomyopathy, has declined considerably given the link to taurine deficiency and subsequent formulation of taurine-enriched commercial diets [35, 36]. Most cats are symptomatic with signs of decreased cardiac output and/or CHF. Dyspnea and tachypnea are commonly seen.

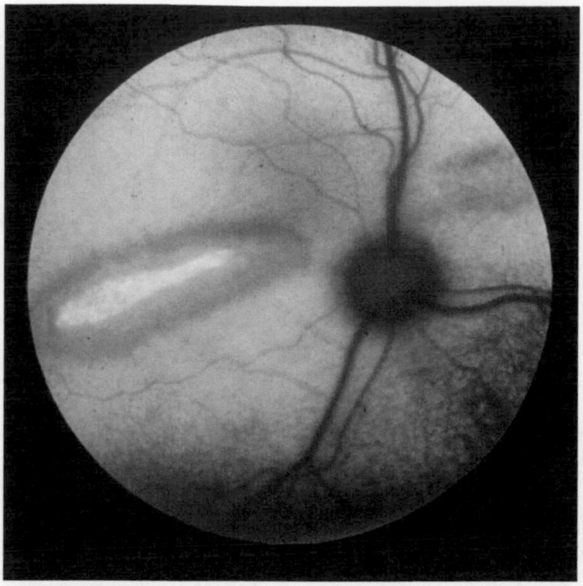

Figure 11.19 Fundus photograph of taurine deficiency retinopathy in a cat. A hyperreflective elliptical area of retinal degeneration is present. (Courtesy of Cecil P. Moore)

Gallops, systolic heart murmurs, muffled lung sounds, or crackles may be auscultated. Additionally, many cats may be hypothermic and have pale mucous membranes. Thorough may reveal retinal lesions in taurine deficient cats (Figure 11.19) [37].

Thoracic radiographs may reveal signs of CHF and cardiomegaly. Echocardiography should reveal an enlarged left ventricle with evidence of systolic dysfunction (Figure 11.20). Left atrial enlargement may also be noted. Plasma and/or whole blood taurine concentrations should be evaluated to document a taurine deficiency.

Treatment is similar as with other cardiomyopathies resulting in CHF. Positive inotropes such as dobutamine may be needed acutely. Taurine supplementation should also be initiated. For chronic therapy oral digoxin or perhaps pimobendan may be considered. Long-term therapy may require antithrombotics and taurine supplementation if indicated. Prognosis of cats with taurine deficient DCM is good with appropriate treatment, as systolic function may improve over time [36]. Prognosis for idiopathic DCM remains poor to guarded. As with other feline cardiomyopathies, a recurrence of CHF is likely.

Feline Arterial Thromboembolism

Systemic arterial thromboembolism is a potential sequela to all feline cardiomyopathies, but may rarely occur with other disease processes. Left atrial enlargement secondary to myocardial disease may allow for thrombus formation and arterial embolization. The most common site of embolization is the aortic trifurcation, but other sites including the renal or brachial arteries can also occur. In addition to restricting blood flow acutely in the affected artery, collateral circulation is compromised as the thromboemboli releases vasoactive mediators. ATE usually results in acute signs due to tissue ischemia and necrosis. Acute hindlimb paresis or paralysis is common. Additionally, the affected limbs

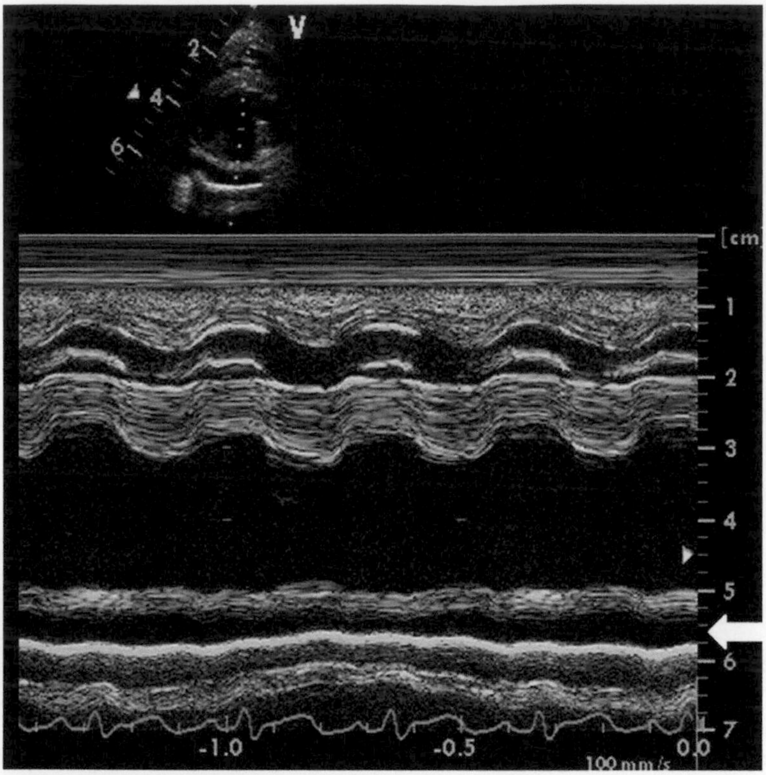

Figure 11.20 An M-mode echocardiogram at the level of the left ventricle in a cat with dilated cardiomyopathy. There is an increase in the left ventricular end-diastolic and end-systolic dimensions consistent with volume overloading and systolic dysfunction, respectively. Pericardial effusion (white arrow) is also evident.

may have absent pulses, appear pale, and cool or painful to the touch. One can remember the "Five Ps" as an aid: Paresis, Pulseless, Palor, Polar, and Pain. Hypothermia may be present and is a negative prognostic indicator, as it may suggest poor systemic perfusion and circulatory shock. A retrospective study found that cats presenting with signs of aortic thromboembolism and rectal temperatures below 98.9 °F have a less than 50% chance of survival and cats with temperatures above a 50% or better chance of survival [38]. Signs of concurrent CHF may also be evident. Radiographs and echocardiography should be performed to diagnose any underlying myocardial disease.

Therapy is mainly supportive, with the goal of providing analgesia, relieving signs of CHF, and preventing further thrombi formation. Anticoagulant therapy with heparin is indicated in the acute management to prevent further thrombi formation. Aspirin and clopidogrel therapy may be initiated once the patients are eating and able to take oral medication. Fibrinolytic therapy and embolectomy are not routinely used as they are associated with an increased risk of reperfusion injury and mortality [39–43]. The prognosis is generally poor, as a significant percentage of cats are euthanized or die from the initial episode. Within weeks, cats may regain some limb function. Full recovery may take months, although residual neurologic or muscular deficits are common. Recurrent thromboembolic events are common and generally occur within a year. Cats may also later develop CHF or have a recurrence of CHF.

Cardiogenic Syncope

Syncope is characterized by a sudden loss of consciousness with an associated loss of postural tone. Syncope most commonly occurs from an acute decrease in cerebral blood flow. Differentiating syncope from seizure can be difficult; however, identifying potential triggers and signs that occur immediately before, during, and after the event can provide clues. Triggers such as exercise or stress are common with syncope due to the increased oxygen demand. Cough, gag, defecation, and micturition can be triggers for situational syncope. A delayed recovery from the episode with an altered mental status is typical for seizures, but can occur with syncope that results in profound hypoxia. Causes of syncope can be divided into cardiac and noncardiac causes. Arrhythmias are the most common cardiac cause of syncope and include tachyarrhythmias (ventricular or supraventricular tachycardias) or bradyarrhythmias (sick sinus syndrome, atrioventricular block, atrial standstill). Other cardiac causes include: structural heart disease such as obstruction of the cardiac outflow (pulmonic and aortic stenosis, pulmonary hypertension, intracardiac neoplasia), obstruction to cardiac filling (cardiac tamponade, constrictive pericarditis), or poor cardiac contractility. Noncardiac causes include metabolic diseases (hypoglycemia, anemia, electrolyte derangements, hypoxemia) and neurocardiogenic or reflex-mediated syncope. Reflex-mediated syncope involves an inappropriate withdrawal of sympathetic tone and an increase in parasympathetic tone leading to varying degrees of hypotension, bradycardia, and reduced cardiac contractility and is a diagnosis of exclusion in veterinary medicine.

Syncope as a result of bradyarrhythmias may be treated with permanent pacemaker therapy, as is neurocardiogenic syncope in humans with a significant bradycardia component. Events related to tachycardias are most often treated with antiarrhythmics. Non-cardiogenic syncope is typically treated by addressing the underlying metabolic disease or condition.

References

1 Fine, D.M., Tobias, A.H. and Bonagura, J.D. (2010) Cardiovascular manifestation of iatrogenic hyperthyroidism in two dogs. *Journal of Veterinary Cardiology*, **12**,141–146.

2 Meurs, K.M., Mauceli, E., Lahmers, S. *et al.* (2010) Genome-wide association identifies a deletion in the 3' untranslated region of striatin in a canine model of arrhythmogenic right ventricular cardiomyopathy. *Human Genetics*, **128**, 315–324.

3 Meurs, K.M., Stern, J.A., Reina-Doreste, Y. *et al.* (2014) Natural history of arrhythmogenic right ventricular cardiomyopathy in boxer dogs: a prospective study. *Journal of Veterinary Internal Medicine*, **28**, 1214–1220.

4 Meurs, K.M., Spier, A.W., Wright, N.A. *et al.* (2002) Comparison of the effects of four antiarrhythmic treatments for familial ventricular arrhythmias in Boxers. *Journal of the American Veterinary Medical Association*, **221**, 522–527.

5 Martin, M.W.S., Stafford Johnson, M.J., Strehlau, G. and King, J.N. (2010) Canine dilated cardiomyopathy: a retrospective study of prognostic findings in 367 clinical cases. *Journal of Small Animal Practice*, **51**, 428–436.
6 Meurs, K.M., Lahmers, S., Keene, B.W. *et al.* (2012) A splice site mutation in a gene encoding PDK4, a mitochondrial protein, is associated with the development of dilated cardiomyopathy in the Doberman pinscher. *Human Genetics*, **131**, 1319–1325.
7 Mausberg, T.B., Wess, G., Simak, J., *et al.* (2011) A locus on chromosome 5 is associated with dilated cardiomyopathy in Doberman Pinschers. *PLoS One*, 6, e20042.
8 Kittleson, M.D., Keene, B.W., Pion, P.D. and Loyer, C.G. (1997) Results of the multicenter spaniel trial (MUST): taurine- and carnitine-responsive dilated cardiomyopathy in American cocker spaniels with decreased plasma taurine concentrations. *Journal of Veterinary Internal Medicine*, **11**, 204–211.
9 Harmon, M.W., Leach, S.B. and Lamb, K.E. (in press) Dilated cardiomyopathy in standard schnauzers: retrospective study of 15 cases (2001–2013). *Journal of the American Animal Hospital Association*, in press.
10 Leach, S.B., Johnson, G.S., Gilliam, D., *et al.* (2014) Dilated cardiomyopathy in standard schnauzers with a homozygous 22 BP deletion in RBM20. Presented at the 32nd Annual ACVIM Forum, June 2014; Nashville, TN. *Journal of Veterinary Internal Medicine*, **28**, 1353.
11 Summerfield, N.J., Boswood, A., O'Grady, M.R. *et al.* (2012) Efficacy of pimobendan in the prevention of congestive heart failure or sudden death in Doberman Pinschers with preclinical dilated cardiomyopathy (the PROTECT study). *Journal of Veterinary Internal Medicine*, **26**, 1337–1349.
12 O'Grady, M.R., O'Sullivan, M.L., Minors, S.L. and Horne, R. (2009) Efficacy of benazepril hydrochloride to delay the progression of occult dilated cardiomyopathy in Doberman Pinschers. *Journal of Veterinary Internal Medicine*, **23**, 977–983.
13 Tidholm, A., Svensson, H. and Sylven, C. (1997) Survival and prognostic factors in 189 dogs with dilated cardiomyopathy. *Journal of the American Animal Hospital Association*, **33**, 364–368.
14 Borgarelli, M., Santilli, R.A., Chiavegato, D., *et al.* (2006) Prognostic indicators for dogs with dilated cardiomyopathy. *Journal of Veterinary Internal Medicine*, **20**, 104–110.
15 Calvert, C.A., Pickus, C.W., Jacobs, G.J. and Brown, J. (1997) Signalment, survival and prognostic factors in Doberman pinschers with end-stage cadiomyopathy. *Journal of Veterinary Internal Medicine*, **11**, 323–326.
16 Monnet, E., Orton, E.C., Salman, M. and Boon, J. (1995) Idiopathic dilated cardiomyopathy in dogs: survival and prognostic indicators. *Journal of Veterinary Internal Medicine*, **9**, 12–17.
17 Gelzer, A.R., Kraus, M.S., Rishniw, M. *et al.* (2009) Combination therapy with digoxin and diltiazem controls ventricular rate in chronic atrial fibrillation in dogs better than digoxin or diltiazem monotherapy: a randomized crossover study in 18 dogs. *Journal of Veterinary Internal Medicine*, **23**, 499–508.
18 Haggstrom, J., Kvart, C. and Pedersen, H.D. (2005) Acquired valvular heart disease, in *Textbook of Veterinary Internal Medicine*, 6th Edition (eds S.J. Ettinger and E.C. Feldman). Elsevier Saunders, St Louis. pp. 1022–1039.
19 Sisson, D., Kvart, C. and Darke, P. (1999) Acquired valvular heart disease in dogs and cats, in *Textbook of Canine and Feline Cardiology*, 2nd Edition (eds P.R. Fox, D. Sisson and N.S. Moïse). WB Saunders Company, Philadelphia. pp. 536–565.

20 Borgarelli, M., Savarino, P., Crosara, S. *et al.* (2008) Survival characteristics and prognostic variables of dogs with mitral regurgitation attributable to myxomatous valve disease. *Journal of Veterinary Internal Medicine*, **22**, 120–128.
21 Atkins, C., Bonagura, J., Ettinger, S. *et al.* (2009) Guidelines for the diagnosis and treatment of canine chronic valvular heart disease. *Journal of Veterinary Internal Medicine*, **23**, 1142–1150.
22 Boswood, A., Haggstrom, J. and Gordon, S. (2016) EPIC trial results. Presented at the 34th Annual ACVIM Forum, June 2016, Denver, CO, USA.
23 Kvart, C., Haggstrom, J., Pedersen, H.D. *et al.* (2002) Efficacy of enalapril for prevention of congestive heart failure in dogs with myxomatous valve disease and asymptomatic mitral regurgitation. *Journal of Veterinary Internal Medicine*, **12**, 80–88.
24 Atkins, C.E., Keene, B.W., Brown, W.A. *et al.* (2007) Results of the veterinary enalapril trial to prove reduction in onset of heart failure in dogs chronically treated with enalapril alone for compensated, naturally occurring mitral valve insufficiency. *Journal of the American Veterinary Medical Association*, **231**, 1061–1069.
25 Kittleson, M.D. (1998) Infective endocarditis, in *Small Animal Cardiovascular Medicine* (eds M.D. Kittleson and R.D. Kienle). Mosby, St Louis. pp. 402–412.
26 Miller, M.W. and Sisson, D. (1999) Infectious endocarditis, in *Textbook of Canine and Feline Cardiology*, 2nd Edition (eds P.R. Fox, D. Sisson and N.S. Moïse). W.B. Saunders Company, Philadelphia. pp. 567–580.
27 MacDonald, K. (2010) Infective endocarditis in dogs: diagnosis and therapy. *Veterinary Clinics of North America Small Animal Practice*, **40**, 665–684.
28 MacDonald, K.A., Chomel, B.B., Kittleson, M.D. *et al.* (2004) A prospective study of canine infective endocarditis in northern California (1999–2001): emergency of Bartonella as a prevalent etiologic agent. *Journal of Veterinary Internal Medicine*, **18**, 56–64.
29 Meurs, K.M., Sanchez, X., David, R.M., *et al.* (2005) A cardiac myosin binding protein C mutation in the Maine Coon cat with familial hypertrophic cardiomyopathy. *Human Molecular Genetics*, **14**, 3587–3593.
30 Meurs, K.M., Norgard, M.M., Ederer, M.M. *et al.* (2007) A substitution mutation in the myosin binding protein C gene in ragdoll hypertrophic cardiomyopathy. *Genomics*, **90**, 261–264.
31 Schober, K.E., Zientek, J., Li, X. *et al.* (2013) Effect of treatment with atenolol on 5-year survival in cats with preclinical (asymptomatic) hypertrophic cardiomyopathy. *Journal of Veterinary Cardiology*, **15**, 93–104.
32 Hogan, D.F., Fox, P.R., Jacob, K. *et al.* (2015) Secondary prevention of cardiogenic arterial thromboembolism in the cat: the double blind, randomized, positive-controlled feline arterial thromboembolism) clopidogrel vs aspirin trial (FAT CAT). *Journal of Veterinary Cardiology*, **17**, S306–S317.
33 Atkins, C.E., Gallo, A.M., Kurzman, I.D. and Cowen, P. (1992) Risk factors, clinical signs, and survival in cats with a clinical diagnosis of idiopathic hypertrophic cardiomyopathy: 74 cases (1985–1989). *Journal of the American Veterinary Medical Association*, **201**, 613–618.
34 Rush, J.E., Freeman, L.M., Fenollosa, N.K. and Brown, D.J. (2002) Population and survival characteristics of cats with hypertrophic cardiomyopathy: 260 cases (1990–1999). *Journal of the American Veterinary Medical Association*, **220**, 202–207.

35 Pion, P.D., Kittleson, M.D., Thomas, W.P. *et al.* (1992) Clinical findings in cats with dilated cardiomyopathy and relationship of findings to taurine deficiency. *Journal of the American Veterinary Medical Association*, **201**, 267–274.

36 Pion, P.D., Kittleson, M.D., Thomas, W.P. *et al.* (1992) Response of cats with dilated cardiomyopathy to taurine supplementation. *Journal of the American Veterinary Medical Association*, **201**, 275–284.

37 Stiles, J. and Townsend, W.M. (2007) Feline Ophthalmology, in *Veterinary Ophthalmology*, 4th Edition (ed. K.N. Gelatt). Wiley–Blackwell, Oxford. pp. 1135–1136.

38 Smith, S.A., Tobias, A.H., Jacob, K.A. *et al.* (2003) Arterial thromboembolism in cats: acute crisis in 127 cases (1992–2001) and long-term management with low-dose aspirin in 24 cases. *Journal of Veterinary Internal Medicine*, **17**, 73–83.

39 Welch, K.M., Rozanski, E.A., Freeman, L.M. and Rush, J.E. (2010) Prospective evaluation of tissue plasminogen activator in 11 cats with arterial thromboembolism. *Journal of Feline Medicine and Surgery*, **12**, 122–128.

40 Moore, K.E., Morris, N., Dhupa, N. *et al.* (2000) Retrospective study of streptokinase administration in 46 cats with arterial thromboembolism. *Journal of Veterinary Emergency Critical Care*, **10**, 245–257.

41 Ramsey, C.C., Riepe, R.D., Macintire, D.K. and Burney, D.P. (1996) Streptokinase: a practical thrombus buster? Proceedings of the International Veterinary Emergency Critical Care Society, San Antonio, TX, USA. pp. 225–228.

42 Whelan, M.R., O'Toole, T.E., Chan, D.L. and Rush, J.E. (2005) Retrospective evaluation of urokinase use in cats with arterial thromboembolism. Proceedings of the International Veterinary Emergency Critical Care Society, Atlanta, GA, USA. p. 8.

43 Reimer, S.B., Kittleson, M.D. and Kyles, A.E. (2006) Use of rheolytic thrombectomy in the treatment of feline distal aortic thromboembolism. *Journal of Veterinary Internal Medicine*, **20**, 290–296.

44 Durack, D.T., Lukes, A.S. and Bright, D.K. (1994) New criteria for diagnosis of infective endocarditis: utilization of specific echocardiographic findings: Duke Endocarditis Service. *American Journal of Medicine*, **96**, 200–209.

12

Pericardial Effusion and Cardiac Neoplasia

Anne Myers

Introduction

Pericardial effusion is defined as an abnormally increased amount of fluid within the pericardial sac that surrounds the heart. Depending on the cause and the size of the animal, anywhere from 15 to over 500 mL can accumulate. It can form acutely or chronically, usually as hemorrhagic fluid containing components of circulating blood, but devoid of coagulation factors. The occurrence of excess fluid in the pericardial sac is relatively rare compared with other heart diseases in the small animal, such as mitral valve degeneration in the dog or hypertrophic cardiomyopathy in the cat, but can occur with either disease as a result of left atrial rupture in dogs, or congestive heart failure in cats.

Pericardial effusion occurs more frequently in the canine than the feline, with the most common cause in the dog being the presence of cardiac neoplasia. A mass growing inside a chamber can erode the wall causing abnormal bleeding into the pericardial sac, or invade the heart base and secrete hemorrhagic fluid into the sac. Build-up of pericardial effusion will cause increased pressure on the outer walls of the heart affecting the well-being of an animal and demonstrating some characteristic physical examination findings. Under the supervision of a veterinary cardiologist, the veterinary technician can assist with imaging techniques to aid in diagnosis of pericardial effusion, determining its cause, and with a *pericardiocentesis* procedure to remove the excess fluid. The causes of pericardial effusion, physical examination findings which indicate its presence, and procedures used to diagnose and treat will be discussed.

Role of the Pericardial Sac

The pericardium is a sac made of collagen and elastic fibers that surrounds almost all of the heart except the base, where the great vessels enter and exit. It normally contains a very small amount (0.25[± 0.15] mL/kg) [1] of serous fluid and an inner visceral layer which lubricates the epicardial surface during contraction and relaxation of the heart muscle. A top parietal layer helps equalize pressure on the outside walls of the heart chambers. Other functions include keeping the heart in a fixed position in the chest cavity and protecting the myocardium. If the pericardium becomes diseased, or is abnormal at birth, it can be partially removed without causing harm to the animal.

Cardiology for Veterinary Technicians and Nurses, First Edition. Edited by H. Edward Durham, Jr.

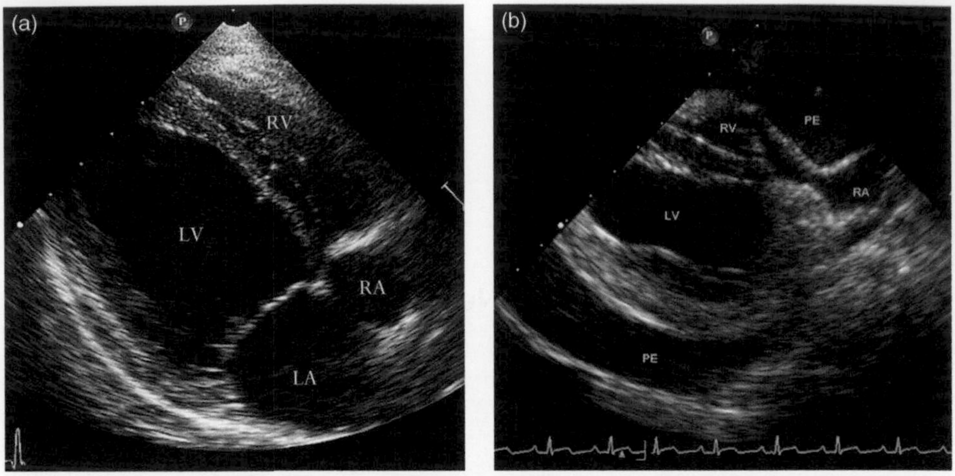

Figure 12.1 (a) Echocardiogram showing a normal heart with a full round right atrium. The larger chambers in the view are the left ventricle and left atrium. (b) Cardiac tamponade caused by hemorrhagic pericardial effusion in a 7-year-old female spayed standard poodle diagnosed, by pleural effusion cytology, with mesothelioma; 500 mL of effusion was removed from the pericardial sac. Note the indentation of the right atrial free wall toward the intra-atrial septum. LV, left ventricle; LA, left atrium; PE, pericardial effusion; RV, right ventricle; RA, right atrium.

However, when the pericardial sac fills with too much fluid, it does not allow the heart muscle to relax and the chambers to fill properly. The thin-walled right atrium (RA) is most affected and will collapse during diastole when receiving venous blood from the anterior and posterior vena cavas. This occurs because the pressure is greater in the pericardial space than inside the RA. Intracardiac pressures in the RA are normally 6/0 mmHg (systolic/diastolic) with a mean of 3 mmHg [2]. Collapse of the RA during diastole (Figure 12.1) caused by pericardial effusion is referred to as *cardiac tamponade* [3]. Tamponade will result in venous congestion, right-sided heart failure, and decreased cardiac output. Because the right heart has difficulty filling due to the tamponade, there is decreased right ventricle (RV) cardiac output leading to decreased preload for the left atrium and ventricle. Consequently, a drop in oxygen-rich blood going out into systemic circulation from the left ventricle occurs. The result can be anything from the discomfort of ascites, to life-threatening forward heart failure, cardiogenic shock, and death.

The amount of effusion does not always relate to the presence of cardiac tamponade. The more important factor is the rapidity of the effusion occurrence. A small amount of effusion can create tamponade if it occurs quickly, whereas large amounts of effusion that occur slowly may not cause tamponade, since they allow time for the pericardium to stretch, accommodating the extra fluid without increasing intrapericardial pressure.

Cardiac Neoplasia

The most common cause of hemorrhagic pericardial effusion in the older large-breed canine is cardiac neoplasia [3]. If a mass forms in the RA, RA/RV groove or right auricle, it is most likely a *hemangiosarcoma* causing erosion and hemorrhage from

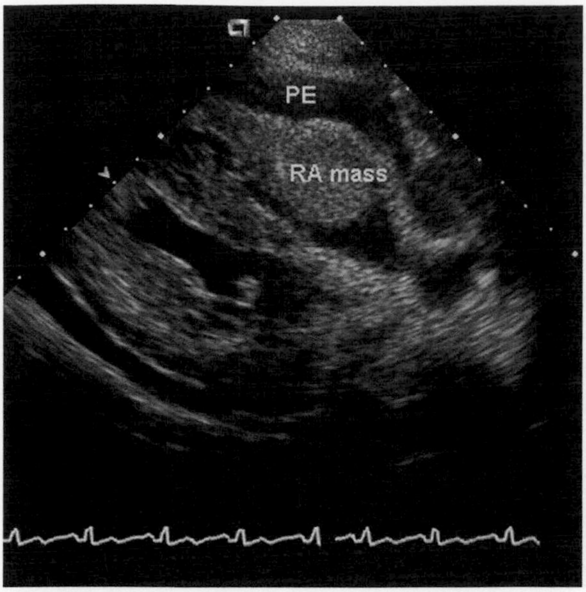

Figure 12.2 Echocardiogram showing a right atrial (RA) mass found in a Labrador retriever that presented with a history of weakness and collapse. The circular mass is located in the right atrioventricular junction. To the right of the mass, the collapse of the right atrial wall is evident. PE, pericardial effusion

the tumor site into the pericardial sac (Figure 12.2). Hemangiosarcomas are locally aggressive, highly metastatic tumors that arise from vascular endothelium and can be primary to the heart or the result of metastasis from the spleen or liver. They tend to cause multiple, acute bleeds and can result in cardiac tamponade rather quickly, by not allowing the fibrous pericardial sac to stretch over a period of time and accommodate excess fluid. Golden retrievers, Labrador retrievers and German shepherd dogs are three breeds commonly affected and usually present with a history of sudden collapse and pale mucous membranes.

If a mass forms at the heart base where the ascending aorta exits the heart, it is typically a *chemodectoma* which arises from neuroepithelial cells within the aortic arch. They tend to be slow growing, only locally invasive and over time can get quite large (Figure 12.3) sometimes causing pericardial effusion and cardiac tamponade by slowly secreting hemorrhagic fluid into the pericardial sac. Because of their location at the heart base, they can also cause compression of the main pulmonary artery leading to right-sided heart failure (hepatic congestion and ascites) [4]. Heart-based masses can be an incidental finding in an older dog with degenerative mitral valve disease and a heart murmur, undergoing a cardiac ultrasound. Brachyocephalic breeds such as the English bulldog and boxer are commonly affected [5]. *Ectopic thyroid carcinomas* have been shown to metastasize and result in heart-based masses also.

Mesothelioma is another neoplastic disease in the dog and cat, which invades the cells lining body cavities and organs. It can occur in the pleura, causing inflammation and pleural effusion, and can metastasize to the pericardium. This cancer can be difficult to diagnose from an effusion sample alone. These patients may undergo more than one centesis procedure to remove both pleural and pericardial fluid, which can lead to inflammation and constriction of the pericardium. Known as *constrictive effusive pericarditis* (discussed in detail later), it presents with only a small amount of pericardial effusion resulting in cardiac tamponade. The optimal method to permanently relieve pericardial

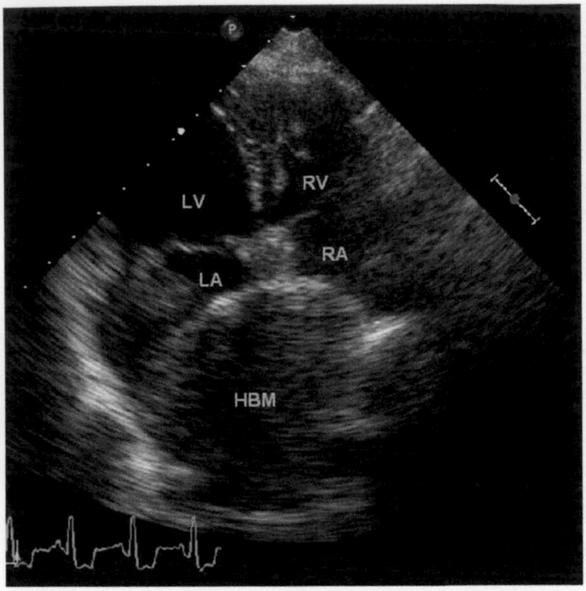

Figure 12.3 Echocardiogram showing a large heart-based tumor invading both the left and right atrium in an English bulldog. HBM, heart based mass; LA, left atrium; LV, left ventricle; RA, right atrium; RV, right ventricle.

effusion and constriction would be a subtotal or total pericardectomy. Some chemotherapeutic agents such as doxorubicin or intracavitary cisplatin or carboplatin may be used to slow progression of this disease. *Lymphoma* can also infiltrate the pericardium, epicardium, and myocardium, in both dogs and cats, resulting in pericardial effusion or constriction and usually responds to chemotherapeutic agents.

Prognosis for Cardiac Neoplasia

The long-term prognosis for patients with right atrial or auricular hemangiosarcoma is poor. They are highly metastatic and tend to cause acute, multiple bleeds into their pericardial sac, or possibly pleural cavity, resulting in low cardiac output from blood loss, shock, and death. This may occur hours, days, or weeks after initial diagnosis and removal of excess fluid. Surgical excision of the mass is risky and may not be curative due to the high incidence of metastasis. Chemotherapy has not been shown to increase life expectancy significantly. When owners are informed of this prognosis, some may choose euthanasia for their pet. Others chose removal of the pericardial fluid once, to relieve the tamponade and if able, take their pet home, knowing that they now have a very limited life expectancy.

The prognosis for a dog with an aortic body tumor (chemodectoma) is much longer, with survival time several months to years, as these tumors tend to be slow growing, only locally invasive, and may not cause pericardial effusion. If these tumors do get large, or secrete fluid into the pericardial sac, they will cause tamponade and venous congestion leading to ascites. If repeated pericardial taps are needed, removal of the pericardium is indicated to avoid inflammation that could lead to constrictive pericarditis. Chemodectomas can also invade the right or left atrium, causing obstruction of venous inflow and either ascites, or pulmonary edema. If ascites occurs from right atrial tamponade or obstruction and accumulates causing patient discomfort, fluid from the abdomen can be removed by performing an abdominocentesis, in which a large gauge over-the-needle catheter is introduced into the abdominal cavity and fluid is removed (see Chapter 16). If pulmonary edema occurs from obstruction of pulmonary venous inflow, the patient can be treated with an angiotensin-converting enzyme inhibitor (ACEI) such as enalapril and a diuretic such as furosemide.

Prognosis for mesothelioma is guarded and owners should be aware the lifespan of their pet will be decreased. As with any cancer, if treatment is to be pursued, thorough staging of the patient's disease is indicated. This would include a complete blood count, chemistry panel, urinalysis, chest radiographs, abdominal ultrasound, and any other testing a veterinary oncologist decides is necessary. Close monitoring with serial complete blood counts is necessary for any animal receiving chemotherapy. Many of these tests can be performed by a veterinary technician.

Idiopathic Hemorrhagic Pericardial Effusion

A common cause of hemorrhagic pericardial effusion, which is more often seen in younger large-breed canines, is of unknown cause or *idiopathic*. No masses are seen in or around the heart or pericardium and cytology of the fluid is nondiagnostic. The effusion tends to form slowly, allowing the pericardium to stretch and accommodate a large amount of fluid before causing cardiac tamponade. If the effusion is persistent, and requires more than one pericardiocentesis to remove the fluid, this may lead to inflammation and constrictive effusive pericarditis. A curative pericardectomy in which most or all of the pericardial sac is removed is indicated. The prognosis for these patients is excellent. Another technique that has been used to prevent recurrent pericardial effusion is a *balloon pericardiotomy* [6] in which the patient is placed under general anesthesia and using fluoroscopy guidance, a catheter with a balloon at its tip is inserted into the pericardium over a guidewire and inflated to create a large hole in which fluid will continue to drain out into the chest cavity.

Other Causes of Pericardial Effusion

Other causes of pericardial effusion in the canine include pericardial cysts, trauma, or foreign bodies. One congenital cause is from a *pericardial peritoneal diaphragmatic hernia*, in which there is an abnormal communication between the pericardial sac and the peritoneal cavity. This results in abdominal viscera migrating into the pericardium, leading to fluid accumulation. Surgery is indicated to correct it. *Left atrial rupture* causing acute bleed of circulating blood into the pericardium can occur in dogs with chronic mitral valve degeneration and severe mitral valve regurgitation into the left atrium [4]. This leads to an extremely enlarged, pressurized chamber that eventually ruptures. This is a life-threatening emergency in which intravenous fluids and supportive care should be administered immediately. If recognized and treated quickly, many of these patients will survive and the area of rupture will close over. Pericardial effusion in the feline is uncommon, but can occur with left-sided congestive heart failure

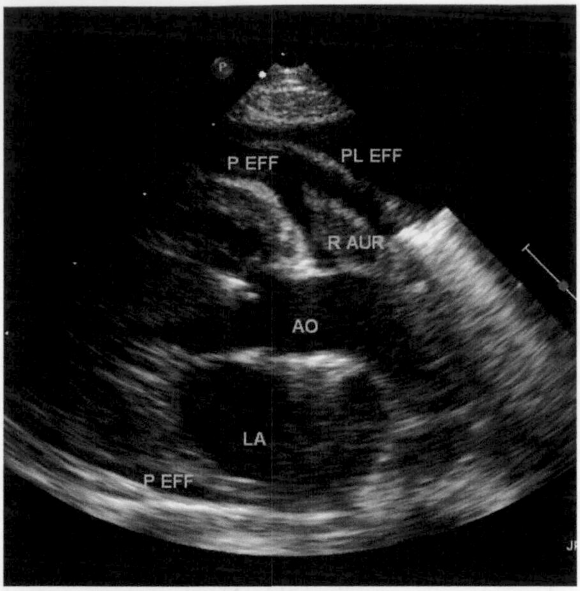

Figure 12.4 Echocardiogram showing pleural and pericardial effusion in a female spayed domestic short-hair cat diagnosed with hypertrophic cardiomyopathy and congestive heart failure. AO, aorta; LA, left atrium; PL EFF, pleural effusion; P EFF, pericardial effusion; R AUR, right auricle.

due to hypertrophic cardiomyopathy causing elevated intracardiac pressures in the left atrium and pulmonary veins leading to transudative fluid accumulation in the pleura and pericardium (Figure 12.4) [3]. Pericardial effusion can also occur as an inflammatory response to feline infectious peritonitis.

Patient History

Frequently the veterinary technician is the first person to see an owner with their pet. The presenting complaint from the owner of a dog with pericardial effusion and with cardiac tamponade can include: exercise intolerance, lethargy, panting, decreased appetite, vomiting, swollen abdomen, or more seriously, sudden collapse with pale gum color. These patients may walk in the door with their tails wagging, or may be recumbent, depending on how long they have been in cardiac tamponade. The last complaint usually indicates acute bleed from a major organ. Physical examination, stabilization of the patient, and diagnostic testing should be started immediately. The history of a cat is usually quite different. When they don't feel well, they usually hide. Most owners will notice abdominal or labored breathing.

Clinical Presentation

There are physical examination findings the veterinary technician should be aware of that can indicate a patient has pericardial effusion and cardiac tamponade. If there is enough fluid to collapse the RA in diastole, there will be signs of venous congestion and right-sided heart failure and usually signs of low cardiac output. The following is a list of possible physical examination findings in a canine or feline [3–5].

Venous Congestion

1) Ascites (fluid in the abdominal cavity, also called peritoneal effusion).
2) Jugular venous distention (may need to shave neck to observe).
3) Subcutaneous or pitting edema in fore- and hindlimbs.
4) Muffled or absent heart sounds (can indicate pericardial or pleural effusion).
5) Positive hepato-jugular reflux test (see Chapter 3).

Forward Failure

1) Poor quality pulses or *pulses paradoxus*: pulse quality weakens during respiratory inspiration due to impaired left ventricular filling caused by increased pericardial pressures. The RV fills more during inspiration and bows into the left ventricle.
2) Sinus tachycardia: the body's response via the sympathetic nervous system to low cardiac output.
3) Tachypnea: from impaired blood flow to and from the lungs.
4) Pale or muddy mucous membrane color: indicates low output.
5) Increased capillary refill time (>2 s).

A veterinarian or veterinary technician can suspect pericardial effusion and by physical examination findings be certain a patient is in cardiac tamponade, but diagnostic imaging should be used for confirmation.

Diagnostics

The Electrocardiogram

The presence of tachycardia warrants diagnostics. One cost-effective diagnostic test that can easily be performed by a veterinary technician and could indicate a patient has pericardial effusion is the electrocardiogram (ECG). It should determine if the tachycardia auscultated is of sinus origin or of ventricular origin, indicating a different problem. Electrocardiography is not a sensitive or specific test for pericardial effusion, but may show *"electrical alternans"* which is associated with pericardial effusion. Electrical alternans is an ECG finding in which every other QRS complex is of lower amplitude than the others, due to the heart swinging in a fluid-filled pericardial sac (Figure 12.5) [3–5]. Low amplitude QRS complexes for the size of a patient can indicate fluid in the pericardium or the pleural cavity, because fluid "dampens" or inhibits the hearts electrical impulses from reaching the electrodes on the patient's skin. However, this can also be a normal finding in a large-chested or obese patient in which the electrical impulse has more tissue to travel through. Sinus tachycardia is commonly noted and arrhythmias can be confirmed with the ECG. Many patients present with ventricular arrhythmias due to poor perfusion of their heart muscle. This occurs because cardiac tamponade causes a decrease in diastolic blood flow through coronary arteries which feed the heart muscle.

Radiography

Veterinary practices that do not have an ultrasound machine to image the heart may rely on radiographs to aid in the diagnosis of pericardial effusion. A dorsoventral

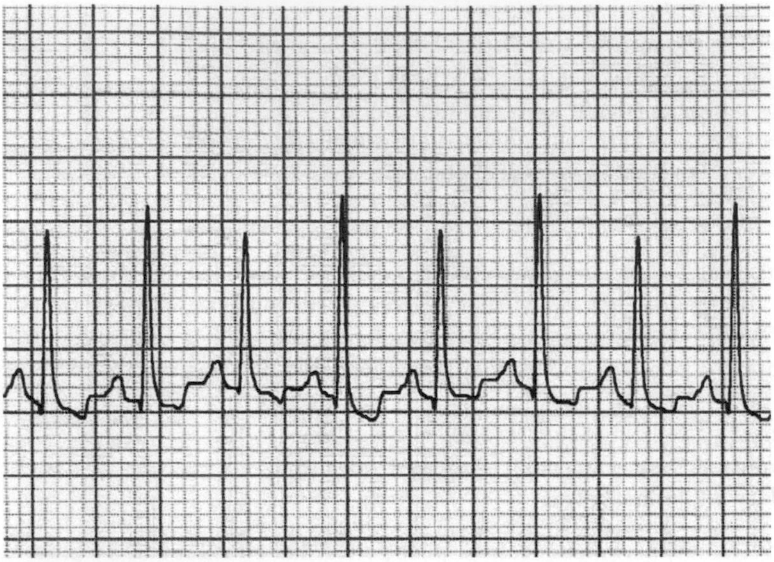

Figure 12.5 Electrocardiogram (50 mm/sec; 10 mm/mv) showing electrical alternans in a Labrador retriever. The patient was subsequently diagnosed with pericardial effusion, a right atrial mass and cardiac tamponade. Note the alternating height of the "R" wave and the tachycardia as indicated by the "P" on "T" phenomenon.

or ventrodorsal and right or left lateral view of the thorax showing a large globoid cardiac silhouette, along with any of the above physical examination findings, can be conclusive (Figure 12.6). Other heart diseases that could display this shape would be dilated cardiomyopathy in which all chambers become dilated and rounded, or chronic mitral valve endocardiosis in the dog causing volume over-loaded heart chambers and an enlarged heart.

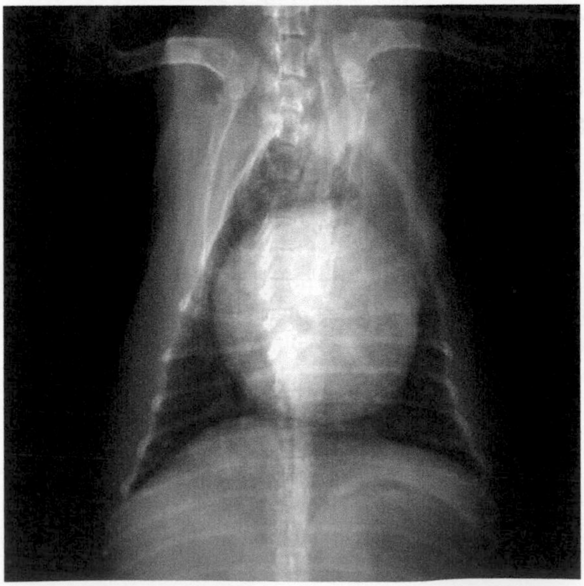

Figure 12.6 Ventral dorsal chest radiographs showing a large globoid heart in a border collie with pericardial effusion. This type of generalized cardiomegaly may also be seen with dilated cardiomyopathy.

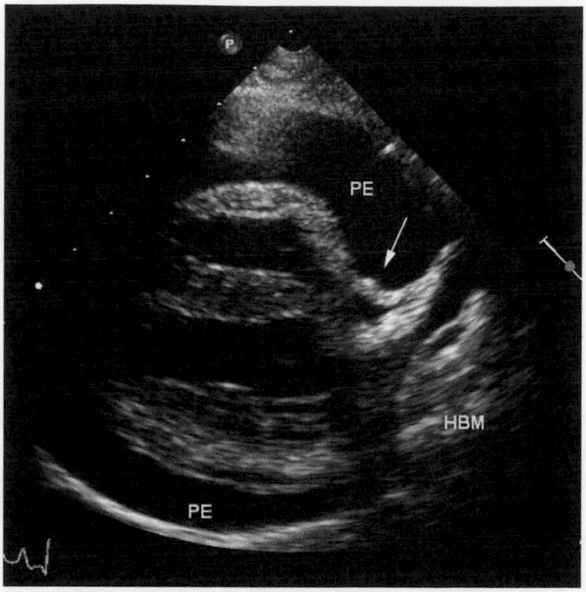

Figure 12.7 Echocardiogram from a dog showing pericardial effusion, cardiac tamponade (collapsed right atrial wall – arrow) and a heart-based mass. HBM, heart-based mass; PE, pericardial effusion.

Echocardiography

Cardiac ultrasound or echocardiography is the preferred diagnostic imaging technique for confirmation of pericardial effusion and cardiac tamponade (Figure 12.7). Echocardiography is an easy and noninvasive procedure used to view the presence and amount of effusion, cardiac tamponade, and any macroscopic masses within the heart or pericardium. It is very important for a sonographer to be able to differentiate between pericardial fluid and pleural fluid, which can also surround the heart, but would never cause cardiac tamponade. If the gain is turned down on the echocardiograph, the pericardium remains the brightest white linear structure of the heart. Fluid remains dark and can be viewed as occurring on the outside (pleural effusion) or the inside (pericardial effusion) of the white line. If a patient is in cardiac tamponade, but stable, it is preferable to perform a full study of all right parasternal and left apical and cranial views before initiating treatment. Fluid around the heart enhances ultrasound images of tissue and makes locating potential masses easier, especially in the RA/auricle. Many veterinarians will also use ultrasound for guidance in selecting a site to drain the fluid and for confirmation they are draining the fluid from the pericardial sac.

Therapy

Veterinarians and their staff may want to start treatment with a diuretic such as furosemide, thinking it will lessen the amount of fluid in the pericardial sac. *Diuretics are contraindicated* because they cause a decrease in overall blood volume and result in even less ventricular filling and cardiac output [4]. This is one example of a heart-failure condition where intravenous fluids can be helpful to the patient by increasing the volume of fluid entering the right heart.

The quickest way to remove effusion is to perform a pericardiocentesis procedure or pericardial tap. The pericardium is entered through the right thorax and fluid is removed

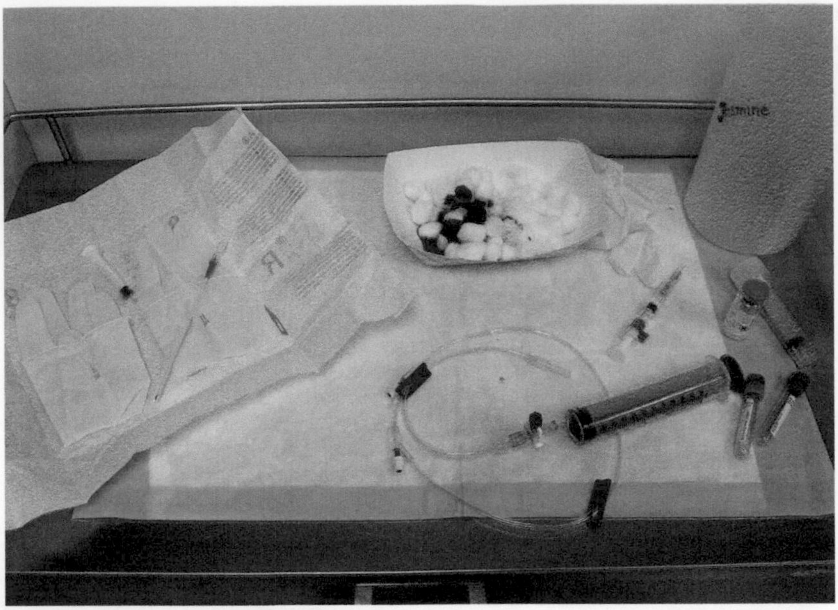

Figure 12.8 Supplies for pericardiocentesis procedure on top of cart showing extension set, large-bore catheter, stopcock and syringe set up for aspirating effusion. Also close by are tubes used for sample collection to submit for histopathological analysis and a syringe of lidocaine to provide local analgesia.

by inserting an over-the-needle catheter into the pericardial sac and gently aspirating. Figure 12.8 shows a typical set-up for pericardiocentesis. A detailed description of the pericardiocentesis procedure is found in Chapter 16.

Constrictive Pericarditis

Infrequently, the pericardial sac itself will become abnormally thick, stiff, and fibrotic and the visceral layer will adhere to the epicardium constricting the myocardium. This is referred to as constrictive pericarditis which inhibits filling of the RA and ventricle during mid-to-late diastole when receiving venous return from the body. The heart chambers begin to relax in early diastole and then the pericardial sac "constricts" late filling. This leads to venous congestion, right-sided heart failure, and can cause cardiac tamponade.

Etiology

The cause of constrictive pericarditis can be idiopathic or the result of an inflammatory response to foreign bodies such as gunshot pellets, infectious agents such as the tick-borne *Bartonella henselae* bacteria, or a systemic fungal infection from an organism such as *Coccidioides immitis*, which lives in the soil of the southwestern USA [7] Repeated pericardiocentesis [4] procedures can also result in an inflamed constricted pericardium.

Clinical Presentation

Many patients present as middle-aged large-breed dogs with a history from the owner of exercise intolerance and a swollen abdomen. This disease is quite rare in felines.

Physical Examination Findings

The most common physical examination finding is ascites. Diagnostics should begin with a complete cardiovascular examination and blood work. If these tests come back normal, the abdomen should be explored with ultrasound, and possibly a computed tomography scan to rule out any masses that could be interfering with venous return to the heart. An intravenous jugular catheter can be placed and a central venous pressure measurement of >15 cm H_2O (normal 0–5 cm H_2O) can confirm elevated right atrial pressures.

Radiographs

Chest radiographs may not be particularly helpful in the diagnosis, because the heart silhouette is generally not enlarged. The descending vena cava may appear enlarged and the liver may be distended due to venous congestion.

Echocardiography

Echocardiography of the heart may show some mild thickening of the pericardium and scant pericardial effusion to the trained eye of a veterinary cardiologist. Cardiac tamponade may or may not be present. The heart chambers and function usually appear normal.

Cardiac Catheterization

If the tests above do not diagnose the cause of ascites, the only way to confirm elevated mid-to-late diastolic pressures in the RA and ventricle caused by pericardial constriction is to perform a right-heart cardiac catheterization [3–5] (see Chapter 8). The dog is placed under general anesthesia, in left lateral recumbency and the area over the right jugular vein is shaved and surgically prepared. A veterinary cardiologist, using the modified Seldinger technique, places a thin-walled entry needle percutaneously into the vein, feeds a wire through it, removes the needle and then feeds an introducing catheter over the wire. They then remove the wire and stabilize the introducer with sutures. An open-ended polyurethane catheter is placed through the introducer and using fluoroscopy guidance, it is fed into the right heart and attached to a pressure transducer via flushed arterial lines. The transducer is calibrated and is then set to "zero" by opening it to room air and keeping it at the level of the patient's heart. Once the transducer is open to the catheter in the right heart, a tracing of intracardiac pressures is generated on a computer screen along with an ECG to time systole and diastole. Elevated diastolic pressures are recorded in both the RA (Figure 12.9) and the RV displaying an early diastolic dip and then an elevated end diastolic pressure of >10 mmHg (Figure 12.10). A trained

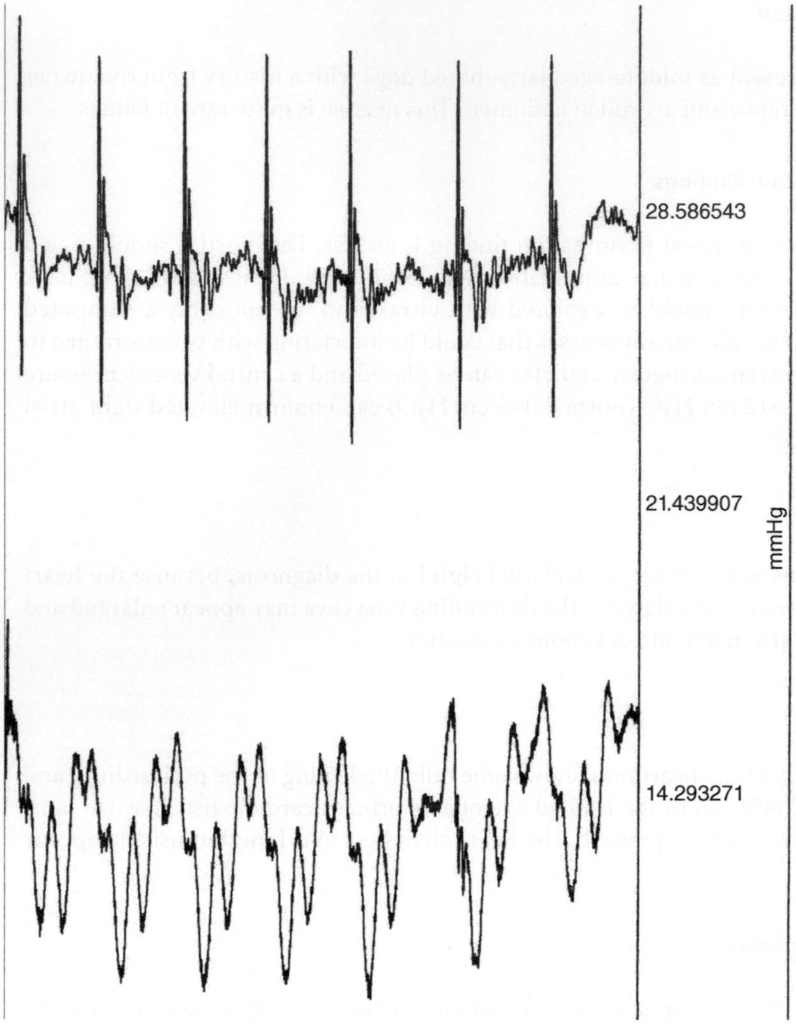

Figure 12.9 Elevated intracardiac right atrial pressures in a female spayed Labrador retriever diagnosed with constrictive pericarditis. The lower tracing shows elevated and spiked pressure waves indicating impaired relaxation and elevated pressures of 17.5/9.2 mmHg with a mean of 13.6 mmHg. Normal systolic and diastolic is 4/2 mmHg. The upper tracing is an electrocardiogram.

cardiology technician plays an important role in organizing and assisting with cardiac catheterization procedures. The following is a list of duties they will perform:

1) Clip and prepare the surgery site using sterile technique.
2) Assist the cardiologist with gloving and gowning for surgery.
3) Set up the surgery table and open catheterization supplies using sterile technique.
4) Set up and assist with operating the fluoroscopy machine.
5) Set up the pressure transducer and assist with obtaining intra cardiac pressure tracings.

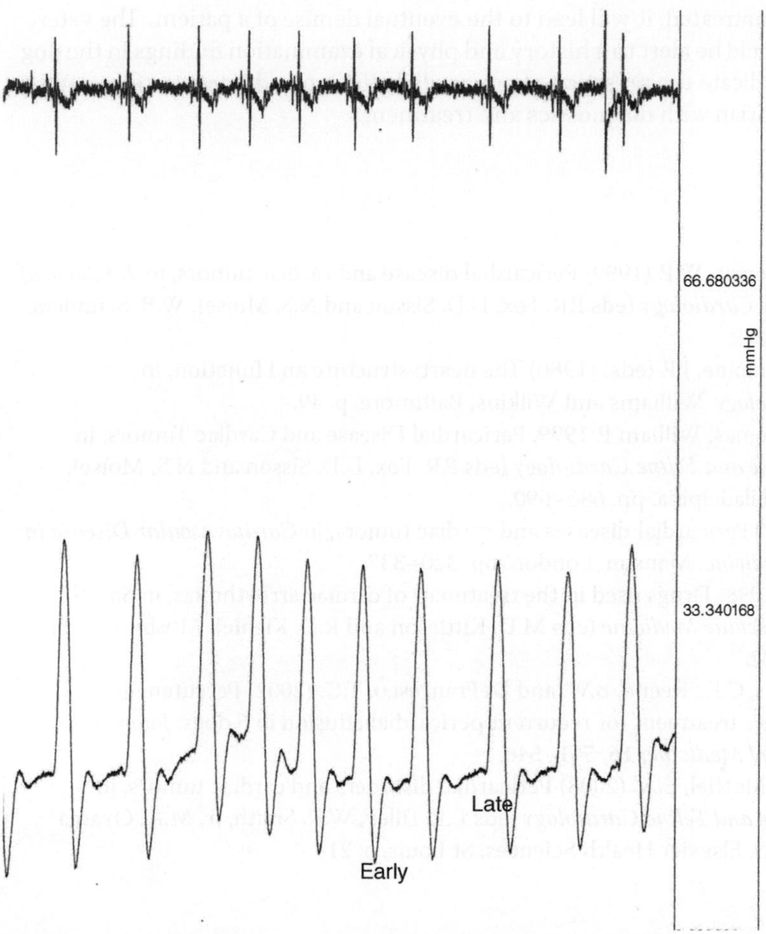

Figure 12.10 Demonstration of intracardiac right ventricular pressures (lower tracing) showing a high systolic pressure of 37 mmHg, an early diastolic dip to 10 mmHg and elevated late diastolic pressures of 17 mmHg in the same dog. The change from the early diastolic to late diastolic wave form demonstrates the so called "square root" sign indicative of constrictive pericarditis. Normal systolic and diastolic in the right ventricle is 20/4 mmHg. The upper tracing is an electrocardiogram.

Therapy

Once the diagnosis is confirmed, constrictive pericarditis can only be treated by performing open chest surgery to remove or "strip" part or all of the pericardium off the epicardium of the heart, also called a pericardectomy. Once the patient has recovered from surgery, they can return to their normal activities and live a normal lifespan.

Conclusion

The occurrence of pericardial effusion is relatively rare in the dog and cat, but as they age, the occurrence of neoplasia causing cardiac tamponade becomes more likely. If left unrecognized and untreated, it will lead to the eventual demise of a patient. The veterinary technician should be alert to a history and physical examination findings in the dog or cat that could indicate the presence of pericardial effusion and be prepared to assist quickly the veterinarian with diagnostics and treatment.

References

1 Sisson, D. and Thomas, W.P. (1999) Pericardial disease and cardiac tumors, in *Textbook of Canine and Feline Cardiology* (eds P.R. Fox, D.D. Sisson and N.S. Moïse). W.B. Saunders, Philadelphia. pp. 679.

2 Smith, J.J. and Kampine, J.P. (eds) (1980) The heart: structure and function, in *Circulatory Physiology*. Williams and Wilkins, Baltimore. p. 49.

3 Sisson, David, Thomas, William P. 1999. Pericardial Disease and Cardiac Tumors, in *Textbook of Canine and Feline Cardiology* (eds P.R. Fox, D.D. Sisson and N.S. Moïse). W.B. Saunders, Philadelphia. pp. 686–690.

4 Ware, W.A. (2007) Pericardial diseases and cardiac tumors, in *Cardiovascular Disease in Small Animal Medicine*. Manson. London. pp. 320–337.

5 Kittleson, M.D. (1998) Drugs used in the treatment of cardiac arrhythmias, in *Small Animal Cardiovascular Medicine* (eds M.D. Kittleson and R.D. Kienle). Mosby, Inc., St Louis. pp. 413–432.

6 Sidley, J.A., Atkins, C.E., Keene, B.W. and DeFrancesco, T.C. (2002) Percutaneous pericardiotomy as a treatment for recurrent pericardial effusion in 6 dogs. *Journal of Veterinary Internal Medicine*, **16**, 541–546.

7 Tobias, A.H. and McNiel, E.A. (2008) Pericardial disorders and cardiac tumors, in *Manual of Canine and Feline Cardiology* (eds L.P. Tilley, W.K. Smith, Jr, M.A. Oyama and M.M. Sleeper). Elsevier Health Sciences, St Louis. p. 210.

Section IV

Therapies and Interventions

13

Pathophysiology of Heart Failure

June A. Boon and H. Edward Durham, Jr.

Definition and Classification

Heart failure is present when the cardiac pump is unable to meet the metabolic and nutritional needs of the body when ventricular filling pressure (preload) is normal or enhanced [1]. The cause of the heart failure is usually related to structural and functional abnormalities within the heart itself but extra cardiac events may also precipitate heart failure. Cardiac causes of heart failure include myocardial failure secondary to cardiomyopathy or ischemic heart disease, and valvular problems leading to regurgitation or obstruction, all of which prevent adequate filling or emptying of the heart. Extra cardiac causes of heart failure include pressure overload secondary to pulmonary or systemic hypertension and high output states caused by metabolic diseases like hyperthyroidism and anemia. High output states result in heart failure because coronary perfusion cannot match the metabolic needs of the myocardium.

Congestive heart failure is the result of elevated pressure in the either the right or left atrial chamber. Increases in left atrial pressure result in congestion of the pulmonary venous system and pulmonary edema. Elevated right atrial pressure results in systemic edema and congestion with eventual effusion of fluid into the abdominal cavity resulting in ascites.

Myocardial failure is the inability of the cardiac muscle to maintain normal cardiac output. Contractility is impaired. Congestive heart failure may not yet be present but animals in congestive heart failure usually have some component of myocardial failure.

Central Venous Pool and Cardiac Output

Venous return from the body into the thoracic veins and right atrium determines the volume in the central venous pool. The central venous pool is the volume contained in the right atrium and great veins within the thorax and central venous pressure (CVP) reflects the pressure within this pool. Under normal conditions venous return equals cardiac output otherwise blood would accumulate in the venous pool or peripheral veins. There are always minor fluctuations in the volume of this pool as cardiac output varies secondary to metabolic needs. This causes changes in CVP.

Peripheral venous pressure must always be higher than CVP otherwise blood would not return to the heart. Peripheral venous pressure is typically around 7 mmHg. Central

Cardiology for Veterinary Technicians and Nurses, First Edition. Edited by H. Edward Durham, Jr.

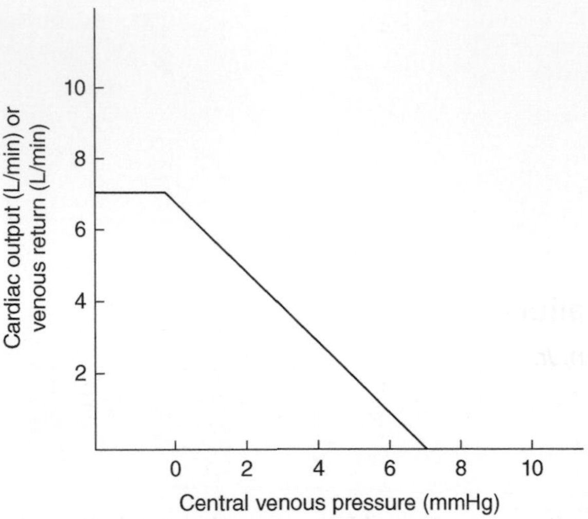

Figure 13.1 The relationship between central venous pressure and cardiac output. As central venous pressure increases, venous return diminishes which in turn diminishes cardiac output. At a low central venous pressure of close to zero, venous return and cardiac output are optimized.

venous pressure approaches 0 mmHg [2]. Flow (Q) from the peripheral venous pool to the central venous pool is determined by the following equation where P = the pressure change between the peripheral pool and the central pool and R equals resistance.

$$Q = \Delta P/R \qquad (13.1)$$

Figure 13.1 shows this relationship graphically. As CVP increases (secondary to decreased cardiac output perhaps), venous return decreases. Notice that at very low CVP, venous return is at its peak and cardiac output is at its peak. Normal CVP should be close to zero for optimal venous return to the heart. Increasing or decreasing peripheral venous pressure relative to the central venous pool also increases or decreases venous return to the heart. Decreases in CVP may be the result of dehydration secondary to vomiting, diarrhea, or blood loss. Increases in peripheral venous pressure may result from fluid retention by the kidneys in response to poor cardiac output. Peripheral vascular tone and pressure is also increased during periods of increased sympathetic stimulus and by external skeletal muscular contraction during exercise.

The right side of the heart and the left side of the heart work together. What is pumped out of the right side of the heart must travel through the lungs and into the left side of the heart in one coordinated effort [3, pp. 355–401]. Flow through each portion of this circuit must be equal. The output from each side of the heart is regulated by the mechanisms that maintain stroke volume and blood pressure. An imbalance between the two sides results in elevated filling pressure of either the right or left ventricle.

The volume and function of the cardiovascular system has been described as a capacitance model. The system is a closed loop which includes the heart, an arterial compartment, a resistance compartment, and a venous compartment. The cross-sectional area of the arterial system is small and holds little volume, while the venous compartment has a large capacity, usually about 30 times that of the arterial component. Total blood volume remains constant and any changes in one compartment must be adjusted for in the other. In other words, the only thing that can change is the allotment of volume between the two compartments.

Pressure between the two compartments varies inversely. Increased arterial pressure and increased arterial volume results in decreased venous volume and pressure. Because venous capacitance is so large, even large changes in arterial pressure and volume result in only small changes in venous volume and pressure. Arterial pressure must also be sufficient to pump blood through the resistance system. Arterial pressure that is too low results in blood collecting in the arterial system until compensatory mechanisms have been put in place, which increase pressure and maintain forward flow.

Influence of Central Venous Presssure on Cardiac Output

Cardiac output is influenced by venous pressure (filling pressure or preload). They are inversely related in that decreased cardiac output corresponds to increased CVP. Decreasing venous pressure must result in increased arterial pressure based upon the closed capacitance system and increased arterial pressure results in increased cardiac output. Increasing venous pressure, however, results in and is the result of low cardiac output and decreased arterial pressure. This of course represents a cycle of adjustments with pressure and output fluctuating between the two compartments. Figure 13.2 shows how cardiac output and venous pressure are related and their relationship at equilibrium (point A). The graph shows that for any increase in cardiac output there is decreased CVP (point B), and any decrease in cardiac output causes CVP to increase (C).

Increased contractility at any left ventricular filling pressure increases cardiac output. Figure 13.3(a) shows how the function curve is shifted to the left. Notice that without any change in filling pressure, cardiac output increases (point B) when sympathetic stimulation is increased (increased contractility). Decreased contractility (decreased sympathetic innervation) decreases cardiac output (point C) when filling pressure is kept constant. This graph also shows how changes in preload affect filling pressure and cardiac output, per the Frank–Starling law of the heart. Without any change in contractility, decreased preload (point E), causes cardiac output to decrease while increased preload increases cardiac output (point D).

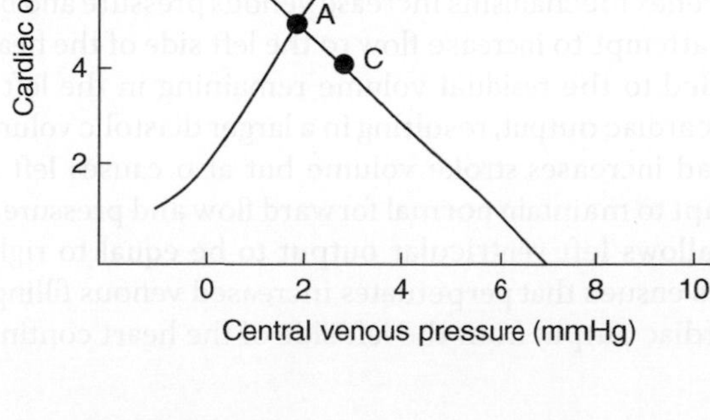

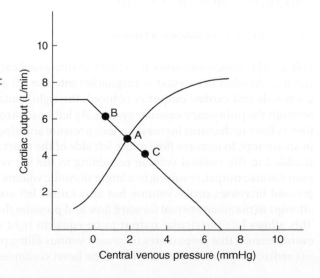

Figure 13.2 Interaction of cardiac output and venous return through central venous pressure (CVP). The intersection of the venous return curve and the CVP curve is shown at optimal conditions for normal cardiac output (point A). As cardiac output increases (B), CVP decreases. As cardiac output decreases (C), CVP increases.

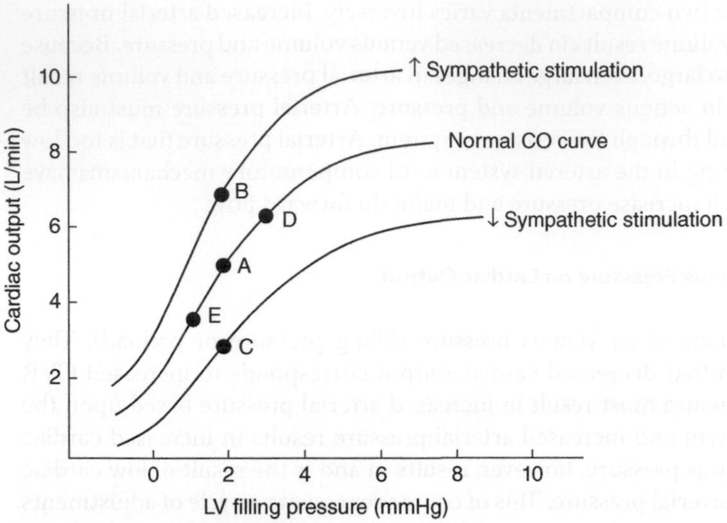

Figure 13.3 Relationship between left ventricular filling pressure, contractility, and cardiac output. At a constant left ventricular (LV) filling pressure, if contractility is increased, cardiac output increases (B) and when contractility is decreased (C), cardiac output decreases. When contractility is held constant, increased preload increases cardiac output (D) and decreased preload decreases cardiac output (E). The x axis can also be central venous pressure or left atrial pressure and the same relationships exist.

We cannot calculate a cardiac output and venous return curves in patients, but we can measure CVP in order to understand a patient's circulatory status. For instance, if CVP is high there must be a decrease in cardiac function or an increase in venous return or both. A patient in congestive heart failure with a high CVP usually has myocardial failure resulting in decreased cardiac output and fluid retention, which shifts the venous return curve to the right (point C in Figure 13.2).

Congestion in Heart Failure

Left Heart Failure – Pulmonary Edema

Left atrial pressure increases secondary to decreased cardiac output from the left ventricular chamber or valvular regurgitation into the left atrial chamber. As the left ventricle fails and cardiac output is reduced, the right ventricle continues to pump blood through the pulmonary vascular system. As left heart stroke volume decreases even further, reflex mechanisms increase venous pressure and blood returns to the right ventricle in an attempt to increase flow to the left side of the heart. The increased venous volume is added to the residual volume remaining in the left ventricular chamber because of poor cardiac output, resulting in a larger diastolic volume (increased preload). Increased preload increases stroke volume but also causes left atrial pressure to increase in an attempt to maintain normal forward flow and pressure through the left side of the heart. This allows left ventricular output to be equal to right ventricular output. A cycle of events ensues that perpetuates increased venous filling pressure and left atrial pressure as cardiac output from the left side of the heart continues to drop.

Peak left atrial pressure typically remains below 10 mmHg [4]. Increases in this pressure causes a back-up of fluid and of course pressure in the pulmonary veins and capillaries. This is called congestion. This may lead to increased respiratory effort because the lungs are heavy and there will be ventilation perfusion abnormalities. Further increases in left atrial pressure will lead to fluid seeping from the pulmonary veins into the interstitial space. If lymphatic drainage cannot keep up, pulmonary edema occurs, which is an accumulation of fluid in the interstitial space and eventually alveoli. This edema leads to partial obstruction of the small airways and the load that the right heart must pump against increases. The resultant poor ventilation leads to myocardial hypoxemia with resultant depression of myocardial function.

Right Heart Failure – Ascites

Right ventricular chambers can accommodate and adapt to large changes in volume without large increases in filling pressure because of its relatively thin-walled structure and compliance. But the thin right ventricle does not handle increases in afterload very well. When the right ventricle is subjected to pressure overload secondary to elevated pulmonary venous pressure (left heart failure), primary pulmonary vascular disease, valvular regurgitation, valvular stenosis or myocardial failure, right atrial pressure increases. Right heart failure resulting from primary pulmonary disease is called cor pumonale. Systemic congestion occurs as a result with eventual peripheral edema. Continued increases in peripheral vascular pressure allow fluid to seep into the abdominal cavity as ascites.

Chronic Congestive Heart Failure

Compensated heart failure is a result of changes in sympathetic activity and peripheral venous and arterial pressure in an effort to maintain normal venous return to the heart and normal cardiac output and organ perfusion. These mechanisms are illustrated in Figure 13.4, which shows the normal cardiac output curve as it relates to CVP and venous return to the heart (point A). As cardiac output decreases from point A to point B there is a compensatory response to increase in sympathetic activity which increases cardiac output to near normal levels (point C) via vasoconstriction. Notice that venous return increases and CVP remains elevated. Sympathetic activity also causes fluid retention via the renin–angiotensin–aldosterone system (RAAS) (as will be detailed below). This eventually allows sympathetic tone to return to normal while increasing CVP and maintaining cardiac output (C > D > E). This compensatory mechanism is important in that normal sympathetic tone is essential in order to maintain normal flow through organs. It also allows myocardial oxygen demand to return to normal and heart rate remains lower as the RAAS system maintains cardiac output.

This compensated state does not maintain cardiac output forever and patients are said to be decompensated when these mechanisms result in congestive heart failure. The elevated CVP (D and E) and fluid retention result in dilation of the heart which, while it increases cardiac output (Frank–Starling law), also increases congestion. The clinical signs of congestive heart failure are the result of these efforts to compensate. Dyspnea and peripheral edema result from congestion and fluid accumulation in the lungs and venous system. Low exercise tolerance and lethargy are the result of poor

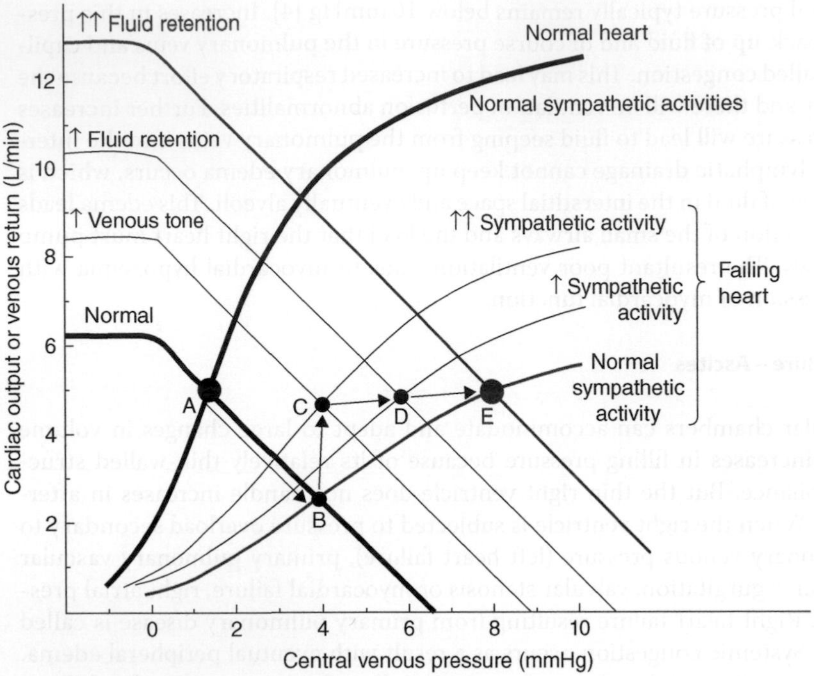

Figure 13.4 Cardiovascular alterations with compensated chronic heart failure. This graph shows how cardiac output and venous pressure are related and their relationship at equilibrium. For any increase in central venous pressure, cardiac output declines, and as cardiac output increases central venous pressure decreases. The intersection of any of the two lines representing central venous pressure and venous return or cardiac output shows equilibrium where there is an optimal relationship between cardiac output and central venous filling pressure. Point A represents this relationship in the normal heart. When cardiac output declines (B) sympathetic activity causes venous constriction increasing venous pressure which increases the venous return curve back to almost normal levels (C). Activation of the renin–angiotensin–aldosterone system promotes fluid retention which increases venous return allowing sympathetic activity to return to normal while maintaining adequate cardiac output (D and E). Source: Mohrman and Heller (2003) [2]. Reproduced with permission of Lange Medical Books.

cardiac output. Treatment of congestive heart failure and low output failure is aimed at balancing cardiac output and fluid retention.

Myocardial Dysfunction

Systolic Dysfunction

Systolic dysfunction or failure results in poor cardiac output secondary to poor contractility or pressure overload. Poor contractility is the result of abnormal myocyte function or destruction. Muscle contraction during systole involves production of energy, utilization of energy and excitation coupling which involves the use and release of calcium during actual fiber shortening. Energy production is generally not impaired in heart failure. However, the conversion of adenosine triphosphate (ATP) to adenosine diphosphate

(ADP) during actin and myosin interaction is reduced in myocardial failure, a direct result of reduced ATPase activity [3, pp. 237–244]. Regardless of other changes in the failing cardiac muscle, there is a definite decrease in cross-bridge formation and there is a direct correlation between contractility and the rate of energy conversion. Changes in myofilament proteins affect the rate of ATPase formation and these proteins play an important role in muscle dysfunction. There is also evidence that the release of Ca^{++} into the sarcoplasmic reticulum is either deficient in heart failure or there is an inadequate ratio of sarcoplasmic reticulum to muscle mass in hypertrophied hearts. Currently there are also studies looking at mitochondrial alterations that may exist in myocardial failure.

Diastolic Dysfunction

Appropriate diastolic function means that the ventricular chamber can fill while maintaining normal filling pressure. If the ventricular muscle does not relax appropriately or does not maintain its elasticity (compliance) then chamber pressure increases above normal as it fills. Diastolic failure of the myocardium involves alterations in relaxation of the myocytes and compliance of the ventricular chambers. Myocardial remodeling that occurs in the presence of cardiac disease resulting from volume or pressure overload causes alterations in the extracellular matrix. The extracellular matrix provides the framework for proper alignment of myofibers during contraction. Remodeling changes the myocardial cells altering systolic function but it also increases fibroblast proliferation resulting in increased interstitial collagen. There is normally a continuous turnover of collagen but an imbalance in this turnover enhances collagen deposition resulting in myocardial fibrosis. The amount of collagen determines myocardial stiffness and increased stiffness results in elevated pressure during left ventricular filling (diastolic dysfunction).

Response to Heart Failure

Hypertrophic Response

Cardiac hypertrophy is a remodeling process that helps the heart maintain its ability to provide adequate flow to the body. The type of remodeling is dependent upon whether the heart is subjected to volume or pressure overload.

Eccentric Hypertrophy

When there are structural or functional abnormalities in the heart leading to decreased forward stroke volume, the body responds with a set of compensatory mechanisms, which promote fluid retention in an attempt to increase venous filling pressure and maintain a normal cardiac output. Fluid retention increases left ventricular or right ventricular chamber size, putting more stretch on the myofibers and increasing preload. Increased preload adds to the heart's workload (area under the pressure volume loop, see Figure 2.5) and increases myocardial oxygen demand. Increased oxygen demand promotes the conversion of ATP in the muscle cells to cyclic adenosine monophosphate (cAMP), which activates protein kinase, which in turn promotes protein synthesis, and muscle hypertrophy (increased number of sarcomeres). This hypertrophic process involves adding sarcomeres in series resulting in elongated myocytes. The result is a dilated ventricular chamber with increased wall thickness and normal wall stress. A heart with volume overload and normal to increased wall thickness is said to be eccentrically hypertrophied. The hypertrophy is the compensatory mechanism that normalizes wall stress (see Figure 2.8). The hypertrophy is just enough to normalize wall stress and the ratio of chamber size to wall thickness remains normal. Chambers that do not hypertrophy adequately to compensate for the increased preload have high wall stress and increased afterload in addition to the increased preload.

Based upon the Frank–Starling law of the heart, increased preload should result in an increase in muscle shortening since there is a greater number of exposed actin and myosin sites for cross-bridge formation. If the muscle does not shorten to the degree expected for the amount of stretch, the muscle is failing. As ventricular volume increases myocardial tension increases. This increase in stiffness (decreased compliance) of the muscle is also thought to contribute to congestive heart failure. Normal ventricular compliance is the ability of the ventricle to fill at normal filling pressure and reduced ventricular compliance (diastolic dysfunction) contributes as much to congestion as systolic myocardial failure.

Concentric Hypertrophy

An increase in afterload (i.e. blood pressure or aortic stenosis) increases myocardial tension. Increased tension starts the process that results in development of concentric myocardial hypertrophy. Increased wall thickness normalizes wall stress and allows the left ventricle to eject a normal amount of blood volume against this high afterload (see Figure 2.8). Concentric hypertrophy involves adding sarcomeres in parallel which thickens the myocyte and therefore is characterized by a normal to small ventricular chamber with increased wall thickness. Hypertrophy in response to pressure overload helps maintain near normal contractility. The increased number of sarcomeres help the heart to contract against the increased pressure. This pressure may be in the form of a stenosis or in the form of hypertension. The tension is spread out over a larger muscle mass and muscle function is preserved.

One of the determinants of myocardial oxygen demand, however, is afterload (contractility and heart rate are the two others). As muscle mass increases, the ability of oxygen to diffuse through its thickness decreases, the number of mitochondria decreases, there is ischemia, myocyte demise and resulting fibrosis. There are limits, in that coronary perfusion is impaired while oxygen demand is increased. Additionally, compliance may also be reduced in this situation which will eventually contribute to the development of congestive heart failure.

Neurohumoral Response

Neurohumoral responses to decreases in cardiac output are compensatory mechanisms by the body in an effort to maintain normal blood pressure, cardiac output, and organ perfusion. These responses include activation of the RAAS and increased adrenergic activity. Unfortunately, these compensatory mechanisms are self-defeating and ultimately lead to the development of chronic congestive heart failure.

Renin–Angiotensin–Aldosterone System Activation

A small decrease in blood pressure associated with decreased cardiac output decreases afferent stimulation to the medulla [3, pp. 512–515; 5]. The response is to increase heart rate via decreased vagal tone and to vasoconstrict the arterial system via stimulation of the α-adrenergic receptors. Decreased cardiac output also reduces renal blood flow. A fall in Na^+ to the juxtaglomerular apparatus causes a release of renin, which converts angiotensinogen to angiotensin I (see Figure 2.11). Angiotensin I is in itself innocuous but it is converted rapidly to angiotensin II.

Angiotensin II stimulates vasoconstriction of vascular smooth muscle (arteries, veins, and capillaries). This increases blood pressure and decreases venous capacitance. Angiotensin II also causes the pituitary gland to produce vasopressin. Vasopressin (antidiuretic hormone) results in increased fluid retention in an effort to maintain cardiac output. Increased fluid retention increases blood pressure further and helps promote cardiac output.

Aldosterone is released from the adrenal medulla, which promotes sodium retention in the distal tubules of the kidney, resulting in fluid retention and decreased urine production. This increases blood volume, increases blood pressure and increases cardiac output. Aldosterone also promotes renal excretion of potassium causing the hypokalemia seen in many patients in congestive heart failure.

Norepinephrine levels increase in this series of events as preganglionic sympathetic ganglia decrease its uptake. Increased norepinephrine results in vasoconstriction of vascular smooth muscle and increases heart rate. Increased heart rate increases cardiac output but it also increases myocardial oxygen demand. Free radicals are released by macrophages and neutrophils during this process leading to cell death (apoptosis).

Neural Response

Decreased cardiac output results in decreased receptor activity in the baroreceptors and decreased signals to the medulla resulting in increased sympathetic stimulation to the heart and peripheral nervous system. Parasympathetic stimulation is decreased. The increased levels of circulating norepinephrine increase the force and velocity of myocardial fiber shortening. Increased catecholamine stimulation also increases heart rate in an effort to increase cardiac output. Additionally, catecholamines also cause vasoconstriction mediated by the α_1-adrenergic receptors in vascular smooth muscle. These mechanisms help maintain blood pressure, cardiac output and perfusion of organs. These compensatory mechanisms in chronic heart failure are self-defeating and over the long term have deleterious results as described above.

Heart Rate

Remembering that cardiac output equals heart rate times stoke volume, when stroke volume declines there must be an adjustment in heart rate in an effort to maintain forward flow. Under normal conditions, changes in heart rate do not affect cardiac output by great degrees. This is because of corresponding changes in venous pressure. As heart rate increases or decreases, venous pressure is altered which in return affects ventricular filling and stroke volume. In heart failure, increased sympathetic stimulation increases heart rate, which decreases the length of the action potential, decreasing the systolic time period and increasing the length of diastole. Improved filling during diastole helps maintain cardiac output. Paradoxically, however, at very high heart rates filling time is again reduced and cardiac output declines.

Nitric Oxide in Heart Failure

Nitric oxide is a potent vasodilator and is released from the endothelium in response to increased stress on the vessel wall. In low output situations nitric oxide levels decrease allowing the vessel to vasoconstrict. This helps maintain blood pressure in the face of low output. Decreased nitric oxide levels in response to low blood pressure also allow endothelin levels to increase. Endothelin is a potent vasoconstrictor. However, nitric oxide may also have deleterious effects. Its presence promotes the formation of a free radical, peroxynitrite, which at low concentration is cardioprotective but at higher levels cause apoptosis (cell death).

Markers of Heart Failure

Natriuretic Peptides

Atrial natriuretic peptide (ANP) is produced in the atria and although brain natriuretic peptide (BNP) was first found in the brain, it is also present in ventricular muscle and to a lesser extent atrial muscle. Atrial muscle normally contains higher levels of ANP than BNP. Very early in the development of congestive heart failure, plasma levels of these peptides elevate, secondary to stretch of the atrial muscle and increased atrial pressure, which stimulates genetic expression for the synthesis and secretion of natriuretic peptides. The levels of BNP to ANP reverse in the presence of atrial stretch and heart failure. Normally, natriuretic peptides counteract the actions of the RAAS causing diuresis by renal afferent arteriolar dilation and efferent vasoconstriction. They also inhibit the sympathetic nervous system. Increasing pressure or volume overloads on the ventricular muscle leads to increased plasma levels of BNP and its precursor amino terminal pro-BNP (NT-pro-BNP). Advancing heart failure with decreased renal perfusion, increased activity of the RAAS system, and depressed receptor activity diminish the diuretic effects of the natriuretic peptides. Advancing heart failure correlates well with increased levels of natriuretic peptides.

Natriuretic peptides are secreted early in the course of heart failure and are used as diagnostic and prognostic aids. Levels of BNP and pro-BNP are now routinely used to evaluate for the presence of heart failure and are often used to differentiate patients with dyspnea secondary to cardiac causes from those with noncardiac causes of dyspnea.

Cardiac Troponin-I

Remember from Chapter 2 that there are three types of troponin, all of which are involved in the actin and myosin interaction during muscle contraction. Troponin C binds calcium and is involved in thin filament function. Once Ca^{++} binds to troponin C conformational changes assuage the inhibitory effect of troponin I, allowing the troponin tropomyosin binding site to be exposed. Troponin T binds troponin to tropomyosin. Troponin I therefore is an inhibitory protein which prevents contraction in the absence of troponin C and calcium. When Ca^{++} levels decline at the end of systole, troponin I is again placed in its inhibitory position initiating diastole. Alterations in the amount or duration of calcium availability within the sarcomere directly affect myocardial contraction. Impaired phosphorylation of troponin I is also thought to increase filament sensitivity to calcium, decreasing the amount of cross-bridge cycling and delaying relaxation. Currently there is investigation into the theory that proteolysis of cardiac troponin I is the initiating event that leads to cardiac hypertrophy.

Troponin I is not found in skeletal muscle and is considered to be very specific for myocardial cell damage. Any amount of myocardial cell damage results in the release of troponin I and troponin T into the circulatory system. Elevated troponin I levels can be seen in conjunction with myocardial strain secondary to volume or pressure overloads, myocarditis, pericarditis, cardiac trauma, infiltrative diseases, tachycardias, and congestive heart failure. Elevated levels, however, may also be seen in patients with renal disease, hypothyroidism, septic shock and sepsis, and pulmonary embolism [6, 7].

References

1 Hamlin, R.L. (1999) Pathophysiology of heart failure, in *Textbook of Canine and Feline Cardiology* (eds P.R. Fox, D.D. Sisson and N.S. Moïse). W.B. Saunders, Philadelphia. pp. 205–215.
2 Mohrman, D.E. and Heller, L. (2003) Central venous pressure: an indicator of circulatory status, in *Cardiovascular Physiology*. McGraw-Hill, New York. pp. 146–156.
3 Opie, L.H. and Perlroth, M.G. (2004) Ventricular function, in *Heart Physiology: From Cell to Circulation*. Lippincott Williams and Wilkins, Philadelphia. pp. 355–401.
4 Smith, J.J. and Kampine, J.P. (1980) The heart: structure and function, in *Circulatory Physiology – The Essentials*. Williams and Wilkins, Baltimore. pp. 48.
5 Guyton, A.C. and Hall, J.E. (2000) Cardiac failure, in *Textbook of Medical Physiology*, 10th Edition. Saunders Elsevier, Philadelphia. pp. 265–273.
6 Korff, S., Katus, H.A. and Giannitsis, E. (2006) Differential diagnosis of elevated troponins. *Heart*, **92**, 987–993.
7 Naik, H., Sabatine, M.S. and Lilly, L.S. (2007) Acute coronary syndromes, in *Pathophysiology of Heart Disease*. William and Wilkins, Baltimore. pp. 182–183.

14

Drugs for Cardiac Therapy

Kathryn J. Atkinson

Editor's Note: as it is not in the technician purview to prescribe medication, this chapter does not include a formulary of drug dosages and the reader is encouraged to consult a reputable formulary for this information as directed by a licensed veterinarian.

Introduction

Many medications are available to treat the various cardiac conditions diagnosed by the veterinary cardiologist. These are grouped into several large categories. The antiarrhythmics are used to control the heart rate or rhythm. Diuretics are used to help remove excess fluid from the body during congestive heart failure. Drugs that suppress the renin–angiotensin–aldosterone system can also be used to manage fluid content. Vasoactive drugs can be used to lower or increase vascular tone to control blood pressure. Positive inotropic medication will be employed to increase the strength of contractility. Antiplatelet drugs are used to reduce thrombus formation. Many of the medications used in veterinary cardiology have multiple effects across these categories. It is necessary to understand the actions and side effects of these commonly used medications. Often these medications are used together for synergistic effects or treating multiple conditions. Knowledge of their interactions is critical for the veterinary technician.

Several other physiological concepts are important for the selection of cardiac drugs in a given patient. The pharmacokinetics of each drug must be considered. Pharmacokinetics is the study of the mechanisms of absorption and distribution of an administered drug, the rate at which a drug action begins and the duration of the effect, the chemical metabolism or changes of the substance in the body and the effects and routes of excretion of the metabolites of the drug. The elimination of the drug from the patient's system might also direct the veterinary cardiologist's selection. The *first-pass* effect is a phenomenon that occurs when the drug is metabolized between the site of its administration and the site of sampling. The liver is usually the first major site that metabolizes many drugs when a drug is administered orally, but other potential sites include the gastrointestinal tract, the vascular endothelium, and the lungs. For some drugs, extensive first-pass metabolism limits their use as oral drugs and they must be given intravenously

Cardiology for Veterinary Technicians and Nurses, First Edition. Edited by H. Edward Durham, Jr.

or via other routes. Other drugs are converted from an inactive form to a pharmacologically active form by first-pass metabolism.

Bioavailability is used to describe the fraction of an administered dose of unchanged drug that reaches the systemic circulation. When a medication is administered through routes other than intravenously, its bioavailability varies. Various factors affect an orally administered drug's bioavailability, including: whether the drug is taken with food, as this affects absorption; disease conditions that affect the gastrointestinal function or hepatic metabolism; other drugs that may be affecting absorption and first-pass metabolism either through enzyme induction or inhibition; intestinal motility; and the physical properties of the drug.

The half-life of a drug is an important pharmacokinetic parameter and it is the time that it takes for the plasma concentration of a drug to reach half of the original concentration. After approximately five half-lives, a drug is 97% eliminated from the body. Steady state exists when the peak, average, and trough plasma concentrations are identical following each administration of a drug during chronic therapy. The half-life is useful to know as the time required to reach steady-state blood concentrations after multidosing is approximately four half-lives. Sometimes loading doses are given to try and achieve a therapeutic drug concentration more rapidly [1].

A review of the physiology of the autonomic nervous system helps in understanding the actions of cardiac drugs (see also Chapter 2). The autonomic nervous system is the body's control system that affects heart rate, digestions, respiratory rate, salivation, perspiration, micturition, sexual arousal, and pupil dilation. It is classically divided into the sympathetic (the "fight or flight"), and parasympathetic (the "rest and digest") nervous systems. The autonomic nervous system has a two neuron efferent pathway; the first or preganglionic neuron will synapse into a second or postganglionic neuron before innervating the effector organ. Acetylcholine is the neurotransmitter released by the preganglionic neurons for both the sympathetic and parasympathetic nervous system and is also released by the postganglionic neurons of the parasympathetic system. Nerves that release acetylcholine are termed cholinergic. Most of the postganglionic neurons of the sympathetic nervous system release norepinephrine and are termed adrenergic. A few postglanglionic neurons of the sympathetic nervous system that release acetylcholine are cholinergic. The adrenal medulla is an important organ in the sympathetic nervous system and secretes both norepinephrine and its metabolite, epinephrine, into the bloodstream [2]. Receptors on a target organ bind to the neurotransmitters to produce an effect on the cell, usually by altering cell membrane permeability or by activating or inactivating enzymes. Acetylcholine activates mainly two types of receptors: muscarinic and nicotinic. Muscarinic receptors are found on target cells stimulated by the postganglionic neurons of the parasympathetic nervous system as well as those stimulated by the postganglionic cholinergic neurons of the sympathetic nervous system. Nicotinic receptors are found at the synapses between preganglionic and postganglionic neurons of both the sympathetic and parasympathetic nervous system and also at many neuromuscular junctions in skeletal muscle. The adrenergic receptors are divided into alpha receptors and beta receptors, and can be further subdivided into alpha$_1$- (α_1), alpha$_2$- (α_2), beta$_1$- (β_1), and beta$_2$- (β_2) receptors. In most regions of the body, α_1- receptors predominate on vascular smooth muscle and stimulation results in vasoconstriction. Vascular smooth muscle also contains β_2-receptors which can produce vasodilation. α_2-receptors are found in the presynaptic membranes of adrenergic synapses and are widely distributed throughout the body, including the CNS. Stimulation can produce sedation/anesthesia and vasoconstriction. Cardiac myocytes can produce an increase in contractility and heart rate when the β_1-receptors are stimulated. Stimulation of β_2-receptors in the lungs produce bronchodilation [2, 3].

Drugs that mimic the actions of the sympathetic nervous system are termed *sympathomimetics* and can be either α- or β-adrenergic receptor agonists. There are also drugs that oppose the sympathetic nervous system that are *sympatholytics* or adrenergic antagonists. Drugs that mimic the action of the parasympathetic nervous system are termed *parasympathomimetics* and can also be termed cholinergic muscarinic or nicotinic agonists. Similarly, there are drugs that oppose the actions of the parasympathetic nervous system termed *parasympatholytics, anticholinergics*, or *vagolytics*.

Anti-Arrhythmics

An arrhythmia is an abnormal heart rhythm that deviates in the rate, regularity, conduction, or site of impulse formation from normal sinus rhythm. Determination of the significance of an arrhythmia depends on accurate electrocardiogram (ECG) acquisition and arrhythmia interpretation. Consideration of the history, clinical signs, physical examination, and complete data base including electrolyte assessment are necessary. Important questions to consider when assessing an ECG include classifying the rhythm as a bradyarrhythmia or tachyarrhythmia, and then deciding whether the rhythm originates from a supraventricular (above the atrioventricular node) or ventricular focus. Any underlying extracardiac factors precipitating an arrhythmia should be identified and resolved, such as thyrotoxicosis, hypoxia, disruption of acid-base status, anemia, trauma, electric shock, drugs, sepsis, high sympathetic tone or pheochromocytoma, uremia, pulmonary disease, splenic masses, gastric dilation/volvulus, CNS disease, or other endocrine disease. Primary cardiac causes should be identified using basic cardiology diagnostics. Cardiac disease or genetic or environmental factors can alter cell electrophysiologic properties, predisposing to arrhythmia development. Remodeling can change the structure or function of ion channels, lead to cardiac myocyte ischemia, fibrosis, or hypertrophy, or change the autonomic nervous system activity. This can lead to abnormal impulse generation (automaticity), abnormal impulse conduction (including re-entry), arrhythmias provoked by a triggering event, or complex arrhythmias involving abnormalities of both automaticity and conduction [4].

Not all arrhythmias need treatment with an anti-arrhythmic agent, and inappropriate therapy has the potential to increase mortality via a pro-arrhythmic effect. Isolated supraventricular and ventricular premature contractions, and accelerated idioventricular rhythms generally do not require specific anti-arrhythmic therapy, but these arrhythmias can serve as markers of underlying systemic or cardiac disease. In general, amongst veterinary cardiologists there is a consensus that therapy is warranted when the arrhythmia causes serious hemodynamic compromise, if it contributes to congestive heart failure, or if it is one that has been associated with sudden arrhythmic death [5, 6]. Few published trials exist documenting specific agents' efficacy in veterinary medicine, and clinical experience, or inference from human medical data, often dictates the anti-arrhythmic choice [7].

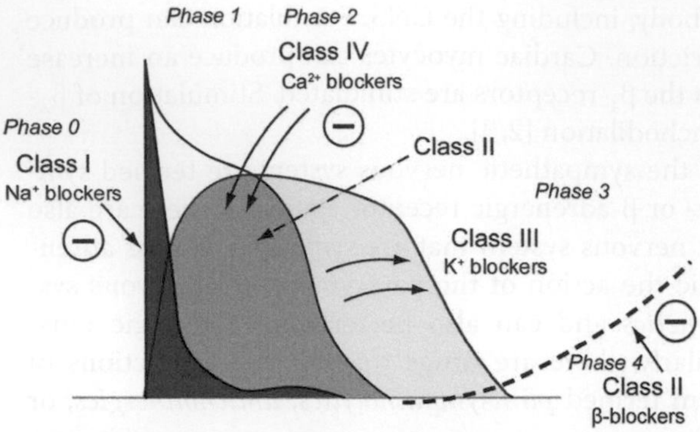

Figure 14.1 The effect of the four classes of antiarrhythmic drugs on the cardiac action potential. Class I agents, as rapid sodium (Na^+) channel blockers, decrease phase 0 or the rapid depolarization phase of the action potential. Class II agents are the β-adrenergic receptor blockers (β-blockers). Their action is complex, including inhibition of the spontaneous depolarization phase (phase 4), and indirect closure of calcium channels. The Class III agents, the potassium (K^+) channel blockers, block the outward potassium channels to prolong the action potential and increase refractoriness during phase III. The class IV agents, as calcium (Ca^+) receptor blockers, all inhibit the sarcolemmal calcium channel. Source: DiMarco, Gersh and Opie (2005) [8]. Reproduced with permission of Elsevier

The Vaughan Williams classification scheme is based on the predominant electrophysiological effects of a drug on the action potential, identifying drugs as blocking either sodium (Na^+), potassium (K^+), or calcium (Ca^{2+}) channels or β-adrenergic receptors [6, 8]. They are identified as Class I, Class II, Class III, and Class IV. This classification scheme has limitations, notably excluding some important drugs used clinically, some drugs having actions relating to more than one class, and not all drugs in the same class having identical effects. Figure 14.1 provides an overview of the effect of anti-arrhythmic drug classes on the cardiac action potential.

Class I Anti-Arrhythmics

Class I drugs are termed the "membrane stabilizers" with a common mechanism of action of blocking myocardial fast sodium channels [1]. By reducing the sodium influx during phase zero (see Figure 14.1) of cardiac cell depolarization, these drugs slow conduction velocity in cells that produce fast response action potentials which are produced by the action of fast sodium channels. This type of action potential is found in non-nodal cardiomyocytes like atrial and ventricular myocytes and Purkinje tissue [6,8]. Class I drugs can also interrupt re-entrant circuits (see Chapter 4). Most Class I agents are ineffective in the hypokalemic patient due to the effects of low potassium on the cell membrane. They are contraindicated in patients with complete atrioventricular block, and avoidance is recommended in sick sinus syndrome, bradycardias, and first or second degree atrioventricular block [9]. In these conditions, the heart is beating due to the automaticity of the ventricular myocytes and suppressing this could decompensate the patient. Class I agents are further subdivided into three subgroups: IA, IB, and IC based on their electrophysiological characteristics. Class IA and IC drugs are considered more pro-arrhythmic than Class IB.

Class IA agents include quinidine, procainamide, and disopyramide. They depress conduction of electrical impulses throughout the heart and slow repolarization by lengthening the refractory period. The refractory period is the time it takes a cell to reset after depolarization (see Chapter 2). These agents suppress the vagal parasympathetic nervous tone (*vagolytic effect*) and can increase the sinus rates.

Quinidine is more commonly used in large-animal rather than small-animal patients especially in the treatment of atrial fibrillation in horses. It treats supraventricular and ventricular arrhythmias. It may increase the risk of digoxin toxicity. Other potential serious side effects include an increased risk of ventricular fibrillation and the polymorphic form of ventricular fibrillation known as Torsades de pointes. Anticonvulsants, and other drugs that induce hepatic microsomal enzymes, can speed its metabolism; hypoalbuminemia and cimetidine can predispose to toxicity. Toxicity is suspected by identifying marked QT prolongation, conduction blocks, or QRS widening >25% of pretreatment values [9,10].

Procainamide is usually preferable in small animals as it has less risk of hypotension, atrioventricular conduction block, and tachycardia than quinidine. Procainamide may be used with other Class I agents or β-blockers. Gastrointestinal side effects and immune-mediated reactions may occur with either quinidine or procainamide. Procainamide may be given as an intravenous bolus, then maintained as a continuous rate infusion, or transitioned over to the oral forms.

Class IB drugs have an affinity for binding to diseased or ischemic tissue preferentially [1, 6, 8]. They work by blocking the fast sodium channels. They have little effect on normal sinus node, atrioventricular node, atrial myocardium or non-diseased ventricular myocardium, so they are usually used in ventricular arrhythmias and are considered ineffective in supraventricular arrhythmias with the notable exception of vagally mediated atrial fibrillation [9, 11]. Class IB drugs have little effect on sinus node rate, AV conduction, and refractoriness. They suppress automaticity, slow conduction, and prolong the effective refractory period in Purkinje fibers and diseased myocardial tissue. Lidocaine, phenytoin, tocainamide, and mexiletine are examples of Class IB drugs.

Lidocaine is commonly used intravenously to halt life-threatening ventricular arrhythmias. An anti-arrhythmic effect occurs within 2 min, and this lasts as long as 10–20 min [5, 9]. A continuous-rate infusion may be utilized to maintain serum concentrations. Lidocaine is also used as a local anesthetic, but these preparations often contain epinephrine to increase the duration of anesthetic effect. Lidocaine with epinephrine should be avoided when treating ventricular arrhythmias. Lidocaine is not effective orally due to extensive first-pass hepatic metabolism. Lidocaine overdose leads to nausea and neurological signs including ataxia, agitation, depression, muscle twitches, and seizures. It usually does not depress contractility. Cats are exquisitely sensitive to lidocaine toxicity, showing neurological signs, bradycardia, respiratory distress, and sudden death, so lower dosages must be used, or an alternative agent selected. Propranolol, cimetidine, and other drugs that decrease blood flow to the liver predispose to toxicity, as does the presence of hepatic disease. Toxicity signs may be treated by discontinuing the lidocaine, and using diazepam if seizures occur. Tocainamide and mexiletine are structurally similar to lidocaine, but unlike lidocaine, they can be used orally. They may cause tremors, vomiting, anorexia, and ataxia.

Class IC drugs are blockers of slow sodium channels in the cell, and strongly suppress conduction, with little effect on refractoriness or sinus rate [6]. Severe hypotension, pro-arrhythmia, and conduction blocks are risks associated with Class IC drugs. Flecainide and propafenone are examples of Class IC drugs.

Class II Anti-Arrhythmics

Class II drugs are the β-adrenergic receptor-blocking drugs or "β-blockers". They inhibit the effects of sympathetic catecholamines like epinephrine and are useful for both supraventricular and ventricular tachyarrhythmias [12]. Increased sympathetic tone can predispose to arrhythmias by increasing abnormal impulse formation, triggered activity, and re-entry. Beta-blockers slow the heart rate (negative chronotropy), reduce contractility (negative inotropy), and increase the atrioventricular nodal conduction time and refractoriness (negative dromotropy) [6]. Cardiac output, myocardial oxygen demand, and the workload of the heart are reduced. They are effective on both supraventricular and ventricular tachyarrhythmias and are often the anti-arrhythmic agent of choice in cats [1]. The anti-arrhythmic effect of β-blockers is indirect, and they blunt catecholamine stimulated initiation or enhancement of a tachyarrhythmia [2].

Beta-adrenergic receptors are located in the vascular system, the heart, and the bronchioles. There are different types of β-adrenergic receptors. The β_1-receptors are mainly found in the myocardium, and stimulation causes increases in heart rate, contractility, automaticity, and an increase in atrioventricular nodal conduction. Receptors specific for β_2 are located in the skeletal muscles, causing vasodilation, and also in the airways, resulting in bronchodilation when stimulated by catacholamines and also mediate insulin and renin release [13]. A small number of β_2 receptors are also found in the heart. There are also α_1-adrenergic receptors in the vasculature that respond to catecholamine stimulation by vasoconstriction.

Some β-blockers are selective for either the β_1- or β_2-receptor, while others act on both sites, and some additionally block the α_1-adrenergic receptor. The nonselective agents that bind to both β_1 receptors and β_2-receptors may result in bronchial smooth muscle constriction. This is a disadvantage in patients with respiratory compromise, and an agent that is "selective" and binds only the β_1-receptors may be more desirable [6, 10].

Examples of β-blockers include atenolol, metoprolol, esmolol, propanolol, sotalol and carvedilol. Atenolol, metoprolol, and esmolol are selective, binding only the β_1-receptor [1, 6]. Propanolol and sotalol are nonselective, binding both the β_1- and β_2-receptors. Carvedilol blocks the β_1-, β_2- and α_1-receptors. Esmolol blocks the β_1-receptor, and is an ultra-short acting intravenous preparation which is used for acute treatment of tachyarrhythmias [10, pp. 194–226]. Notice the ending of "lol" is commonly used in the drug name to identify β-blockers pharmacologically.

The common side effects of all β-blockers include bradycardia, lethargy, hypotension, exacerbation of heart failure, anorexia, vomiting, diarrhea, and atrioventricular block. Hypoglycemia and bronchoconstriction may occur with nonselective β-blockers. Beta-blockers are contraindicated in high-grade atrioventricular block, sick sinus syndrome, or fulminant congestive heart failure (CHF). When CHF is present the patient may decompensate if a reduction in heart rate or contractility occurs.

When using β-blockers slow up-titration of the β-blocker is the best way to avoid side effects. The initial dose should be at the low end of the dose range and frequency for that drug for 7–10 days [10, pp. 164–193]. Blood pressure and heart rate should be monitored during the up-titration process. Providing the patient tolerates the β-blocker, gradual increases in dosage and frequency are instituted approximately every 7–10 days until the therapeutic dose is reached. Patients may show some signs of lethargy during the titration process. If significant negative side effects are observed then the drug may need to be prescribed at a lower dose, a slower up-titration may be needed or the drug may be discontinued. Chronic oral use β-blockers leads to increased numbers of β-receptors or increased affinity of the β-receptors, known as up-regulation, so abrupt discontinuation should be avoided. Abrupt cessation of the drug may lead to systemic hypertension or cardiac arrhythmias [5]. Concurrent use of a β-blocker and a calcium channel blocker should be avoided or used cautiously [12]. Both of these classes of drugs have negative inotropic and chronotropic effect and could lead to decompensation due to depressed heart rate and contractility leading to CHF.

Class III Anti-Arrhythmics

Class III drugs inhibit the repolarizing potassium channel, prolonging the action potential duration and refractory period. They are very effective in suppressing ventricular arrhythmias, and they are used to decrease the risk of fibrillation in atrial and ventricular tissue [8, 12].

Examples of Class III agents include sotalol, amiodarone, ibutilide, dofetilide, and bretylium. Sotalol is traditionally classified as a Class III anti-arrhythmic, but it is also a weak nonselective β-blocker. Amiodarone also has some β-blocking ability in addition to sodium and calcium channel-blocking ability. Because of their potential to further depress contractility, Class III agents should be used cautiously in the setting of fulminant congestive heart failure and systolic dysfunction. The use of an up-titration protocol is recommended. Pro-arrhythmia effects are a risk with all Class III drugs, and they can have potential interactions with other anti-arrhythmics. Other adverse effects of sotalol include hypotension, depression, nausea, vomiting, diarrhea, and bradycardia, although these side effects are rare, and this drug has been widely used in both dogs and cats to control ventricular arrhythmias. Steady state of sotolol is reached within 2–3 days.

Veterinary experience with amiodarone is still limited, but increasing [6, 9, 12]. It is available in an intravenous and an oral form. It is a complex drug, with a prolonged duration of action and an extremely long time to steady state and elimination. Many potential side effects occur with long-term use, including hepatotoxicity, gastrointestinal upset and anorexia, pneumonitis leading to pulmonary fibrosis, neutropenia, thrombocytopenia, and thyroid dysfunction [14]. Hypotension and acute hypersensitivity reactions may occur with intravenous use [15]. Serial monitoring of serum biochemistry profiles is necessary to monitor the hepatic parameters. Bretylium is not available in the USA.

Class IV Anti-Arrhythmics

Class IV drugs block the L-type calcium channels in cardiac cell membranes and vascular smooth muscle, blocking the slow inward calcium current. Collectively they are referred to as calcium channel blockers. Their primary anti-arrhythmic effect targets the sinus node and atrioventricular junction, making these drugs most effective for treating supraventricular tachyarrhythmias (SVT) [1, 12]. They decrease spontaneous depolarization in the sinus node and atrioventricular junction, slow conduction times, and can suppress arrhythmias dependent on abnormal calcium fluxes. Their effects on the vasculature may also lead to vasodilation.

These agents are often classified into the dihydropyridines, and the non-dihydropyridines, based on structure and binding sites [6, 8]. The non-dihydropyridine drugs form the anti-arrhythmics agents in this class, having an anti-arrhythmic effect on the cardiac nodal tissue. Verapamil and diltiazem are examples of non-dihydropyridine calcium-channel blockers. The dihydropyridines are more vascular specific, leading to vasodilation, with minimal effects on nodal tissue. Agents such as nifedipine and amlodipine belong to this subtype, and are chiefly used for therapy of systemic hypertension.

Side effects of the non-dihydropyridines include hypotension, lethargy, vasodilation, and gastrointestinal disturbances. Like β-blockers, they should be used cautiously in the setting of fulminant congestive heart failure and systolic dysfunction, as they depress contractility and to some degree heart rate. They are also contraindicated in the setting of bradycardia, sick sinus syndrome, high-grade atrioventricular block, and pulmonary edema. Verapamil is more likely than diltiazem to cause severe hypotension and cardiovascular collapse when administered rapidly intravenously.

Up-titration of calcium-channel blockers is not as necessary as with β-blockers; however, careful monitoring of blood pressure is recommended and the dose adjusted accordingly.

Other Drugs for Arrhythmia Therapy

Both atropine and glycopyrrolate are anticholinergics used to increase the sinus rate and atrioventricular conduction when vagal tone is increased. They are used to treat sinus bradycardia. An atropine response test may be utilized to see if a bradyarrhythmia is vagally induced and if the patient may be responsive to oral anticholinergics. This test is discussed in Chapter 15. These drugs are commonly used during anesthesia or cardiac resuscitation to increase the heart rate. Propantheline bromide and hyosyamine sulfate are oral anticholinergics that may be used to increase heart rate. Anticholinergics may cause drying of ocular, oral, and respiratory secretions. They may also cause vomiting, increased intraocular pressure, and constipation [9].

Edrophonium is a short-acting anticholinesterase, which results in acetylcholine accumulation and stimulation of both muscarinic and nicotinic cholinergic receptors. Muscarinic stimulation in the heart slows atrioventricular conduction and the heart rate, and is uncommonly used to help treat or diagnose SVTs. It is also used in the diagnosis of myasthenia gravis [5, 9]. It may cause vomiting, diarrhea, salivation, bradycardia, hypotension, bronchospasm, and muscle twitching.

Sympathomimetics are also used to treat bradycardias. Isoproteronol stimulates β_1- and β_2-adrenergic receptors. It is given intravenously, but caution must be used as β-receptor activation in the systemic arterioles can produce vasodilation and resultant hypotension. Many of the oral bronchodilators increase the heart rate. The bronchodilators most commonly used in veterinary medicine include the methylxanthine derivatives such as aminophylline, theophylline, and the β_2 -adrenergic receptor agonists like terbutaline. These drugs have been used for oral treatment of sinus bradycardia and sinus arrest.

Phenylephrine is an α-adrenergic agonist that causes intense vasoconstriction and systemic hypertension which is sensed by the baroreceptors and results reflexively in an increase in vagal tone which slows atrioventricular conduction [5,6].

Ivabradine is a highly selective funny current (I_f) inhibitor that acts directly in the sinoatrial node to cause a decrease in the heart rate without any effects on contraction, relaxation, or conductivity. Its use in cats with cardiomyopathy is under investigation [16].

Digoxin

Digoxin is probably the oldest drug used in cardiology and has several uses. It is a cardiac glycoside that binds to the myocardial membrane Na^+/K^+/ATPase pump, inhibiting its function as shown in Figure 14.4 [1, 17]. Intracellular sodium accumulates, and this promotes an influx of calcium into the cell via the sodium–calcium exchanger. The end result is increased cytosolic calcium-ion concentration with enhanced contractility and positive inotropy. As an anti-arrhythmic drug, it is useful as a negative chronotrope. The slowing of the heart rate is mediated by digoxin's activation of the parasympathetic nervous system and its inhibition of the sympathetic nervous system. This slows atrioventricular conduction, and prolongs the atrioventricular nodal refractory period, making digoxin useful in the therapy of supraventricular arrhythmias by slowing the ventricular response rate. However, combination therapy is often needed to attain adequate rate control, and it should not be used in cases where ventricular pre-excitation is suspected [6, 17, 18].

Dosing digoxin must be done carefully. Digoxin has an extremely narrow therapeutic–toxic range. There are numerous drug interactions that can potentiate the risk including quinidine, verapamil, amiodarone, and any drugs that inhibit microsomal enzymes (tetracyclines, chloramphenicol, erythromycin). The technician must be aware of the signs of digoxin toxicity. This often initially appears as gastrointestinal signs such as anorexia, vomiting, and diarrhea. This will progress to CNS signs and myocardial toxicity, which manifests as virtually any cardiac arrhythmia, severe depression, and death. The risk of digoxin toxicity is greater in patients with kidney or liver disease, hypothyroidism, and hypokalemia. It should be dosed based on lean body weight, with reductions in dose if ascites or any of the above is present. Dosing strategies and ideal blood levels in veterinary and human medicine appear to be following the trend of giving lower doses than in the past. Therapeutic blood levels occur within 2–4.5 days in dogs when using twice daily dosing. An 8–10 h post-pill serum measurement should be taken 7–10 days after the initiation of digoxin, or after any dosage changes [9; 10, pp. 164–193]. The serum level 8–10 h post-treatment or "trough level" should be 0.8–1.2 ng/dL in dogs. Cats vary wildly in their half-lives for digoxin, and the steady state is often achieved within 10 days when utilizing a dosing frequency of every 48 h [19]. Although intravenous digoxin may be used to treat supraventricular arrhythmias, or to achieve a steady state sooner, this carries risk, and often other therapies are chosen. Digoxin elixir has a greater bioavailability, but it should not be used in cats as they dislike the taste and will salivate heavily. Digitoxin may be used in place of digoxin in dogs when renal dysfunction is present, but it should be avoided in cats due to a prolonged half-life [19].

Should digoxin toxicity be identified, mild gastrointestinal signs may be managed by discontinuation of the drug and correction of fluid or electrolyte disturbances. More serious signs may require hospitalization with anti-arrhythmic therapy, or in severe cases, digoxin-specific antigen-binding fragments. Electrocardiographic changes may help diagnose digoxin toxicity. Ventricular premature complexes, prolonged P–R interval, decreased Q–T interval and ventricular pre-excitation have all been linked to digoxin toxicity [1].

Other Anti-Arrhythmic Considerations

A vagal maneuver is often performed in patients with sustained supraventricular tachycardias; gentle massage of the carotid sinus or firm bilateral pressure on the eyes increase vagal tone. This may slow a sinus tachycardia, or abruptly terminate an arrhythmia dependent on the atrioventricular node for re-entry. Bypass tracts of re-entry supraventricular tachycardia are often best treated with radiofrequency catheter ablation [20].

Periodic monitoring is necessary for all patients receiving an anti-arrhythmic agent. Dosage adjustments or therapy with alternative agents is often necessary, and adverse drug effects need to be identified. Ambulatory ECG monitoring (Holter monitor) is a very useful tool for assessing anti-arrhythmic therapy.

Some arrhythmias are not amenable to medical therapy. Sick sinus syndrome, high-grade second-degree atrioventricular block, or third-degree atrioventricular block generally are poorly responsive to oral therapy and usually require placement of a permanent pacemaker in symptomatic patients [5].

Interventional procedures including pacemaker implantation, catheter ablation procedures, and synchronized electric cardioversion are important and efficacious anti-arrhythmic therapies discussed elsewhere in this text.

Drugs for Heart Failure Therapy

Diuretics are critical in heart failure treatment as they are the sole agents that quickly reduce the fluid retention causing clinical signs in heart failure. Other drugs such as angiotensin-converting enzyme (ACE) inhibitors, and inodilators are useful to decrease maladaptive neurohormonal activation during heart failure, improve cardiac function, and minimize cardiac remodeling. In 2009, the American College of Veterinary Internal Medicine issued a consensus statement with recommended protocols for diagnosing and treating congestive heart failure in dogs with chronic valvular heart disease [21].

Diuretics

To discuss the diuretics mechanism of action, it is necessary to review kidney physiology [2, pp. 279–294]. Blood enters the kidney through the glomerular capillaries located in the cortex (outer zone) of the kidney. Red blood cells and plasma proteins are retained in the capillary while glomerular hydrostatic pressure filters water and electrolytes into Bowman's capsule and the proximal convoluted tubule, forming the filtrate, which is urine. The proximal convoluted tubule is the site of the majority of sodium, water, and bicarbonate resorption. The tubule dives into the medulla, or middle zone of the kidney, then turns and forms a loop (the loop of Henle). The interstitium of the medulla is hyperosmotic, and water is reabsorbed from the loop of Henle, concentrating the urine. The thick ascending loop of Henle is impermeable to water, and is a major site of electrolyte reabsorption through ion transporters. From here, the urine flows into the distal convoluted tubule, which is impermeable to water and is another site of sodium reabsorption. Finally, the tubule dives back into the medulla as the collecting duct, and joins with other collecting ducts in the kidney to form the ureters. The distal segment of the distal convoluted tubule and the proximal collecting duct have transporters regulated by aldosterone that reabsorb sodium while exchanging it for potassium and hydrogen ions, which are excreted in the urine. Activity of this transporter increases when the tubular concentration of sodium is high, or when more aldosterone is secreted by the adrenal gland. Pores in the collecting duct allow for further water reabsorption, which is regulated by the action of antidiuretic hormone, also known as vasopressin.

Diuretics increase urine flow often by inhibiting the reabsorption of sodium. More sodium excretion by the kidney leads to more water excretion. As heart failure worsens, often the combination of two diuretics can be more effective than one agent alone. The major classes of diuretics include the loop diuretics, the thiazide diuretics, and the potassium-sparing diuretics. See Figure 14.2 for the sites of action of the diuretic drugs.

The loop diuretics inhibit the sodium, potassium, chloride cotransporter on the ascending loop of Henle. This class of diuretic includes furosemide, as well as the lesser utilized torsemide, bumetanide, and ethacryanic acid [22]. The result is that sodium, potassium, chloride, and hydrogen ions remain intraluminally in the loop of Henle, and

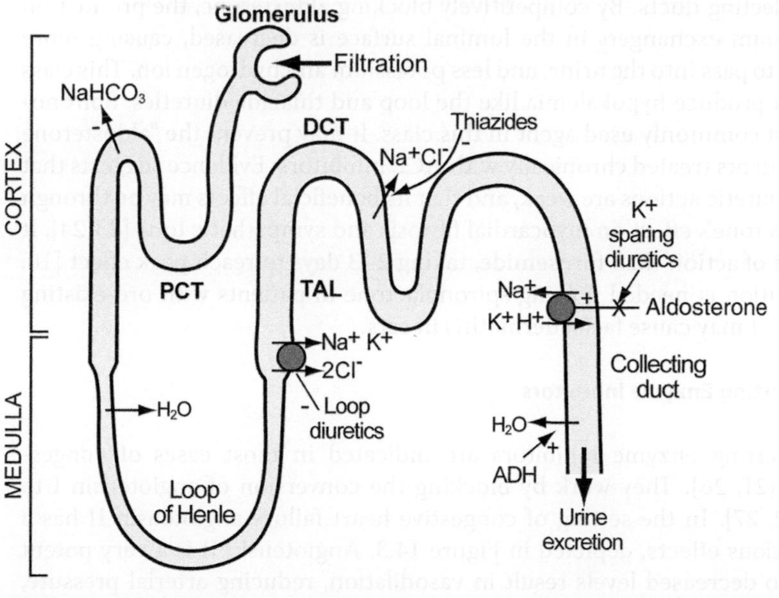

Figure 14.2 The site of action of the different classes of diuretic drug on the nephron. Each class of diuretic has a specific site of action. By blocking the reabsorption of water (H_2O), and sodium (Na^+), diuresis is induced. The loop diuretics work by blocking a receptor on the thick ascending loop of Henle (TAL). Thiazide diuretics block reabsorption of sodium in the early distal convoluted tubule (DCT). The potassium (K^+) sparing diuretics block the action of aldosterone (Aldo) on the collecting duct and distal tubule. ADH, antidiuretic hormone; $NaHCO_3$, sodium bicarbonate; PCT, proximal convoluted tubule. Source: Courtesy of Klabunde. http://www.cvpharmacology.com/diuretic/diuretics.htm

are lost in the urine, resulting in electrolyte wasting and alkalosis. Furosemide may also cause venodilation.

Intravenous administration has an onset of action of 5 min, peaks at 30 min, with a duration of effect of 2 h [9, 22]. Intermittent boluses may be administered, or a constant rate infusion may be chosen to maintain serum levels. Oral doses have an effect within 1 h of administration, and last about 6 h. As a general rule, the goal of therapy with furosemide is to give as much as needed to control pulmonary edema symptoms, and as little as possible to minimize side effects. Thus doses vary widely between patients, and must be titrated to the individual patient's response. Side effects include azotemia, electrolyte imbalances, and dehydration. Patient receiving furosemide therapy need to have serum blood chemistry periodically to monitor these side effects. Furosemide is rarely given as a sole agent, as it potentiates neurohormonal activation, including the renin–angiotensin–aldesterone system [10, pp. 164–193].

The thiazide diuretics block the sodium–chloride transporter in the distal tubule, resulting in reduced sodium and chloride absorption and increased calcium absorption [22]. The increased delivery of sodium to the collecting duct enhances urinary secretion of potassium and hydrogen, predisposing the patient to hypokalemia and metabolic alkalosis. They are weaker diuretics than loop diuretics. They reduce renal blood flow, and should not be given to azotemic patients. Examples of agents in this class of diuretics include hydrochlorthiazide and chlorothiazide.

The potassium-sparing diuretics antagonize the actions of aldosterone on the distal tubule and collecting ducts. By competitively blocking aldosterone, the production of sodium–potassium exchangers in the luminal surface is decreased, causing more sodium and water to pass into the urine, and less potassium and hydrogen ion. This class of agents does not produce hypokalemia like the loop and thiazide diuretics. Spironolactone is the most commonly used agent in this class. It may prevent the "aldosterone escape" seen in patients treated chronically with ACE inhibitors. Evidence suggests that spironolactone's diuretic actions are weak, and that its beneficial effects may be through modulating aldosterone's effect on myocardial fibrosis and sympathetic tone [23, 24]. It has a slower onset of action than furosemide, taking 2–3 days to reach peak effect [10, pp. 164–193]. Caution is needed if using spironolactone in patients with pre-existing hyperkalemia, and it may cause facial dermatitis in cats.

Angiotensin-Converting Enzyme Inhibitors

Angiotensin-converting enzyme inhibitors are indicated in most cases of congestive heart failure [21, 26]. They work by blocking the conversion of angiotensin I to angiotensin II [22, 27]. In the setting of congestive heart failure angiotensin II has a number of deleterious effects, depicted in Figure 14.3. Angiotensin II is a very potent vasoconstrictor, so decreased levels result in vasodilation, reducing arterial pressure, preload, and afterload [2, pp. 195–209]. By decreasing the formation of angiotensin II, ACE inhibitors block its action on the kidney, facilitating renal excretion of sodium and water, producing a mild diuresis. Decreased angiotensin II levels decrease the activation of the sympathetic nervous system. Aldosterone release is decreased from the adrenal glands, and less antidiuretic hormone is released from the pituitary, thus reducing blood volume. The cardiac fibrosis and remodeling caused by aldosterone and angiotensin II is

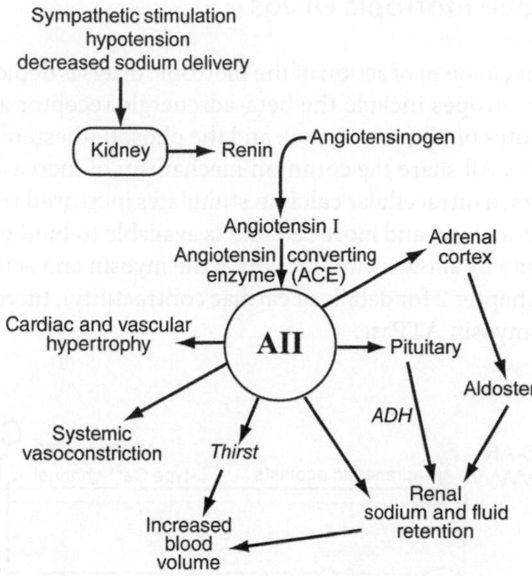

Figure 14.3 The stimulus for production of angiotensin II (AII), and its mechanisms of action. The release of renin by the kidney promotes conversion of angiotensinogen to angiotensin I. Angiotensin-converting enzyme (ACE) catalyzes the cleavage of angiotensin I to angiotensin II. This molecule has a number of physiologic effects, including vasoconstriction directly and also by its activation of the sympathetic nervous system, cardiac remodeling, and increases in aldosterone and antidiuretic hormone (ADH) which promote sodium and fluid retention.

decreased by the use of ACE inhibitors. Angiotensin-converting enzyme inhibitors also block the breakdown of bradykinin, and by increasing bradykinin levels, vasodilation occurs.

Examples of ACE inhibitors include enalapril, benazepril, captopril, lisinopril, and ramipril. Evidence shows they prolong life, while improving the quality of life, and blunt pathological remodeling of the heart in humans and animals [26]. While indicated once patients are in congestive heart failure, enalapril has failed to definitively delay the onset of heart failure in asymptomatic cases of mitral regurgitation, or to confer only a modest benefit [28, 29]. Adverse effects of ACE inhibitors include systemic hypotension, azotemia, gastrointestinal upset and hyperkalemia (especially if used concurrently with a potassium-sparing diuretic). Angiotensin-converting enzyme inhibitors release the angiotensin II-mediated constriction of the efferent renal artery, and so can reduce glomerular filtration rate. They also promote increased sodium and water excretion by decreasing aldosterone levels. These effects may result in acute azotemia. Commonly, baseline biochemical renal parameters are evaluated before therapy, and then repeated 5–14 days after the initiation of therapy to monitor for this complication, and the owners are instructed to watch for any anorexia or vomiting [19, 27]. Benazepril has less excretion by the kidneys than enalapril, but the significance of this clinically is unknown [30].

Angiotensin-converting enzyme inhibitors do not always completely prevent the formation of angiotensin II as there are alternative production pathways. A phenomenon called aldosterone escape or breakthrough is seen in patients on chronic ACE inhibitor therapy [31]. This could be minimized by utilizing spironolactone or angiotensin II receptor blockers (such as valsartan, losartan, or telmisartan) in the treatment of congestive heart failure or systemic hypertension, but current clinical data is lacking in veterinary medicine. An angiotensin II receptor blocker inhibits the action of angiotensin at the angiotensin I receptors.

Positive Inotropic Drugs

The mechanism of action of the inotropic drugs is depicted in Figure 14.4. Classes of positive inotropes include the beta-adrenergic receptor agonists, the digitalis compounds (see notes on digoxin above), and the phosphodiesterase III inhibitors/calcium sensitizers [17]. All share the common mechanism of increasing intracellular calcium [27, 32]. Increased intracellular calcium stimulates increased release of calcium by the sarcoplasmic reticulum, and more calcium is available to bind to troponin-C. This increases contractility by allowing interaction of the myosin and actin filaments of the cardiac muscle (see Chapter 2 for details of cardiac contractility). Increased calcium increases the activity of myosin ATPase.

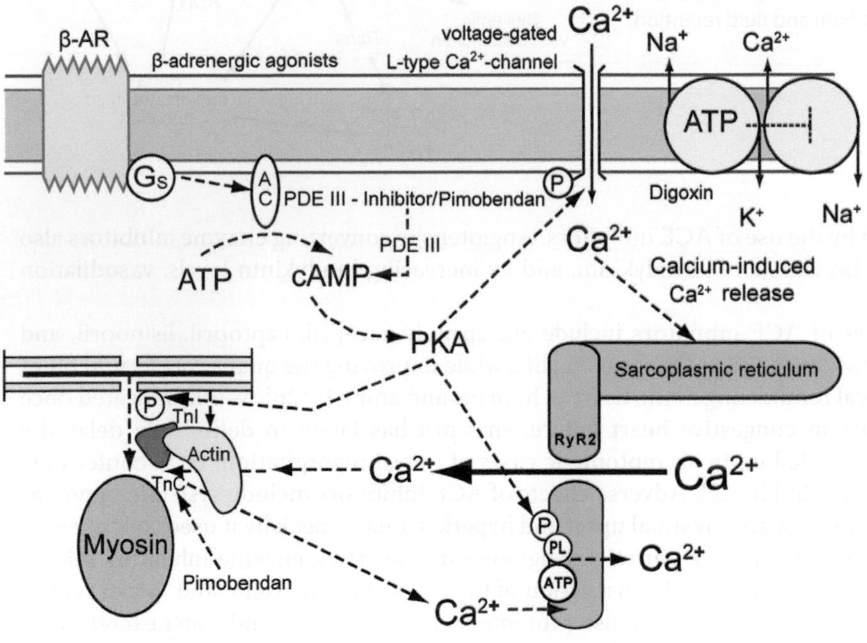

Figure 14.4 Schematic illustration of the mechanism of action of the commonly utilized positive inotropic drugs. β-adrenergic receptor (β-AR) stimulation or phosphodiesterase III (PDE III) inhibition increase levels of cyclic adenosine monophosphate (cAMP). This will activate protein kinase A (PKA) to phosphorylate calcium channel protein, phospholamban (PL), and troponin I (TnI). Phosphorylation (P) of calcium channel protein increases calcium movement into the cell, which will subsequently increase calcium release from the sarcoplasmic reticulum through a calcium release channel (RyR2). Digoxin works to increase calcium levels inside the cell by inhibiting a pump on the sarcolemma, the sodium/potassium/adenosine triphosphate (Na^+/K^+/ATPase) pump. Calcium movement into the cell increases through the action of the sodium/calcium (Na^+/Ca^+) exchanger. Increases in cytosolic calcium through any mechanism results in more calcium binding troponin C (TnC), initiating contraction, and increasing inotropy. Relaxation is enhanced by phosphorylation of phospholamban increasing the re-uptake of calcium back into the sarcoplasmic reticulum, and by phosphorylation of TnI. Of the inotropic drugs, pimobendan has a unique action of calcium sensitization. It binds to TnC during systole and increases the sensitivity of the contractile apparatus of the cardiac cell to calcium. AC, adenylate cyclase; Gs, stimulatory guanine nucleotide binding proteins. Source: Toller and Stranz (2006) [36]. Reproduced with permission of Anesthesiology.

Pimobendan and levosimendan have an additional mode of action by enhancing myocardial contractility through increasing the sensitivity of troponin-C for calcium, so that more calcium becomes bound to troponin-C, facilitating contraction [32, 33]. Pimobendan also may inhibit proinflammatory cytokines and have platelet inhibitory effects [34, 35]. The beta-adrenergic receptor agonists such as dobutamine, dopamine, isoproterenol, norepinephrine and epinephrine simulate the effect of the sympathetic nervous system on the heart. Beta$_1$- and β_2-adrenoreceptor binding increases intracellular cyclic adenosine monophosphate (cAMP) levels. Phosphodiesterase III inhibitors such as pimobendan, levosimendan, and milrinone also act by increasing cAMP through decreasing its degradation. Increased cAMP increases the activity of the enzyme protein kinase A, with numerous intracellular effects [33, 36]. Intracellular protein phosphorylation by protein kinase-A results in increased intracellular calcium, and enhanced calcium uptake by the sarcoplasmic reticulum, with subsequent greater release of calcium in systole. This results in increased inotropy. Other effects of protein kinase-A enhance relaxation. In summary, compounds which work via increasing cAMP result in increased heart rate, contractility, conduction velocity, relaxation rate, and cardiac output. All positive inotropes are usually contraindicated in cases of ventricular outflow obstruction [9].

As discussed in the section on anti-arrhythmic drugs above, digoxin inhibits the sodium/potassium-ATPase pump, which increases intracellular calcium through the action of the sodium–calcium exchanger [12, 18]. It produces mild positive inotropy and negative chronotropy. Digoxin has additional actions that promote its use in heart failure since it restores baroreceptor sensitivity in addition to increasing contractility. It decreases renin release, and also has a mild diuretic effect [9].

Epinephrine and norepinephrine are sympathomimetics that can stimulate contractility but because they are arrhythmogenic and increase the myocardial oxygen demand these agents are not used in congestive heart failure, and are instead reserved for patients in shock [27]. Norepinephrine chiefly stimulates α_1-receptors in the periphery with minor β_1-receptor stimulation in the heart. Epinephrine is mostly β_1- and β_2-stimulatory, with some α effects at higher doses.

Dopamine is a norepinephrine precursor, and stimulates dopaminergic, β-adrenergic, and at high doses, α_1-adrenergic receptors. At low doses it causes vasodilation of several circulatory beds, but at higher doses, it results in systemic arteriolar vasoconstriction. Dobutamine is a synthetic analog of dopamine, stimulating primarily the β_1-adrenergic receptor, but also the β_2- and α_1-adrenergic receptors weakly [17, 27]. It has the advantage of being less arrhythmogenic and causing less afterload increase than dopamine, although the potential for arrhythmias exists, especially at higher dosages. It is often the agent of choice in heart failure patients needing increased contractility with little change in the heart rate or afterload [22]. Potential adverse effects of dobutamine and dopamine include nausea, vomiting, and tachycardia. Cats may become agitated and seizure, so careful monitoring is important. All of these sympathomimetic agents have short half-lives, and need to be administered intravenously, often as constant rate infusions that may be titrated to effect.

Beta-receptors are downregulated by the body in heart failure, which decreases the inotropic effect of the β-adrenergic receptor agonists over time [17, 27]. The phosphodiesterase inhibitors and digoxin work downstream from the β-receptor, and remain efficacious as positive inotropes chronically.

Phosphodiesterase III-inhibiting agents include milrinone, amrinone, levosimendan, and pimobendan. They are inodilators, producing positive inotropy and vasodilation.

While positive intotropy may be beneficial in the short term, milrinone and amrinone, like the beta-adrenergic agents, increase myocardial oxygen consumption long term, and increase the risk of arrhythmias, leading to increased mortality when used chronically [17]. Pimobendan and levosimendan are phosphodiesterase inhibitors, but they also sensitize the cell to calcium. Pimobendan increases survival times in dogs with symptomatic heart failure due to dilated cardiomyopathy or chronic degenerative mitral valve disease [33, 37]. Side effects are minimal, with gastrointestinal upset and diarrhea reported. Placebo-controlled, prospective studies using pimobendan off-label in feline heart failure have not been published, but case reports have been published with good tolerance [38]. It is contraindicated in left ventricular outflow tract obstruction such as subaortic stenosis or hypertrophic obstructive cardiomyopathy [9].

Vasoactive Drugs

Vasoactive drugs include all medication that change vascular compliance by dilating the vasculature to increase vessel size or constrictors that decrease vessel size. Dilating a vessel will reduce the pressure in the vessel and constricting it will increase the pressure. The pure vasodilator drugs may relax the smooth muscle of the veins (venodilators), the arterioles (arterial vasodilators), or both (balanced vasodilators) [27]. Venodilators increase venous capacitance, reducing pulmonary edema and preload (the volume of blood within the left ventricle before contraction). Arterial dilators can be used to reduce the arteriolar vasoconstriction produced by activation of the sympathetic nervous system and the renin–angiotensin–aldosterone system in CHF. In the failing heart, these agents decrease the afterload, or resistance to left ventricular ejection. Use of arterial dilators increases forward stroke volume, and reduces the volume of mitral regurgitation by reducing the pressure difference between the left atrium and left ventricle. Arterial dilators are also used in the therapy of systemic hypertension. Arteriolar vasodilators should be avoided in animals with outflow obstructions, as afterload reduction may worsen the degree of obstruction [22].

Amlodipine is a dihydropyridine calcium-channel blocker that is vascular selective, resulting in arteriolar vasodilation, with minimal cardiovascular depression or effect on atrioventricular conduction [10, pp. 164–193, 19]. It has a long duration of action. It is usually very well tolerated, but the patient should be monitored for hypotension, vomiting, and renal dysfunction. This drug is commonly used to treat systemic hypertension in cats.

Hydralazine is an arteriolar vasodilator, likely working via increasing prostacyclin [19]. It commonly produces side effects, including hypotension, reflex tachycardia, and gastrointestinal upset. It has a faster onset of action than amlodipine, and dosing is usually started at the low end of the dose range, with careful titration based on monitoring of the systemic blood pressure.

Phenoxybenzamine is an alpha-receptor antagonist with no effect on the beta-adrenergic receptors or on the parasympathetic nervous system. It is often used in the management of pheochromocytomas, often in combination with beta-blockers [9].

The nitrates include nitroglycerin transdermal paste, isosorbide, and nitroprusside. They share a common mechanism of action by producing nitric oxide, a potent endogenous vasodilator which increases cyclic guanosine monophosphate (cGMP) levels [19]. Whereas intravenous nitroprusside is a balanced vasodilator, the other compounds in this class are chiefly venodilators. Although a standard drug used in the treatment of acute congestive heart failure, the efficacy of nitroglycerin paste and oral isosorbide is questionable, and the chronic use of these nitrates is limited by the development of nitrate tolerance [19]. Gloves must be worn when applying nitroglycerine paste to avoid transdermal absorption by the technician.

Nitroprusside is a potent drug used intravenously in the therapy of severe hypertension or fulminant congestive heart failure. Nitroprusside is used in the acute phase of CHF therapy. Careful monitoring of blood pressure is needed to avoid drastic decreases in systemic blood pressure. Typically, the use of nitroprusside requires direct arterial blood pressure monitoring since the effect is so rapid and profound. Cyanide toxicity is also a concern when using nitroprusside, so long-term use should be avoided. It is commonly co-administered with dobutamine in dogs with dilated cardiomyopathy and fulminant pulmonary edema. It should be protected from light, and not infused with other medications through the same intravenous catheter [9].

Sildenafil is a drug used to reduce pulmonary hypertension that enhances pulmonary vasodilation through inhibition of breakdown of cGMP by phosphodiesterase type V [9, 39].

Thromboembolic Agents

Primary hemostasis involves the formation of a platelet plug as a response to blood vessel injury. Von Willebrand's factor mediates adhesion between the exposed vessel wall and platelets, triggering platelet adhesion, activation, and aggregation. This is followed by secondary hemostasis, a series of enzymatic reactions which stabilize the plug with fibrin. Fibrin breakdown (fibrinolysis) is a result of plasmin-degrading fibrin [40].

Arterial thromboembolism is commonly seen in cats with underlying heart disease, and infrequently in dogs. Fibrinolytic therapy may be used in some cases of recent vascular occlusion to break down the clot. The reader is cautioned to review the publications detailing the use of these agents as there are dosage uncertainties, the potential for serious complications, as well as a lack of clear survival advantage.

Streptokinase is a nonspecific plasminogen activator that promotes the breakdown of fibrin and fibrogen, and degrades some clotting factors. Recombinant tissue plasminogen activator has a more specific affinity for fibrin within thrombi and a low affinity for circulating plasminogen [40]. Both of these compounds have a risk of mortality from reperfusion injury, and acute hemorrhage. They are expensive, and must be administered intravenously, with intensive monitoring.

Antiplatelet and anticoagulant therapies are more commonly used, with the goal of reducing the growth of existing thrombi and reducing platelet aggregation while collateral circulation develops, or as a prophylactic agent in patients with an increased risk. Aspirin (acetylsalicylic acid), clopidogrel, and heparins are commonly used. Warfarin is rarely recommended due to the high risk of acute hemorrhage and necessitation of close monitoring with serial blood collection.

Aspirin irreversibly inhibits platelet cyclooxygenase, preventing the formation of thromboxane A_2, a platelet-aggregating substance. The optimal dose is unclear, and its efficacy in preventing thromboembolic events has been questioned. However, it is widely used at low doses in cats that have evidence of potential thrombus formation on echocardiogram [40].

Clopidogrel inhibits adenosine diphosphate binding at platelet receptors, and thus decreases aggregation [41]. A study is currently examining whether it is more effective than aspirin in preventing a future thromboembolic event in cats that have had an initial arterial thromboembolism/"saddle thrombus" event (see Chapter 11). Both aspirin and clopidogrel have a risk of side effects that include stomach ulceration, anorexia, vomiting, and diarrhea.

Unfractionated heparin binds thrombin as well as antithrombin III, thus inhibiting factors IX, X, XI, and XII of the clotting cascade. Low-molecular-weight heparins exert their anticoagulant activity by binding to antithrombin III and preferentially inhibiting clotting factor X, with minimal inhibition of thrombin. Low-molecular-weight heparins include enoxaparin and dalteparin [42]. Optimal doses and dosing intervals are uncertain, although low molecular weight heparins are thought to have a longer half-life than unfractionated heparin when given subcutaneously [43].

References

1 Muir, W.M., Sams, R.A. and Moïse, N.S. (1999) Pharmacology and pharmacokinetics of antiarrhythmic drugs, in *Textbook of Canine and Feline Cardiology* (eds P.R. Fox, D.D. Sisson and N.S. Moïse). W.B. Saunders, Philadelphia. pp. 307–330.

2 Guyton, A.C. and Hall, J.E. (2000) *Textbook of Medical Physiology*, 10th Edition. Saunders Elsevier, Philadelphia.

3 Klabunde, R.E. (2005) Neurohormonal control of the heart and circulation, in *Cardiovascular Physiology Concepts.*, 1st Edition. Lippincott Williams & Wilkins, Philadelphia. pp. 117–139.

4 Dangman, K.H. (1999) Electrophysiologic mechanisms for arrhythmias, in *Textbook of Canine and Feline Cardiology* (eds P.R. Fox, D.D. Sisson and N.S. Moïse). W.B. Saunders, Philadelphia. pp. 291–306.

5 Moïse, N.S. (1999) Diagnosis and management of canine arrhythmias, in *Textbook of Canine and Feline Cardiology* (eds P.R. Fox, D.D. Sisson and N.S. Moïse). W.B. Saunders, Philadelphia. pp. 331–385.

6 Côté, E. and Ettinger, S.J. (2005) Electrocardiography and cardiac arrhythmias, in *Textbook of Veterinary Internal Medicine*, 6th Edition (ed. S. J. Ettinger). W.B. Saunders, Philadelphia. Vol. **2**. pp. 1040–1076.

7 Meurs, K.M., Spier A.M., Wright, N.A. *et al.* (2002) Comparison of the effects of four antiarrhythmic treatments for familial ventricular arrhythmias in boxers. *Journal of the American Veterinary Medical Association*, **221**, 522–527.

8 DiMarco, J.P., Gersh, B.J. and Opie, L.H. (2005) Antiarrhythmic drugs and strategies, in *Drugs for the Heart*, 7th Edition (eds L.H. Opie and B.J. Gersh). W.B. Saunders, Philadelphia. pp. 235–292.

9 Plumb, D.C. (2011) *Plumb's Veterinary Handbook*, 7th Edition. Wiley-Blackwell, Oxford.

10 Ware, W.A. (2007) Management of arrhythmias. *Cardiovascular Disease in Small Animal Medicine*. Manson, London. pp. 194–226. [old 14] pp. 164–193.

11 Moïse, N.S., Pariaut, R., Gelzer, A.R. *et al.* (2005) Cardioversion with lidocaine of vagally associated atrial fibrillation in two dogs. *Journal of Veterinary Cardiology*, 7, 143–148.

12 Kittleson, M.D. (1998) Drugs used in the treatment of cardiac arrhythmias, in *Small Animal Cardiovascular Medicine* (eds M.D. Kittleson and R.D. Kienle). Mosby, Inc., St Louis. pp. 502–524.

13 Kittleson, M.D. and Kienle, R.D. (1998) Normal cardiovascular physiology, in *Small Animal Cardiovascular Medicine* (eds M.D. Kittleson and R.D. Kienle). Mosby, Inc., St Louis. pp. 11–35.

14 Kraus, M.S., Thomason, J.D., Fallaw, T.L. and Calvert, C.A. (2009) Toxicity in Doberman Pinschers with ventricular arrhythmias treated with amiodarone (1996–2005). *Journal of Veterinary Internal Medicine*, **23**, 1–6.

15 Cober, R.E., Schober, K.E., Hildebrandt, N. *et al.* (2009) Adverse effects of intravenous amiodarone in 5 dogs. *Journal of Veterinary Internal Medicine*, **23**, 657–661.

16 Reisen, S., Schober, K.E., Cervennec R.M. and Bonagura, J.D. (2011) Comparison of the effects of ivarabine and atenolol on heart rate and echocardiographic variables of left heart function in healthy cats. *Journal of Veterinary Internal Medicine*, **25**, 469–476.

17 Poole-Wilson, P.A. and Opie, L.H. (2005) Digitalis, acute inotropes, and inotropic dilators. Acute and chronic heart failure, in *Drugs for the Heart*, 7th Edition (eds L.H. Opie and B.J. Gersh). W.B. Saunders, Philadelphia. pp. 149–183.

18 Gelzer, A.R., Kraus, M.S., Rishniw, M. *et al.* (2009) Combination therapy with digoxin and diltiazem controls ventricular rate in chronic atrial fibrillation in dogs better than digoxin or diltiazem monotherapy: a randomized crossover study in 18 dogs. *Journal of Veterinary Internal Medicine*, **23**, 499–508.

19 Kittleson, M.D. (1998) Management of heart failure, in *Small Animal Cardiovascular Medicine* (eds M.D. Kittleson and R.D. Kienle). Mosby, Inc., St Louis. pp. 149–194.

20 Wright, K.N., Mehdirad, A., Giacobbe, E. *et al.* (2008) Radiofrequency catheter ablation of atrioventricular accessory pathways in 3 dogs with subsequent resolution of tachycardia-induced cardiomyopathy. *Journal of Veterinary Internal Medicine*, **13**, 361–371.

21 Atkins, C., Bonagura, J., Ettinger, S. *et al.* (2009) Guidelines for the diagnosis and treatment of canine chronic valvular heart disease. *Journal of Veterinary Internal Medicine*, **23**, 1142–1150.

22 Sisson, D.D. and Kittleson, M.D. (1999) Management of heart failure: principles of treatment, therapeutic strategies, and pharmacology, in *Textbook of Canine and Feline Cardiology* (eds P.R. Fox, D.D. Sisson and N.S. Moïse). W.B. Saunders, Philadelphia. pp. 216–250.

23 Riordan, L. and Estrada, A. (2005) Diuretic efficacy of oral spironolactone when used in conjunction with furosemide in healthy adult greyhounds. Abstract. *Journal of Veterinary Internal Medicine*, **19**, 451.

24 Bernay, F., Bland. J.M, Häggström, J. *et al.* (2010) Efficacy of spironolactone on survival in dogs with naturally occurring mitral regurgitation caused by myxomatous mitral valve disease. *Journal of Veterinary Internal Medicine*, **24**, 331–341.

25 Macdonald, K.A., Kittleson, M.D., Kass, P.H. and White, S.D. (2008) Effect of spironolactone on diastolic function and left ventricular mass in Maine coon cats with

familial hypertrophic cardiomyopathy. *Journal of Veterinary Internal Medicine*, **22**, 335–341.
26 Ettinger, S.J., Benitz, A.M., Ericsson, G.F. *et al.* (1998) Effects of enalapril maleate on survival of dogs with naturally acquired heart failure. The long-term investigation of veterinary enalapril (LIVE) study group. *Journal of the American Veterinary Medical Association*, **213**, 1573–1578.
27 Bulmer, B.J. and Sisson, D.D. (2005) Therapy of heart failure, in *Textbook of Veterinary Internal Medicine*, 6th Edition (ed. S. J. Ettinger). W.B. Saunders, Philadelphia. Vol. 2. pp. 948–972.
28 Kvart, C., Häggström, J., Pederson, H.D. *et al.* (2002) Efficacy of enalapril for prevention of congestive heart failure in dogs with myxomatous valve disease and asymptomatic mitral regurgitation. *Journal of Veterinary Internal Medicine*, **16**, 80–88.
29 Atkins, C.E., Keene, B.W., Brown, W.A. *et al.* (2007) Results of the veterinary enalapril trial to prove reduction in onset of heart failure in dogs chronically treated with enalapril alone for compensated, naturally occurring mitral valve insufficiency. *Journal of Veterinary Internal Medicine*, **231**, 1061–1069.
30 King, J.N., Strehlau, G., Wernsing, J. and Brown S.A. (2002) Effects of renal insufficiency on the pharmacokinetics and pharmacodynamics of benzepril in cats. *Journal of Veterinary Pharmacology Therapy*, **25**, 371–378.
31 Bomback, A.S. and Klemmer, P.J. (2007) The incidence and implications of aldosterone breakthrough. *Nature Clinical Practice Nephrology*, **3**, 486–492.
32 Lee, J., Ruegg, J. and Allen, D.G. (1989) Effects of pimobendan, a novel inotropic agent on intracellular calcium and tension in isolated ferret ventricular muscle. *Clinical Science*, **76**, 609–618.
33 Luis-Fuentes, V. (2004) Use of pimobendan in the management of heart failure. *Veterinary Clinics of North American Small Animal Practice*, **34**, 1145–1155.
34 Saniabadi, A.R., Lowe, G.D., Belch, J.J. and Forbes, C.D. (1989) Platelet aggregation inhibitory effects of the new positive inotropic agents pimobendan and UD GC 212 in whole blood. *Cardiovascular Research*, **23**, 184–190.
35 Iwasaki, A., Matsumori, A., Yamada, T. *et al.* (1999) Pimobendan inhibits the production of proinflammatory cytokines and gene expression in inducible nitric oxide synthase in a murine model of viral myocarditis. *Journal of the American College of Cardiology*, **33**, 1400–1407.
36 Toller, W.G. and Stranz, C. (2006) Levosimendan, a new inotropic and vasodilator agent. *Anesthesiology*, **104**, 556–569.
37 Häggström, J., Boswood, A., O'Grady, M. *et al.* (2008) Effect of pimobendan or benazepril hydrochloride on survival times in dogs with congestive heart failure caused by naturally occurring myxomatous mitral valve disease: the QUEST study. *Journal of Veterinary Internal Medicine*, **22**, 1125–1135.
38 MacGregor, J.M., Rush, J.E., Laste, N.J. *et al.* (2011) Use of pimobendan in 170 cats. *Journal of Veterinary Cardiology*, **13**, 251–260.
39 Bach, J.F., Rozanski, E.A., MacGregor, J. *et al.* (2006) Retrospective evaluation of sildenafil citrate as a therapy for pulmonary hypertension in dogs. *Journal of Veterinary Internal Medicine*, **20**, 1132–1135.
40 Smith, S.A. and Tobias, A.H. (2004) Feline arterial thromboembolism, an update. *Veterinary Clinics of North American Small Animal Practice*, **34**, 1245–1271.

41 Hogan, D.F., Andrews, D.A., Green, H.W. *et al.* (2004) Antiplatelet effects and pharmacodynamics of clopidogrel in cats. *Journal of the American Veterinary Medical Association*, **225**, 1406–1411.

42 Smith, C.E., Rozanski, E.A., Freeman, L.M. *et al.* (2004) Use of low molecular weight heparin in cats: 57 cases (1999–2003). *Journal of the American Veterinary Medical Association*, **225**, 1237–1241.

43 Alwood, A., Downend, A., Brooks, M.B. *et al.* (2007) Anticoagulant effect of low-molecular weight heparins in healthy cats. *Journal of Veterinary Internal Medicine*, **21**, 378–387.

15

Treatment of Cardiac Disease

Robert J. Schutrumpf III

Editor's Note: while it is not in the purview of the veterinary technician to direct therapy for heart disease or CHF, if the cardiology veterinary technician understands the concepts of therapy and the drugs in treatments of common heart conditions, they will become valuable members of the cardiac team with an advanced ability to administer medications and monitor patients. The following is ***not*** intended to guide a veterinary technician to initiate therapy without the direct supervision of a licensed veterinarian.

Introduction

Treatment of cardiac disease often falls into two major categories: congestive heart failure (CHF) or arrhythmia. These major areas can further be subdivided into acute therapy and chronic therapy, which often encompass different immediate goals. For example, acute treatment of CHF is generally aimed at resolving the incidence of life-threatening pulmonary edema or pleural effusion. On the other hand, chronic therapy goals are to prevent the recurrence of edema or effusion in addition to maintaining renal health, preventing development of arrhythmias, prolong lifespan, and promote a good quality of life for the pet. As such, treatment strategies will differ depending on the clinical situation and manifestation of symptoms.

Indications for Arrhythmia Treatment

The decision to begin therapy to treat an arrhythmia should never be taken lightly. Any drug that can beneficially decrease the incidence of an arrhythmia can also increase the occurrence and possibly worsen the clinical state of the patient. This should always be considered when asking if therapy will improve the clinical state of a patient. Several criteria can be helpful in making an informed decision regarding anti-arrhythmic therapy.

The most obvious indication for anti-arrhythmic treatment is if the patient is exhibiting clinical signs related to the arrhythmia. If a boxer dog presents for apparent syncope and has a history of arrhythmogenic right ventricular cardiomyopathy (aka boxer cardiomyopathy), the treatment is appropriate after other possible causes of collapse are ruled out. Other clinical indicators that anti-arrhythmic therapy is indicated include lethargy, weakness, and a decreased blood pressure.

Cardiology for Veterinary Technicians and Nurses, First Edition. Edited by H. Edward Durham, Jr.

Tachycardias, originating from the atria or ventricles that are markedly increased above normal rates, often need treatment to maintain hemodynamic stability. Normal heart rates for dogs vary depending on body size and level of excitement, with higher rates being appropriate for smaller dogs or dogs that are excessively stimulated. Cats generally have a more consistent range of heart rates due to their more uniform body size, and any rate greater than 200 bpm can be considered tachycardic. Any dog with a heart rate greater than approximately 180 bpm should be considered tachycardic; however a large-breed patient may be tachycardic at much lower rates. Clinical judgment must be used to assess the appropriateness of each heart rate.

In addition to physical examination and historical findings there are many electrocardiographic (ECG) findings that can warrant the initiation of therapy. Further information on heart rate can be gained by ECG analysis based on the origin of the rate. When evaluating a rapid ventricular rhythm it is essential to rule out accelerated idioventricular rhythm, which is a benign arrhythmia often seen with severe disease of other body systems such as abdominal disease or trauma. The rate is often slower than a true ventricular tachycardia, usually less than 180 bpm, and regular. This arrhythmia does not result in hemodynamic compromise and often will not respond to treatment.

The presence of a true ventricular tachycardia does not immediately indicate that treatment is needed. Hemodynamic stability should always be assessed first; which can be quickly done by measuring systemic blood pressure noninvasively. However, certain QRS morphology changes warrant therapy. If R-on-T phenomenon or multifocal ventricular depolarizations are noted then therapy is indicated to reduce the risk of ventricular fibrillation [1, p. 483].

True supraventricular tachycardia also does not necessitate immediate treatment; often an underlying cause can be identified and addressed. Evaluation of the heart rate, rhythm, and hemodynamic stability is critical. Very rapid rates may require treatment if a decrease in blood pressure results from the tachycardia. The rhythm noted on physical examination and ECG is one of the most important criteria in diagnosing atrial fibrillation, a common arrhythmia seen in veterinary medicine.

A 24-hour ambulatory ECG monitor (Holter monitor) is often necessary to evaluate the need for treatment in cases of sporadic arrhythmia, with the best example being arrhythmogenic right ventricular cardiomyopathy. Instances of greater than 1000 ventricular premature contractions in a 24-hour period may be considered an indication for anti-arrhythmic therapy even if the patient is not showing symptoms of the disease [2]. The inherent risk of anti-arrhythmic drug therapy is outweighed by the risk of sudden death at this frequency of ectopic activity.

Lastly, slow heart rates (bradycardia) can also be an indication for therapy. However, often this involves pacemaker therapy instead of medical management. Cases of vagal mediated bradycardia or atrioventricular block can usually be addressed by treating the underlying cause of parasympathetic stimulation. Rare cases of bradycardia may be treated with medical therapy to increase baseline heart rates.

Strategies for the Management of Arrhythmias

Prior to treatment of an arrhythmia the clinician must determine if the arrhythmia is supraventricular or ventricular in origin. Although some medications are used to treat both classes of arrhythmia, others may have no effect or even be detrimental in certain cases. An ECG should be performed to determine the origin of the arrhythmia. In some cases it is not possible to determine whether an arrhythmia is a supraventricular tachycardia with aberrant conduction or a true ventricular tachycardia. In these situations, best judgment must be used when deciding upon therapy.

Supraventricular Tachycardia

Acute treatment of any tachyarrhythmia is aimed at slowing the heart rate, usually through an intravenously administered medication. Intravenous administration allows rapid delivery of the medication for optimal rate management. In veterinary cardiology the most commonly used injectable drugs for treatment of supraventricular tachycardia are ß-blockers and calcium channel blockers [1, pp. 463, 466]. Ideally, left ventricular function is assessed before administration of either of these classes of drugs due to their potentially negative inotropic effects.

The predominant injectable calcium channel blockers in veterinary medicine are verapamil and diltiazem, which are also available in an oral formulation. Acute therapy for both drugs consists of a single injection of 0.05 mg/kg given slowly, which can be repeated every 5 min up to 0.15 mg/kg (three total doses) [1, pp. 463, 466]. Calcium channel blockers may be preferable as a first therapy in the patient that is not stable for echocardiographic evaluation due to a lower level of negative inotropic action when compared with ß-blockers. The one caveat to this is that calcium channel blockers can be detrimental in the face of ventricular tachycardia due to their ability to lower blood pressure. The ventricular tachycardia makes it more difficult for the heart to compensate for this decrease which can result in severe hypotension.

Esmolol is the main injectable ß-blocker used in veterinary medicine. This is given in the range of 0.2–0.5 mg/kg as a bolus and can then be administered as a constant rate infusion (CRI) at 25–200 µg/kg/min if it is initially effective [3]. A ß-blocker can be effective against both supraventricular and ventricular arrhythmias due to its adrenergic blocking action. However, the main concern regarding this class of drug is its negative inotropic effect which is considered more potent than a calcium channel blocker.

Supraventricular tachycardia can present with some of the most rapid tachycardias seen in veterinary medicine. Effective and rapid response is important for successful treatment; however, the practitioner must be careful to always optimize care. This includes attempting to determine the origin of the arrhythmia and if underlying disease is present. With these considerations treatment can be instituted to restore optimal hemodynamics. After stabilization of the emergent patient and appropriate evaluation for underlying cardiac disease one can begin to consider options for long-term treatment.

Chronic treatment of supraventricular tachycardia is centered on similar drugs as acute treatment (i.e. ß-blockers and calcium channel blockers) with the addition of cardiac glycosides predominantly in the form of digoxin. The drugs used for chronic treatment of supraventricular tachycardias can be remembered by the acronym ABCD (A, atrial for "atrial tachyarrhythmias are treated with"; B, ß-blockers; C, calcium channel blockers; D, digoxin). The major change between acute and chronic treatment is the transition to oral therapy. Many oral formulations are not the same medications used acutely so titration is sometimes necessary.

The major oral ß-blocker is atenolol, which is dosed at 0.2–1.0 mg/kg twice daily orally [3]. This medication is preferable when compared to other ß-blockers due to its selective β_1-inhibitory properties. Propranolol is still used sometimes but is less favorable due to its combined β_1-β_2 properties which can lead to bronchoconstriction. As with injectable ß-blockers it is advisable to evaluate systolic function prior to institution of atenolol therapy. Systemic blood pressure and heart rate should be monitored initially to assess for efficacy of therapy and to avoid excessive bradycardia and hypotension.

While verapamil is available in an oral formulation the predominant oral calcium channel blocker is diltiazem. Diltiazem is given orally at a dosage of 0.5–1.5 mg/kg three times daily [3], and also is available in an extended-release formulation for use in many cases. As with the injectable form of calcium channel blockers, blood pressure should be assessed during institution of therapy. Again, systolic function should be assessed prior to the initiation of therapy.

Digoxin is a unique medication in the treatment of supraventricular arrhythmias in that it is a negative dromotropic drug, slowing conduction through the atrioventricular (AV) node, in addition to being a positive inotrope. These features make digoxin an especially attractive treatment option for atrial fibrillation. In some cases this medication is sufficient to slow the rate of AV nodal conduction. However, there are instances where an additional anti-arrhythmic is needed to achieve adequate rate control. A combination of digoxin and diltiazem for combination treatment of atrial fibrillation has come into favor with excellent results [4]. Doses for this combination are typically diltiazem at 3 mg/kg and digoxin at 0.05 mg/kg.

Digoxin exhibits a high rate of complications, which predominantly manifest as gastrointestinal signs but can progress to arrhythmias and neurologic signs. As such, digoxin is dosed very carefully when used at increased doses compared with what is described above, taking into consideration factors such as lean body weight, renal and hepatic function, and the presence of ascites or pleural effusion that does not absorb digoxin. Digoxin is often disregarded as an anti-arrhythmic drug due to its potential side effects, but with proper administration this classic cardiac medication still has a place in modern therapy.

Other drugs are used throughout the veterinary cardiology community to treat supraventricular arrhythmias, such as amiodarone for treatment of atrial fibrillation. These medications are beyond the scope of this text but may be investigated further under the guidance of a senior clinician.

Once a chronic anti-arrhythmic drug is started it must be closely monitored for efficacy and/or detrimental side effects. This is best accomplished through recheck examinations looking at heart rate, blood pressure, and ECGs to assess for the presence of arrhythmias. Depending on the disease present, advanced diagnostics such as repeat echocardiograms or Holter monitoring may also be indicated. Lastly, the cardiology staff must make every effort to optimize treatment of underlying diseases, both cardiac and otherwise.

Ventricular Tachycardia

As with supraventricular tachycardia, primary treatment for ventricular tachyarrhythmias center around intravenous medications that have the potential to rapidly convert the rhythm to a sinus origin. The first line medication in this case is the sodium channel inhibitor lidocaine (2 mg/kg bolus potentially followed by a CRI due to the short half-life of the drug). The majority of ventricular rhythms will be eliminated or improved with lidocaine administration; however, frequent repeat boluses can lead to signs of toxicity such as nausea, vomiting, ataxia, seizures, and exacerbation of arrhythmias. These potential side effects are an indication for continuous low dose infusion (0.025–0.08 mg/kg/min) [3].

In the event that lidocaine is ineffective in converting to a sinus rhythm another sodium channel blocker, procainamide, is often the next step in potential therapy. Although this drug is in the same class as lidocaine, it has a slightly different mechanism of action that causes it to be effective in some instances where other drugs have failed. In an emergent situation procainamide is administered intravenously at a dose between 5 and 15 mg/kg followed by a CRI of 0.025–0.05 mg/kg/min [3]. Procainamide can also be administered orally for chronic management of arrhythmias. However, it is no longer being commercially produced so must be acquired through a compounding pharmacy.

As with supraventricular tachycardias there is a handy acronym to help remember the main oral antiarrhythmics that are used to treat ventricular arrhythmias chronically: SPAM. This stands for *S*otalol, *P*rocainamide, *A*tenolol, and *M*exiletine. These medications encompass three classes of antiarrhythmics: sodium channel blockers (procainamide and mexiletine), ß-blockers (atenolol), and potassium channel blockers (sotalol). These drugs can be used individually or in some combinations to optimize management of the arrhythmic patient.

Mexiletine is now the predominant oral sodium channel blocker available due to cessation of production of oral procainamide. Mexiletine is in the same subclass as lidocaine and is administered at a dose of 4–10 mg/kg three times daily [3]. Mexiletine can be combined with a ß-blocking agent, usually sotalol or atenolol, to increase the spectrum of antiarrhythmic therapy. This combination has been shown to be one of the effective strategies for reducing the incidence of ventricular premature contraction in dogs suffering from arrhythmogenic right ventricular cardiomyopathy [5].

Atenolol is the major ß-blocker used in veterinary medicine for treatment of arrhythmias and as a negative chronotrope in management of hypertrophic disease in cats. Dosage is from 0.2 to 1 mg/kg twice daily [3] and dosing may be started low and titrated upward to avoid hypotension and lethargy. As stated above, atenolol can be combined with a sodium channel blocker, such as mexiletine, to broaden the spectrum of therapy. Beta-blockers in general, especially atenolol, is the one drug that can be used regularly in therapy for both supraventricular and ventricular arrhythmias.

Sotalol is an antiarrhythmic drug with multiple mechanisms of action. The predominant mechanism is inhibition of the potassium channels on the sarcolemma. However, beta blockade is also a significant mechanism of treatment. Sotalol is administered at 1–3 mg/kg twice daily [3] and is an effective drug for reducing the incidence of ventricular activity in arrhythmogenic right ventricular cardiomyopathy patients [5]. As discussed above a sodium channel blocker (i.e. mexiletine) may be added to this regimen for better control.

With all of these medications it is often necessary to titrate to an effective dose. Institution of chronic oral therapy is best done while the patient is still hospitalized and intravenous medication can be administered if needed. The combination of multiple drugs is also a necessary step in the ideal chronic treatment of arrhythmias and can be undertaken as it becomes apparent that monotherapy is not effective. There are a small number of treatment options that do not require the administration of medication. These are discussed below.

Cardioversion/Defibrillation

One of the options for emergent treatment of a severe tachycardia (supraventricular or ventricular) or fibrillation is to attempt to restore sinus rhythm via mechanical or electrical conversion. It is important to note that conversion of a tachycardia to a sinus rhythm is called cardioversion, while conversion from fibrillation of a sinus rhythm is termed defibrillation. The difference is not just in terminology as cardioversion carries the risk of inducing a more serious arrhythmia, i.e. fibrillation.

Mechanical conversion, or a precordial thump, is simply a brisk blow to the chest at the point of the apex beat. This can cause spontaneous depolarization of the myocardium which allows the normal conduction system to resume control of the cardiac rhythm after a brief pause in electrical activity. This technique is effective for cardioversion but is unlikely to have any effect on atrial fibrillation or ventricular fibrillation. There is inherent risk with the pericardial thump in that if the blow comes during the relative refractory period there is a chance that ventricular fibrillation could occur.

Electrical conversion is more demanding in its application. The most common form of electrical restoration of sinus rhythm is defibrillation. In this application a large electrical shock is directed through the heart to depolarize all the cells of the myocardium simultaneously. As with mechanical conversion this allows the natural cardiac rhythm to be restored. The initial shock delivered is dependent on the patient size (50 J for small animals, 100 J for medium-sized animals, and 200 J for large dogs) [1, p.483] and can be increased if initial shocks are ineffective. It is also possible to convert a tachyarrhythmia via electrical cardioversion by delivering a shock timed on the R wave of the QRS complex. This avoids depolarization during the relative refractory period and eliminates the risk of ventricular fibrillation. This is a technique that is relatively new in veterinary medicine and may become an important part of veterinary cardiology practice in the future for treatment of arrhythmias such as atrial fibrillation [6].

Bradyarrhythmia

Bradycardia often occurs due to underlying disease of other body systems and as such does not require primary treatment. Disease of the brain/eye, thorax, or abdomen can cause a pronounced bradycardia, even to the degree of atrioventricular block, through stimulation of the vagal nerve. If it is not clear whether or not a bradyarrhythmia is due to underlying disease an atropine test can be administered. A resulting increase in heart rate is indicative of parasympathetic (vagal) disease. Atropine is administered at 0.04 mg/kg intravenously or subcutaneously and an ECG recorded 15–20 min post-injection. A positive atropine response will show an increase in the heart rate in the 150–160 bpm range [7]. Medical therapy is usually not necessary in these patients if successful treatment of their underlying disease can be achieved.

If bradycardia is due to primary cardiac disease it is often related directly to the specialized conduction system, an example being atrioventricular block. Medical treatment for primary conduction system disease is usually unsuccessful, as can be demonstrated by the lack of response to atropine administration. Definitive treatment usually requires the use of a pacemaker to allow for appropriate myocardial stimulation. In the emergent situation it is possible to use a temporary pacemaker (either an intravenous or transthoracic unit). This is usually a bridge to a permanent pacemaker. However, in some situations, such as toxicities or infection, a patient may recover to the point of not needing permanent pacing. The details of pacemaker implantation will be covered in Chapter 16.

Acute Treatment of Congestive Heart Failure

When treating the acute heart failure patient the veterinarian and veterinary technician must always remember the fragile nature of the patient. It is imperative to perform diagnostics and provide therapy in an efficient manner so as to reduce stress to the patient. It can be a difficult balance between providing optimal care and overexerting the patient resulting in worsening CHF or inducing cardiac arrest.

Once a diagnosis of CHF has been made the choices of first-line therapies is quite small. The drugs used can be remembered by thinking of the phrase "FON a friend," which stands for *F*urosemide, *O*xygen, and *N*itroglycerine paste.

Oxygen therapy is the first treatment administered to most animals presenting for dyspnea because it is easily provided and often of rapid benefit. Therapy may be provided via the "flow by" method with a bare oxygen line, oxygen mask, nasal cannula, or oxygen cage. If a patient is severely dyspneic, oxygen therapy and a quiet environment may be the most efficacious treatment for stabilization prior to further diagnostics. Smaller patients can be placed in an oxygen cage to provide a high concentration of oxygen, but larger dogs often require a nasal cannula. If oxygen alone does not stabilize the patient for further diagnostics then an initial dose of furosemide may be indicated.

Furosemide is the first-line drug for treatment of CHF in both the acute and chronic phases. It is preferentially administered intravenously in the acute phase at a dose of 2–4 mg/kg [3]. However, if the patient is critical it can be given intramuscularly. Intramuscular administration is less desirable due to the slower absorption, and a higher dose is usually given to compensate for this drawback. After initial administration the patient should be closely monitored for urine production and changes in the respiratory rate within an established period of time, often 30–60 min. If the initial dose is not effective, another injection of the same dose or an increased dose may be administered in 1–2 h, depending on the clinical needs of the patient. Alternatively, a CRI may be administered which can allow for greater titration of the dose based on clinical signs. This can be initiated with a loading dose then followed at a rate of 0.66 mg/kg/h, and may in fact be a more effective way to encourage diuresis.

Nitroglycerine paste is applied cutaneously to reduce preload via venodilation. This medication is often applied to the pinna of the ear; however, peripheral vasoconstriction may limit absorption in the extremities. It may be more efficacious to apply the paste to the trunk or the inguinal area for better absorption. Veterinary personnel should wear examination gloves when applying nitroglycerine paste since this medication can be absorbed through the skin and cause vasodilation in veterinary staff.

Some patients will be refractory to FON therapy alone and will require additional support to get them through the initial crisis. Dobutamine is a synthetic adrenergic agonist which has varying dose-dependent effects and is administered as a CRI. At low doses

(2.5–10 μg/kg/min) this drug acts as a positive inotrope without significantly increasing heart rate or peripheral resistance [1, p. 168]. At higher rates of infusion tachycardia may develop. Dopamine, which is a precursor for the adrenergic neurotransmitter norepinephrine, is not often used for treatment of CHF due to the typical increase in heart rate and peripheral vascular resistance. Lastly, the vasodilator nitroprusside can be employed, via a CRI, for combined venodilation and arteriodilation to decrease preload and afterload respectively. These drugs are very potent in their actions and should only be administered in an intensive care setting.

The patient in acute CHF should be managed with oxygen therapy and injectable furosemide until their respiratory rate has decreased to less than 40 breaths/min. At this point it is appropriate to taper oxygen therapy by incrementally decreasing the flow rate into the oxygen cage or through nasal cannulas. Some patients will exhibit an increased respiratory rate that necessitates increasing the oxygen rate again. In these cases it is important to reassess therapy for potential optimization; however, often a patient simply needs to be tapered more slowly off oxygen therapy for successful weaning.

Once a patient has begun eating and drinking they may be considered for transition to oral maintenance therapy and discontinuation of nitroglycerine paste therapy. Transitioning to oral medications involves switching to an oral form of diuretic which is almost always accompanied by an angiotensin-converting enzyme (ACE) inhibitor. Additional drugs may also be initiated at this time depending upon the disease causing the CHF.

Chronic Treatment of Congestive Heart Failure

A standard maxim of chronic therapy is that it takes more to get an animal out of heart failure than it does to keep them out of heart failure. This is what allows for aggressive treatment in the acute phase which can then be reduced to manageable oral therapy chronically. The number and type of medications used depends on the severity and type of disease.

The cornerstone of therapy in the chronic phase of treatment remains furosemide, albeit administered orally at a reduced frequency and possibly reduced dose. Furosemide administration is usually started at approximately 2 mg/kg orally twice a day. The dose and/or frequency can be increased as needed based upon clinical signs. An ACE inhibitor is also a mainstay of chronic therapy in all forms of CHF. This medication helps to blunt the body's natural response to the reduction in circulating blood volume that is caused by diuretic therapy. Enalapril and benazepril are the most common ACE inhibitors used and have approximately equal efficacy. Many veterinarians choose benazepril due to the fact that it is partly excreted by the liver so may be less harmful to the kidneys. However, no studies are available that show a clinical benefit of one drug over the other.

Pimobendan is a third drug that is often used as a component of chronic therapy. This drug has been shown to increase survival time significantly in dogs with myxomatous mitral valve degeneration leading to CHF [8]. Benefit in other forms of heart disease is extrapolated or shown through smaller studies. Pimobendan acts as an "inodilator", essentially increasing contractility (positive inotrope) and decreasing afterload (arteriodilator). Pimobendan is contraindicated in patients with pure hypertrophic diseases, feline obstructive cardiomyopathy, or outflow tract stenosis.

Often anti-arrhythmic therapy is needed in addition to treatment of CHF. The most common arrhythmia needing treatment is atrial fibrillation. This, and all other arrhythmias, can be addressed as described in the anti-arrhythmic section of this chapter.

Additional drugs are added to the treatment regimen as needed. Beta-blockers may be indicated in patients with obstructive disease after resolution of acute heart failure. Spironolactone, which is an aldosterone-inhibiting agent, is classified as a potassium-sparing diuretic. This is thought to act as an antifibrotic drug and is used in pre- and postclinical dilated cardiomyopathy to prevent further myocardial remodeling in addition to its mild diuretic properties. It is also gaining widespread use in the chronic treatment of mitral valve disease based on new evidence of improved long-term survival [9]. Spironolactone is available in combination with a second diuretic, hydrochlorothiazide, and may be useful in refractory cases which are already on high doses of furosemide.

Regardless of the combination of drugs used it is essential that the patient be monitored for recurrence of CHF. The simplest method for monitoring is teaching the client how to take a daily respiratory rate, which should typically be below 40 breaths/min while the patient is asleep. This easy parameter allows for early detection of a recurrence of CHF and may allow for changes to the medical protocol that prevents hospitalization. Monitoring of serum renal chemistry values is also indicated to assess the effect of therapy on kidney function. If blood-urea-nitrogen and creatinine are increased relative to pretreatment blood work then a decision must be made as to whether the doses of furosemide or the ACE inhibitor must be decreased. A modest increase in blood-urea-nitrogen and creatinine is usually considered to be acceptable. However, if clinical signs of renal disease are present a change must be considered.

Pulmonary Hypertension

Pulmonary hypertension (PHT) is a condition in which the right heart must generate an increased pressure in order to eject blood through the pulmonary artery to the lungs. This results from an increase in pulmonary vascular resistance and can be due to many causes. Causes include obstructive diseases (heartworm infection, pulmonary thromboembolism), alveolar hypoxia (interstitial disease, pulmonary fibrosis, airway disease, and pneumonia), pulmonary overcirculation due to congenital shunting, or increased pulmonary venous pressure due to cardiac disease leading to increased left atrial pressure. The heart failure patient that does not fully respond to standard treatment (i.e. Lasix, ACE inhibitors, and pimobendan) should be evaluated for pulmonary hypertension. Treatment for PHT will fall into two categories: generic treatment of PHT itself and specific treatment for the underlying cause.

Indications for Treatment of Pulmonary Hypertension

The mere presence of PHT does not mean that treatment is needed. PHT is can be diagnosed noninvasively via the echocardiographic measurement of tricuspid regurgitation flow velocity (see Chapter 6). A scale has been assigned to help with decisions regarding whether or not to treat the underlying disease process, the pulmonary hypertension itself or a combination of both. Mild PHT is classified as tricuspid regurgitation jet velocities from 2.9 m/s to 3.5 m/s (35–50 mmHg), moderate as between 3.6 m/s and 4.3 m/s

(51–75 mmHg), and severe >4.4 m/s (>75 mmHg) [10,11]. Measurements of maximum pulmonic valve regurgitation velocities can also be used to assess pulmonary arterial diastolic pressure noninvasively. Invasive measures are rarely practical in the veterinary field.

Treatment for mild disease is rarely, if ever, needed although assessment for underlying causes is definitely warranted. Primary treatment of moderate disease is often based on severity within the range and the presence of clinical signs such as coughing, dyspnea or ascites. Moderate disease should always trigger a search for underlying causes and assessment as to whether treatment would benefit the patient. Severe disease often requires primary treatment to alleviate symptoms and treatment of underlying disease if possible. Severe pulmonary hypertension that progresses to the symptomatic stages often carries a guarded prognosis even with treatment of underlying causes.

Treatment of Pulmonary Hypertension

In the acute phase of treatment of PHT, oxygen can often be the best option for initial treatment. Oxygen is a potent vasodilator of pulmonary vessels and allowing a patient to relax in an oxygen cage prior to initial diagnostics is often necessary if dyspnea is the presenting complaint. Once a diagnosis of pulmonary hypertension is made and the decision is made to treat, oral medications are the easiest option for chronic medication.

The most successful medication for treatment is sildenafil. Sildenafil is often fast acting and effective for a period of time in alleviating symptoms of PHT such as coughing, dyspnea, and exercise intolerance [12]. Ascites may be alleviated by sildenafil therapy alone but often addition of diuretics and ACE inhibitors is needed also. Angiotensin-converting enzyme inhibitors, or typical other vasodilators, may be used as part of standard treatment to help sildenafil with opening up pulmonary blood vessels. Little information is available about their overall efficacy though. Pimobendan is a medication which has shown potential as an additional option for treatment. However, its place in preheart failure patients is still unclear [13].

In cases where underlying cardiac disease is increasing pulmonary venous pressure and causing PHT, treatment to reduce the left atrial pressure can be helpful. In preheart failure patients ACE inhibition may help slightly with this through vasodilation and mild diuretic properties. In patients that have developed CHF, treatment is always recommended with standard triple therapy (furosemide, ACE inhibitor, and pimobendan). The resulting decrease in left atrial pressure allows increased pulmonary blood flow and a reduction in resistance in addition to reducing hypoxia caused by pulmonary edema.

Pulmonary hypoxia due to primary diseases of the respiratory system is the second most common cause of PHT, and underlying treatment can be more diverse due to the higher number of disparate issues that can contribute. Even in issues involving airway disease, treatment may be further divided into upper and lower airway disease. Disease of the upper airway (larynx, trachea, and mainstem bronchi) may require more direct management to open collapsing areas such as laryngeal tie-back surgery or tracheal stenting. In cases such as these, intervention is usually a last resort due to the many potential complications. Treatment of lower airway disease is often aimed at reducing inflammation, promoting bronchodilation, and addressing secondary infections. Treatment of these disease processes would require a separate chapter and the reader should refer to sources on respiratory disease for further information.

Interstitial diseases also fall into the category of hypoxic causes of PHT. Infectious processes such as pneumonia are addressed with antibiotic therapy and the need for continued therapy after resolution depends on residual damage. One of the more common diseases causing PHT is idiopathic pulmonary fibrosis, and this can be one of the most frustrating causes to try to address. The underlying cause of the replacement of normal pulmonary tissue is unknown and specific treatment is often limited to trying to reduce inflammation through steroids. This is rarely successful and treatment continues on a symptomatic basis.

Obstructive diseases can cause some of the most severe PHT seen and can occur on an acute basis. Thromboembolic disease, in the form of pulmonary thromboembolism, is a severe and life-threatening disease process. Treatment is often focused on support (oxygen and fluid therapy), pulmonary vasodilation (sildenafil) and prevention of further embolization (heparin, clopidogrel, or aspirin). If the patient survives the initial phase, identification of the underlying problem, such as coagulopathies or endocrine disease, should be pursued vigorously. The other common obstructive disease seen in veterinary medicine is heartworm infection. Underlying treatment in this case often focuses on relieving inflammation to allow improved blood flow followed by adulticide treatment to remove the cause of the problem. As with other diseases damaging the tissue of the lungs, the need for chronic treatment depends of recovery of the pulmonary arteries.

An uncommon cause of pulmonary hypertension is chronic overcirculation due to congenital shunts such as patent ductus arteriosus, and septal defects of the atria or ventricles. Treatment of these defects depends upon the degree of the pulmonary hypertension itself. If severity is mild to moderate, closure of the defects through catheter-based intervention can be very rewarding. If changes in the pulmonary circulation have advanced to the point that the pressures of pulmonary and systemic circulation have equalized, then occlusion is not an option and the focus of treatment shifts to the primary management of PHT and polycythemia via phlebotomy or bone marrow suppression.

Treatment of pulmonary hypertension has advanced greatly in recent years with the advent of sildenafil therapy in veterinary medicine. However, this disease still remains a negative prognostic indicator, with worsening outcomes as severity worsens. In all cases an attempt to identify the underlying cause and to eliminate it should be made to slow or arrest progression of pulmonary hypertension.

Treatment of Congestive Heart Failure in the Feline Patient

The basic tenants of pharmacologic treatment of acute CHF in the cat are the same as described in the dog. However, doses must be adjusted in consideration of an increased sensitivity to the renal side effects of diuretics. A starting dose of approximately 1 mg/kg for furosemide is appropriate, with re-administration if needed based upon clinical signs. Several other factors must also be assessed when treating the feline patient in CHF.

Unlike the canine patient, cats may manifest heart failure by the accumulation of pleural fluid in addition to or instead of pulmonary edema. Thoracic auscultation may reveal muffled lung sounds if the amount of fluid is significant. The presence of pleural effusion may be found via thoracic radiographs (Figure 5.19), echocardiography, or a diagnostic thoracentesis. If present, as much fluid as possible should be removed via thoracentesis with a small gauge needle or butterfly catheter (see Chapter 16). A three-way stopcock can be employed to allow for emptying of the syringe without detachment from the line. The thorax should always be shaved and prepared in an aseptic manner prior to tapping. Fluid should always be saved for analysis and culture; however, fluid analysis consistently yields an interpretation of a modified transudate or chylous effusion. Small amounts of pericardial effusion are often found on echocardiogram but is rarely addressed due to small volumes and the difficulty in feline pericardiocentesis.

Chronic treatment is again based upon furosemide and ACE-inhibitor therapy, albeit at reduced doses. Furosemide dosing is typically maintained at the previously described 1 mg/kg dose twice daily, while the ACE inhibitor is dosed at approximately 0.25 mg/kg once to twice daily. Pimobendan has been found to be safe for use in cats [14] and studies to assess for clinical benefits are ongoing at this time. This medication is often reserved for cats with heart disease with a component of systolic dysfunction, not pure hypertrophic cardiomyopathy.

Another manifestation of severe heart disease in the cat is the occurrence of aortic thromboembolism (ATE). This often manifests as extreme pain and paralysis of the hind limbs after a thrombus that has formed in the left atrium lodges at the aortic trifurcation. In the acute phase of treatment it is vital to assess the patient for signs of shock and concurrent CHF, and to treat accordingly. This can be very challenging as therapy for shock (i.e. fluid therapy or pressors such as dopamine) can precipitate or exacerbate CHF. For the stable ATE patient the main component of acute therapy is pain medication. An opioid such as buprenorphine or hydromorphone is appropriate in cases of extreme discomfort. As the patient recovers, nursing care and physical therapy become more important to prevent further complications and to optimize recovery of mobility.

Removal of the clot via surgery or thrombolytic drugs is an option, but carries several important limitations. Surgical removal (embolectomy) is a challenging procedure that requires general anesthesia. Unfortunately, the majority of ATE patients are poor anesthesia candidates. Medical dissolution of the embolus can be attempted through the use of drugs such as tissue plasminogen activator, streptokinase, or urokinase, all of which act by increasing the conversion of plasminogen to plasmin to break down fibrin [1, pp. 544–545]. These medications are exceedingly expensive, often thousands of dollars per patient, and must be administered in the acute phase of the disease for optimal effect.

Regardless of the method of embolus removal, a common sequelae is reperfusion injury, in which electrolytes and waste products that have accumulated in the extracellular space of the affected limbs are flushed into the systemic circulation. This can lead to rapid increases in potassium and hydrogen ion concentration, resulting in hyperkalemia and a metabolic acidosis. These complications must be monitored for and addressed via cardioprotective measures and fluid therapy. Recent studies have shown a decreased survival in patients undergoing clot removal/dissolution compared with more conservatively managed patients [15].

At this time clot removal/dissolution is rarely pursued and may in fact be considered detrimental. Therapy often focuses on pain control and nursing care. This involves nutritional support and bladder and bowel management in addition to range of motion exercises. Passive flexion and extension of the joints of the affected limbs and massage of the muscles is essential to prevent fibrosis and limb rigidity after the affected vessels have been recannulated. With proper management and a dedicated owner, approximately 40% of ATE patients will survive to discharge and many regain use of the affected limb to some degree [16].

Prophylactic measures to prevent the formation of clots in patients with an enlarged left atrium are available and a standard component of therapy in cats. The most common drug used is aspirin, similar to regimens in human medicine. Aspirin can be given as one-quarter of an 81 mg tablet or in a compounded form that delivers 5 mg per cat. Both dosage methods are effective and are administered every third day. Another medication that is currently gaining increased usage is clopidogrel. This is another medication often used in the human field and has been shown to work well as a feline platelet inhibitor *in vitro* [17]. Current studies are underway to determine the clinical efficacy of this medication relative to aspirin, and it will likely become more common in the chronic treatment of heart disease in cats (see Chapter 11).

Management of cardiac disease in the feline patient is different from management of the dog due to the different presentations that can occur. As stated before, a finer control on therapeutics is often needed due to the more fragile balance between helping and harming the patient. With careful attention treatment can be successful and the patient rescued from their disease.

Nutrition and Nutraceuticals

Nutritional management of heart disease in the dog and cat is far easier than dietary restrictions in the human heart disease patient. Our pets do not have the problem of coronary artery disease or cholesterol imbalance so fat modification is not typically needed. The only nutrient which may need to be restricted in the veterinary patient is sodium. Several cardiac diets are available but may be unpalatable to some animals. Certain sodium restrictive diets have been shown to decrease the size of the heart in cardiac patients, but increased survival has not been proven at this time [18]. It is also important for the patient to receive adequate caloric intake to prevent weight loss, and as such dietary changes must be undertaken with care not to cause inappetence.

Taurine is an essential amino acid involved in energy transport within the cell [19]. In the feline patient it cannot be produced from other amino acids. Taurine is naturally produced by the body in other animals, including most dogs. When taurine is not supplemented in cat food, some individuals will develop taurine-deficient cardiomyopathy, which is clinically identical to dilated cardiomyopathy. Other body systems can also be affected with retinal degeneration and blindness also sequelae of taurine deficiency. This is rarely seen today because of standard supplementation in commercial pet food, but can occur in patients who are fed a non-traditional diet. Whenever a cat is diagnosed with dilated cardiomyopathy a full dietary history should be taken. Addition of taurine to the diet may help to arrest or reverse the changes found in the heart to some degree.

A small percentage of dogs with dilated cardiomyopathy will also respond to taurine supplementation. It has been speculated that some dogs lack the ability to produce taurine from other, nonessential amino acids and can therefore become deficient. A blood test can be performed to assess for circulating taurine concentrations or a trial of supplementation can be tried. Breeds that are "nontraditional" for dilated cardiomyopathy should always be tested. Labrador retrievers, Newfoundland dogs, and cocker spaniels are all reported to be predisposed to taurine deficiency [19].

A second amino acid, L-carnitine, has been implicated in causing dilated cardiomyopathy in a limited number of cases. A case series reported a family of boxer dogs (a bitch, a sire, and two offspring), who all developed severe dilated cardiomyopathy which resolved with administration of L-carnitine [19]. A blood test is also available for L-carnitine but is less reliable because myocardial levels do not correlate well with blood levels. At this time L-carnitine deficiency induced dilated cardiomyopathy is of unknown prevalence and supplementation is often not pursued due to a potential increase in gastrointestinal side effects.

There are several nutritional supplements which may benefit the chronic heart failure patient. The most commonly used is fish oil supplements, which are thought to be beneficial due to the high content of free radical scavenging omega-3 fatty acids. One study showed a significant reduction in ventricular activity in patients with arrhythmogenic right ventricular cardiomyopathy when compared with placebo when supplemented with fish oil [20]. These supplements may be helpful and are unlikely to cause side effects beyond gastrointestinal upset. When giving any nutritional supplement it is important to use products from reputable manufacturers. In the case of fish oil it is essential to get products with the content of omega-3 fatty acids (such as EPA and DHA) listed. A general rule of thumb for supplementation is one capsule per every 4.5 kg of patient weight. Other supplements, such as coenzyme Q_{10}, are sometimes used but there is no evidence to support a benefit in the veterinary patient at this time. As research continues into the efficacy of supplements, other useful substances will surely be found, while others may fall out of favor. Nutrition and supplementation is an area that warrants close scrutiny in the future.

References

1 Kittleson, M.D. and Kienle, R.D. (1998) *Small Animal Cardiovascular Medicine*, 1st Edition. Mosby, St Louis.

2 Meurs, K.M. (2004) Boxer dog cardiomyopathy: an update. *Veterinary Clinics of North America*, **34**, 1235–1244.

3 Plumb, D.C. (2011) *Plumb's Veterinary Drug Handbook*, 7th Edition. PharmaVet, Stockholm, WI.

4 Gelzer, A.R., Kraus, M.S., Rishniw, M. *et al.* (2009) Combination therapy with digoxin and diltiazem controls ventricular rate in chronic atrial fibrillation in dogs better than digoxin or diltiazem monotherapy: a randomized crossover study in 18 dogs. *Journal of Veterinary Internal Medicine*, **23**, 499–508.

5 Meurs, K.M., Spier, A.W., Wright, N.A. *et al.* (2002) Comparison of the effects of four antiarrhythmic treatments for familial ventricular arrhythmias in Boxers. *Journal of the American Veterinary Medical Association*, **221**, 522–527.

6 Bright, J.M., Martin, J.M. and Mama, K. (2005) A retrospective evaluation of transthoracic biphasic electrical cardioversion for atrial fibrillation in dogs. *Journal of Veterinary Cardiology*, **7**, 85–96.

7 Ware, W.A. (2007) *Cardiovascular Disease in Small Animal Medicine*. Manson, London.

8 Häggström, J., Boswood, A., O'Grady, M. *et al.* (2008) Effect of pimobendan or benazepril hydrochloride on survival times in dogs with congestive heart failure caused by naturally occurring myxomatous mitral valve disease: the QUEST study. *Journal of Veterinary Internal Medicine*, **22**, 1124–1135.

9 Bernay, F., Bland, J.M., Häggström, J. *et al.* (2010) Efficacy of spironolactone on survival in dogs with naturally occurring mitral regurgitation caused by myxomatous mitral valve disease. *Journal of Veterinary Internal Medicine*, **24**, 331–341.

10 Barst, R.J., McCoon, M., Torbicki, A. *et al.* (2004) Diagnosis and differential assessment of pulmonary arterial hypertension. *Journal of the American College of Cardiology*, **43**, 40S–47S.

11 Johnson, L., Boon, J. and Orton, E.C. (1999) Clinical characteristics of 53 dogs with Doppler-derived evidence of pulmonary hypertension: 1992–1996. *Journal of Veterinary Internal Medicine*, **13**, 440–447.

12 Brown, A.J., Davison, E. and Sleeper, M.M. (2010) Clinical efficacy of sildenafil in treatment of pulmonary arterial hypertension in dogs. *Journal of Veterinary Internal Medicine*, **24**, 850–854.

13 Atkinson, K.J., Fine, D.M., Thombs, L.A. *et al.* (2009) Evaluation of pimobendan and N-terminal probrain natriuretic peptide in the treatment of pulmonary hypertension secondary to degenerative mitral valve disease in dogs. *Journal of Veterinary Internal Medicine*, **23**, 1190–1196.

14 Macgregor, J.M., Rush, J.E., Laste, N.J. *et al.* (2011) Use of pimobendan in 170 cats (2006–2010). *Journal of Veterinary Cardiology*, **13**, 251–260.

15 Welch, K.M., Rozanski, E.A., Freeman, L.M. and Rush, J.E. (2010) Prospective evaluation of tissue plasminogen activator in 11 cats with arterial thromboembolism. *Journal of Feline Medicine and Surgery*, **12**, 122–128.

16 Smith, S.A. and Tobias, A.H. (2004) Feline arterial thromboembolism: an update. *Veterinary Clinics of North America*, **34**, 1245–1271.

17 Hogan, D.F. and Ward, M.P. (2004) Effect of clopidogrel on tissue-plasminogen activator-induced in vitro thrombolysis of feline whole blood thrombi. *American Journal of Veterinary Research*, **65**, 715–719.

18 Rush, J.E., Freeman, L.M., Brown, D.J. *et al.* (2000) Clinical, echocardiographic, and neurohormonal effects of a sodium-restricted diet in dogs with heart failure. *Journal of Veterinary Internal Medicine*, **14**, 513–520.

19 Sanderson, S.L. (2006) Taurine and carnitine in canine cardiomyopathy. *Veterinary Clinics of North America*, **36**, 1325–1343.

20 Smith, C.E., Freeman, L.M., Rush, J.E. *et al.* (2007) Omega-3 fatty acids in Boxer dogs with arrhythmogenic right ventricular cardiomyopathy. *Journal of Veterinary Internal Medicine*, **21**, 265–273.

16

Interventional Therapies

Anna McManamey, Anne Myers and H. Edward Durham, Jr.

Introduction

This chapter will discuss the details of performing various procedures common to cardiology veterinary technicians. It should be understood that the descriptions included are only one way of approaching the procedure indicated. Each facility will have variations that work best with their equipment and staff expertise. The procedures as described should not be seen as the definitive "correct" method, but simply as a starting point for the cardiology veterinary technician to begin. With the skills contained herein, the author hopes that the reader will develop an understanding of how these procedures may be done, and be able to apply this foundation in their facility. The procedure should be read through completely *before* attempting to perform the procedure. This chapter will cover common procedures performed in the intensive care unit or cardiology treatment area. These procedures include: abdominocentesis, thoracocentesis, and pericardiocentesis. Additionally, the more complex procedures included are: occlusion of a patent ductus arteriosus (PDA) with an Amplatz® Canine Ductal Occluder (Infiniti Medical Supply, Menlo Park, CA, USA. http://infinitimedical.com/index.html) (ACDO), balloon valvuloplasty in pulmonic stenosis, and permanent endocardial pacemaker implantation; all performed in the cardiac catheterization suite.

As part of the veterinary healthcare team, the cardiology veterinary technicians play a vital role and it is incumbent upon them to be intimately familiar with these procedures. Knowledge of the supplies necessary can add efficiency to the procedure. During cardiac catheterization the veterinary technician fills the role of circulating nurse and possibly anesthesia technician, and therefore knowing what supplies are needed when becomes important. Lastly, in emergency situations the veterinary technician may be called upon to scrub in for portions of the cardiac catheterization, or may need to perform a body cavity centesis if allowed by relevant state regulation.

It should be understood that all the procedures described here are considered aseptic procedures. Body cavity centesis may be performed with sterile gloves and aseptic technique, but usually does not require full sterile gown and gloving. Complete removal of hair and aseptic preparation with an antiseptic scrub and rinse solution is required. A sterile field should be maintained at all times. It is beyond the scope of this chapter to discuss the advantages and disadvantages of various scrub solutions and protocols; in general, all will work well when applied correctly.

Cardiology for Veterinary Technicians and Nurses, First Edition. Edited by H. Edward Durham, Jr.

Pacemaker implantation, PDA closure, and balloon valvuloplasty should be done with surgical sterility including full cap, mask, gown, and gloves. Sterile instrument packs, surgical drapes, and perioperative antibiotics are also needed, especially when a device such as a pacemaker or an ACDO is to be left in the patient's body. Additionally, fluoroscopy is often required and thus appropriate radiation safety protocol must be followed including the provision of lead aprons for all personnel in the cardiac catheterization suite.

Body Cavity Centesis

Abdominocentesis

The following procedure description is specifically for a therapeutic abdominocentesis. A diagnostic abdominocentesis can be performed quickly with a 20–22 gauge needle attached to a 3–5 mL syringe inserted into a clipped and aseptically scrubbed abdomen. A small sample can be collected for diagnostic fluid analysis.

Abdominocentesis is indicated whenever free fluid is present in the abdomen contributing to dyspnea. This may be noted with visible abdominal distention or ultrasound evidence. Causes of ascites include right heart failure, pericardial effusion, hypoalbuminemia, cancer, or hemorrhage. In the case of hemorrhage from tumor rupture or trauma, it may be advisable to not remove the fluid until surgical intervention is available to stop the source of the hemorrhage [1].

Equipment [2, p. 1178]

- Clippers with a #40 blade
- Sterile gloves
- Sterile surgical preparation scrubs, solutions, and supplies
- Needles/catheter approximately 2 inches long (20, 22, or 25 gauge based on patient's size). Many options are available: a large bore over-the-needle catheter is useful. For large dogs a 14 gauge × 2 inch catheter works well
- Intravenous extension set
- 3 or 5 mL syringe
- Red and lavender-top sterile tubes for fluid analysis
- 30–60 mL syringe (optional)
- Ultrasound guidance (optional)

Procedure [2, p. 1178; 3]

1) The patient is positioned in left lateral recumbency. Some doctors prefer dorsal or ventral recumbency. Left lateral recumbency is preferred if dyspnea is present.
2) The bladder may be emptied prior to the procedure to avoid accidental perforation.
3) An area caudal to the umbilicus and just left of the midline is clipped and then scrubbed using aseptic technique.
4) The needle/catheter is affixed to a 3–5 mL syringe and is advanced into the skin and body wall while directing the needle slightly downward into the abdomen. Needle placement may be lateral to the midline or inserted directly through the linea alba.
5) Once the tip of the needle is under the skin the plunger is pulled back to observe for a flash of fluid. If an over-the-needle catheter is used, the whole system is advanced

a couple of millimeters, then the catheter is advanced over-the-needle into the abdomen.

6) When fluid flow is obtained the desired amount of fluid is aspirated. This can be accomplished by manual aspiration, suction, or passive gravity drainage. One limitation of aspiration and suction is a tendency for omentum or organs to be pulled to the catheter. With passive gravity drainage, fluid free-flows into a basin easily with little interference from abdominal contents.
7) The needle is withdrawn from the abdomen smoothly and quickly.
8) Some of the fluid is placed into a lavender-top tube (EDTA tube) and a red-top tube (sterile glass tube). The two tubes are submitted for standard fluid analysis and cytology.
9) A sample is saved on a sterile swab so that it may be submitted for a culture if needed.

Postprocedure Patient Care

The patient may experience subcutaneous pooling of ascitic fluid after the procedure. This is common when large volumes of ascites are partially drained. Seepage of ascitic fluid may be reduced by inserting the drainage cannula through the linea alba. The pooling may resolve spontaneously or may require an abdominal wrap. Other complications include internal or external hemorrhage, infection, organ trauma, or rarely uroabdomen.

In cases of right-side heart failure as much fluid as possible should be removed to provide the greatest amount of relief on the diaphragm.

Thoracocentesis

Thoracocentesis is indicated for the presence of pleural effusion sufficient to cause dyspnea. Dogs rarely develop pleural effusion from congestive heart failure, but will from cancer, lymphatic disease (chylous effusion), pyothorax, or pneumothorax. Cats may develop pleural effusion from all the above plus congestive heart failure, and repeated thoracocentesis may be needed as it recurs.

Equipment [2, pp. 1308–1309]

- Clippers with a #40 blade
- Sterile gloves
- Sterile surgical preparation scrubs, solutions, and supplies
- 10–60 mL syringe
- Four-way stopcock
- Intravenous extension tubing
- An appropriate sized needle, catheter, or butterfly catheter (Table 16.1)

Table 16.1 Appropriate sizes for needles, catheters, and butterfly catheters.

Large dogs	18–22 gauge × 1.5 inch needle or catheter
Medium dogs	18–22 gauge × 1 inch needle or catheter
Cats and small dogs	19–22 gauge × 0.75 inch butterfly catheter
Diagnostic sample only	25–22 gauge needle 5/8 to 1 inch

- Basin for collecting fluid
- Red and lavender-top sterile tubes for fluid analysis

Procedure [2, pp. 1308–1309]

1) The patient may be standing or placed in sternal recumbency.
2) The area between the fifth and tenth intercostal space at the level of the costochondral junction is clipped and aseptically prepared. If a pneumothorax is the expected reason for the thoracocentesis the area between the eighth and ninth intercostal space at the level of the costochondral junction and dorsally is clipped and aseptically prepared.
3) The appropriate size needle or butterfly catheter is attached to the extension set, four-way stopcock, and syringe while wearing sterile gloves.
4) Ultrasound is useful for locating the optimal centesis site. If ultrasound is not available, the needle/catheter is usually inserted between the seventh and eighth ribs or the eighth and ninth ribs.
5) The first operator inserts the needle slowly into the thorax, on the cranial aspect of the caudal rib of the intercostal space selected.
6) When the needle is through the skin and the bevel of the needle is no longer visible aspiration is initiated by a second operator. The appropriate amount of negative pressure is applied for the size of the animal: a few tenths of a millilitre for small patients and 1–2 mL for larger patients; never more than 5 mL for any animal.
7) The hub of the needle is observed for the flash of fluid.
8) If blood is obtained, it is evaluated for clotting. The blood from a hemothorax should not clot. If the aspirated blood clots it may be from the heart or a blood vessel, and the procedure is stopped.
9) If another kind of fluid is obtained aspiration is continued until no more fluid can be removed. Effusions may be a serosanguinous transudate, chylous effusion, hemorrhagic, purulent, or air.
10) Samples of the fluid are placed in a lavender-top tube (EDTA tube) and a red-top tube (sterile glass tube) for standard fluid analysis and cytology as desired. A third sample is taken and kept for a bacterial culture if necessary.
11) If air is aspirated the tubing will become foggy due to the warm air inside the thoracic cavity. Aspiration is continued until negative pressure is obtained.

Postprocedure Patient Care [2, pp. 1308–1309]

The patient should be monitored for evidence of returning respiratory distress. This could indicate the return of an underlying pleural disease. Respiratory distress may also be indicative of an iatrogenic pneumothorax or hemothorax. Iatrogenic pneumothorax may be caused by air leaking during the procedure or by lung puncture. Hemothorax may be caused by lung puncture or damage to a vessel or heart. Infection is a rare complication.

Pericardiocentesis

Pericardiocentesis is indicated for significant effusion of the pericardial space. Some cases with even lesser degrees of effusion should be tapped if cardiac tamponade is present. A detailed description of pericardial disease is given in Chapter 12.

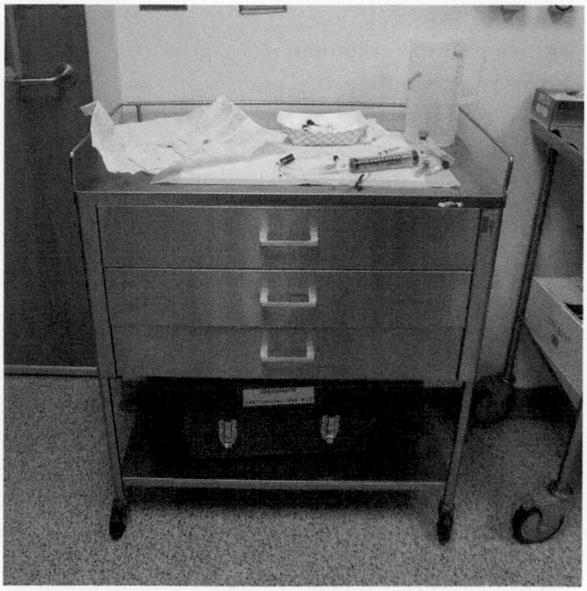

Figure 16.1 A typical pericardiocentesis set up showing the necessary equipment laid out on a clean work surface. This institution keeps all the supplies in the cart ready for emergency deployment. Source: Courtesy of North Carolina State University Veterinary Teaching Hospital Cardiology Service.

There are several protocols the veterinary technician should follow when assisting with this procedure. Ideally, there should be three staff members assisting a veterinarian performing the pericardiocentesis. To help ensure a favorable outcome for the patient veterinary technicians will assist with stabilizing the patient, watching the electrocardiogram (ECG) for arrhythmias, and obtaining fluid samples. It is recommended to have all the necessary supplies in a ready-made kit, along with a description of the procedure ready for rapid deployment. The use of a cart on wheels (Figure 16.1) that contains all supplies and a work surface that is ready to wheel up to the patient on the examination table is helpful. The veterinary technician plays an important role in set up and organization, and may be called upon to perform every aspect, except the actual pericardiocentesis.

Equipment

- Clippers with a #40 blade
- Sterile surgical preparation scrubs, solutions, and supplies
- Sterile surgical gloves
- Fenestrated drape (pre-wrapped)
- #11 scalpel blade
- 2% lidocaine
- Sterile probe cover
- Red-top tube
- Lavender-top tube
- 5 cm^3 culture vial
- Gray-top tube with diatomaceous earth
- 16 or 14 gauge × 2″ or 14 gauge × 3.25″ over-the-needle catheter
- 60 mL syringe
- 20 mL syringe (for feline patients)

- Four-way stopcock
- Intravenous extension set
- 3 mL syringe (optional)

Procedure [2, pp. 1308–1309; 4]

1) The patient should be placed in left lateral recumbency or sternal recumbency. Echocardiography can be used to identify the optimal intercostal space to perform the procedure. If echocardiography is not available using the fourth or fifth intercostal space slightly dorsal to the costochondral junction is recommended [4] to avoid laceration of the left extramural coronary artery. The right-side approach is also recommended due to the larger cardiac notch in the right lung lobes where the pericardium is located adjacent to the body wall. In order to avoid the thoracic artery and vein that run along the back of each rib, the thoracic cavity should be entered from the front of a rib.
2) It is always good practice to place a peripheral intravenous catheter before proceeding with a pericardiocentesis. Quick intravenous access is essential for a patient to receive any type of cardiopulmonary resuscitation drugs or fluids, and to treat any ventricular arrhythmias that may occur. Saline flush and a dose of lidocaine at 2.2 mg/kg [4] should be drawn up and ready to give if needed for ventricular arrhythmias. If the patient presents recumbent and in cardiogenic shock, an intravenous fluid bolus is administered as needed.
3) Always have the patient connected to an ECG and have one person closely monitor the ECG during the tap procedure. Ventricular premature complexes and ventricular tachycardia can occur if the catheter comes into contact with an irritable myocardium.
4) It is of utmost importance that the patient remains still during the procedure. If stable, mild sedation with a narcotic such as buprenorphine at 0.005–0.02 mg/kg in dogs and 0.005–0.01 mg/kg intravenously in cats is recommended [5, p. 113] or butorphanol at 0.2–0.4 mg/kg intravenously in the dog and cat [5, p. 118].
5) The right lateral thorax is shaved and surgically prepared with an accepted protocol between the second and eighth intercostal spaces; starting at the tap site and moving to the outside. If the patient is stable, the scrub solution should have a minimum of 3 min of contact time with the skin.
6) After one surgical scrub, either the operator or the veterinary technician should numb the tap site using 2% lidocaine. You may buffer the lidocaine with a small amount of sodium bicarbonate at a ratio of 10:1; usually a total of 1 cm^3 of solution is sufficient administered with a 25 or 22 gauge needle. Always change the needle after entering the rubber stoppers of solutions before administering the medication to the patient as the needle will be dulled by the bottle stoppers.
7) Start by carefully placing the needle into the thoracic cavity while applying negative pressure to the syringe and then infiltrate the area by slowly backing out of the body wall, subcutaneous tissue, and into the skin, or start by blocking subcutaneously, intramuscularly, and into the pleura. A region of at least 2 cm that spans the entire thickness of the chest wall should be infiltrated
8) The catheter selected is prepared with two small fenestrations near the tip, if not already present. The first is placed 1 cm from the tip of catheter, then the catheter is rotated 90 degrees to place a second fenestration another centimeter down

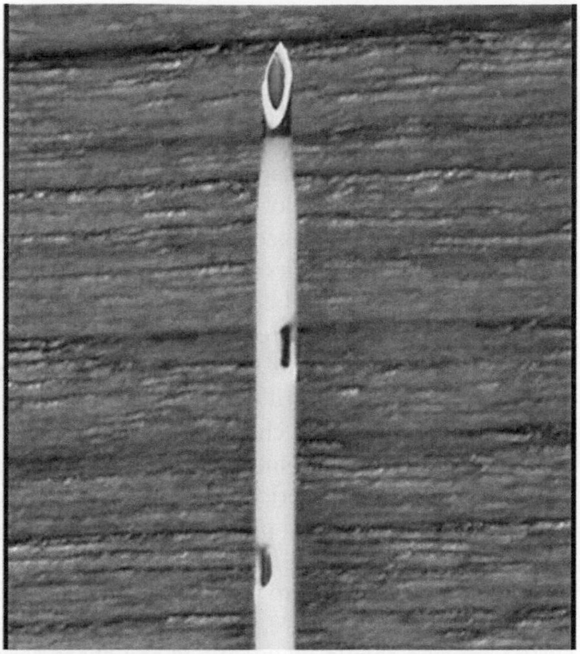

Figure 16.2 A pericardiocentesis catheter with fenestrations. Notice that the fenestrations are positioned so as not to weaken the catheter linear strength. The fenestrations should be placed at a 90 degree angle to each other, not on opposite sides of the catheter which could create a "hinge point" between them that could collapse during the procedure occluding the catheter.

(Figure 16.2). This allows for the fluid to be aspirated quickly. In an emergency, this step may be skipped or pre-fenestrated catheters can be used. Typically a 14 gauge by 3.25″ or 5.25″ catheter is used in large dogs, and a 16 gauge 3.25″ catheter in small dogs and cats.

9) A stab incision is made with a #11 surgical blade into the skin at the location of the lidocaine block, before entering with the catheter. This allows for smooth entry of the catheter into the thoracic cavity without causing a bur at the tip of the catheter. If the patient reacts to the stab incision negatively, then more lidocaine or more sedation may be necessary.
10) The selected catheter is inserted through the skin into the thoracic cavity and is slowly advanced toward the pericardium. A 3 mL syringe may be attached to the end of the tap catheter. Negative pressure is applied when the operator enters the thorax. The operator should get a flash of fluid as the catheter is advanced to signal they are in the pericardium. Pericardial fluid is typically hemorrhagic in color and does not clot. If pleural effusion is present, clear serosanguinous fluid may be seen. The needle should be advanced until a flash of pericardial fluid is seen. The catheter assembly is advanced another 2–3 mm, and then the catheter is advanced over the needle and into the pericardium. One technician should watch the ECG for arrhythmias while the catheter is being advanced. Once the catheter is positioned in the pericardium the needle/stylet is removed from the thorax.
11) An extension set is attached directly to the end of the catheter in the pericardium by the person performing the tap. This is followed by a four-way stopcock and a 60 mL syringe which can be attached by a technician. This allows for some distance between the catheter and the movement caused by operating the stopcock and syringe. As a note the catheter may need to be repositioned during the

procedure to remove the maximum amount of fluid. Approximately 10 mL of fluid is aspirated for culture, fluid analysis, and cytology as desired.

12) As mentioned earlier, pericardial effusion does not coagulate. To verify placement of the catheter in the pericardium and not directly into the right ventricle, a sample of the effusion is placed in the grey-top tube (activated clotting time [ACT] tube with diatomaceous earth) to assess for clot formation. The use of the ACT tube quickly assesses clot formation, although in the absence of such tubes a plain red-top tube can be substituted. If a red-top is used, more time should be allowed for clot formation to occur before serious fluid aspiration begins. The ACT tube should be warmed to body temperature before the sample is instilled, and then kept at body temperature for 2 min. The tube is then checked for clot formation. If no clotting is evident, then aspiration may begin in earnest. If clotting occurs, this means the myocardium has been penetrated and circulating blood is being aspirated from a heart chamber. The catheter should be removed and the patient re-evaluated by ultrasound. The centesis procedure can then be repeated to place the catheter in the pericardium rather than the ventricle as needed. A packed cell volume can also be performed on hemorrhagic effusion to make sure a heart chamber has not been entered. The packed cell volume of hemorrhagic effusion should be low, anywhere from 4 to 10%, when compared with that of the systemic blood.
13) The effusion should be quantified and characterized. A sample of the fluid should be submitted for fluid analysis and cytology to allow for the best diagnosis. Sometimes patients have both pleural and pericardial fluids that need removal. Typically, the veterinarian will remove the more life-threatening hemorrhagic pericardial fluid first, and then back out and remove the pleural fluid which is normally a modified transudate. The amount of fluid removed should be measured and recorded.

Occasional scans with the ultrasound probe should confirm that the pericardial fluid is disappearing, the collapse of the right atrium has ceased, the heart rate is decreasing, and the heart itself can relax and fill again.

In review, veterinary technicians can help obtain the echo, set up for the pericardial tap, place an intravenous catheter, sedate the patient if needed, attach ECG leads and monitor for arrhythmias, administer the local block and aseptically prepare the site while the veterinarian is opening sterile items, donning sterile gloves, and fenestrating the tap catheter. Once the centesis has begun, the technician may be called on to operate the aspiration syringe and/or use the ultrasound to verify catheter placement and evaluate the therapeutic effect.

Postprocedure Patient Care [2, pp. 1298–1299]

Post procedure, the patient should be observed for signs of discomfort or dyspnea. There is a small risk of pneumothorax when entering the thoracic cavity with a catheter. If a pneumothorax occurs, a thoracocentesis should be performed to remove the air. A recheck echocardiogram should be performed immediately and then 12–24 h after the procedure to assess the amount of fluid present in the pericardium. If re-accumulation of the fluid is rapid it suggests malignancy, atrial rupture from stretch, or coagulopathy. This is especially important for patients thought to have hemangiosarcoma. Ascites that was caused by cardiac tamponade should resolve spontaneously within 12–36 hours following the procedure. Providing sterile technique has been observed, postcentesis antibiotics are usually not necessary.

Unlike dogs, cats can develop pericardial effusion from congestive heart failure. Most often it does not cause cardiac tamponade and can often be controlled with diuretic therapy. However, occasionally pericardiocentesis is necessary in cats. The procedure is identical to dogs with the following caveats [4]

1) A 22 gauge 1 or 1.5 inch needle or butterfly should be used and can be attached to an extension set and 20 mL syringe.
2) It is recommended to perform pericardiocentesis only under echocardiographic guidance due to the small pericardial effusion volumes and low safety margin.
3) Sedation is necessary in many feline patients.

Cardiac Catheterization Procedures

This section will cover the basic steps in performing the common cardiac catheterization procedures in veterinary medicine. Details of angiography equipment, supplies and concepts are covered in Chapter 8. There the reader will find information regarding cardiac catheters, introducers, and guidewires; their sizing and uses as well as a discussion on intracardiac pressure measurement common to the procedures are listed here in greater detail. This section is designed to be a quick reference checklist and is not to be considered exhaustive or definitive.

Patent Ductus Arteriosus

Transcatheter occlusion of PDA has been attempted since the early 1990s in children [6] and since the late 1990s in dogs [7,8]. Transcatheter occlusion promised the opportunity to close the PDA without performing a thoracotomy (see Chapter 8). Early transcatheter occlusion was done by placing an embolization coil in the ampulea of the PDA. The embolization coil's Dacron fibers would induce a thrombus in the PDA thereby closing off blood flow. This procedure was successful, but the embolization coils had significant drawbacks.

In 2007 the ACDO became clinically available [9]. This device was specially designed to fit in the canine PDA and occlude it. The ACDO is a nitenol mesh device that will collapse to allow it to be passed through a cardiac catheter, be deposited into the PDA, and upon deployment from the catheter will reform into its nominal shape. The ACDO has simplified transcatheter occlusion of the PDA as well as decreasing the time of the procedure compared with coil occlusion.

Equipment

The following list is a simple check list of basic supplies. The sizes of the catheter introducer, catheters (angiography and device deployment) and guidewires will be dictated by the patient size and chosen by the veterinary cardiologist. A wide size range of catheterization catheters and introducers should be kept on hand. The method described herein is for using a guiding catheter as the ACDO deployment catheter. An alternative method uses a 45 cm or longer catheter introducer sheath through which to deploy the ACDO.

The long introducer sheath comes with an integral hemostatic valve, so a Cook® (Cook Medical Bloomington, IL, USA.
http://www.cookmedical.com/) Tuohy-Borst adapter is not needed.

- Physiological monitoring equipment: direct pressure transducers, SpO_2, electrocardiogram, etc.
- Surgical masks, surgical caps, and surgical shoe covers
- Surgical hand scrub brushes, surgical gowns, and sterile gloves
- Lead aprons and radiation safety gear
- Sterile surgical preparation scrubs, solutions, and supplies.
- Patient drapes
- Large table drape
- Four towel pack
- Small (24″ × 24″) extra drapes
- Image intensifier cover
- Cardiovascular instrument pack
- 1 L heparinized saline solution (~1500 IU/liter)
- mL syringes (with or without Luer-lock as surgeon prefers)
- Two basins and two stopcocks
- Scalpel blades; #10, #11
- Power injector with syringe and pressure injection line
- Iohexol radiographic contrast (4–5 mL/kg max dose)
- Catheter introducer with appropriate guidewire and arterial needle (aka vascular access sheath)
- Angiography catheter: Arrow-Berman™ (Arrow International/Teleflex, Research Triangle Park, NC, USA. http://www.arrowintl.com/) catheter or pigtail catheter (typically 4–7 F × 75–100 cm)
- Absorbable 2-0 suture for vessel retraction/ligature
- 0.035″ × 150 cm J-tipped guidewire
- Assorted sizes of Amplatz® Canine Ductal Occluder (ACDO)
- Multipurpose guiding catheter (with size based on ACDO size)
- 0.035″ × 150 cm angled or straight hydrophilic guidewire
- Cook® Tuohy-Borst adapter or similar hemostatic device
- Suture: absorbable 2-0, absorbable 3-0, and nonabsorbable 3-0 for closing incision

Procedure [9]

This procedure is performed using fluoroscopic guidance and/or transesophageal echocardiography.

1) After following routine protocols for anesthesia the patient is positioned in right lateral or dorsal recumbency. The left rear leg is secured away from the right inguinal area.
2) An area from the umbilicus to the femorotibial joint is clipped. The area extends lateral and medial approximately 3–6 cm past the anterior and posterior edge of the each leg such that the entire inguinal area from the knee to the umbilicus is clipped. The right or left femoral artery is then surgically scrubbed and prepared following hospital.

3) The femoral artery is cannulated with a catheter-introducer sheath. This may be done surgically via a "cut down" technique or percutaneously using the modified Seldinger technique (see Chapter 8). The size of the sheath (4–9F) should be selected so that it will accommodate all the angiographic and guiding catheters used during the procedure. This size will be determined by the size of the ductal aperture as measured by echocardiogram. An ACDO device will need to be twice the size of the aperture; therefore, the sheath selected should be large enough to accommodate catheters necessary to deliver the ACDO estimated to be used. If the echocardiographic estimate is dramatically erroneous, the sheath may be exchanged for the correct one if necessary, but should be avoided if possible.
4) A nonselective pigtail catheter or Berman™ angiographic catheter is advanced under fluoroscopic guidance through the femoral artery and into the aorta just cranial to the junction of the aorta and the PDA. A 0.035″ × 150 cm J-Tipped guidewire is used to assist in advancing the catheter. Remember the mantra: *never lose sight of the wire.*

   Note: a calibrated radiographic marker needs to be in the field of interest during the angiogram to allow for accurate measurements of the PDA from the angiogram. Such markers are available as a built in feature of some catheters and guidewires. If a calibrated radiographic marker catheter or guidewire is unavailable, then another radiographic marker of known size must be placed in the field as a reference.
5) The patient is moved to right lateral recumbency if not already positioned so. To appropriately size the PDA, an aortogram is performed by injecting the radiopaque contrast at a rate appropriate for the intrinsic rate of flow (0.5–1.0 mL/kg of contrast solution at 20 mL/s) [10] with the power injector.
6) The images from the aortogram (Figure 16.3) are examined to determine if the anatomy of the ductus is suitable for transcatheter occlusion. The pulmonic ostium, which is the minimal ductal diameter at the aperture into the main pulmonary artery, is measured. The angiography catheter is then removed from the patient.

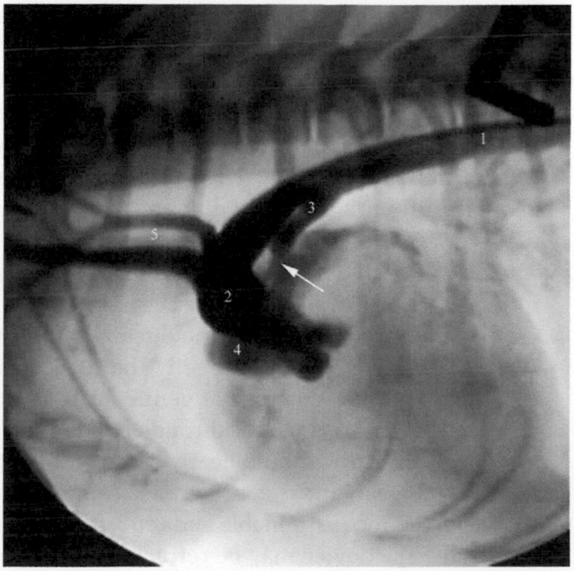

Figure 16.3 Lateral projection angiographic image is of the aortic arch, patent ductus arteriosus (PDA), and main pulmonary artery. The patient's head is toward the left and the sternum is toward the bottom. A cardiac catheter has been advanced from the femoral artery (1) to the ascending aorta for the radiopaque contrast injection (2). The aortic arch is predominantly highlighted with the pulmonary artery (4) just behind it. The PDA is noted in the descending (3) extending ventral to the pulmonary artery. The brachiocephalic trunk and common carotid arteries can be seen leading cranial (5). Careful examination of the PDA will reveal a thin "jet" of contrast streaming into the pulmonary artery. This contrast indicates the size of the ductal aperture. (arrow)

7) The appropriate ACDO is selected based on the diameter of the pulmonic ostium of the PDA measured by the aortogram. The waist of the selected device should be 1.5–2.0 times the determined size of the pulmonic ostium of the PDA.
8) Using the included product specification chart, a multipurpose angled tip guiding catheter (end hole with no side holes) is selected. This will be used to deliver the device. The product specification chart will indicate the minimum inner diameter of guiding catheter the ACDO will pass through.
9) A braided steel delivery cable comes attached to the ACDO that is used to advance the ACDO through the catheter and ensures the device can be recaptured if necessary without deforming the catheter. The delivery system is used only once as this will ensure that it has enough integrity to withstand deployment and recapture of the device without deforming.
10) Utilizing the vascular access sheath, a hydrophilic angled or straight guidewire is advanced across the PDA. The use of the multipurpose guiding catheter may facilitate the passage of the guidewire to the PDA.
11) The guiding catheter and guidewire are advanced together across the PDA into the main pulmonary artery. It may be necessary to advance the wire alone initially, which will often be carried by blood flow through the PDA; the catheter is then advanced over the wire into the pulmonary artery.
12) The guidewire is removed and a Cook® Tuohy-Borst hemostasis valve is connected to the end of the guiding catheter.
13) To prepare the device the hoop dispenser and loader are flushed thoroughly with saline.
14) The distal end of the loader is placed through the hemostatic valve and is seated into the hub of the guiding catheter.
15) The device is advanced by feeding the delivery cable forward. Care is taken to ensure the end of the loader is fully advanced through the hemostasis valve and seated in the hub of the catheter to prevent partial deployment of the device in the hemostatic valve. If the device does not load easily into the catheter make certain the device is compatible with the delivery catheter and the loader was properly positioned.
16) The device is advanced within the delivery system by pushing the attached delivery cable forward while under fluoroscopic guidance. The device is advanced until the flat distal disk is deployed in the main pulmonary artery.
17) The partially deployed device, guiding catheter, and delivery cable are retracted as a single unit until the distal disk engages in the pulmonic ostium of the ductus. A tugging sensation should be perceived during retraction.
18) The delivery cable is held in a fixed position while the guiding catheter is retracted to deploy the waist of the device across the pulmonic ostium of the ductus and the cupped proximal disk within the ductal ampulla (Figure 16.4).
19) If the device is deployed correctly the device should assume its native shape. To test proper positioning further gentle push–pull motions on the delivery cable are used and contrast is injected through the delivery system with the delivery cable still attached. PDA flow should nearly cease within 10 min. A small amount of residual flow may be seen and is considered acceptable. Residual flow ceases within 24 h.
20) The device is reconstrainable and repositionable until it is detached from the delivery cable. The device may be retracted into the catheter and then redeployed if it

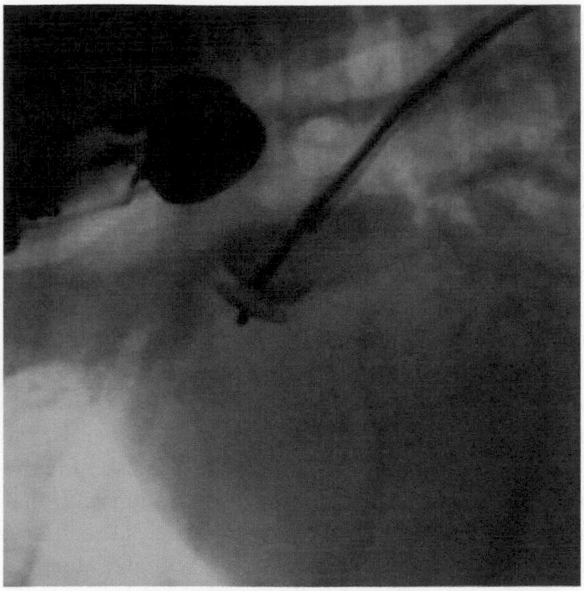

Figure 16.4 The Amplatz® Canine Ductal Occluder fully deployed. The delivery cable remains attached and the delivery catheter is noted caudal to the device with the cable passing through it. The distal disk (furthest from the delivery cable) sits in the main pulmonary artery, and the proximal cup sits in the ductal ampulea with the "waist" of the device crossing through the ductal aperture to the pulmonary artery.

is malpositioned. To recapture the device, the guiding catheter is stabilized and the delivery cable is withdrawn to pull the ACDO back inside the catheter.

21) Once proper positioning has been confirmed, the device is released. The device is released by rotating the delivery cable in a counterclockwise direction. An aortogram is repeated.
22) The delivery cable and delivery system are removed together.
23) The vascular access is closed routinely and then bandaged.

Postprocedure Patient Care

1) The patient should be restricted to a crate or small area to minimize activity for the first 2 weeks. The patient may be taken out on a leash to go to the bathroom but then should be confined again.
2) The patient should not be allowed to take stairs, play with other dogs, run off a leash, or have access to furniture during the first 2 weeks. Extra motion will increase the risk of the ACDO becoming dislodged.
3) The patient should wear an E-collar to prevent them from licking or chewing at the sutures. Licking or chewing can lead to premature removal of the sutures or infection of the surgical site.
4) The sutures should be removed by a veterinarian 10–14 days after the surgery. After the sutures are removed the patient may be taken on leash walks and move freely about the home; but free running and playing with other dogs should still be prohibited.
5) The patient should be re-examined 3 months after the surgery and an echocardiogram should be performed to evaluate for residual flow through the PDA. After the 3-month recheck the patient may slowly return to normal activity levels. Running and playing with other dogs may now be allowed.

Balloon Valvuloplasty for Pulmonic Stenosis

Balloon valvuloplasty is an interventional procedure performed in the cardiac catheterization suite for the treatment of valvular pulmonic stenosis (see Chapter 8). In this procedure, an interventional balloon catheter (Figure 8.10) is inserted into the main pulmonary artery straddling the pulmonic valve. The balloon catheter is then inflated to dilate the valve leaflets to increase flow through the pulmonic valve thereby reducing the obstruction and decreasing the pressure gradient between the right ventricle and main pulmonary artery.

Balloon valvuloplasty can be performed from either a jugular vein access or femoral vein access. Once vascular access has been achieved, the overall procedure is identical. The choice of one site over the other is dictated by operator preference, size of introducer required, and patient size. First, a brief description of each vascular access will be presented, and then the balloon valvuloplasty procedure itself will be described.

Often smaller catheter introducers are used for the beginning of the procedure and exchanged for larger ones to accept the interventional balloon catheter. The final introducer size used is determined by the size of the interventional balloon selected. A measurement from an echocardiogram will give the veterinary cardiologist an estimated range of interventional catheters they wish to use. Generally, the final catheter introducer will be large enough to accept the largest interventional catheter the veterinary cardiologist may select. This will impact the selection of the vascular access site as related to patient body size and the size of interventional catheter potentially needed. The femoral vein may be too small to accept the largest catheter introducer required, and the jugular vein is therefore a better option.

Equipment

- Physiological monitoring equipment: direct pressure transducers, SpO_2, electrocardiogram, etc.
- Surgical masks, surgical caps, and surgical shoe covers
- Surgical hand scrub brushes, surgical gowns, and sterile gloves
- Lead aprons and radiation safety gear
- Sterile surgical preparation scrubs, solutions, and supplies
- Patient drapes
- Large table drape
- Four towel pack
- Small (24″ × 24″) extra drapes
- Image intensifier cover
- Cardiovascular instrument pack
- 1 L heparinized saline solution (~3000 IU/L)
- 10 mL syringes (with or without Luer-lock as surgeon prefers)
- Two basins, and two stopcocks
- Power injector with syringe and pressure injection line
- Iohexol radiographic contrast (4–5 mL/kg max dose)
- Scalpel blades: #10, #11
- Catheter introducer with appropriate guidewire and arterial needle (aka vascular access sheath)
- Absorbable 2-0 suture for vessel retraction/ligature

- 0.035″ × 150 cm J-tipped guidewire
- Suture: absorbable 2-0, absorbable 3-0, and nonabsorbable 3-0 for closing incision
- Angiography catheter: Berman™ catheter or pigtail catheter (typically 4–8F × 75–100 cm)
- or 7F PA flow-directed catheter accepting a 0.035″ guidewire
- 0.035″ × 200 or 260 cm J-tipped full exchange guidewire
- Assorted sizes of Tyshak® balloon valvuloplasty catheters

Vascular Access to the Femoral Vein [11]

The following is a description of the transcutaneous (Seldinger) technique (see Chapter 8). For the purposes of completeness, this description includes an explanation of "upsizing" in which a small vascular sheath is used first, then once vascular access is securely obtained, the small introducer is exchanged for one of an appropriate size to carry the interventional catheter. This "upsizing" step is not necessary; yet some cardiologists may choose to employ it. A surgical cut-down procedure may also be used for femoral vein access as described in the PDA section above.

1) After following routine protocols for anesthesia the patient should be placed in lateral or dorsal recumbency. Lateral recumbency may be adequate. However, dorsal recumbency may be preferred if larger introducers are required for the procedure.
2) The inguinal region of the selected leg is shaved and then surgically prepared in accordance with hospital protocols.
3) The femoral arterial pulse is palpated using the index and middle finger of one hand. Then using the other hand a 21 gauge arterial needle connected to a 3 cm^3 syringe filled with 1–2 cm^3 of saline is directed at a 45 degree angle medial and caudal to the palpated pulse and into the femoral vein.
4) After a flash of blood is seen, the syringe is detached from the needle. The flash should be a gentle flow of blood, not a pulsatile ejection of blood, which would indicate arterial puncture.
5) The introducer and all guidewires are flushed with heparinized saline. A 0.018″ guidewire from a 4F micropuncture set is selected to advance into the lumen of the femoral vein. The guidewire should advance with minimal resistance. If excessive force is used to advance the guidewire the wire may become kinked or curled. Remember the mantra: *never lose sight of the wire.*
6) With the guidewire in place the needle is removed and a #11 blade is used to make a small nick to allow room for advancement of the introducers.
7) The 4F micropuncture set is advanced over the guidewire and into the lumen of the femoral vein. The inside dilator of the 4F micropuncture set is removed and a 0.035″ guidewire is placed.
8) With the 0.035″ guidewire in place the 4F introducer is removed and a larger size introducer is advanced over the guidewire. The size of the larger introducer is guided by the expected size required for the interventional catheter. The larger introducers may meet more resistance at the entry point into the vessel but they should never be forced into the lumen of the vessel [6]. The guidewire and dilator of the large introducer are removed. The larger introducer is secured into place. To determine if the introducer was placed properly, negative pressure is applied to the side

port which should produce venous blood. The introducer is then flushed with heparinized saline.

Pulmonic Stenosis via the Jugular Vein [12,13]

The following description is for a cut-down procedure of the jugular vein for vascular access. A transcutaneous (Seldinger) technique described above and in Chapter 8 for the introduction of smaller bore introducers may also be used in the jugular vein.

1) After following routine protocols for anesthesia the patient should be placed in left lateral recumbency. Catheterization of the right jugular is generally preferred since the presence of a persistent left cranial vena cava would direct the catheter into the coronary sinus rather than the right atrium. The right jugular vein rarely has anomalous venous drainage.
2) The area over the right jugular vein is shaved from the base of the skull to the point of the shoulder and from the left jugular vein to the dorsal midline. The clipped area is surgically prepared in accordance with hospital protocols.
3) The jugular vein is accessed via a surgical cut-down technique followed by ligation of the jugular vein once the procedure is completed.
4) The introducer and all guidewires are flushed with heparinized saline.
5) The jugular vein is dissected. Two pieces of 2-0 absorbable suture or moistened umbilical tape are passed behind the vessel with right angle forceps to isolate the vein.
6) A #11 blade is used to make a small incision parallel to the long axis of the jugular vein.
7) The J-tipped introducer guidewire is inserted into the jugular vein with the J-tip going in first. It is advanced until at least 5 or 6 cm of the guidewire is passed into the lumen.
8) A vein dilator and introducer that will accommodate the size of the balloon catheter are advanced over the guidewire until the guidewire passes through the hub of the vein dilator and can be grasped. Always maintain a hold on the guidewire. Remember the mantra: *never lose sight of the wire*. Then, the vein dilator and introducer can be inserted into the vein together.
9) The caudal ligature may need to be loosened to allow the introducer to pass. Once the introducer is secure retighten the ligature over the introducer.
10) The vein dilator and guidewire are removed. To determine if the introducer was placed properly, negative pressure is applied to the side port which should produce venous blood. The introducer is then flushed with heparinized saline.

Balloon Valvuloplasty Procedure

1) Once vascular access has been achieved, a 5–6F flow-directed pulmonary capillary wedge pressure (Swan–Ganz) catheter is advanced into the right atrium from the vena cava (cranial or caudal depending on vascular access), through the tricuspid valve and into the right ventricle. From the right ventricle the catheter is pushed into the main pulmonary artery across the pulmonic valve.
2) The proximal end of the catheter (the part in the operator's hand) is connected to a direct pressure transducer via a saline flushed line and the pressure of the main pulmonary artery is recorded. The catheter is retracted into the right ventricle to record

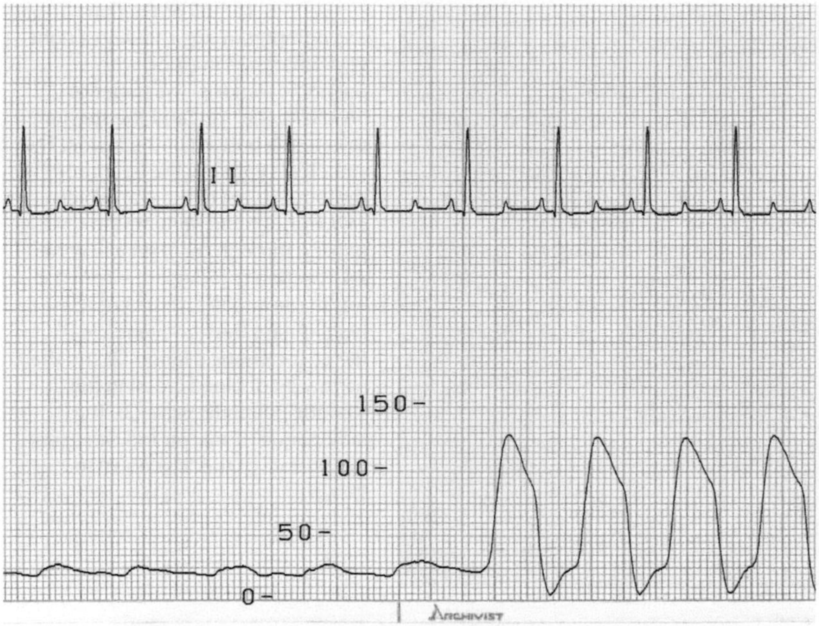

Figure 16.5 A direct pressure trace taken from the main pulmonary artery (PA) and the right ventricle (RV) in a dog with pulmonic stenosis. The top line shows the electrocardiogram. The lower line shows the pressures recorded in the main PA. As the catheter is withdrawn, the tracing demonstrates the pressure in the RV, as indicated by the classic waveform and increase in the difference in the systolic and diastolic pressures. The main PA the pressure reads 25/20 mmHg and in the RV 130/0 mmHg which indicates a RV to PA pressure difference of 105 mmHg. The normal pressure difference is approximately 10–15 mmHg.

the pressure there. The catheter is retracted into the right atrium and the pressure is recorded (Figure 16.5). The difference between the right ventricular pressure and the main pulmonary artery pressure equals the *pressure gradient.* The catheter is then completely withdrawn.

Note: some institutions have moved away from this step. Intraoperative transesophageal echocardiography Doppler is being used to assess the pressure gradient before and after the intervention. Transesophageal echocardiography can also be used to help align the interventional balloon through the pulmonic valve.

3) A 5–6F angiographic catheter is placed through the introducer and advanced into the right ventricle. This could be a Berman^{TM} catheter or a pigtail catheter. To obtain the best angiographic image, the thorax of the patient should be placed in lateral recumbency. This position will provide a better view of the hinge points of the pulmonary valve so as to obtain a more accurate measurement of the annulus.
4) A contrast ventriculogram is performed by injecting the radiopaque contrast at a rate appropriate for the intrinsic rate of flow (0.5–1.0 mL/kg of contrast solution at 20 mL/s) [10] with the power injector (Figure 16.6). A calibrated radiopaque marker or calibrated guidewire should be in the field of view. The pulmonic valve annulus should be measured during systolic frames.

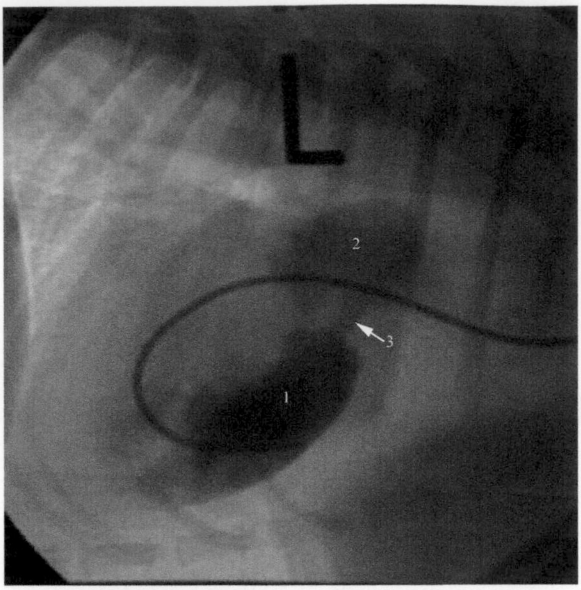

Figure 16.6 Lateral projection angiographic image showing a right ventriculogram in a dog with pulmonic stenosis. The patient's head is to the right and the sternum toward the bottom of the image. The catheter is entering the heart from the jugular vein to the cranial vena cava through the right atrium passing through the tricuspid valve. An injection of radiopaque contrast was made into the right ventricle highlighting the right ventricle (1), the post stenotic dilation (2) and the narrow jet of blood crossing the stenotic pulmonic valve (3). The radiopaque "L" marker indicates size; the bottom of the "L" is equal to 10 mm.

5) The interventional balloon is selected based on the measured size of the annulus. The balloon diameter should be 1.2–1.5 times the size of the measured annulus.
6) The ventriculography catheter is withdrawn from the patient.
7) A Swan–Ganz catheter is advanced back into the main pulmonary artery. A 200 or 260 cm 0.035″ full exchange guidewire is advanced through this catheter into the pulmonary artery. The exchange wire is advanced well into the pulmonary artery to prevent the exchange wire from sliding back into the right ventricle.
8) The catheter is slowly removed while the guidewire is slowly and simultaneously advanced to prevent movement of the guidewire tip from its position in the pulmonary artery. This step must be done under fluoroscopic guidance. The goal is to remove the catheter without changing the location of the guidewire.
9) The interventional catheter should be pre-inflated before crossing the pulmonic valve. Contrast is necessary to observe the balloon function via fluoroscopy; but contrast agents tend to be viscous. Rapid inflation and deflation is important so contrast dilution is recommended. The balloon is inflated to ensure proper inflation and the absence of bubbles. This may be accomplished by inflating the balloon while it is in the caudal vena cava using a dilute saline and contrast mixture of 3:1 [11] or 1:1 [12, 13]. This may also be done at the instrument table before passing the catheter into the patient. The protective sheath is pulled toward the operator on the catheter shaft to expose the balloon. The balloon is inflated with the dilute contrast, air is removed and the contrast is completely removed to collapse the balloon. The sheath is replaced and the catheter is ready to be advanced into the patient.
10) With the Swan–Ganz catheter removed and the guidewire maintained in place; a Tyshak® balloon valvuloplasty catheter is slowly advanced over the guidewire and across the stenosis. The balloon catheter is slowly advanced while the guidewire is slowly and simultaneously withdrawn to prevent distal movement of the guidewire deeper into the pulmonary vasculature.

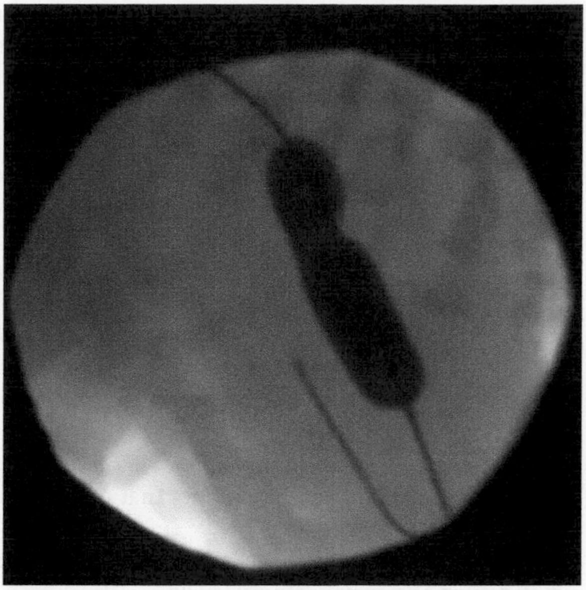

Figure 16.7 The interventional balloon valvuloplasty showing the waist created as the balloon straddles the stenosis during the inflation. At complete balloon inflation the waist will disappear and the full diameter of the balloon will be evident.

11) The balloon is advanced over the guidewire until it is across the pulmonic valve. The midpoint of the balloon is positioned across the stenosis and then the balloon is rapidly inflated while being held in place. The balloon is inflated until a definite "waisting" and subsequent loss of a waist is observed (Figure 16.7). The balloon is left inflated for approximately 6 s and then is rapidly deflated. It is possible that while the balloon is inflated the patient will have arrhythmias on its ECG. Upon deflation of the balloon the ECG should return to normal. If the arrhythmias persist a subsequent inflation should not be performed and the balloon should be retracted into the right ventricle. Two following inflations are performed to ensure no residual waist is seen.
12) The balloon catheter is slowly and carefully retracted while the exchange wire is slowly advanced to keep its position in the pulmonary artery until the catheter is completely removed. The exchange wire is then removed.
13) The Swan–Ganz catheter is returned to the pulmonary artery and the pressure gradient re-assessed. The therapy may be repeated with a larger interventional balloon not to exceed 1.5 times the annulus diameter, or with the same balloon as necessary. In a successful procedure the pressure gradient across the stenosis should be reduced by 50% [11–13].
14) The catheter and guidewire are removed.
15) If a percutaneous Seldinger technique was used, then constant pressure is applied to the puncture site for 10–15 min to avoid hematoma formation as the introducer is pulled from the vessel. A bandage is applied as needed.
16) For a surgical cut-down procedure, the jugular vein is ligated cranial to the incision in the vein before the introducer is removed. A loose suture knot is placed caudal to the incision around the vessel and introducer shaft. The introducer is removed slowly and the knot is tightened immediately. Double ligation may be appropriate

above and below the incision site. The vessel is inspected for hemorrhage before closing the incision. The vascular access site is closed routinely and bandaged.

Postprocedure Patient Care

1) The patient should be given a recheck echocardiogram 24 h after the procedure. The maximal transpulmonic pressure should be measured to determine the benefit derived from the procedure. Anesthesia tends to lower pulmonary arterial pressures so the pressure gradient will likely be greater than what was recorded during the procedure. If the gradient is still 50% of the original pre-anesthesia gradient, then the procedure is considered beneficial. A normal pressure gradient is very rarely achieved.
2) The bandages may be removed 24–48 h after the procedure and the patient should be monitored for any signs of swelling or bleeding from under the bandage.
3) During the first 10–14 days following the procedure the patient's activity should be restricted to allow the incision site and vein to heal sufficiently. The patient may go on walks and go out to the bathroom but excessive play should be prohibited. A harness is recommended for those patients that experienced jugular access until healing is complete.
4) Sutures may be removed 10–14 days after the procedure. After this period the patient may return to normal activity levels.
5) The patient should be seen again in 3 months and then 6–12 months after that for an echocardiogram to re-evaluate the pressure gradient across the pulmonic valve as this can change over time after the procedure.
6) Further evaluations will depend on the severity of the disease, progression of the disease, and owner compliance [13].

Pacemaker Therapy

Implantation of permanent pacemaker systems is a common procedure for veterinary cardiologists. Permanent pacemakers are used to treat symptomatic, pathologic bradycardias like sick sinus syndrome and third degree atrioventricular block. These rhythms are discussed more completely in Chapter 4. Pacemaker implantation is more commonly performed in dogs since they are more apt to develop bradyarrhythmias and have a slower ventricular escape rate. Although cats may develop third degree atrioventricular block, their ventricular escape rate is often over 100 bpm and a pacemaker is generally not necessary. The first reported use of cardiac pacing in veterinary medicine was in a horse in 1967 [14]. The first use of a cardiac pacemaker in a dog was just a year later.

The pacemaker system consists of two main components: the pulse generator and the pacing lead. The pulse generator delivers the electrical impulse through an electrode in the pacing lead to depolarize the myocardium, causing the heart to contract. Either the ventricle alone (single chamber pacing) or the ventricle and the atrium (dual chamber pacing) can be paced (Figures 16.8 and 16.9). In recent years, dual chamber physiological pacing has become more common. The pulse generator is powered by a lithium iodide battery that has a life expectancy of 8–10 years when new. The pulse generators used in veterinary medicine are usually human units that have exceeded their shelf life for human implantation. These pulse generators have 6–8 years of battery life when acquired for veterinary use, which meets the needs of most veterinary patients.

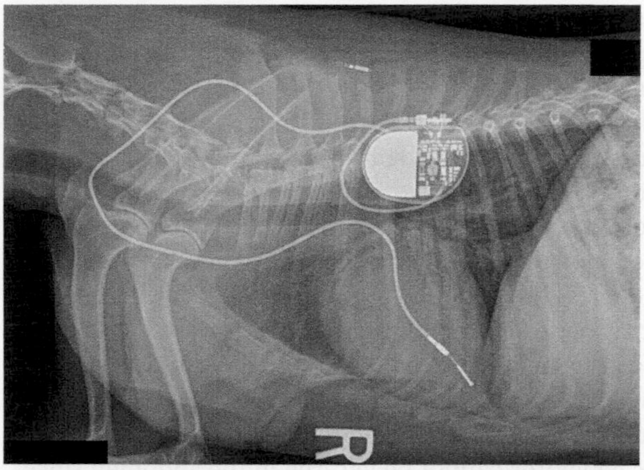

Figure 16.8 A right lateral radiograph of a single chamber pacemaker system. The pulse generator is located in the subcutaneous tissue caudal to the scapula. The pacemaker lead is tunneled under subcutaneous tissue to the jugular vein; traveling through the vein to the cranial vena cava, right atrium then to the right ventricle. The two electrodes of the lead can be seen at the end; one on the tip and another about 1 cm proximal. No helix can be seen indicating this as a passive fixation lead.

There are two types of pulse generators available, unipolar and bipolar. A bipolar system uses a lead with two electrodes at the tip. Current is delivered through one electrode and returns to the generator via the other electrode and the pacing lead. Unipolar systems use the patient's body as the return conduction system. The bipolar system is preferred because it is less likely to cause muscle fasciculation as the impulse returns to the pulse generator through the pacing lead and is less likely to have sensing errors due to external stimulation.

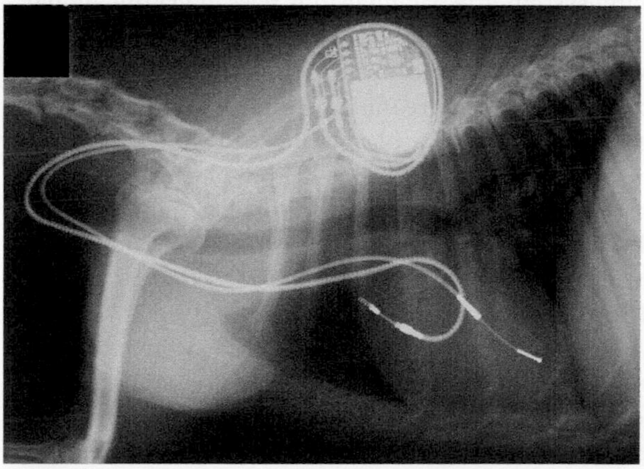

Figure 16.9 A right lateral radiograph of a dual chamber pacemaker system. The pulse generator is located in the subcutaneous tissue caudal to the scapula. The pacemaker leads are tunneled under subcutaneous tissue to the jugular vein; traveling through the vein to the cranial vena cava. The ventricular lead continues through the right atrium then to the right ventricle, while the atrial lead turns back to the right auricle. In this example the atrial lead is an active fixation and the ventricular is a passive fixation lead; both are bipolar.

There are also two basic lead placement systems available for cardiac pacing: endocardial and epicardial. Epicardial pacing systems consist of a generator with a pacing lead that is attached to the *left ventricular epicardium* or outer surface of the left ventricle. This system is implanted using an abdominal incision with a transdiaphragmatic approach to the pericardium. A small opening is made in the diaphragm right where the heart is situated. The pericardium is then opened to expose the apex of left ventricle. The lead is literally screwed into the epicardium of the left ventricular apex with a corkscrew-type tip on the lead or plunged in the myocardium with a barbed hook type of lead. Both of these types then have a suture ring around the electrode to further secure the lead to the myocardium. The lead is then brought through the diaphragm and attached to the generator, which is generally placed within the muscle layers of the abdominal wall, or in the subcutaneous tissue outside the abdominal cavity. It is preferable to have the pulse generator near the body wall for more feasible interrogation of the pulse generator later. The pulse generator cannot be left free in the abdomen since this may allow the lead to create strangulation on the liver, bowel, or spleen and the pulse generator to move in the abdomen. The pulse generator must be secured in place and any extra lead secured with it. The pericardium is closed, adding another layer of tension to hold the lead in place. The diaphragm is closed, followed by the abdominal incision.

Epicardial pacing is most commonly used in very small patients (e.g. cats and ferrets), when vascular access is a problem, when there is another reason for a celiotomy (e.g. abdominal tumor), or when training and equipment for transvenous endocardial pacing is lacking. Epicardial pacing requires surgical skill and positive pressure ventilation since the thorax is opened at the diaphragm. Epicardial leads are typically unipolar, but newer bipolar leads are becoming available.

Endocardial transvenous pacing is less invasive than epicardial pacing since it does not require the opening of a body cavity. Endocardial leads can be either unipolar or bipolar. In the endocardial transvenous pacing system, the pacing lead is passed via the jugular vein (transvenous), through the right atrium and into the apex of the right ventricle. Either jugular vein may be used, but the right is typically chosen to avoid any undiagnosed persistent cranial left vena cava. This procedure must be done with fluoroscopic guidance to ensure proper placement of the lead. Once placed, the lead is either actively screwed into the endocardium with a corkscrew-like tip or is held in place passively by grappling hook-type projections or *tines* that snag the trabeculae of the right ventricle (Figure 16.10). These systems hold the lead tip in place until scar tissue surrounds the lead tip, anchoring it more securely.

The jugular vein is ligated distal to the lead insertion point and the lead is secured with the proximal portion of the vessel. Surgical ligation of the jugular vein causes no problems in dogs due to their excellent collateral vascularization. The remaining distal portion of the lead is then tunneled under the superficial muscles of the neck and connected to the pulse generator (Figure 16.11). The lead is secured to the pulse generator with set screws. These tiny screws are essential for establishing a secure attachment and electrical contact between the lead and the generator. The pulse generator is sutured into a pocket under the superficial muscles on the dorsolateral aspect of the neck. Currently, the endocardial pacing system is most commonly used due to equipment availability, ease of placement, lower morbidity, and decreased anesthetic complication rate compared with epicardial pacing [15].

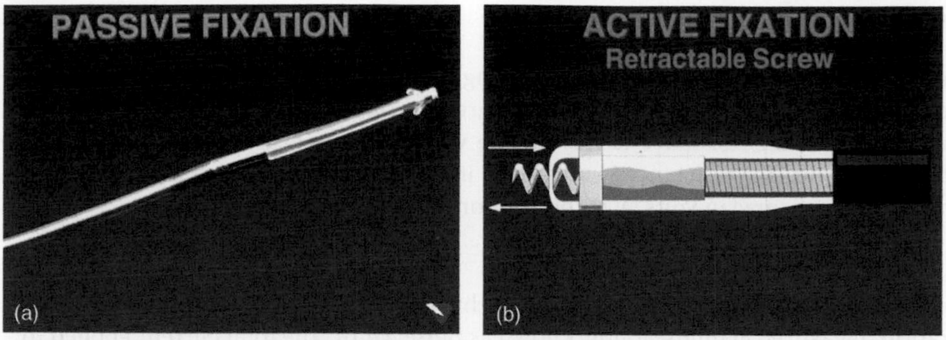

Figure 16.10 A close-up view of the pacemaker lead fixation types. (a) Passive fixation lead with small projections that "grapple" to the right ventricular endocardial trabeculae securing the lead until scar tissue formation occurs. (b) Active fixation lead shows the "corkscrew" style projection that is twisted into the right ventricular endocardium to secure in place.

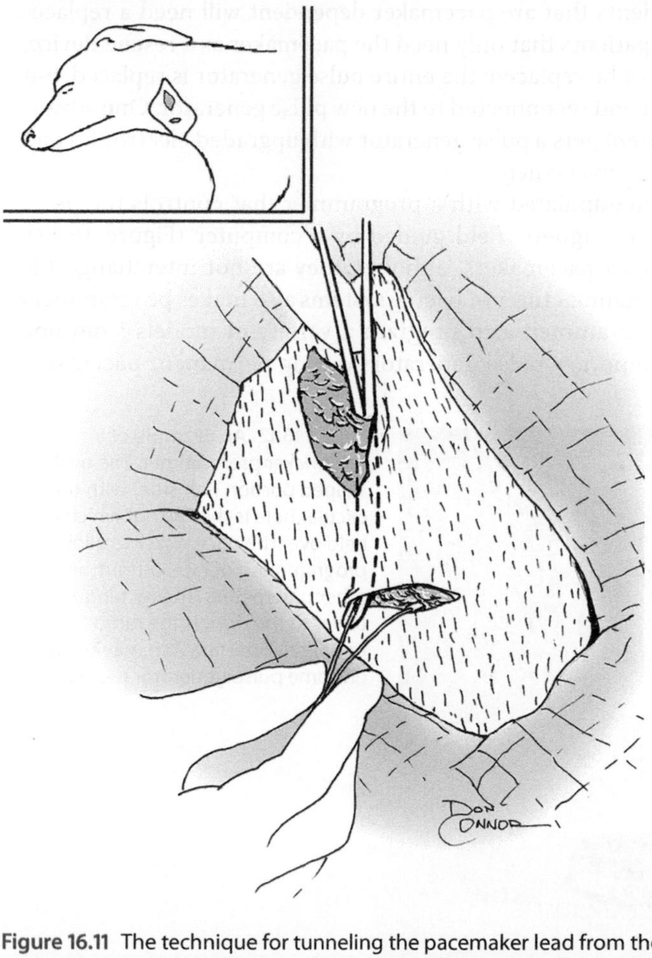

Figure 16.11 The technique for tunneling the pacemaker lead from the venotomy site to the dorsal neck where the pulse generator can be placed. The pulse generator may be positioned in the dorsal neck or behind the scapula depending on the patient size. Source: Courtesy of Don Conner.

Electrical Theory of Pacemakers

The lithium iodine pacemaker batteries, though only about 3 volts, are capable of producing sufficient energy to depolarize the heart. The *current* (I) delivered by the battery must overcome the resistance to flow of the voltage to the heart created by the lead and heart tissue. The resistance is measured in *ohms* (Ω), and the output of the pulse generator is measured in volts (V). The relationship (Ohm's Law) is:

$$I = V/\Omega \qquad (16.1)$$

The volts delivered are known as *amplitude*. This voltage is delivered as a "pulse" of brief duration, measured in milliseconds, known as *pulse width*. The total current applied to the myocardium is the amplitude multiplied by the pulse width.

The current needs to be controlled such that sufficient energy is delivered to depolarize the heart, but battery strength is not wasted. The pacemaker discharge rate (i.e. the heart rate) also must be controlled. Pacemaker batteries deplete faster the more they are used, so high heart rates and high currents will deplete a battery faster than low currents and slow heart rate. Patients that are pacemaker dependent will need a replacement pacemaker sooner than patients that only need the pacemaker as a rescue device. Pulse generator batteries cannot be replaced; the entire pulse generator is replaced, but the lead may be left in the heart and reconnected to the new pulse generator. One advantage of this approach is the patient gets a pulse generator with upgraded electronics and functionality when they need a replacement.

Pacemaker settings can be manipulated with a programmer that controls the pulse generator noninvasively with a magnetic field guided by a computer (Figure 16.12). A programmer is available for all pacemakers, although they are not interchangeable between manufacturers. Each manufacturer of pacing systems also makes programmers for their systems. Modern programmers can program a variety of models from one manufacturer and serve as temporary pulse generators during permanent pacemaker

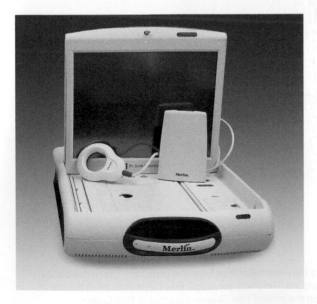

Figure 16.12 An example of a pacemaker programmer. The oval shaped portion (left side) with the circular hole is the "wand" which is held over the pacemaker to allow programming of rate, output, and other parameters. The rectangular tower to the right is the radio frequency antenna that may be used on some pulse generator models.

implantation. The available parameters that are programmable vary with the model of pulse generator, but all pacemakers allow control of the pulse (heart) rate, voltage amplitude, pulse width, and level of sensing native heartbeats and pacing mode. Newer pulse generators are highly programmable allowing for programming of sleep modes, variable rates depending on patient activity, automatic threshold tests, and arrhythmia recording.

Pacemaker Programming

Pacing Modes

To understand programming of a pacemaker one must first understand pacing *mode* (Table 16.2). Pacemakers may be set to a variety of pacing modes. These modes determine the overall function of the pacemaker. Pacemakers will not only pace the heart, but they will also sense native cardiac activity. The sensing feature provides two functions: the first is a safety feature to keep the pacemaker from firing during repolarization; the second is to allow for sensing of one chamber then subsequent pacing of a different

Table 16.2 Common examples of pacing modes. This list is not exhaustive, but will give the reader a basis for deciphering pacing modes they may encounter.

MODE	Chamber paced	Chamber sensed	Trigger/inhibited	Rate responsive
VOO	Ventricle	None	None	No
VVI	Ventricle	Ventricle	Inhibited	No
VVIR	Ventricle	Ventricle	Inhibited	Yes
AOO	Atria	None	None	No
AAI	Atria	Atria	Inhibited	No
DDD	Atria/ventricle	Atria/ventricle	Inhibits/triggers*	No†
VDD	Ventricle	Atria/ventricle	Inhibits/triggers*	No†
DDDR	Atria/ventricle	Atria/ventricle	Inhibits/triggers*	Yes

V, ventricle. A, atria. I, inhibited. D, dual. R, rate responsive.

*Dual trigger and inhibiting means that if a native complex is sensed in either chamber the pacing is inhibited in that chamber. If an atrial native complex is sensed but no ventricular complex is sensed, then the pacemaker will fire in the ventricle only. If no atrial complex is sensed within the set heart rate interval, then the pacemaker will fire in the atria; if no subsequent ventricular complex is sensed within the pre-set time, the pacemaker will fire in the ventricle as well. This represents the "dual" function of triggering when needed and inhibiting when needed.

†VDD and DDD modes will have some native rate change. True rate responsiveness is programmed into the pulse generator; these modes use the intrinsic rate of the sinoatrial node to drive ventricular pacing. VDD differs from DDD in that VDD uses a special lead and that the atria can only be sensed, and not paced. A pacemaker set in these modes will sense the ventricle and pace if needed in response. If a native ventricular impulse is sensed the pacemaker does not fire until the next atrial sense or the lower limit of pace rate is reached. These modes are particularly useful for third degree atrioventricular block because the ventricular pacing rate will be driven by the native atrial depolarizations, thereby allowing the patient to maintain a more physiological heart rate. These modes are considered more physiologic because the heart rate will change with sympathetic nervous system tone; if the atrial rate increases due to stimulation the ventricle will respond accordingly.

chamber. The modes allow for complicated sensing and pacing and synchronization of atrial and ventricular depolarization to achieve a more physiological function.

Pacing modes are identified by a four letter code system. This system designates the first letter to be the chamber paced, the second letter is the chamber sensed, the third letter indicates the pulse generator function when a native beat is sensed, and the final letter is optional and indicates if a pacemaker is *rate responsive* (Table 16.2). Rate responsive pulse generators increase the pacing rate in response to patient activity. The abbreviations used are: V, ventricle; A, atria; D, dual(atrial and ventricular); O, nothing; I, inhibit; T, trigger; R, rate responsive. The most basic mode is VOO or ventricle paced; nothing sensed and because there is no sensing, there is nothing done. This mode paces at the programmed rate regardless of the native activity of the heart. There is the danger of pacing "on the T wave", inducing ventricular fibrillation.

Most systems are programmed to VVI mode and fire only when the patient's heart rate drops below a preset value (aka demand mode). In VVI mode the designation indicates that the ventricle is paced, the ventricle sensed, and the pulse generator is inhibited from firing when a native beat is detected. If the pacemaker is set for 80 bpm and the patient's native heart rate is 90 bpm, the pacemaker simply monitors. When the patient's heart rate drops to 60 bpm the pacemaker starts firing at 80 bpm. It will continue to fire until the patient's heart rate increases above 80 bpm.

As pulse generators available to the veterinary market have become more sophisticated, rate responsive pacing has become more popular since it provides for some physiological heart rate variability. A good example is VVIR pacing. This mode is identical to VVI pacing with the added feature of an upper and lower rate setting. The pacemaker will stop the heart rate from going below the lower limit, and when the patient exercises the pacing rate will increase based on the patient's activity as sensed by an accelerometer in the pulse generator. The pacemaker will not sense sympathetic nervous system signals, however, so an adrenaline rush will not cause a pace rate increase, only the activity will. The pacemaker will still be inhibited by any native impulses.

Other pacing modes, including dual chamber pacing to achieve a more physiologic contraction, are now available. By placing a pacing lead in the atria as well as the ventricle, the atria can be sensed and/or paced with the ventricle set to follow at a physiological interval. This works particularly well in case of third degree atrioventricular block where the atria depolarize normally, but the impulse is not conducted to the ventricle. In dual chamber pacing, the pacemaker can be set to DDD or VDD modes.

Threshold Testing

A standard evaluation done at every recheck for any pacing system is the *threshold* test. The threshold test is used to determine the minimum amount of current necessary to depolarize the heart and cause a myocardial contraction. The threshold test is performed by attaching the patient to an ECG, then using the pacemaker programmer to gradually reduce the amplitude until *capture* is lost; capture referring to sufficient energy to cause contraction. The amplitude is restored to its previous setting and the test is repeated by reducing the pulse width until capture is lost. The points at which capture is lost for amplitude and pulse width can be plotted into a graph, and a threshold determined (Figure 16.12). Modern pacemaker programmers have functions to run a threshold test that, once started, will automatically drop the current and restore the previous setting immediately after capture is lost.

Once the threshold is determined the pacemaker output is set to be at least twice the threshold to allow a margin of safety. During the initial healing and maturation of the lead contacting the myocardium, the *impedance* or resistance (Ω) usually increases. The increase in resistance means less current reaches the myocardium and the threshold increases. The margin of safety is important to ensure capture during healing. The output should not be set much higher than twice the threshold because it will more rapidly deplete the battery.

Other Pacemaker Functions

Many other parameters such as sensitivity, rate responsive functions, automatic threshold tests, and arrhythmia event recording can be programmed. The pulse generator can even be programmed to switch mode if necessary due to an arrhythmia. The sensitivity setting of the pacemaker indicates the minimum amplitude of a native depolarization is necessary for the pulse generator to count it as beat. For example, if the sensitivity is set for 2.0 mV then the pacemaker will disregard any electrical activity it senses less than 2.0 mV. Setting the pacemaker sensitivity correctly allows the pacemaker to not be "fooled" by T waves, mistaking them for ventricular depolarizations. Incorrect sensing will usually lead to incorrect pacing rates.

Another important parameter of pacemaker function is the *refractory period.* The refractory period is the time after any depolarization the pulse generator senses that it waits before it begins to count the time for the next beat. This period ensures that the pacemaker does not fire on the T waves. When programming the pacemaker it is important to set the refractory period longer than the normal Q–T interval of the patient, usually about 300–325 ms. A feature similar to refractory period is the *blanking period.* The difference is that during the refractory period the pacemaker is sensing for another depolarization, but during the blanking period no sensing occurs. The blanking period is generally very short. In dual chamber pacing there are atrial and ventricular blanking periods. The atrial blanking ensures that the atrial lead does not mistake ventricular activity as atrial, and may be set to start *after* the ventricular depolarization. Known as the *postventricular atrial blanking period,* it allows for proper synchronization of the atria and ventricular activity of the pacemaker.

Hysteresis is a function that allows extra time for native activity to occur before the pacemaker rescues the heart. Hysteresis is particularly useful in pacing for sick sinus syndrome. For example, with the hysteresis turned on, the pacemaker may be set to let the heart pause for a time equal to 40 bpm, and when the time limit is reached, the pacemaker paces at a rate of 60 bpm.

Rate responsive functions control how quickly the pulse generator increases or decreases rates; factors such as the amount of motion before the rate is prompted to increase, how fast the rate increases once it starts, and how fast it recovers to the base rate can all be controlled. Each pacemaker manufacturer has different control for each model, and the operator must familiarize themselves with the function of each model they interrogate.

A particularly useful feature of modern pacemakers is the automatic threshold test. The system can be programmed to run a threshold test at a set time; usually during the sleep cycle at night. The pacemaker can either store that data for later retrieval or can actually change the current to maintain the margin of safety. Parameters can also be programmed into the pulse generator to record high or low heart rate events and store an ECG for later viewing. This can be useful in diagnosing tachyarrhythmias that may occur or a loss of capture.

Because of the sophisticated nature of the modern pacing systems, it is beyond the scope of this text to cover all possible programming features. The operator should take the time to learn features of each programmer at their disposal, and the different model of pulse generators they use. A pacemaker does not have to be implanted to be interrogated, and one can practice with any model of pulse generator their programmer will interrogate by simply placing the magnet wand over the pacemaker in the sterile packaging. You can then see what functions a particular model has and can manipulate them to learn how to use the programmer. All pacemaker companies provide 24-h technical supports for their systems. The technical support phone number can be posted with the programmer for quick reference. Technical support can usually answer any questions regarding the function of the pacemaker. They will not be able to give answers regarding arrhythmias or patient care.

Trouble Shooting a Pacing System

There are several potential problems that can be seen with pacemaker systems that are not complications of the implantation. Eventually the batteries will exhaust, pacing function may cease or be intermittent, and/or expected rate of pacing may be incorrect. Dual chamber systems increase the potential problems twofold. This section will address some of the more common malfunctions of single chamber pacing and their corrections. Due to the complex nature of dual chamber pacing, the reader is referred to a pacemaker specific text [16].

One question commonly asked by clients is "What happens when the battery runs out?" Generally speaking, a pacemaker battery will last 8–10 years when new; most pulse generators implanted in veterinary patients have reached their "shelf-life" for human implantation and have 6–8 years of battery life left. All pulse generators are preprogrammed not to suddenly turn off as the battery weakens. When the battery is within 9 months of expiring on the current settings it reaches the *elective replacement indicator.* The indicator appears during interrogation to inform the cardiology staff to schedule a replacement within 6 months. The final stage is the *end of life* (EOL) indicator. During this time the pulse generator will automatically change its mode and output setting to conserve battery life. Each manufacturer programs this slightly differently, but a common function is to have the pulse generator switch modes to a VVI mode at a lower rate than previously set; for example, if the base rate was 100 bpm, the pacemaker will reduce the rate to 70 bpm. If the pacemaker cannot be changed within a specified time, the pulse rate may drop to 50 bpm. This keeps the patient safe until a new system can be implanted.

One of the most serious problems is a loss of capture. There are several causes. First, the operator needs to determine if the loss of capture is complete or intermittent and if there is still a pacing stimulus but no capture.

Lead dislodgement is a common cause of both intermittent and complete loss of capture. This means the lead is no longer in contact with the endocardium and the paced impulse cannot depolarize the tissue. In some instances, the lead may be in sufficient proximity to cause occasional capture, yet in both instances the lead will need to be surgically replaced.

In some cases of capture loss there may simply be an increase in the pacing threshold. This is sometimes termed *exit block*. Reprogramming the pacemaker to a greater current may correct this problem. Some patients may develop such profound increases in threshold that very high current is required, exhausting the battery much sooner than is typical. In such cases a new lead should be placed when the pulse generator is changed and threshold testing should be performed at implantation to locate the optimal position.

Lead fracture can also cause loss of capture and is usually seen to be complete. If the metal wire component of the lead breaks then no electrical impulse can be transmitted to the heart. During interrogation, the operator will notice the impedance will be infinitely high indicating a loss of conduction. Sometimes the break in the lead can be seen on a radiograph. The lead must be changed to correct this issue.

Another reason for loss of capture similar to lead fracture is fracture of the insulation of the lead. During an insulation fracture, the electrical impulse will "leak" from the wire out into the surrounding tissue and fail to be transmitted to the heart. In this case the operator will see extremely low impedance, usually less than 300 Ω. Once again the lead will need to be replaced to correct the problem.

During an intermittent loss of capture one should consider a poor connection at the pulse generator to the lead interface. If the lead is not seated completely into the pulse generator, or the set screws are not securely tightened the circuit may be interrupted causing capture loss. This problem may also be seen on a radiograph and can be corrected by surgically approaching the pulse generator and securing the connection. Finally, reaching the EOL indicator may reduce the rate to preserve battery life and appear to be a loss of capture. Interrogation of the pacemaker should diagnose this problem and the pulse generator can be changed.

If during the evaluation of a capture loss event no pacing stimulus can be noted on the ECG, then the most common cause is lead fracture. This may also be seen during the implantation of a unipolar pacing system before the cardiologist places the pulse generator in contact with the patient. Since a unipolar pacemaker relies on the patient body as part of the circuit, the pulse generator must be touching the patient to complete the circuit. Simply placing the pulse generator in contact with the patient will correct this problem.

Another problem seen with pacing systems is the programmed rate not being achieved or being inconsistent. Usually this is simply due to sensing of native beats and does not need to be corrected. Other times it may be due to improper pacemaker settings. Sensing of T waves is the most common problem. The pacemaker may sense T waves as native activity and reset its beat to beat interval starting point. This may be due to the sensing setting being too low or the refractory period set too short. If the T wave has significant amplitude, the sensing setting may need to be increased. If the T wave is under the sensing threshold, then the refractory period should be increased. The pacemakers usually come with a preset refractory period of 275 ms, which is often too short for most canine patients. This will allow the T wave to occur after the refractory period, tricking the pacemaker into thinking another native beat has occurred. This will reset the refractory period and will make the next paced beat occur later than it should thereby reducing the overall rate per minute. To correct this problem the refractory period should be set to 300–325 ms.

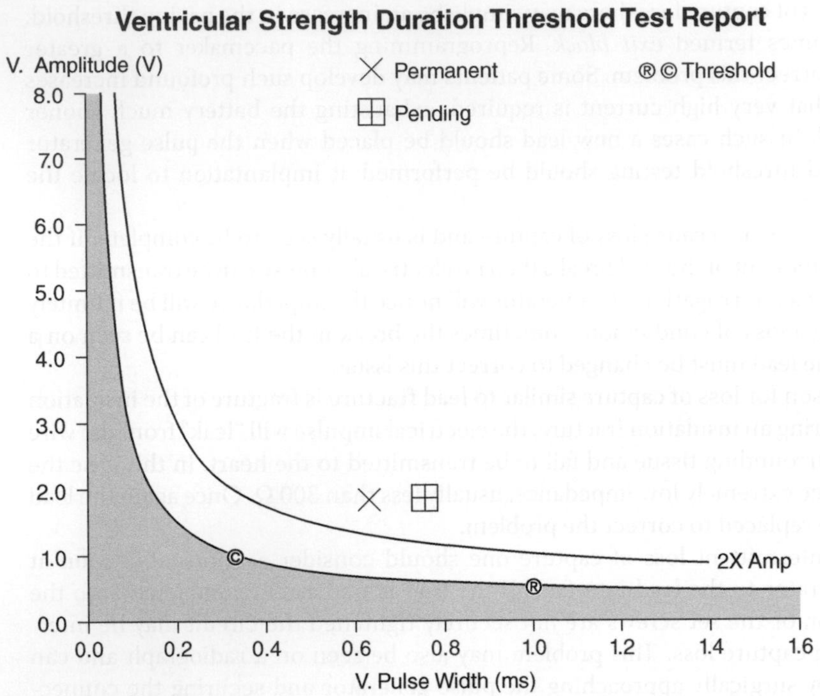

Figure 16.13 A printout of the strength duration curve of a pacemaker threshold test showing the amplitude on the y axis and the pulse width on the x axis. The shaded area under the curve represents the output setting below the pacing threshold. The line labeled "2X Amp" indicates the setting equal to two times the pacing threshold or the margin of safety. The "X" indicates the current settings of the pacemaker, and the box with a cross indicates the proposed setting calculated by the computer; the ® and the © indicate the measurements from which the threshold was calculated. Any setting above the "2X Amp" line will ensure safe pacing.

Temporary Pacing

Patients with sick sinus syndrome or third degree atrioventricular block are often poor candidates for anesthesia due to their decreased heart rate. Application of temporary pacing systems can be used to control the heart rate during the anesthesia required for permanent pacemaker implantation. Two systems are available to accomplish temporary pacing: transthoracic and transvenous. Temporary transthoracic pacing is done by means of adhesive pads attached to the patient's chest over the heart on the left and right sides of the thorax. The pads are connected to a transthoracic pacer via cables (Figure 16.13). The temporary pacer is similar to a cardiac defibrillator, but delivers a much lower output of energy at a preset rate. The electrical current stimulates the heart to contract as current passes through the chest. Transthoracic pacing is simple to use, quickly applied, and will provide a margin of safety during the implantation. The disadvantage is that the patient will twitch on each depolarization since the thoracic muscles are also stimulated by the current impulse. Transthoracic temporary pacing is best used at the lowest rate to keep the patient hemodynamically stable and at the lowest output necessary to generate a pulse. To assure capture of the temporary pacemaker, direct arterial blood pressure measurement is preferred since the technician can see a pulse trace; however, Doppler blood flow detection or digital palpation of the femoral pulse will suffice as a substitute method.

Temporary transvenous pacing may be done with special pacing catheters. These catheters are approximately 100 cm long and have two electrodes at the tip. The catheter is typically introduced into the venous system via the femoral or saphenous vein, and then advanced through the caudal vena cava, the right atrium, the tricuspid valve and into the right ventricle where it makes contact with the endocardium. The proximal end of the catheter has two connections for attachment to an external temporary pulse generator. The catheter is temporarily secured in place for the implantation procedure described below. Transvenous temporary pacing provides stable heart rate control, with no patient movement as seen with transthoracic temporary pacing. The disadvantages include the need for sedation or general anesthesia to insert the pacing catheter, potential arrhythmias from the catheter residing in the heart, and increased time before implantation of the permanent system while the temporary catheter is being placed.

Both temporary pacing systems are reliable and in the hands of experienced operators can be done with minimal complication. Their benefit of controlled heart rate during the surgical implantation of a permanent pacing system vastly outweighs any disadvantages they possess.

Equipment

- Physiological monitoring equipment: direct pressure transducers, SpO_2, electrocardiogram, etc.
- Surgical masks, surgical caps, and surgical shoe covers
- Surgical hand scrub brushes, surgical gowns, sterile gloves
- Lead aprons and radiation safety gear
- Sterile surgical preparation scrubs solutions and supplies
- Patient drapes
- Large table drape
- Four towel pack
- Small extra drapes pack
- Image intensifier cover
- Cardiovascular instrument pack
- 1 L saline solution
- 10 mL syringes (with or without Luer-lock as surgeon prefers)
- One basin
- Scalpel blades; #10, #11
- Suture: 2-0 absorbable, 3-0 absorbable, 3-0 non-absorbable
- Umbilical tape
- Vein pick (usually supplied with new pacing leads)
- Permanent pacemakers
- Permanent pacemaker lead: atrial and ventricular as needed
- Pacing lead stylet
- Pacemaker programmer for model being implanted
- Temporary pulse generator and cables
- Bandage materials including 2″ cast wrap padding, 4″ cast wrap padding, 2″ vet wrap, and 4″ vet wrap

Preparation of the Pacemaker [17]

1) Read the manufacturer's instructions for the pulse generator and lead.
2) Note and record the preprogrammed values for the pacemaker. These settings can be reprogrammed if a programmer is available to allow for optimal performance when necessary.

After Donning Sterile Attire On Sterile Field:

3) Make a curve in one of the stylets by grasping the stylet approximately 5 cm from the tip and then with the other hand pull the wire between the thumb and the index finger. The curve is to prevent the lead from advancing into the caudal vena cava. The curve of the arch in the stylet should therefore match the arch taken to enter the right ventricle.
4) When using an active fixation pacemaker lead the mechanical function should be verified before implanting the device. Within a sterile field insert a straight stylet into the lead. Then use the most distal hole of the fixation tool to grasp the connector pin of the lead. Rotate the fixation tool clockwise until the coiled electrode is completely exposed (1.5–2 coils). The maximum number of rotations is stated in the instructions for each lead. Care should be taken not to make excessive rotations as this may damage the lead. Disconnect the fixation tool from the connector pin to release the lead. This relieves any residual torque on the lead. After this test is completed attach the fixation tool and rotate the tool counter-clockwise to retract the coil back into its protective sheath.

Pacemaker Implantation Procedure [17]

1) After following appropriate protocols for anesthesia the patient should be placed in left lateral recumbency. A rolled towel or gauze roll should be placed under the neck for support. The head should be positioned so that the jugular vein is easily seen and the skin of the neck is mildly taught.
2) Shave and surgically prepare the cervical region. Be sure to include enough room for the pulse generator pocket. The clipped area generally extends from the base of the skull to the shoulder and beyond the midline both ventrally and dorsally toward the left side. The right external jugular vein and location for the pulse generator are surgically scrubbed and prepared following hospital protocol.
3) Drape the prepared area with sterile drapes.
4) A 5–8 cm long incision should be made at the base of the neck slightly dorsal to the jugular vein.
5) The subcutaneous tissue should be bluntly dissected to expose and free up approximately 3–4 cm of the jugular vein.
6) Curved hemostats or right angle forceps are used to slip two strands of absorbable suture under the jugular vein so that the cranial and caudal loop can be grasped to raise the vein manually from the surrounding structures. The cranial ligature is tied and the caudal ligature is held somewhat taught to allow blood to enter and distend the vein while also controlling hemorrhage.
7) Atraumatic thumb forceps are used to pinch one-third to one-half of the diameter of the vein perpendicular to its long axis to cause the vein to tent along its axis.
8) A #11 surgical blade is used to perform a horizontal venotomy. The incision is deep enough to reach the lumen but not deep enough to sever the vein.

9) A curved stylet is inserted into the lumen of the lead, prior to making the venotomy. The lead and the stylet are inserted through the venotomy into central venous circulation. The use of a vein pick may be helpful during this step.
10) Under fluoroscopic guidance the lead and stylet are guided through the jugular vein, cranial vena cava, right atrium, tricuspid valve and finally into the right ventricle. The lead is positioned in the middle of the right ventricle and the curved stylet may be exchanged for a straight stylet to facilitate lead placement in the right ventricular apex.

    Note: If a passive fixation lead is used, skip steps 11 and 12.
11) If using an active fixation lead, the fixation tool is positioned on the connector pin as described in the pacemaker preparation. The lead tip with the straight stylet is gently pressed against the endocardium.
12) Rotate the fixation tool clockwise until the coil is completely extruded and the torque is released. Complete coil extraction is verified via fluoroscopy. When the coil is fully retracted, the two radiopaque crimp sleeves are separated. When the coil is fully extended the two sleeves come together.
13) The stylet is carefully withdrawn once full extension is confirmed.
14) A pacemaker system analyzer is used to obtain initial thresholds. The typical pulse duration in canine patients is 0.5 ms for measuring capture threshold. The maximum acute amplitude should be 1.0 V with a resistance of 300–1200 Ω. The minimum acute sensing amplitude should be 5.0 mV. Values will vary depending on the lead type and cardiac tissue condition. If acceptable values are not initially found, wait 10 min and repeat. If the thresholds are still too high the lead needs to be repositioned.
15) An intracardiac electrogram is recorded through the implanted lead to identify the current of injury and to determine if good contact has been made.
16) With an active fixation lead, a "tug test" is performed with the stylet in place. The lead is gently tugged while the heart is observed with fluoroscopy. If the lead is secured properly resistance will be felt and the lead will move with the heart as it contracts. If the lead is not secure the coil is retracted and repositioned. A passive fixation lead is simply secured into place snugly against the endocardium.
17) Once the lead is securely in place and good contact is made, the permanent lead may be connected to an external pulse generator (Figure 16.14). The temporary external pulse generator is attached by means of a sterile cable dropped from the table to be attached (Figure 16.15). The patient's heart rate can now be controlled while the pocket is made for the permanent pulse generator.

    Alternatively, the stylet is removed and the connector pin is inserted into the permanent pulse generator. Care is taken to ensure the pin is completely in the connecting port and the end of the lead is secured in the pulse generator.
18) A hex wrench tool is inserted through the rubber slit of the grommet to engage the set screw in the connector block. To secure the lead the hex wrench tool is turned clockwise until resistance is felt. Many lead systems come with a "torque" wrench that will click when the correct amount of tightening is reached. Care is taken not to overturn the set screw.

    Note: if the pulse generator is a bipolar system, pacing will begin automatically. If the pulse generator is a unipolar system, pacing will begin when the noninsulated side of the pulse generator contacts the tissue.

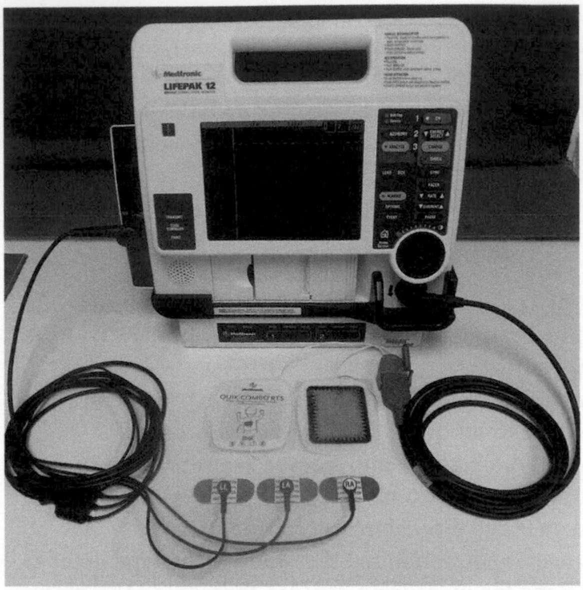

Figure 16.14 A transthoracic pacing system. This device will also function as a defibrillator. The small blue patches shown will provide an electrocardiogram for the system; the larger electrodes just above them are placed on either side of the thorax over the heart. Each side of the pacing patch is shown. The transthoracic pacing system allows control of rate and amplitude only and is for short-term temporary use.

19) Once pacing begins through the permanent lead any other (either transthoracic or transvenous) temporary pacemaker is turned off to avoid complications of two competing pacing systems.
20) A subcutaneous pocket is prepared by digital dissection in the dorsal neck or just caudal to the scapula. The size of the pocket should be large enough to snugly fit the pulse generator and any residual lead but not so large that there is excess space around the generator. Care is taken not to make the pocket too large to prevent

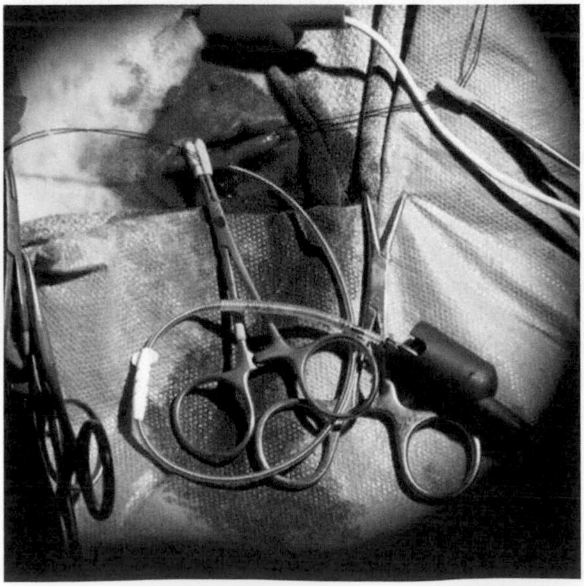

Figure 16.15 The temporary pacing lead wires attached to the permanent pacing lead to control the heart rate while the pocket for the pulse generator is incised. The black clip attaches to the end of the permanent pacemaker lead and the red clip is attached to the patient to complete the circuit. The permanent pacemaker lead can be seen entering the jugular vein, with the white securement collar visible to the left. The collar will be slid along the lead until it can be partially introduced into the vein to allow for circumferential sutures to be secured around the vein, lead, and collar. This collar protects the lead insulation from potential damage caused by the suture.

seroma formation and excess movement of the pulse generator nor too small or the pacemaker may erode through the skin. A small amount of lead slack is allowed and it is pushed into the jugular vein. The remainder of the lead is loosely wrapped in a circle and placed under the pulse generator in the pocket.

21) The permanent lead is disconnected for a very short time while the lead is tunneled under the skin from the jugular incision site to the pulse generator pocket then immediately reattached. Pacing will be disrupted during this process and external temporary pacing may need to be re-established for a short time. The lead is resecured to the pulse generator and the set screws tightened as described in step number 18. The pulse generator is attached to surrounding tissues by placing nonabsorbable sutures through the suture hole located in the pulse generator connector assembly.
22) The lead is secured in the vein with the aid of the grooved anchoring sleeve that fits over the lead. The sleeve is pushed caudally down the lead until it enters the vein. At this point sutures are placed around the sleeve and fascia and tightened securely. Care is taken not to place sutures directly around the bare lead as this could damage the lead insulation.
23) The pulse generator pocket is carefully sutured closed to eliminate any extra space.
24) The subcutaneous tissues are closed routinely.
25) The incision sites are bandaged with gauze, cast padding, and elastic self-adherent bandage material.

Postprocedure Patient Care

Transvenous endocardial pacing is the primary method of pacing today. The surgical site is small and postoperative pain is less than with epicardial pacing. Postimplantation care for epicardial pacing is typically the same as with any abdominal surgery. The pacemaker settings are interrogated the same as with an epicardial pacing system. Postimplantation care of an epicardial pacing system involves analgesia, sedation, and continuous electrocardiographic monitoring. Antibiotics are given peri-operatively and continued postoperatively 12–24 hours parenterally then orally for 1–2 weeks. Opiate sedation/analgesia also keeps the patient quiet after surgery to avoid dislodging the lead thereby necessitating surgical repositioning. The amount and type of sedation/analgesia will be customized to each patient. A bandage is generally placed around the neck to protect the surgical site and reduce seroma formation.

The following day, radiographs are taken in the right lateral and dorsoventral views to confirm the lead placement. Avoid positioning the patient on its back during the first 2 weeks following implantation as this may dislodge the lead. *Neck leads or collars should NEVER be used on a dog with a transvenous pacemaker system*; they should always wear a harness thereafter.

An ECG is used to verify pacemaker function and rate. Pulse generator parameters are programmed to a base setting and the patient is released from the hospital 1–3 days after implantation. At discharge, the client is instructed how to take the patient's heart rate and asked to check it daily until the next visit. If the patient's heart rate goes below the pacing rate, the client is instructed to call the clinic immediately.

The clients are asked to return for suture removal 10–14 days from discharge. At this visit an ECG and thoracic radiographs are performed. The pulse generator is also evaluated with the programmer. As the endocardium develops a reaction around the pacemaker lead tip where it contacts the heart, increased resistance to the pacing impulse can develop. The minimum current the pulse generator needs to "capture" the ventricle, causing it to depolarize and contract, is determined. To verify capture, a continuous ECG is performed while programming the pacemaker while the current is gradually reduced until capture is lost. When this "threshold" is determined, the pacemaker is programmed at a sufficiently high output to assure capture in the event that resistance increases. Typically, an output setting of two times the threshold is programmed to allow a sufficient margin of safety.

A similar follow up visit is scheduled about 1 month postimplant and again at 3 months postimplant at which time radiographs and pulse generator evaluation are performed. Unless complications arise, the client is asked to see their local veterinarian for biannual radiographs and to visit the cardiologist annually for pacemaker system evaluation. At all follow-up visits an ECG, echocardiogram, and pacemaker programming are repeated. Other tests may be added as indicated.

It is recommended to keep conspicuous records of pacemaker details in the patient's chart. The information included should be: pacing mode, rate settings, along with the pacemaker system's location in the patient. When the patient comes into the clinic for follow-up visits the cage ID card should include a "pacemaker" sign or indicator. It is a good idea for these guidelines to be followed at the referring veterinarian's office as well.

Although the stable pacemaker patient can resume a substantially normal life, there are details of patient care that must be remembered. In epicardial pacing, the pacemaker generator is usually located in the abdomen or in between abdominal muscle layers. It must be remembered where the pacemaker is located during palpation so as not to mistake it for a mass. For endocardial transvenous systems the generator and leads are more superficial and greater care must be exercised. During the physical examination the generator is usually palpable and should not be moved, rotated, or mistaken for a mass. Likewise, the lead in the jugular vein is easy to feel. In obtaining blood for laboratory analysis, it is crucial to know where the pacemaker and lead are located. *One should NEVER attempt venipuncture in the jugular vein that carries the pacing lead.* Striking the lead with a hypodermic needle could cause damage to the insulation around the lead or the actual metallic core of the lead resulting in immediate malfunction of the system and potential life-threatening complications for the patient.

The veterinary technician should become acquainted with the electrocardiogram of pacemaker patients [4]. Patients with pacemakers have a distinctive electrocardiogram pattern that shows a "pacing spike" and typically demonstrate wide QRS complexes. Knowing the pacemaker rate setting can also alert the technician to depletion of battery life in a pulse generator. Modern pacemakers are not susceptible to interference from microwave ovens, garage door openers, or pet identification microchip readers. Patients with pacemakers should remain clear of strong magnetic fields such as magnetic resonance imaging or children playing with magnets. Patients that have pacemakers implanted cannot wear electric shock collars like those used with invisible fencing systems.

Although it should be avoided if possible, electrocautery may be used carefully in patients with pacemakers. The safest way to accomplish this is by placing the pacemaker in VOO mode for the duration of the electrocautery use. The patient should also have the electrocautery ground placed such that the pulse generator is *not* between the ground plate and the surgical site. For example, if surgery is done on the knee, then the electrocautery ground plate must be placed under the pelvis. This keeps the electrical current of the cautery from passing over the pacing system.

Complications of Implantation

Complications of pacemakers have been well documented [1; 2, pp. 1308–1309] and can range from mild to serious. The most common complications seen are seroma, or hematoma around the pulse generator, dislodgment of the pacing lead from the heart, congestive heart failure from concurrent heart disease or subsequent myocardial failure, tissue reaction sufficient to prevent pacing capture, and malfunctions of the pacing system.

Infections occur infrequently, and can be months after the implantation, from hematogenous spread. Extreme care should be taken during the procedure to maintain sterility. In the event of pulse generator infection, aggressive antibiotic therapy may be tried, but often removal of the pulse generator is necessary. The pulse generator should be removed, the pocket irrigated thoroughly, and a drain placed and allowed to heal. The new pulse generator should be placed in a new incision and only attached to the existing lead if the surgeon is confident the infection has not invaded the lead. If there is a question about the sterility of the lead, or the infection tracks along the lead, then the entire system will need to be replaced. If possible, the infected lead is removed from the heart and a new lead placed down the other jugular vein and the new pulse generator implanted. In cases where the infection is at the pulse generator and the lead near the pulse generator, the lead may be excised where it enters the jugular vein, then cut and capped and left in place. This can only be done if the infection does not track below the venotomy.

Seroma formation over the pulse generator is also a potential complication. In the event of a seroma forming, the best course is referral back to the cardiologist for treatment. The seroma may be drained under surgical style sterile procedure to avoid infection of the system. A bandage is recommended and antibiotics are prescribed. Erosion of the pulse generator is a rare complication and is avoided at surgery by making a subcutaneous pocket large enough to accommodate the pulse generator, but not so large to create dead space that could lead to seroma formation.

References

1 Silverstein, D.C. and Hopper, K. (2009) *Small Animal Critical Care Medicine.* Saunders-Elsevier, St Louis. pp. 669.

2 Côté, E. (2007) *Clinical Veterinary Advisor: Dogs and Cats.* Mosby, St Louis.

3 Rick, A.A. (2003) Abdominal, thoracic, and pericardial effusions. *The Veterinary Clinics of North America: Small Animal Practice*, **33**, 89–118.

4 Gidlewski, J. and Petrie, J.-P. (2005) Therapeutic pericardiocentesis in the dog and cat. *Clinical Techniques in Small Animal Practice*, **20**, 151–155.

5 Plumb, D.C. (2008) *Plumb's Veterinary Drug Handbook*, 6th Edition. Wiley-Blackwell, Oxford.

6 Rao, P.S., Wilson, A.D., Sideris, E.B. and Chopra, P.S. (1991) Transcatheter closure of patent ductus arteriosus with buttoned device: first successful clinical application in a child. *American Heart Journal*, **121**, 1799–1802.
7 Miller, M.W., Bonagura, J.D. and Meurs, K.M. Percutaneous Catheter Occlusion of Patent Ductus Arteriosus. *Proceedings 13th Annual ACVIM Forum*. pp. 308.
8 Glaus, T.M., Gardelle, O., Bass, M. and Kiowski, W.K. (1999) [*Closure of a persistent ductus arteriosus of Botallo in two dogs using transarterial coil embolization*]. *Schweiz Arch Tierheilkd* [Article in German] Klinik für Kleintiermedizin, Universität Zürich **141**, 191–194.
9 Nguyenba, T.P and Tobias, A.H. (2007) The Amplatz® canine duct occluder: a novel device for patent ductus arteriosus occlusion. *Journal of Veterinary Cardiology*, **9**, 109–117.
10 Kittleson, M.D. and Kienle, R.D. (1998) *Small Animal Cardiovascular Medicine*. Mosby, St Louis. pp. 70.
11 Estrada, A., Moïse, S.N. and Renaud-Farrell, S. (2005) When, how and why to perform a double ballooning technique for dogs with valvular pulmonic stenosis. *Journal of Veterinary Cardiology*, 7, 41–51.
12 Bright, J.M., Jennings, J., Toal, R. and Hood, M.E. (1987) Percutaneous balloon valvuloplasty for treatment of pulmonic stenosis in a dog. *Journal of the American Veterinary Medicine Association*, **191**, 995–996.
13 Schrope, D.P. (2005) Balloon valvuloplasty of valvular pulmonic stenosis in the dog. *Clinical Techniques in Small Animal Practice*, **20**, 182–195.
14 Taylor, D.H. and Mero, M.A. (1967) The use of an internal pacemaker in a horse with Adams-Stokes syndrome. *Journal of the American Veterinary Medical Association*, **151**, 1172–1176.
15 Bonagura, J.D., Helphrey, M.L. and Muir, W.W. (1983) Complications associated with permanent pacemaker implantation in the dog. *Journal of the American Veterinary Medical Association*, **182**, 149–155.
16 Moses, H., Weston Miller, B.D. Moulton, K.P. and Schneider, J.A. (2000) *A Practical Guide to Cardiac Pacing*, 5th Edition. Lippincott, Williams & Wilkins, Philadelphia.
17 Fox, P.R., Sisson, D. and Moïse, N.S. (1999) *Textbook of Canine and Feline Cardiology: Principles and Clinical Practice*, 2nd Edition. W.B Saunders Company, Philadelphia. pp. 416–417.

Section V

Large Animal Cardiology

17

Equine Cardiology

H. Edward Durham, Jr.

Introduction

Cardiac disease is a less common clinical problem in equine patients compared with small animals. Although congestive heart failure (CHF) does occur in horses, it is uncommon. Arrhythmias are an important cause of reduced exercise performance, and valvular disease is more common in older horses. Infections in the heart or pericardium are typically fatal and a number of toxic substances can be lethal due to their cardiac effects. However, primary myocardial disease is rare, as are aortic and pulmonic stenosis.

The basic anatomic structure, physiologic, and pathophysiologic principles are similar to those in small animal medicine, yet important species differences do exist. This chapter seeks to review those cardiac conditions common to horses.

Anatomy and Physiology

One of the defining characteristics of mammals is the four chamber quadra-valved heart. Chapter 1 discusses the anatomic features of the mammalian heart. Structurally, the equine heart is exactly the same as that of all mammals. The biggest difference when compared with small animals is the conduction system of the equine heart. Mammalian cardiac conduction systems can be divided into two categories: those in which the Purkinje fibers penetrate to the subendocardium only (type A) and those with Purkinje fibers that penetrate the myocardium completely from endocardium to the epicardium (type B). The type B conduction system allows for nearly simultaneous depolarization of the complete myocardium and is seen in horses, ruminants, and pigs. This conduction system may give a slight physiologic advantage at high heart rates (HR). A significant limitation of type B from the diagnostic point of view is the absence of a "depolarization wave" that moves through the heart, enabling electrocardiographic detection of cardiac chamber enlargement using the mean electrical axis. Since the depolarization is conducted directly throughout the entire myocardium there is no mean electrical axis to measure. Therefore electrocardiography in horses is limited to evaluation of HR and rhythm.

Myocardial function and hemodynamics are similar to small animals. The most striking feature of horse hemodynamics is their relatively large capacity for increases in cardiac output during exercise.

Cardiology for Veterinary Technicians and Nurses, First Edition. Edited by H. Edward Durham, Jr.

Exercise Physiology

Exercise physiology is an important component of equine cardiology because so much of human interaction with horses is a result of their athletic ability. In addition to the general health question, assessing the athletic ability of horses as a predictor of future performance is an area of ongoing research. Many cardiovascular indices have been evaluated or are being actively investigated, but no single parameter has been identified that will accurately predict a horse's athletic performance.

Perhaps one of the simplest indices to measure for exercise performance is evaluation of HR. It is generally accepted that the better an athlete's conditioning the lower their HR for any given level of exercise. The relationship of HR to work effort in horses is linear at submaximal exercise. By comparing the HR of a horse at known submaximal exercise level to other horses at the same level of exercise, some predictions may be made regarding future performance.

The resting HR of a healthy horse is 24–48 bpm, but at peak exercise the HR may reach 240–260 bpm, which is about an approximately eight- to tenfold increase. This increase is perhaps the greatest increase in HR in the animal kingdom. The typical human athlete, for example, has a peak HR of 170–200 bpm; assuming a resting HR of 60-70 bpm this represents about a 2.5–2.8 times increase in HR during peak exercise.

Heart-rate recovery is another method to evaluate fitness. Rapid postexercise HR recovery implies better cardiovascular conditioning. In horses, the HR falls quite quickly following exercise to a steady-state (50–70 bpm), slightly higher than the resting HR for a short recovery period then gradually decreases to normal. Horses with a higher postexercise HR tend not to perform as well as those with lower postexercise HR. Research has demonstrated that in endurance horses with HRs of greater than 65 bpm after 30 min of recovery were more likely to not finish or to finish poorly compared to horses with a HR 60 bpm after 30 min of rest. Those horses also showed less echocardiographic evidence of dehydration during a rest period [1]. When prolonged submaximal work is undertaken, HR tends to plateau and stabilize until a higher level of work is performed. Some HR drift or a gradual upward trend may occur, especially in dehydrated animals (as seen with prolonged exercise).

A more standardized method of evaluating performance is the V_{140} and V_{200} or the horse's running velocity at a HR of 140 or 200 bpm as measured during treadmill exercise. Simply stated, this test asks the question, how fast is the horse running when HR reaches 140 or 200 bpm? By running a horse on a treadmill and attaching an ambulatory ECG monitor, one can record the velocity of the treadmill when the HR reaches the target HR. A better performer should have a higher V_{140} or V_{200}. This method is very useful for tracking the response to training in an individual animal. One limitation of V_{140} or V_{200} is that it does not take into account individual horse's preferences for running on varying surfaces, so results when comparing two different animals may not present a complete picture.

A third method of assessing cardiovascular performance is to calculate the maximal uptake of oxygen (O_2) possible for an individual athlete as a volume. This index, called VO_2 max, also has a linear relationship with HR at submaximal exercise, which makes HR monitoring useful since VO_2 max is so closely linked with O_2 demand. VO_2 max is calculated by acquiring a venous and arterial blood sample for blood gas analysis, calculating the difference of oxygen content then multiplying by the cardiac output. The final product is expressed in liters per minute (L/min) of oxygen with normal being around 50–60 L/min for the average horse, with high-performance horses nearing or exceeding 100 L/min.

In healthy horses, the O_2 exchange across the lungs is fairly constant. Changes in the VO_2 max are mostly affected by components of cardiac output, not the oxygen exchange rate (see Chapter 2 for an explanation of cardiac output). Cardiac output can be estimated invasively by the thermodilution method or noninvasively using Doppler echocardiography [2]. Since both HR and stroke volume (SV) can be measured noninvasively (unlike obtaining blood gas samples), measuring HR and SV by echocardiography and using a formula, estimates of VO_2 max can be performed, which do not require the acquisition of blood samples.

In racehorses, cardiac output increases from about 20 L/min at rest, to nearly 300 L/min during peak exercise. Interestingly, SV reaches its maximum at about 40% of VO_2 max. Additional increases of cardiac output are a result of increases in HR alone. Stroke volume is significantly related to the absolute size of the heart of course; the bigger the heart the greater the SV therefore the greater cardiac output at a given HR. An average-sized horse heart weighs about 4.5–6 kg. When compared with the heart weights of historically renowned racehorses, we can see the importance of heart size to speed performance. The 1970s racehorse Sham would have likely been one of the most winning horses of all time (had he not been running against Secretariat); he had a heart weight of 8.2 kg when he died. At an estimated racing HR of about 200 bpm his calculated cardiac output was about 430 L/min. Secretariat's heart, although not actually weighed, was estimated (by the same pathologist that weighed Sham's heart) to be a full 10 kg, giving him a calculated cardiac output of 540 L/min and a VO_2max of 120 L/min [3, pp. 699–727]. Consequently, a great deal of research emphasis has been placed on the assessment of heart size in racehorses.

The use of ECG changes to predict performance in racehorses has been evaluated. The so-called "heart score" is the mean of the QRS durations measured in milliseconds as recorded in the frontal plane bipolar leads. Heart score is obtained by recording an electrocardiogram (ECG) using limb electrode placement in the frontal plane to acquire standard bipolar leads I, II, and III. The recording is mostly undertaken at 50 mm/s paper speed to obtain the most accurate measurement. Using calipers, measurements of the duration of the QRS complex in all three leads are taken and the values averaged. The resulting number is the heart score. Changes in T-wave morphology were once thought to be predictive of performance but this avenue also proved inconsistent. At this time, the ECG is not thought to give much information on performance other than ruling out clinical arrhythmias that might reduce performance and to assist in measurement of HR during recovery from exercise or standardized exercise tests.

Echocardiography is both a diagnostic tool and is used for performance prediction. Measurements of heart size by echocardiography have been evaluated as related to performance. An echocardiogram allows for accurate measurements of cardiac dimensions. Consistent estimations of heart size and SV can be made by using standard imaging protocols. Doppler echocardiography can also provide hemodynamic information related to SV and cardiac output. Several studies have been conducted in which better performing horses also showed slightly larger cardiac size by echocardiography. However, other research has not always found similar results and the predictive value may be limited. The best correlations have been reported for equine endurance athletes.

One interesting finding from 2000 demonstrated that mild valvular regurgitation had no significant negative effect on racehorse performance [4]. The horses of this study (526 in total) were assessed by cardiac auscultation, color Doppler echocardiography, and evaluated by an objective racehorse performance index common in England (Timeform rating).

Exercise physiology continues to be an area of interest and research in horses. The techniques used to examine exercise performance are also used for diagnostic purposes, particularly when performance is judged to have diminished.

Physical Examination

Exercise intolerance, poor performance, and identification of arrhythmias and/or murmurs are the most common justifications for a complete cardiac evaluation. Horses may present with ventral subcutaneous edema, fever of unknown origin, loss of bodily condition, or rarely present with coughing. Murmurs are commonly detected during routine veterinary care or prepurchase examinations. When a significant cardiac condition is suspected, a complete physical examination should be performed, with attention to those aspects of the examination specific to the cardiovascular system. Before the horse is excited due to handling, the examiner should observe the horse's respiratory effort and rate, and look for jugular pulses. Although cardiac disease is an uncommon cause of disturbed ventilation increases in respiratory rate and effort may be associated with CHF. Actual disease of the lungs, pleura, and airways are more commonly identified as causes of increased respiratory rate and effort.

Observation of the patient's jugular veins for distension or pulsation give indications of right heart disease or cranial mediastinal mass (see Chapter 3). Jugular distension is an indication of elevated right atrial pressures. Jugular pulsations extending higher than the lower third of the neck are abnormal, implying tricuspid regurgitation. Care must be given in this assessment not to confuse carotid pulses under the jugular vein as jugular pulsations. This false positive finding is especially common in thin horses, horse who are recumbent, or have their heads down.

Peripheral arterial pulses should be assessed. Arterial pulses can easily be felt in the facial artery under the rostral third of the mandible in horses. Hypokinetic pulses are associated with conditions that cause hypotension like dehydration or hypovolemia. Hyperkinetic pulses can be detected with significant aortic valve regurgitation. Arterial pulses feel extra strong because of the increased pulse pressure created by a decrease in diastolic pressure due to aortic regurgitation. The facial artery can also be palpated during auscultation to evaluate for pulse deficits associated with arrhythmias. Just as with small animals, blood pressure cannot accurately be determined by arterial pulse quality alone. Indirectly assessed blood pressure measurements can be undertaken using the Doppler method at the tail using the coccygeal artery (see Chapter 7).

Cardiac Auscultation

Cardiac auscultation is a key component of the cardiovascular examination. A good quality stethoscope should be used in a quiet area for proper auscultation. The stethoscope should have a diaphragm approximately 2 inches (4.5 cm) in diameter and tubing no more than 25 inches (62.5 cm) in length. Comfortable ear pieces and thick-walled tubing will improve the sound quality of the stethoscope.

To begin the auscultation, one should palpate the ventral aspect of the left hemithorax (intercostal spaces 3–6) for the presence of palpable vibrations or *thrills* associated with murmurs. During the palpation the apical impulse should be located. The apical impulse is the point on the chest wall where the heart makes contact during systole.

Auscultation typically begins over the mitral valve area, which is located at about the fifth to sixth intercostal space just caudal to the left elbow near the apical impulse. The S_1 sound is best heard in this area. Proceed with the auscultation by moving the stethoscope cranially and dorsally approximately one intercostal space where the aortic valve may be evaluated for murmurs. The S_2 sound is best heard over the aortic valve. From the aortic valve, moving the stethoscope cranial and ventral approximately one intercostal space will allow for auscultation over the pulmonic valve. Note the HR and rhythm for arrhythmias. Before ausculting the right hemithorax, it should also be palpated for thrills. The tricuspid valve is best heard directly across the thorax from the mitral valve. One should also auscult the right base of the heart near the right axillary region for a murmur associated with ventricular septal defects (VSD).

Normal HR for healthy adult horses is 24–48 bpm. Foals have higher resting HR than adults; around 80–120 bpm that gradually slows during the first few weeks of life. Typically, the HR of foals will begin to decrease at about 2 weeks, and be the normal adult HR by weaning or about 6 months of age.

With experience, during cardiac auscultation of healthy horses, it is common to ascult all of the four sounds of the cardiac cycle: the first and second heart sounds, S_1 and S_2; the so called "lub" and "dub" typically heard in all mammals and the third and fourth heart sounds, labeled S_3 and S_4 respectively. The third heart sound is the sound associated with early ventricular filling and the S_4 sound, also called the "atrial contraction sound" denotes the atrial systolic phase of ventricular filling (see Chapter 3 for more detail on heart sounds). Any combination of these sounds is considered normal in the equine species.

In some instances, a "dropped" beat may be detected in which the S_4 sound is heard but lacks the normally following S_1 and S_2. A pulse deficit will also be noted when performing simultaneous arterial pulse palpation. This finding is almost always a normal physiologic variation of horses that is due to a transient second degree atrioventricular (AV) block that will be discussed later in this chapter. Exercise should abolish this arrhythmia if it is caused by physiologic second degree AV block.

A number of murmurs may be detected in horses (see Chapter 3 for details on murmur type, grading, and classification). The point where a murmur is heard the loudest is termed the *point of maximal intensity* and is abbreviated *PMI*. The two most common murmurs are functional murmurs, which occur in a structurally normal heart, and mitral regurgitation murmurs due to valvular degeneration (endocardiosis). Functional murmurs are usually systolic murmurs which reportedly occur in approximately 66% of horses [5, 6]. Differentiating between functional murmurs and mitral regurgitation murmurs by auscultation is a useful clinical skill. Functional murmurs are best auscultated near the aortic and pulmonic valves. They are typically grade 3 or less in loudness but may increase with exercise. With prolonged exercise appropriate to the patient's fitness, some functional murmurs may disappear. A functional systolic murmur is often present in cases of colic, and vanishes once the colic problem has been resolved. The

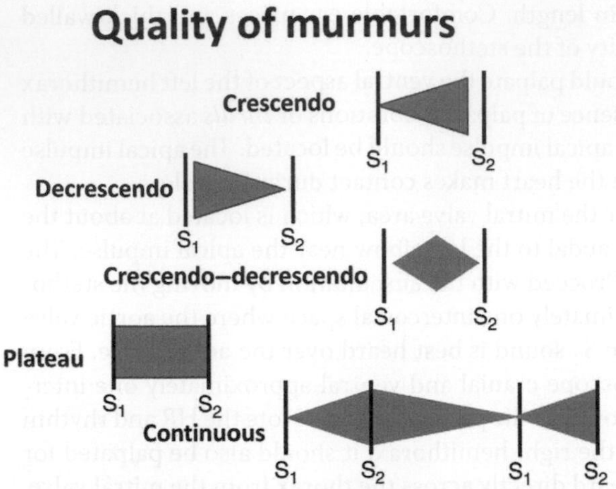

Figure 17.1 Murmur sound representations. The vertical line labeled S_1 and S_2 mark the acoustic borders of systole; S_1 being the beginning and S_2 the end of systole. Murmur types are drawn by the shape the intensity of their sound makes over the course of the cardiac cycle. The *crescendo* murmur increases in loudness and intensity through systole; the *decrescendo* murmur decreases. The *crescendo–decrescendo* murmur initially increases then decreases in intensity. The *plateau* murmur maintains the same intensity throughout systole. The *continuous* murmur increases in systole to a peak at end-systole then decreases throughout diastole to rise again at the onset of systole. A purely diastolic murmur (not shown here) would be drawn as the same shape seen in the continuous between S_2 and the next S_1, with no portion shown in systole.

timing of the murmur will provide clues to its origin. Functional murmurs tend to start in mid-to-late systole and stop just prior to the S_2 sound.

Murmurs of mitral regurgitation are commonly appreciated in older horses and are most often due to chronic valvular degeneration. Mitral regurgitation murmurs are typically ausculted best near the apical impulse at the left hemithorax. The murmur timing is holosystolic, starting in early systole near S_1 and continuing to or through S_2. The quality of the mitral regurgitation murmur is band- or plateau-shaped as opposed to a functional murmur which is more crescendo or crescendo-decrescendo (Figure 17.1). Echocardiography is the best diagnostic tool to identify the cause and significance of a murmur.

Another common cause of systolic murmurs, especially in young horses, is VSD. This murmur generally radiates toward the right sternum. The murmur is described as pansystolic starting before S_1 and lasting beyond S_2 and is typically grade 4–6 in loudness. The clinical prognosis is best determined by echocardiography. If the size of a VSD is small, then the horse may suffer no serious cardiac effects and may still be useful for pleasure riding, but may not be suited for competitive performance.

Diastolic murmurs are most commonly due to aortic valvular regurgitation and are also commonly identified in the clinically normal animal. They are generally longer in duration than systolic murmurs and have a decrescendo quality. In some instances they may be described as a "dive bomber" sound. Diastolic murmurs can be an incidental finding in young healthy horses. In older horses aortic regurgitation is commonly due to endocardiosis and large volume regurgitation often leads to myocardial failure. An echocardiogram is indicated to assess the degree of regurgitation and the volume load effect on the left ventricle.

One can sometimes hear a systolic–diastolic combination murmur or "to-and-fro" murmur. This unusual murmur can be heard in healthy horses with functional murmurs or in aged horses with valvular degeneration. The quality of this murmur is similar to the sound of hand sawing wood, with a characteristic break in the sound at S_2 as the direction of flow changes when the heart changes from systole to diastole. This feature is used to distinguish it from a continuous murmur. In the case of a healthy athletic animal, a functional systolic murmur may be combined with an innocent diastolic murmur. Likewise, if an older horse has degeneration of both the mitral and aortic valves they may both be insufficient and be the cause of a systolic–diastolic combination murmur.

Continuous murmurs are typically ausculted in foals with patent ductus arteriosus. This continuous murmur can be appreciated during examination of young foals less than a week old but is extremely rare in adult horses. The continuous murmur is ever present though it waxes and wanes in intensity throughout the cardiac cycle, being loudest in systole. It is best auscultated on the left hemithorax over the base of the heart high in the axillary region. There is always the potential for a systolic and diastolic murmur to occur in the same animal creating the "to-and-fro" murmur. The sound of this murmur is distinguished from the continuous by a short cessation of the sound at end-systole.

Very rarely, presystolic S_4 and S_3 filling murmurs may also be detected in clinically normal animals, but these murmurs are usually soft and difficult to hear. These murmurs are generated as blood rushes into the left ventricle during ventricular filling. If audible, they are usually heard in the left hemithorax.

Diseases of the pericardium can produce rubbing, or knocking sounds. These sounds can occur at any time during the cardiac cycle when the heart is in motion. In the presence of pericardial effusion, these sounds, and all heart sounds, are often difficult to ascult.

During the auscultation, arrhythmias may also be appreciated. Atrial fibrillation is the most common pathologic arrhythmia heard in the horse. It is characterized as irregular with no discernable pattern, yet resting HRs in horses with atrial fibrillation are often normal. More details of atrial fibrillation will be discussed later in the chapter.

Atrial and ventricular premature beats also occur in horses and can be heard during auscultation. They are noted as heart sounds occurring early in the expected rhythm and are typically followed by a pause as the heart "resets". The determination of the origin (atrial vs ventricular) can only be made by electrocardiography. Although rare, ventricular tachycardia (VT) can be seen in horses and will be auscultated as a rapid regular rhythm and is an indication for an electrocardiogram.

Ancillary Diagnostics

Radiography

A number of ancillary diagnostic modalities are available for evaluating the cardiac system of horses. Thoracic radiography may be employed for foals, small-breed horses, and ponies, but is usually unhelpful for most adult horses. Thoracic radiography is useful in these smaller patients for diagnosing CHF and assessing the overall size and shape of the cardiac silhouette.

Electrocardiography

The standard method of recording the electrocardiogram in horses entails the base-apex lead (Figure 17.2). The base-apex lead requires only three electrodes. It is created by setting the electrocardiograph to record lead II, then attaching the negative right arm (white) electrode at the right jugular furrow, a positive left leg electrode (red) at the left hemithorax apical impulse and the remaining ground electrode (black) attached in an unobtrusive place. A normal equine ECG recorded in this fashion demonstrates a positive P wave, negative QRS complex and positive T wave (Figure 17.3) for which the normal durations are provided in Table 17.1. Due to a lack of a mean electrical axis, waveform amplitudes are not typically diagnostic or measured.

Before echocardiography was available, some advanced evaluation of the electrical activity of the horse was performed using vector electrocardiography. Extensively researched by Dr J.R. Holmes, this method uses electrodes placed in the orthogonal planes identified as X, Y, and Z (Figure 17.4). By tracing the electrical depolarization

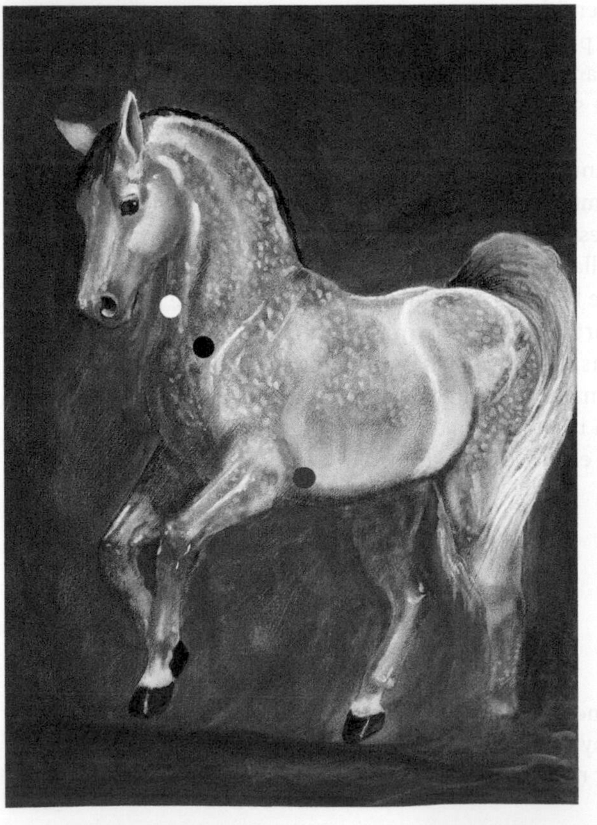

Figure 17.2 The proper electrode placement for obtaining the base-apex lead in horses. With the electrocardiograph set to record lead II, the negative right arm (RA-white) electrode goes near the right jugular furrow, the positive left leg (LL-red) electrode goes on the left hemithorax near the apical impulse of the heart, the left arm (LA-Black – which in a three electrode system will serve as the ground) can be attached anywhere on the horse that is convenient, typically on the right withers or near the left apex also. Note that with the LL and LA electrodes near the left apex, the electrocardiograph may be set to record lead I or lead II for the same result. When set to lead I the machine will use the RA and LA as the active electrode and the LL as a ground; in lead II the RA and LL will be active and the LA becomes the ground electrode. Source: painting by Judy D. Heim

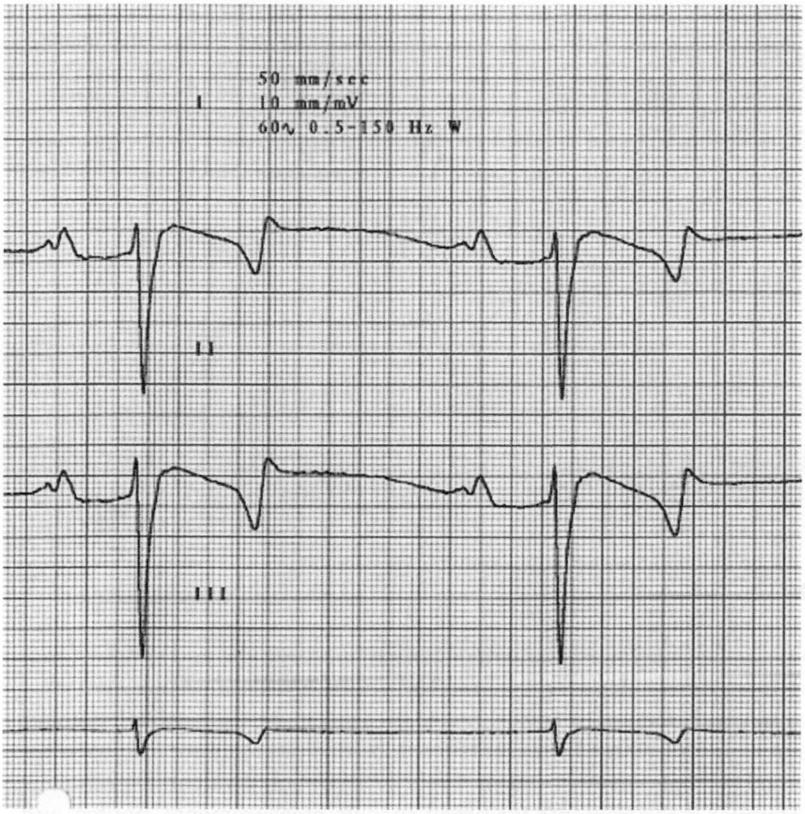

Figure 17.3 Electrocardiogram illustrating the normal cardiac depolarization in the horse. The P wave is positive, and may or may not show the notching seen here. A small positive R wave, deep negative S wave and negative T wave is normal from the base-apex lead. Lead III is of low amplitude because the vector of lead III is almost completely perpendicular to the mean electrical axis of the depolarization wave. Paper speed: 50 mm/s. Calibration: 1 cm/ mV. Leads I, II, III shown.

Table 17.1 Normal horse electrocardiographic measurements (base-apex lead).

Measurement	Value
P wave duration [15]	≤160 ms
P wave amplitude [27]	0.04–0.32 mV*
P-R interval [15]	≤ 500 ms
QRS complex duration [15]	≤ 140 ms
Q-T interval [15]	≤ 600 ms

Durations and interval are presented in milliseconds (ms).
Amplitudes are reported in millivolts (mv).
*May not represent all equids; only one species of donkey. Equid P waves are commonly bifid, with P_1 tending to be in the lower half of the range and P_2 in the upper. Range quoted includes entire value for P_1 and P_2.

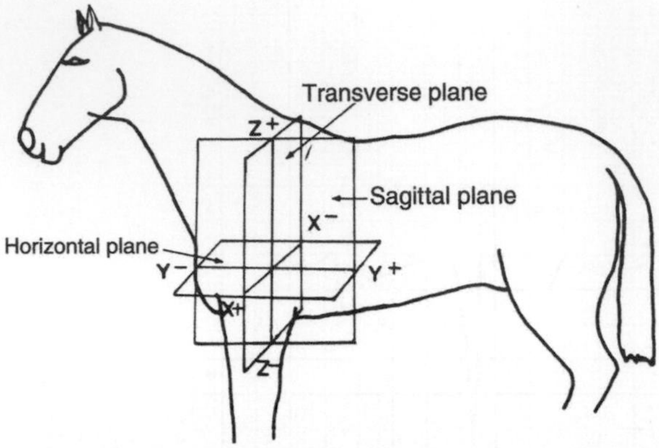

Figure 17.4 The horizontal (x), sagittal (y) and transverse (z) planes in which electrocardiograms can be recorded. Before echocardiography was common, these planes were used to assess the vector cardiogram as a diagnostic tool.

wave as it traveled through the various chambers of the heart over time, cardiac chamber enlargement could be identified. Echocardiography replaced vector electrocardiography as a more accurate, less labor-intensive method of assessing cardiac enlargement.

Echocardiography

Echocardiography can be used for assessment of cardiac chamber size and systolic function. By imaging from both sides of the horse the entire heart can usually be visualized using the standard imaging planes. Precise measurements of cardiac chamber size can be obtained. The same measurements used in small animals are also used for horses, with reference range values listed in Table 17.2. Detailed values for echocardiographic and Doppler measurements for breed specific measurements, ponies, and other equine species may be found in Boon's *Veterinary Echocardiography*, 2nd Edition [7]. The source of murmurs can be located and quantified using color-flow Doppler. The experienced sonographer can also calculate pressure differences in the cardiac chambers using spectral Doppler echocardiography (see Chapter 6). Cardiac masses and pericardial effusion can be identified. An echocardiogram can be useful for horses with atrial fibrillation. Atrial fibrillation can be found in horses with otherwise normal hearts and those with cardiac disease. The echocardiogram is the best tool for distinguishing the two. Horses with atrial fibrillation about to undergo electrical cardioversion or quinidine therapy should have an echocardiogram to assess systolic function before initiating therapy which may suppress cardiac contractility.

Cardiac Biomarkers

Several biochemical markers have been utilized in the past to attempt to differentiate cardiac disease from other conditions. Biochemical substances like creatine kinase and lactate dehydrogenase have been replaced with more cardiac specific biomarkers such as cardiac troponin-I and natriuretic peptides. These compounds are still being investigated for the diagnosis of equine heart disease. Current research has shown that cardiac troponin levels are low in normal and healthy racehorses and elevated in horses with myocardial disease [8, 9]. Mild elevation is also seen in horses undergoing treadmill training and endurance horses [8–12].

Table 17.2 M-mode reference values in adult horses.

Parameter	Dressage (Mean ± SD mm)	Show jumping (Mean ± SD mm)	Untrained (Mean ± SD mm)	Endurance (Mean ± SD mm)	Unconditioned (Mean ± SD mm)	THB and FRH (Mean ± SD mm)	Mixed breed (Mean ± SD mm)	STD (Range mm)
RVd (mm)	39 ± 8	41 ± 5	42 ± 8	–	–			
RVs (mm)	35 ± 6	38 ± 5	38 ± 6	–	–			
LVd (mm)	116 ± 7	121 ± 10	115 ± 7	101 ± 2	95 ± 3	11.06 ± 1.34	11.2 ± 0.8	111.5–121.2
LVs (mm)	82 ± 6	86 ± 8	82 ± 7	60 ± 2	52 ± 3	6.11 ± .9	7.3 ± 0.8	70.3–78.2
%FS	29 ± 5	29 ± 5	28 ± 5	42 ± 1	46 ± 2	44.1 ± 6.4		34.7–37.7
LVET (s)	–	–	–	0.44 ± .01	0.40 ± .02			
PEP (s)	–	–	–	0.08 ± .01	0.50 ± .01			
Vcf (cir/s)	–	–	–	0.91 ± .05	1.16 ± .07			
VSd (mm)	35 ± 4	30 ± 3	33 ± 5	28 ± 1	27 ± 1	3.06 ± .6	2.8 ± 0.2	29.4–32.5
VSs (mm)	43 ± 7	40 ± 5	40 ± 6	45 ± 1	44 ± 1	4.81 ± .7	4.6 ± 0.5	43.5–46.2
VSexc(mm)	–	–	–	20 ± 1	19 ± 1			
VS%Δ	–	–	–	59 ± 3	66 ± 4			
LVWd(mm)	30 ± 3	26 ± 4	27 ± 6	24 ± 1	18 ± 1	2.92 ± .49	2.5 ± 0.3	24.2–26.9
LVWs(mm)	36 ± 5	32 ± 5	32 ± 6	36 ± 1	33 ± 1	4.45 ± .59	3.8 ± 0.3	34.4–38.3
LVWexc(mm)	–	–	–	24 ± 1	26 ± 1			

(*continued*)

Table 17.2 *(Continued)*

Parameter	Dressage (Mean ± SD mm)	Show jumping (Mean ± SD mm)	Untrained (Mean ± SD mm)	Endurance (Mean ± SD mm)	Unconditioned (Mean ± SD mm)	THB and FRH (Mean ± SD mm)	Mixed breed (Mean ± SD mm)	STD (Range mm)
LVW % Δ	–	–	–	53 ± 5.4	86 ± 7			
VS/LVW	–	–	–	1.22 ± .1	1.57 ± .07			
AO(mm)	78 ± 6	74 ± 9	75 ± 6	64 ± 1	58 ± 1	7.31 ± .83	7.5 ± 0.6	76.2–79.7
LA(mm)	56 ± 5	60 ± 4	58 ± 8	43 ± 1	41 ± 1			
LA/AO	–	–	–	0.68+.02	0.71 ± 0.2			
EPSS(mm)	–	–	–	15 ± 1	10 ± 1			5.1–6.7
Age (year)	10.1 ± 1.8	8.8 ± 1.7	8.3 ± 2.9	6–208	1–25		4–16	
kg	602 ± 38	587 ± 40	549 ± 44	329–523	186–636	X = 445	454–620	
n	15	15	15	53	32	100	16	
Two-dimensional guided	Y	Y	Y	N	N		Y	Y

THB, thoroughbred; FRH, French riding horses; STD, standardbred; mixed breed horses, 3 warm bloods; 1 Shire; 7 thoroughbreds; 5 thoroughbred mixes; SD, standard deviation; SE, standard error; mm, millimeter; cm, centimeter; s, systole; d, diastole; RV, right ventricle; LV, left ventricle; FS, fractional shortening; LVET, ventricular ejection time; PEP, pre-ejection period; Vcf, velocity of circumferential shortening; VS, ventricular septurm; exc, excursion; LVW, left ventricular wall; AO, aorta; LA, left atrium; EPSS, E point to septal separation.
Source: Data from Boon, J. (2011) *Veterinary Echocardiography*, 2nd Edition.Wiley-Blackwell, Ames.

It may also be useful for diagnosing the rare case of viral myocarditis. Brain natriuretic peptide is unavailable at this time. Existing assays do not detect equine brain natriuretic peptide and investigations of atrial natriuretic peptide have not yielded clinically useful data.

Congestive Heart Failure

Congestive heart failure is the term used for the inability of the heart to maintain forward cardiac output in the presence of normal or elevated preload (see Chapter 13). Congestive heart failure may be primarily due to failure of the left ventricle (LV), so called *left heart failure,* the right ventricle (RV) called *right heart failure* or both simultaneously known as *biventricular failure.* Congestive heart failure may be caused by any of the heart conditions listed in this chapter.

Horses with left heart failure may develop pulmonary edema and signs such as exercise intolerance, lethargy, tachypnea, dyspnea, coughing, or hemoptysis. Some horses will show a white or blood-tinged froth around the nares. Horses with right heart congestive failure have increased pressure in the RV and right atrium (RA) leading to systemic venous congestion, including jugular distension and peripheral edema, particularly on the ventral aspect. Biventricular failure may result from chronic left heart failure creating pulmonary vasoconstriction and pulmonary vascular remodeling creating increased afterload on the RV leading to its failure. Because of this, occasionally the first signs of chronic left heart failure is venous distension.

Treatment of heart failure in horses is typically limited to the use of diuretics, digoxin and, recently angiotensin-converting enzyme inhibitors. The standard diuretic used in horses is furosemide which can be administered at 1–2 mg/kg either intravenously or intramuscularly two to three times daily as needed. Oral furosemide is not used due to a lack of absorption in the equine gut. Digoxin has several potential benefits in the treatment of CHF. As in small animals, it is a positive inotrope and negative chronotrope (see Chapter 14). By lengthening the refractory period of the AV node and suppressing sympathetic tone, digoxin is particularly attractive for the treatment of supraventricular arrhythmias such as atrial fibrillation. The recommended dose can be found in Table 17.3. Digoxin has a variable half-life in horses and assessment of serum concentrations is recommended for accurate dosing. Adverse reactions include anorexia, depression, and ventricular arrhythmias.

Angiotensin-converting enzyme inhibitor drugs have been used in canine and human medicine for many years now, but present research shows poor oral bioavailability and has not been shown to provide significant clinical benefit [13]. Hydralazine may be of value but must be carefully used since it may induce severe hypotension. These drugs can be used to relieve the symptoms of CHF but will not repair the damaged heart. Consequently, most horses that develop CHF are euthanized.

Disease Conditions

In 2014, a group of noted veterinary cardiologists with extensive equine experience published recommendations for managing horses with cardiac abnormalities [14]. The

Table 17.3 Anti-arrhythmic drugs used in horses.

Drug	Indications	Dose
Amiodarone	AF, VT	5 mg/kg/h for 1 h then 0.83 mg/kg/h for 2 h*
Atropine	Sinus bradycardia AV block	0.005–0.01 mg/kg IV
Bretylium tosylate	Life-threatening VT and VF	3–5 mg/kg IV, can repeat up to 10 mg/kg*
Digoxin	SVT	0.0022 mg/kg IV twice daily 0.011 mg/kg PO twice daily
Diltiazem	SVT	0.125 mg/kg IV over 2 min, may repeat every 12 min*
Dopamine	Advance and complete AV block	3–5 μg/kg/min CRI
Epinephrine	Sinus bradycardia	0.01 mg/kg IV
Flecainide	AF	4.1 mg/kg every 2 h up to maximum dose of 4–6 doses then every 4–6 h* *DO NOT USE INTRAVENOUSLY*
Isoproterenol	Advance and complete AV block	0.05–0.2 μg/kg/min CRI
Lidocaine	VT	0.02–0.05 mg/kg/min; 0.25–0.5 mg/kg slow IV, can repeat in 5–10 min *OR* loading dose of 1.3 mg/kg IV over 5 min followed by CRI of 0.05 mg/kg/min
Magnesium sulphate	VT	2.2–4.4 mg/kg slow IV, can repeat in 5 min to a total dose of 55 mg/kg*
Phenytoin	Digoxin toxicity; supraventricular and ventricular arrhythmias	7.5–8.8 mg/kg IV single bolus Loading dose of 20 mg/kg PO, then modify twice daily dose to keep phenytoin plasma level at 5–10 mg/L
Procainamide	AF,VT supraventricular and ventricular arrhythmias	1 mg/kg/min IV to a total dose of 20 mg/kg 25–35 mg/kg PO three times daily
Propafenone	VT, AF, supraventricular and ventricular arrhythmias	0.5–1.0 mg/kg in 5% dextrose IV over 5–8 min 2 mg/kg PO three times daily*
Propranolol	SVT, VT	0.03–0.1 mg/kg IV 0.38–0.78 mg/kg PO three times daily
Quinidine gluconate	AF, VT	0.5–2.2 mg/kg IV every 10 min to a total dose of 12 mg/kg
Quinidine sulphate	AF	22 mg/kg via nasogastric tube until converted, toxic or quinidine plasma levels = 3–5 mg/L, usually 4–6 doses, then every 6 h until converted or toxic
Verapamil	SVT	0.025–0.05 mg/kg IV every 30 min to a total dose of 0.2 mg/kg*

*There are limited data to support these dosage regimens. The reader is encouraged to consult recent literature for modifications or other recommendations.

AF, atrial fibrillation; CRI, constant rate infusion; IV, intravenously; PO, per oram; SVT, supraventricular tachycardia; VT, ventricular tachycardia.

Source: Marr and Bowen (2010) [15]. Reproduced with permission of Elsevier.

article provides a group of assessment and diagnostic recommendations sorted by the most common cardiac conditions presented in equine athletes. A summary of their recommendations can be found in Table 17.4.

Arrhythmias

Arrhythmia detection and characterization represent an important part of equine medicine as arrhythmias are commonly associated with poor performance. Many arrhythmias detected in horses are physiologic and manifest no clinical signs nor require any treatment. Abnormal rhythms such as transient postexercise sinus arrhythmia, first and second degree AV block, sinus bradycardia, sinoatrial block, wandering pacemaker, and occasional supraventricular and ventricular premature depolarizations have no impact on athletic performance. These rhythms are rarely associated with cardiac disease. Arrhythmias such as atrial fibrillation, supraventricular tachycardia, and VT are more likely to be associated with clinical problems. These arrhythmias may be the cause of exercise intolerance, and more likely to be associated with cardiac disease, but not always.

Perhaps the most common arrhythmia reported in horses is second degree AV block. This physiologic arrhythmia is related to the strong parasympathetic vagal tone present in horses and abates with excitement or exercise (higher HR). Second degree AV block results from the fact that occasional impulses from the sinoatrial node are extinguished in the AV node (when the horse is calm and sympathetic tone is low). When stimulated, sympathetic nervous system tone increases and overrides the parasympathetic vagal tone causing the block to disappear. On the electrocardiogram this arrhythmia is characterized by a normal sinus rhythm at a resting HR with an occasional P wave occurring with no subsequent QRS complex (Figure 17.5). These atrial contractions can usually be detected on auscultation during the "dropped" contraction as S_4 sound without a following S_1 and S_2. Premature atrial depolarizations on an electrocardiogram are often detected in horses affected with gastrointestinal disease.

Supraventricular Arrhythmias

Atrial premature complexes (APC) occur as abnormal depolarizations arising from the atrial tissue before the sinus node depolarizes. When four or more APCs occur together, the term supraventricular or atrial tachycardia is used. Atrial premature complexes are associated with systemic disease, abnormalities of autonomic tone, electrolyte imbalances, systemic inflammation, and atrial myocarditis.

During the physical examination, APCs will be detected as an early beat in the expected rhythm. Without an ECG it is not possible to distinguish them from a ventricular premature complex (VPC).

An electrocardiogram will show a normal-appearing QRT and T wave close to a previous beat. The P wave of the APC may be seen immediately after the preceding T wave or it may be buried in the T wave, making it "hidden".

Isolated APCs are typically not a clinical problem unless linked to serious myocardial disease. An echocardiogram may be used to rule out underlying heart disease. If no structural disease can be detected, an ambulatory exercise ECG can be utilized to determine if the arrhythmia worsens with exercise. Electrolytes should be assessed and

Table 17.4 Recommendations for management of equine athletes with cardiovascular abnormalities.

Key recommendation for mitral regurgitation (MR)	
	Determine most likely etiology
	Assess severity based on combined assessment of performance history, exercise testing, clinical examination, and echocardiographic findings
	Re-examine at least annually or, for mild MR every other year
	Ensure that HR and rhythm are monitored on a regular basis in horses with moderate to severe MR
	Perform ECG exercise test in: (1) all horses with moderate to severe MR; (2) if AF becomes established; (3) if MR progresses more rapidly than expected in the absence of CHF signs
	Manage complications of advanced disease. Limited data have been published about ACE inhibitors and no consensus could be reached regarding their use in horses with MR in the absence of CHF
Key recommendation for aortic regurgitation (AR)	
	Determine most likely etiology
	Assess severity based on combined assessment of performance history, exercise testing, clinical examination, and echocardiographic findings
	An exercise ECG is indicated in horses with moderate to severe AR
	Re-examine twice yearly when there is moderate to severe AR (including echocardiography and exercise ECG test) and at least annually thereafter if progression has been minimal. Similarly, longer follow-up intervals are appropriate for horses with mild AR after the first re-evaluation
	If AF develops in a horse with mild to moderate AR, a re-examination is indicated this time including an exercise ECG
	Ensure that HR and rhythm are monitored on a regular basis in horses with moderate to severe AR; an increase in resting HR or an irregularly irregular rhythm suggestive of AF or PVCs indicates progression
	The detection of exercise induced VA is considered an important negative prognostic indicator
	Horse with AR and PVCs during exercise are considered less safe to ride or drive than their age-matched peers
Key recommendation for ventricular septal defects (VSD)	
	Perform comprehensive clinical and echocardiographic examinations
	Re-examine annually

(*continued*)

Table 17.4 (*Continued*)

	Perform exercise ECG testing of horses with moderate to large VSDs, in prepurchase situations or when performance is suboptimal Consider horses with a small VSD and minimal cardiomegaly as safe to compete; evaluate larger VSDs on a case by case basis in consultation with a specialist experienced in equine cardiology Consider affected horses as unsuitable for breeding
Key recommendation for premature atrial complexes (PACs)	
	A continuous 24 hour ECG is recommended to assess frequent PACs Horses with occasional PACs that are overdriven during exercise and those with occasional PACs during exercise are considered as safe to ride or drive as their age-matched peers Underlying causes should be sought The risk of AF should be appreciated
Key recommendation for high grade second degree atrioventricular block (2° AVB)	
	Horses with high grade 2° AVB that disappears with exercise should only be ridden or driven by an informed adult, and the HR and rhythm should be frequently monitored Horses with high grade 2° AVB during exercise or after atropine administration should be rested and re-evaluated; they are considered less safe to ride or drive than their age-matched peers Horses with symptomatic bradyarrhythmias generally have a poor prognosis and are *not* safe to ride or drive
Key recommendations for premature ventricular complexes (PVCs) and ventricular tachycardia (VT)	
	Underlying causes should be sought and managed if possible Horses with occasional PVCs at rest or during exercise or with sustained AIVR that is overdriven by exercise can be ridden or driven with caution by an informed adult. Owing to ongoing concerns about underlying myocardial or electrical disease and increased risk of exercise-induced collapse and SCD, these horses should not be used by a child or as a lesson horse. Horses with sustained monomorphic VT should be rested and treated. Normal sinus rhythm should be present for at least 4 weeks before re-evaluation is performed. A continuous 24-h

(*continued*)

Table 17.4 (*Continued*)

	ECG is indicated before returning the horse to work. If normal, an exercising ECG should be performed, followed by another exercising ECG once the horse has returned to full work. Horses affected by a single episode generally have a favorable prognosis, but on occasion monomorphic VT can recur. Horses with symptomatic or complex VA should be rested and treated. Follow-up examinations are similar as for horses with sustained monomorphic VT although the safety of these horses remains uncertain. These horses should only be ridden or driven by an informed adult Rigorous athletic work is not recommended for horses that showed VA in the setting of moderate or severe structural heart disease, including echocardiographic lesions suspected to indicate myocardial fibrosis or scar, and moderate to severe AR. These horses should only be ridden or driven by an informed adult because of the risk of possible recurrence of VT. These horses are not safe to be used by a child or as a lesson horse. For horses with a history of VT that remain in work follow-up 24-h and exercising ECGs should be performed at least annually
Key recommendations for atrial fibrillation (AF)	Select the most appropriate method of cardioversion based on risk factors for pharmacologic cardioversion or TVEC Perform continuous 24-h ECG and ideally evaluate LA function after cardioversion Return to training within 1 week with paroxysmal AF or short-duration lone AF if normal after cardioversion; rest horses with long-standing AF for 4–6 weeks Avoid the use of furosemide, supplements containing sodium bicarbonate and thyroid hormones after cardioversion Supplement oral potassium chloride to horses administered furosemide before racing or demonstrating low fractional excretion of potassium Because safety is a concern with persistent AF, the horse should be cardioverted or retired when the exercising HR during sustained maximal exercise exceeds 220 bpm or if concurrent VA are detected during exercise or with SNS stimulation Horses with persistent AF should only be ridden or driven by an informed adult and limited to an exercise level considered relatively safe based on an exercising ECG. The use of a heart rate monitor might be useful to track HR during exercise and modify the rigor of the work performed

ACE, angiotensin-converting enzyme; AIVR, accelerated idioventricular rhythm, CHF, congestive heart failure; ECG, electrocardiogram; HR, heart rate; SCD, sudden cardiac death; SNS, sympathetic nervous system; TVEC, transvenous electrical cardioversion; VA, ventricular arrhythmia.

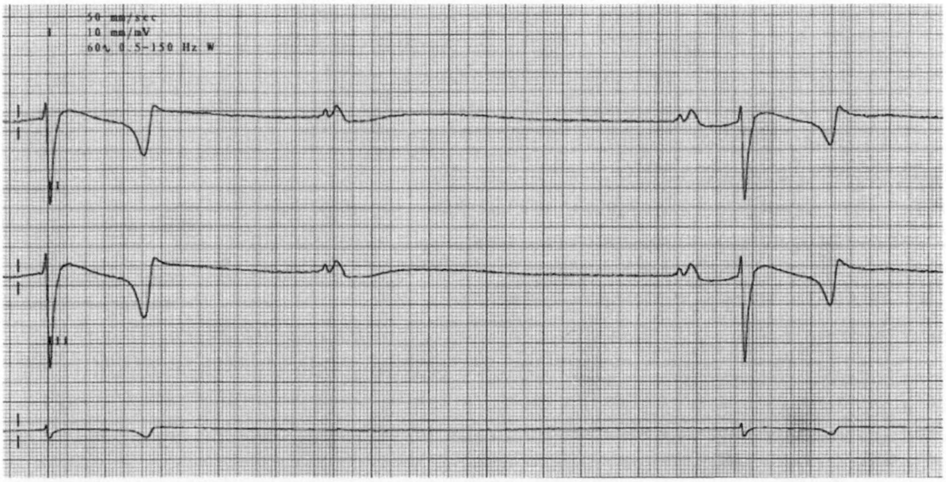

Figure 17.5 Electrocardiogram demonstrating a physiological atrioventricular (AV) block in a horse. The first and third QRS complexes are normally conducted through the AV node but the center of the figure shows a P wave with no subsequent QRS complex. After exercise the sympathetic nervous system overrides this vagally mediated AV block and all P waves are normally conducted. This is a normal finding in healthy horses. Paper speed: 50 mm/s. Calibration: 1 cm/ mV. Leads I, II, III shown

assays such as cardiac troponin-I may help distinguish a cardiac cause from other systemic conditions. Other circulating plasma biomarkers such as serum amyloid-A and plasma fibrinogen may also be helpful by indicating an inflammatory process.

Treatment of supraventricular arrhythmias is typically unnecessary unless it is felt that they may degenerate into a more malignant arrhythmia or has marked consequences on cardiac output. Since inflammation (myocarditis) is a common cause of APCs some horses may respond to anti-inflammatory medications. Correction of any electrolyte disturbances also is recommended. Atrial premature beats or tachyarrhythmias resulting from underlying gastrointestinal disease usually resolve if the primary condition can be resolved. If cardiac disease is present, appropriate therapy will often resolve the atrial arrhythmia. In cases of sustained atrial tachycardia, drugs like digoxin or diltiazem may be recommended (see Table 17.3).

Atrial Fibrillation

Atrial fibrillation (AF) is the most common pathologic arrhythmia in horses. It can occur with structurally normal hearts related to the relatively large atrial size of the horse. AF is classified as a supraventricular tachyarrhythmia. It may also occur as a result of chronic mitral regurgitation and left atrial enlargement. Atrial fibrillation is important because it is a leading cause of non-lameness performance reduction, behind airway disease and lameness.

In AF there is no organized atrial contraction leading to a loss of the atrial component of ventricular filling. Instead, the AV node is bombarded with atrial depolarization "wavelets" emerging from multiple foci within the atria. The horse will appear normal at rest, but the normal atrial contribution to end diastolic volume is necessary for peak cardiac output at high HRs and athletic performance. The abnormal atrial impulses bombarding the AV node cause the ventricle to depolarize with irregularity. This rhythm does not allow for consistent filling during the early diastolic period disrupting stroke volume further. Paradoxically, using ambulatory ECG monitors has shown that AF may occur transiently during or after exercise with no clinical signs or decrease in performance [15]. The pathology occurs when the AF is sustained or occurs frequently enough to reduce exercise performance.

In the absence of heart disease, AF is called *idiopathic atrial fibrillation or "lone a. fib"*, and the prognosis is quite good with medical therapy. Longstanding AF has a less positive prognosis. If the horse has been affected with AF for more than 4 months, then therapy is less effective and the horse is more likely to revert back to AF. In the presence of heart disease, the prognosis becomes guarded to poor. Horses that have AF with cardiac disease rarely return to their performance activity. If they show signs of CHF then athletic performance is out of the question. Reports of exercise intolerance or reduced athletic performance are often the reason for presentation by the client. Horses with AF may also be asymptomatic, have epistaxis, ataxia, or collapse when exercised.

Physical examination of horses in AF will usually reveal a markedly irregular rhythm with an absent S_4 sound. The arterial pulses are typically chaotic in rhythm and intensity. The HR may be within the normal reference range or show a tachycardia depending on the state of underlying cardiac disease. In the absence of cardiac disease, normal vagal tone allows the slowing and accelerating effect at the AV node. On auscultation this allows for the heart rhythm to somewhat mimic second degree AV block, making it possible to miss AF during auscultation (hence the value in detecting the presence or absence of the S_4 heart sound). The other heart sounds may also be abnormal. S_1 and S_2 are often highly variable in noise intensity and S_3 may be quite loud in some horses. These changes are due to the variable states of ventricular filling during AF. A cardiac murmur may be heard, especially when chronic valvular disease or VSD is present, that may also vary in intensity and regularity.

On the base-apex ECG, AF is characterized by the lack of P waves and normal morphology in the QRS complex (Figure 17.6). Often there are undulations of the trace baseline ("f" waves), but a flat baseline may also be evident (Figure 17.7). If concurrent heart disease is present, the HR is usually elevated, otherwise it is normal. Occasionally, premature ventricular complexes may also be noted.

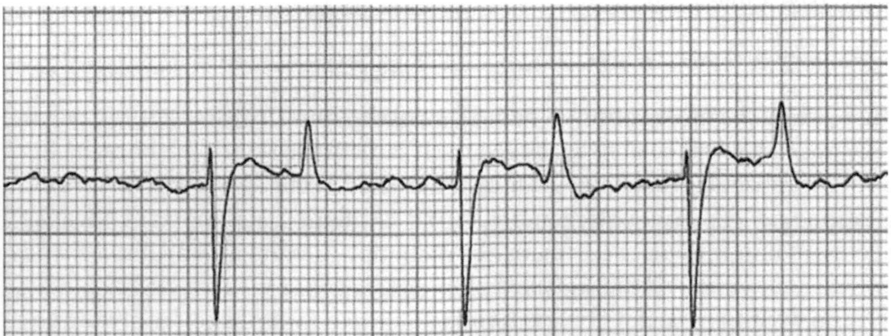

Figure 17.6 Base-apex lead showing atrial fibrillation. The baseline has no distinct P waves but shows fine undulation or "F" waves. The overall heart rate is approximately 60 bpm which is a tachycardia and irregular. Paper speed: 50 mm/s. Calibration: 1 cm/mV.

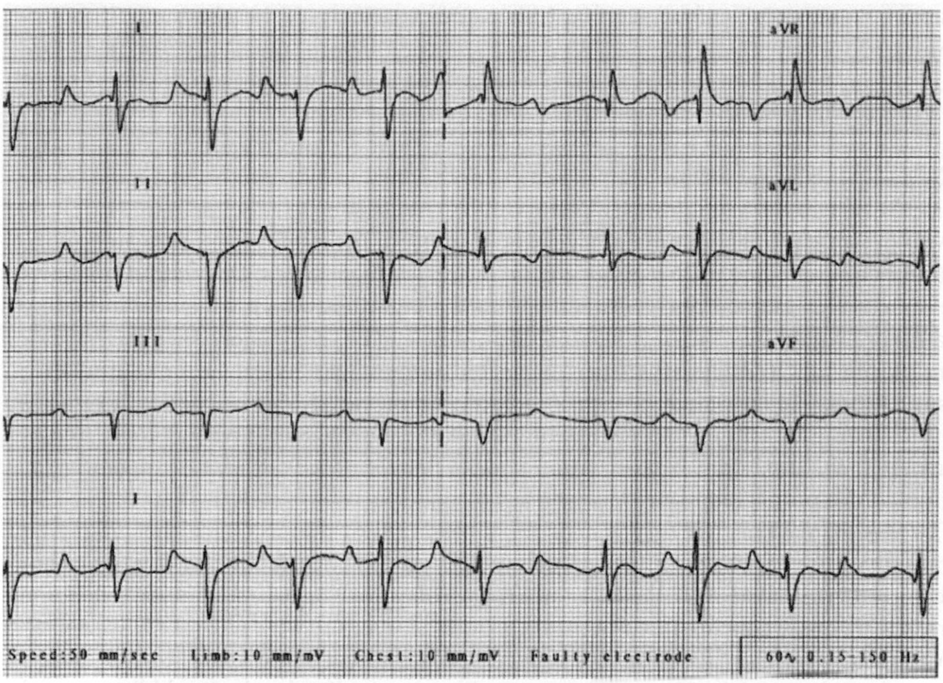

Figure 17.7 The baseline has no distinct P waves (no F waves present). The overall heart rate is approximately 120–140 bpm; which is a tachycardia and irregular. Notice that the QRS morphology is normal indicating normal supraventricular conduction distinguishing this from ventricular tachycardia. Paper speed: 50 mm/s. Calibration, 1 cm/mV. Multi-lead ECG showing atrial fibrillation.

Treatment strategies for AF involve either converting the rhythm back to a normal sinus rhythm or controlling the ventricular response rate. Since idiopathic AF in horses occurs in ostensibly normal myocardial tissue, treatments that convert back to sinus rhythm are preferred. In patients with concurrent cardiac disease, cardioversion to a normal rhythm is less successful and, even if effective, is usually unsustainable. An echocardiogram will help rule out heart disease as the underlying cause of AF. Treatment of AF in this situation focuses on reducing the ventricular response rate.

Since AF in healthy horses is often self-limiting, simple observation for 72–96 h is recommended [3, pp. 699–709]. Any therapy begins with correcting electrolyte or acid-base balances that may be identified. This treatment alone may abolish the arrhythmia.

The most commonly employed treatment of idiopathic AF in horses is quinidine sulfate therapy. In recent years, electrical cardioversion has been used with success for refractory AF. Quinidine sulfate is administered via nasogastric tube to minimize mucous membrane irritation. Quinidine has a narrow limited therapeutic range of only 2–5 μg/mL. Several cardiovascular side effects have been reported including alterations of conduction, hypotension, tachycardia, CHF, and sudden death. Non-cardiovascular toxic signs include colic, diarrhea, ataxia, laminitis, nasal/laryngeal edema obstructing airways, urticaria and/or wheals, and depression. Continuous ECG monitoring is recommended to observe for prolongation of the QRS complex, ventricular arrhythmias or supraventricular tachycardia.

Before treatment begins, a standard base-apex ECG should be obtained. The QRS complex duration should be measured and recorded before initiating therapy. Before each subsequent dose the QRS should be measured again. Increases in the duration of the QRS complex of 25% are associated with quinidine toxicity. This will indicate predisposition of the patient to life-threatening ventricular arrhythmias. Treatment should be halted if this occurs. Once the QRS duration has returned to pretreatment measurement; treatment with quinidine sulphate can be tried again.

A couple of treatment regimens have been proposed. The reader is encouraged to consult an equine specific text or publications for the latest protocol. One limitation, however, is a lack of concordance between specialists regarding which of several quinidine treatment protocols is the most reliable. Quinidine can be administered at a dose of 20–22 mg/kg every 2 h until the rhythm is converted, signs of toxicity appear, or a cumulative dose of 120 mg/kg is reached. Serum blood quinidine levels should be checked to ensure that the therapeutic range has been achieved but not surpassed. If AF has converted to sinus rhythm, quinidine administration should be stopped. Stall rest is imperative as quinidine is a potent hypotensive agent.

One protocol [3, pp. 699–709] calls for a cessation of therapy once the 120 mg/kg cumulative dose has been reached even if conversion was not achieved. A 24 h treatment free period is initiated, and then a second round of every 2 h treatment is started. Some horses will convert during this drug-free period.

An alternative plan [16] proposes reducing doses to every 6 h at the end of the 2 h protocol until conversion or toxicity occurs. Blood quinidine levels should be assessed if signs of toxicity occur.

If AF persists after 2 days of oral quinidine therapy, additional treatment with oral digoxin (0.01 mg/kg) may be implemented every 12 h. This protocol requires extreme care since quinidine and digoxin compete for the same receptor site and can predispose the patient to digoxin toxicity. Toxic side effects of digoxin overlap those of quinidine, so the assault to the gastrointestinal system and the cardiovascular system is especially severe. Ventricular or supraventricular arrhythmias are also a risk using this approach. Continuous monitoring and prompt treatment of side effects is essential.

Once sinus rhythm has been restored, a convalescence period is recommended [3, pp. 699–709]. Refraining from training for 3–4 months is ideal to allow for the atrial myocardium to remodel to more normal tissue. Due to the financial pressures placed on owner/trainers, this is often not done. The return to training should be gradual after the longest recovery period feasible. A minimum of 5–7 days should be allowed for any residual effects of therapy to be cleared. The owner should be instructed on methods for monitoring HR at the stable especially after exercise.

Recently, new anti-arrhythmics such as flecainide and amiodarone have been evaluated for converting AF to a sinoatrial rhythm in horses [17]. Research is ongoing, with amiodarone holding promise; however, flecainide may be limited to use in acute AF. Neither has proven to be successful enough to replace quinidine at this time.

Perhaps the boldest therapy for AF is transvenous electrical cardioversion. During this cardiac catheterization procedure, special electrode-tipped catheters are advanced into the right side of the heart, one into the main pulmonary artery and the other into the right atrium, using two different sites along the length of the jugular vein. This configuration allows the electrical current applied to travel through the atrial tissue, but minimally through the ventricles. Once the catheters are placed, an electrical defibrillation shock is administered to convert the arrhythmia back to a sinus rhythm.

This therapy requires special equipment, knowledge of cardiac catheterization and general anesthesia. Currently only a few veterinary colleges in the USA and Canada provide this service. The success rate for electrical cardioversion in horses is approximately 65–90% as compared with 90–93% with quinidine therapy [14]. However, electrical cardioversion is still a new procedure in equine medicine and has been tried in considerably fewer animals; consequently, further research is required and long-term follow-up data acquired. Since quinidine therapy also has a greater than 90% success rate and is much less expensive to perform, medical therapy is still undertaken in most cases, with referral for electrical cardioversion being reserved for those cases that are refractory to quinidine therapy.

Ventricular Arrhythmias

Premature ventricular complexes, VT, and complete or third-degree AV block are also seen in horses. Horse with ventricular arrhythmias present a special concern since these arrhythmias can lead to collapse of the horse leading to potential injury to the horse and/or a rider.

Third-degree AV block is a bradyarrhythmia that rarely occurs in horses but has a profound effect on performance. As with small animals, third-degree AV block is a complete blocking of the atrial depolarization wave at the AV node and the patient subsists on a ventricular escape beat arising from the Purkinje system (see Chapter 4). Horses with complete AV block may present with collapse (syncope) and/or profound exercise intolerance. Since the AV node is blocking all depolarizations from above, the horse cannot appropriately elevate its HR in response to exercise. Any exertion will cause weakness and collapse.

On physical examination of horses affected with third-degree AV block, a bradycardia is noted with a faster rate S_4 sound "in the background". A murmur may also be present. The ECG will show AV dissociation with P waves and ventricular depolarizations not appropriately related to each other. The QRS-T complexes have no association with the P waves. The ventricular rate will be very slow, less than 20 bpm and long pauses (>30 s) may be present. Permanent pacemaker implantation is the only effective therapy. Due to the expense, lack of availability to return to performance work, and the limited access to pacemaker leads of sufficient length to permanently pace a horse, it is rarely done, even though the first pacemaker used in veterinary medicine was actually implanted in a horse [18].

Ventricular premature complexes are not always associated with heart disease. Ventricular arrhythmias might be noted with ventricular dilation or inflammation. They are often seen with electrolyte and acid-base imbalances, postexercise, with other systemic diseases, induced hypoxia or conditions that alter autonomic tone. Isolated or multiple VPCs that are associated with recovery from exercise rarely are associated with cardiac disease. Usually they will show no clinical signs or require treatment. If the number of VPCs increases during exercise then the likelihood that they result from heart disease increases and should be investigated.

Ventricular premature complexes can be detected on palpation and auscultation as an early beat as compared with the overall rhythm. The difficulty is that, by auscultation

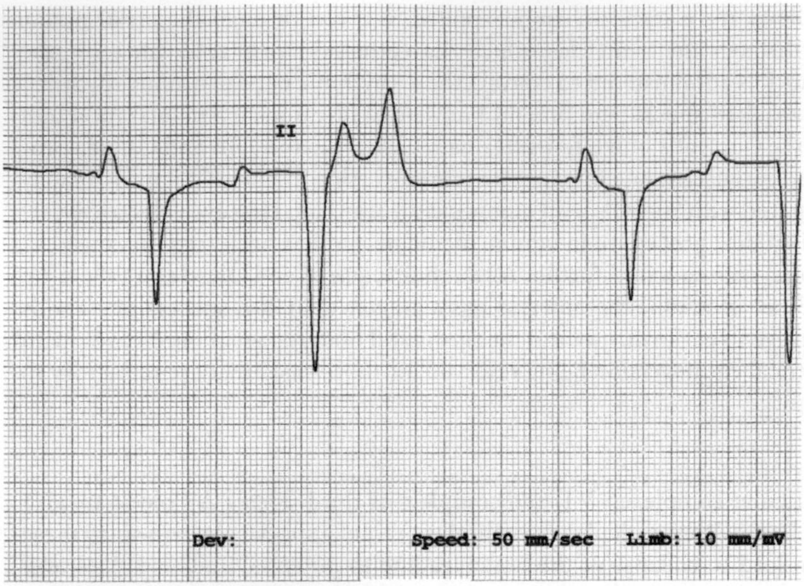

Figure 17.8 Electrocardiogram showing a ventricular premature complex (VPC) between two normal sinus complexes. The first complex on the page demonstrates a positively deflected P wave, negative QRS complex and a diphasic T wave characteristic of a normal sinus beat. The following negative deflection and two positive deflections are the QRS and T waves of the VPC; subsequently followed by another normal sinus complex. Paper speed: 50 mm/s. Calibration, 1 cm/mV. Lead II.

alone, the listener cannot ascertain whether the premature beat is of atrial or ventricular origin and an ECG is therefore recommended.

Ventricular premature complexes usually occur as single depolarizations (Figure 17.8). They also occur in pairs or triplets. If they occur in groups of four or more, they are termed VT. These "runs" of VT may be sporadic, paroxysmal, or sustained. Sporadic runs appear for very short periods of time and occur infrequently over several minutes. Paroxysmal VT seemingly turns "on" and "off" and may be present up to 50% of the time over several minutes. "Sustained VT" is diagnosed when no other sinus rhythm is seen over several minutes.

Ventricular tachycardia is most often associated with primary heart disease, but may be caused by many other abnormalities. Conditions such as bacterial endocarditis, hypoxia, electrolyte abnormalities, drugs, rattlesnake envenomation, septic shock or even aortic root tears have all been associated with VT.

The characterization of VT begins with an ECG. The origin of the ectopic ventricular complexes may be in one location (*monomorphic*) or from multiple locations within the ventricles (*polymorphic*). A monomorphic VT will be regular with rates over 100 bpm. The ventricular complexes on the ECG will all have the same morphology. Polymorphic VT will have an irregular rhythm and variability in the QRS complex morphology. The different foci have different rates of depolarization and therefore the irregular pattern. More severe clinical signs are associated with polymorphic VT, which have a greater chance of degenerating into a fatal arrhythmia such as ventricular fibrillation. Long-standing monomorphic VT will also lead to signs of CHF.

Clinical signs often seen with VT include a rapid rhythm on auscultation, which is irregular with polymorphic VPCs and more regular with monomorphic VPCs. A murmur may be present. *Bruit de cannon* or extra loud heart sounds are heard as a result of AV dissociation. Pleural effusion, ventral subcutaneous edema, jugular pulses, generalized venous distension, and ascites may all be present on physical examination. Additionally, the presence of paroxysmal VT may lead to sustained VT which will lead to horses presenting with signs of weakness, delirium, and even syncope.

Diagnosing and managing any underlying cause is the primary treatment for VT. Lidocaine can be useful for acute management of VT until the underlying cause can be ameliorated. Lidocaine may cause anxiety and neurologic signs in horses so must be used carefully. Diazepam may be needed to help control anxiety in horses receiving lidocaine. Most anti-arrhythmic drugs are administered as a bolus or a constant-rate infusion. Other anti-arrhythmic drugs such as quinidine gluconate, procainamide, amiodarone, and propafenone have been used in the management of VT in horses. See Table 17.3 for anti-arrhythmic doses and treatment regimens. Part of any assessment for ventricular arrhythmias should include blood biochemical analysis including magnesium and acid-base balance. Magnesium sulphate has been used in refractory VT in conjunction with other medications.

Congenital Heart Disease

Congenital cardiac defects are often recognized in horses. They are similar to those seen in small animal patients with some notable exceptions. Certain defects common to small animals, such as aortic stenosis, are virtually never seen in horses.

Although not strictly a congenital defect the aortic–cardiac fistula is a continuously shunting fistula from the aorta to another part of the heart. The etiology of this rare defect is unknown. It could be a true congenital defect or an acquired condition of a degeneration of the media of the aorta. The fistula starts in the right aortic sinus of Valsalva near the ostium of the right coronary artery extending into the right atrium, RV directly, or through the interventricular septum exiting into the RV. This shunt allows blood volume to flow freely from the aorta to the RV, either directly or via the RA. This shunt causes a drop in the aortic diastolic pressure causing hyperkinetic pulses and volume loading of the ventricles. First the RV is directly volume loaded, then the extra volume load is pumped through the lungs then back to the LA, which in turn adds a volume load to the LV.

It is most often seen in stallions greater than 10 years old, but has been reported in gelding and occasionally mares [19]. The presenting complaint is often acute pain or distress (sometimes confused with colic signs), collapse, or exercise intolerance. Physical examination findings include a right-sided continuous murmur, tachycardia, and hyperkinetic pulses. Many horses with aortic–cardiac fistula will demonstrate a VT during an ECG.

Echocardiography is recommended which will show continuous flow by color Doppler exiting the aortic root toward the RV or RA. If a dissecting track is present it appears as an anechoic space with the interventricular septum. Ventricular dilation, rounding of the ventricles and decreased contractility may also be seen. In some cases, the myocardial function can be preserved leading to hyperkinetic contractility. Occasionally an aneurysmal bulge may be seen along the aortic root.

Outcomes for horses with aortic–cardiac fistula are variable. Ventricular arrhythmias pose the most immediate cause of sudden death. Emergency treatment of ventricular arrhythmias is warranted for HRs greater than 120 bpm. Rarely, horses will have ruptures of the aortic root which may also lead to sudden death, but can be survivable. Myocardial failure can lead to CHF, which may be treated with diuretics. Typically, survival times are measured in weeks or months, but cases have been reported of greater than 12 months [19]. In all cases horses diagnosed aortic–cardiac fistula with should be removed from breeding or working programs.

Pulmonic stenosis is very rare and usually diagnosed as part of another more complex abnormality such as tetralogy of Fallot. Pulmonic stenosis may be so severe that virtually no blood flow proceeds from the RV to the lungs via the PA, so blood shunts from the RA to the LA and from the aorta to the main PA through the ductus arteriosus. *Pulmonary atresia* is a lack of communication between the RV and the PA, in which a VSD may or may not be present. Foals with pulmonary atresia are short lived and benefit from various systemic to pulmonary shunts that develop. Pulmonary atresia, along with the critically severe form of pulmonic stenosis, is apparent from birth and survival is unlikely.

Other defects such as VSD are considerably more common than in small animals. Serious congenital heart defects (such as a large VSD) are usually identified shortly after birth and warrant euthanasia. The clinical signs, however, may mimic other treatable conditions. In poor-thriving neonatal foals an echocardiogram may diagnose serious congenital cardiac disease, preventing expenditure of resources treating other suspected conditions when cardiac disease is present.

Ventricular Septal Defects

Ventricular septal defects are the most commonly reported congenital defect in horses [15, p. 196]. Ventricular septal defects can range in prognosis from incidental to life-threateningly severe. Many VSDs are small and restrictive, meaning the diameter is small enough that flow through the defect is hemodynamically inconsequential. It is not uncommon to find a restrictive VSD as an incidental finding during an echocardiogram in an otherwise normal horse. If the defect is large, the added volume passing through the VSD out of the pulmonary artery can cause overcirculation of the lungs and the left atrium and ventricle which can ultimately lead to CHF. These large defects are usually noticed when the horse is a foal and may contribute to a failure to thrive.

The VSD develops as a result of incomplete closure of the ventricular septum during the late stages of cardiac development in the fetus. These defects are in the membranous region of the septum just under the aortic valve. Additionally, the aortic valve apparatus may be deformed and serious aortic insufficiency may contribute to left ventricular volume overload and lead to CHF.

Murmurs of VSD are typically grade 3 or higher systolic murmurs heard best from the right hemithorax and radiate toward the sternum. This radiation is due the shunted blood moving down toward the right ventricular apex during early systole. The additional volume will be expelled with ventricular contraction. As a result of this extra volume, a left basilar systolic murmur of relative pulmonic stenosis may be appreciated in some patients.

A less common VSD can be seen in the infundibular region near the pulmonic valve. This defect is interesting in that the resulting murmur sounds like pulmonic stenosis;

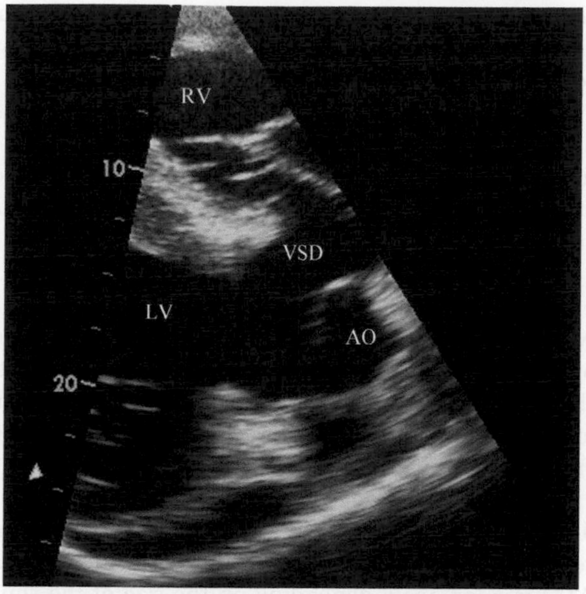

Figure 17.9 Echocardiographic image of a right parasternal long axis view of a horse with a ventricular septal defect. RV, right ventricle; LV, left ventricle; AO, aortic valve; VSD, ventricular septal defect. The tricuspid valve can be seen just above the VSD in the RV.

however, since pulmonic stenosis and aortic stenosis are quite rare in horses (unless they are seen as part of a more complex set of congenital defects) it can be easily misdiagnosed by auscultation alone. Even with echocardiography the infundibular VSD can be difficult to diagnose.

Definitive diagnosis of congenital cardiac defects requires echocardiography (Figures 17.9 and 17.10). It is extremely helpful in evaluating the severity and hemodynamic consequences. Therefore, echocardiography is critical in determining the prognosis of

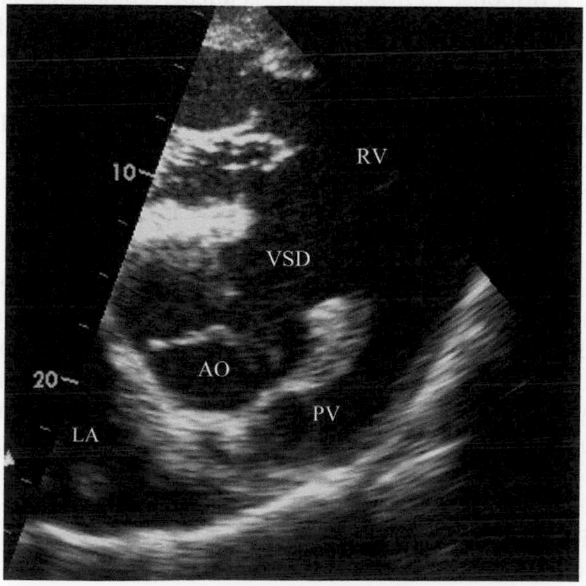

Figure 17.10 Echocardiographic image of a right parasternal short axis view of a horse with a ventricular septal defect. RV, right ventricle; LA, left atrium; AO, aortic valve; VSD, ventricular septal defect; PV, pulmonic valve. In this image the aortic valve in seen end-on with a large VSD emptying into the RV.

congenital cardiac disease. The echocardiographic features of a VSD include a visible opening between the LV and the RV, high velocity flow between the LV and RV seen by color Doppler, and a dilated LV if the VSD is >1 cm.

There is no specific treatment for a VSD and therapy is focused on managing the hemodynamic consequences. Specifically, this means treating any resulting CHF with furosemide and digoxin. Restrictive VSDs will not require any intervention and large (>1 cm) VSDs will make the horse unsuitable for riding, even if surgical correction is attempted.

Atrial Septal Defect

Atrial septal defects are uncommon as a single cardiac congenital defect and are most often associated with other defects. They lead to right ventricular volume overload, as shunted blood typically flows from the left atrium to the right atrium. The volume overload in the RV can lead to signs of ventral edema, ascites, jugular distension, and other signs of right-sided heart failure.

Echocardiography again is the diagnostic test of choice to identifying the ASD and determining its severity. In neonatal foals, the foramen ovale may remain patent for several days and should not be confused with an ASD. Typically, the prognosis for an ASD is poor, again depending on the size of the shunt. A small ASD will allow only a small amount of shunting and less hemodynamic derangement. Furosemide therapy can be used to palliate clinical signs, but once CHF is diagnosed, performance work will never be regained.

Patent Ductus Arteriosus

Unlike dogs, a left-to-right shunting patent ductus arteriosus (PDA) is rarely be seen in horses past the first few days of life, and is usually closed by approximately 7 days. In some instances, a reversion to fetal flow may occur. This maladaptive condition leads to right-to-left shunting of blood, decreased oxygenation of the caudal body, polycythemia as a response to hypoxia, and is uncorrectable (see Chapter 1 for information on fetal circulation.). Euthanasia is usually recommended in a foal with persistent fetal flow.

When a PDA is seen, it is common for it to be associated with other cardiac defects. Left untreated, the PDA ultimately has the same consequences as the PDA in other species, namely left ventricular volume overload and ultimately CHF and possibly spontaneous rupture of the main pulmonary artery caused by pulmonary arterial hypertension.

Tricuspid Atresia

Tricuspid atresia is a rare yet serious congenital defect recognized in foals, in which the tricuspid valve fails to form. Tricuspid atresia may present with cyanosis, sign of right ventricular heart failure, and a murmur most prominent on the right hemithorax. Echocardiographically, the right atrium often enlarges, and the RV will be diminished. A VSD will be noted providing blood to the lungs via the RV. There is no cost-effective treatment for tricuspid atresia and these foals are typically euthanized.

Tetralogy of Fallot

Tetralogy of Fallot (TOF) is a congenital heart malformation more commonly seen in ruminants than horses which consists of four distinct developmental defects in the heart: a VSD, a dextropositioned aorta, pulmonic stenosis, and RV hypertrophy. This condition causes the blood of the RV to shunt into the aorta leading to peripheral cyanosis. In very rare instances TOF may be accompanied with an ASD creating the so called "pentalogy of Fallot". The degree of severity is generally dictated by the relative obstruction of the pulmonic stenosis. In cases of mild stenosis the horse may live to maturity, but is rarely suitable for work. Horses with severe stenosis usually die as foal, or are euthanized. Clinical signs are hypoxemia, cyanosis of the mucous membranes, exercise intolerance, a systolic murmur (from the pulmonic stenosis), polycythemia, and hyperviscosity of the blood. The four defects are visible by echocardiography making it the best diagnostic test for diagnosing TOF.

Glycogen-Branching Enzyme Deficiency

Glycogen-branching enzyme deficiency is not actually a congenital heart defect in the classical sense. It can, however, lead to sudden cardiac death. It is really a genetic defect that leads to stillbirth, limb deformities, seizures, and respiratory and/or cardiac failure caused by an enzyme needed to form glycogen to be missing in the affected foals. Without the formation of glycogen, muscle and brain tissue is lacking in the fuel necessary for metabolism. It is suggested that this mutation may occur in as many as 10% of all Quarter Horses. Bloodlines related to Quarter Horses are also at risk.

The defect is an autosomal recessive trait and carriers can be identified using mane or tail follicles by several licensed veterinary genetic laboratories [20]. Biopsy samples of liver and skeletal muscle are the best way to diagnose the condition in affected foals. There is no treatment for glycogen-branching enzyme deficiency.

Acquired Heart Disease

Horses may develop several forms of acquired heart disease: valvular degeneration and dilated cardiomyopathies from idiopathic and toxic causes, pericardial effusion and endocarditis.

Acquired Valve Disease

Valvular Degeneration

As horses age they may develop a chronic myxomatous valvular degeneration (valvular endocardiosis) that primarily affects the aortic and mitral valves. This degeneration can lead to valve incompetency, murmurs and, if regurgitation is severe enough, CHF. Mitral regurgitation from valvular degeneration is one of the most common causes of murmurs in horses. It is also a common cause of heart failure and can lead to pulmonary rupture and sudden death.

The most common presenting complaint for a horse with valvular degeneration is exercise intolerance, shortness of breath especially after exercise, tachycardia, or a murmur heard during a routine physical. Occasionally, a horse will present to the veterinarian in heart congestive failure with signs of respiratory issues with left ventricular heart failure and ventral subcutaneous edema with right ventricular heart failure.

Echocardiograms may reveal thick valve leaflets that may prolapse into the left atrium, increased left atrial and left ventricular size. Color-flow Doppler demonstrates large color jets of mitral regurgitation crossing into the left atrium during systole creating

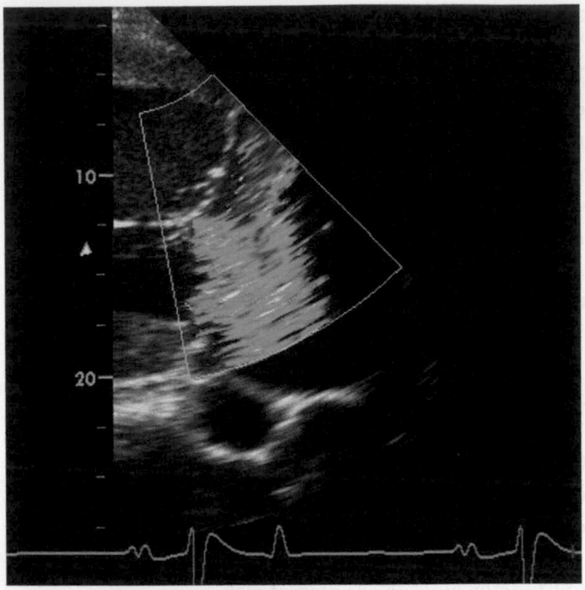

Figure 17.11 Echocardiographic image of a right parasternal long-axis view of a horse with a ventricular septal defect showing the color-flow Doppler signal of the left ventricle flow into the right ventricle. The yellow–green mosaic indicates turbulent blood flow and blood approaches the septal defect. The red signal indicates flow toward the transducer (located at the top of the screen) as blood enters the right ventricle.

a systolic murmur (Figure 17.11). Degeneration that affects the aortic valve may cause a diastolic murmur. As the aortic valve degenerates and more leakage occurs, the volume overload from blood moving back from the aorta eventually causes the left ventricle to fail. One would expect to see a large left ventricle during an echocardiogram, and unless mitral regurgitation is also present a normal-sized left atrium.

Valvular Bacterial Endocarditis

Infectious/inflammatory conditions such as endocarditis and myocarditis are also seen in horses. Endocarditis is an infection of the heart valves and endocardium typically presenting with either an intermittent or continuous fever, lethargy, shifting limb lameness, tachycardia, anorexia, or respiratory signs associated with CHF. Arrhythmias are also noted in some cases due to inflammation of the myocardium. Vegetative lesions on the heart valve may lead to regurgitation creating a murmur. Depending on the valve affected, the murmur may be systolic or diastolic; AV valves causing systolic murmurs and semilunar valves causing diastolic murmurs. Typically the left heart valves are most often affected, but the right heart valves are also susceptible.

The diagnosis of bacterial endocarditis is difficult, but aided by echocardiography and blood culture. Vegetative lesions on the heart valves due to endocarditis may be apparent by echocardiography, thereby supporting the clinical diagnosis and helping to assess damage to the heart. Incidence of volume load due to valvular regurgitation will be apparent if present. Blood cultures and clinical signs are all part of the diagnostic scheme. Collection of a blood culture sample is identical to that in small animals (see Chapter 16). A number of organisms have been implicated in infective endocarditis in horses. *Streptococcus* spp. and *Actinobaccillus* spp. are the most common, but fungi like *Aspergillus* and *Candidia* spp. and *Borrelia burdorferi* have been cultured or identified by serology in some cases.

Aggressive treatment with targeted antibiotics (following blood culture to identify infectious agent and susceptibility) is indicated. Treatment is prolonged and broad-spectrum antibiotics should be initiated while blood cultures are pending. Antibiotic therapy can be tailored based on the organism susceptibility report. Standard therapy for CHF may also be indicated if damage to the heart is severe; unfortunately the prognosis with bacterial endocarditis is grave for left heart infection and guarded at best for right heart infections.

Pericarditis

Pericarditis has traditionally been thought of as a fatal condition, yet in recent years more success has been achieved in treating this serious condition. The exact cause of pericarditis can be elusive and often considered idiopathic; however, it can be associated with infections which worsens the prognosis. If not idiopathic, the causes of pericarditis leading to effusion in horses include bacterial infection, viral infection, and ingestion of eastern tent caterpillars. Unlike dogs, cardiac neoplasia in horses is uncommon as a cause of pericardial effusion. Pericarditis in horses may be classified into three types: (1) effusive – effusion in the pericardial space; (2) fibrous – excessive fibrin in the pericardium; and (3) constrictive – there may or may not be a small amount of effusion present but the heart is compressed. Respiratory conditions such as pneumonia and pleuritis can often been seen in conjunction with pericarditis although an exact link is not known. Often a history of respiratory disease is reported or is the reason for presentation.

Ingestion of the eastern tent caterpillar is associated with mare reproductive loss syndrome, a syndrome that includes early fetal loss, late fetal loss, fibrinous pericarditis, unilateral uveitis, and in a few rare cases *Actinobacillus* meningoencephalitis. This serious health condition is speculated to be caused by migrating setae: the "hairs" on a caterpillar that carry pathologic bacteria can spread throughout the mare hematogenously causing clinical signs.

Horses with pericardial effusion will typically present to the veterinarian for exercise intolerance, fever, depression or lethargy, and tachycardia. Often clinical signs at presentation could be either respiratory or pericarditis. Careful examination of the respiratory system is warranted since pleuritis may be seen in conjunction pericarditis. Occasionally horses with pericarditis/pleuritis may present with anorexia or colic. During the physical examination one may see ventral edema, venous distension and weak arterial pulses. During auscultation the heart sounds may be muffled, murmurs may be present and a pericardial friction rub may be auscultated. Pericardial friction rubs are the tissue of the visceral and epicardial surfaces of the epicardium rubbing on each other creating an audible sound during the cardiac cycle. The sound has been described as "creaking leather", "crunching of snow" or a "wood sawing" sound. Pericardial rubs are usually biphasic, or triphasic, meaning they occur in systole and diastole and even sometimes are presystolic. Rarely are they monophasic.

Radiographs are difficult to take in large horses, and usually yield little information. The electrocardiogram may show a tachycardia, diminished QRS complex size, electrical alternans and occasionally S–T segment changes. Serum chemistry and complete blood count are generally nonspecific but may show anemia, leukocytosis, or hyperfibrinogenemia. If heart failure is present, then azotemia, hyponatremia, or hyperkalemia could also be present.

In suspected cases of constrictive pericarditis, right heart catheterization is useful for making the diagnosis. With a pressure reading catheter system (see Chapter 8) advanced to the RV, a characteristic "dip and plateau" or "square root" sign can be seen on the RV pressure trace which can be seen in Figure 12.11 in Chapter 12.

In suspected cases of pericardial effusion, echocardiography is the best diagnostic tool for making a positive diagnosis. Pericardial effusion can be detected readily by ultrasonography as an anechoic space between the pericardium and the myocardium. In cases of septic pericarditis, the fluid will appear to have large amounts of fibrin. Compression of the right atrium can be seen in cases of tamponade. The RV may also compress in early diastole when pericardial pressure is greater than the RV pressure. The left ventricle may show decreased internal diameter due to decreased output from the right heart and decreased indices of systolic function. Doppler evaluation of left ventricular filling will also be impaired. Echocardiography can also be used to guide placement of the cannula for fluid retrieval and intrapericardial antibiotic administration.

Treatment for pericarditis and pericardial effusion requires removal of the effusion from the pericardial sac. Often the cannulae to remove such fluid can be maintained for 24–48 h until the effusion subsides. This approach also allows for administration of antibiotics directly into the pericardium in the case of infective pericarditis. Lavage with antibiotic-laden 0.9% saline has been used to aid in recovery by flushing bacteria, cellular debris and fibrin from the pericardial space. With aggressive treatment, cases of idiopathic pericardial effusion have a guarded prognosis, but may return to normal function and performance. Horses with a septic effusion have a more guarded prognosis, but recovery is possible. Horses with mare reproductive loss syndrome-induced pericarditis are reported to have favorable outcomes with treatment.

Partial pericardectomy is often used in small animal patients to treat constrictive pericarditis. Only one such case has been reported in a horse which was unsuccessful [21].

Myocardial Disease

Unlike dogs, cats, and humans, myocardial diseases of horses are comparatively uncommon. Dilated cardiomyopathy (DCM) is virtually the only cardiomyopathy seen in horses and has been associated with CHF with the accompanying clinical signs thereof. Echocardiographically, DCM has the same hallmarks as seen in dogs and humans; a dilated left ventricle with poor contractility. The wall thickness of the left ventricle is normal but the chamber size is markedly increased. The prognosis is poor for DCM in horses, as associated heart failure may be treated but the cardiomyopathy cannot be cured and the horse will never return to performance. Cardiac troponin-I is usually elevated in horses with DCM.

A condition known as atypical myocarditis (AM) or multiple acyl-CoA dehydrogenase deficiency has been reported in horses [22–25]. The first reports of this condition were seen in Europe in the early 1980s, but some publications from the 1940s suggest myopathy outbreaks in pastured horses. No single definitive cause for AM has been described, but some early investigations have shown a correlation to clusters of cases in the late fall, particularly associated with "wet and no frost" weather. Noted also was the presence of many trees and shed leaves leading some to speculate about a toxic cause from an unknown source [22]. Two more recent publications link AM to ingestion of maple leaves containing European tar spot (*Rhytisma acerinum)* and *Clostridium sordellii* [23, 24].

Atypical myopathy is a condition in which some or all of the acyl-CoA dehydrogenase molecules in the mitochondria necessary for fatty acid metabolism to supply fuel for muscle tissue are lacking. The lack of multiple acyl-CoA dehydrogenase impairs mitochondrial aerobic metabolism in the muscles, leading to weakness, recumbency, respiratory distress, myocardial failure, and death. Other clinical signs include myoglobinuria, pain, tachycardia with congested mucous membranes, and less commonly icterus, paddling, hemorrhage, diathesis, laminitis, and signs consistent with CHF. Diagnosis of AM can be difficult since it mimics many other conditions such as postexercise rhabdomyolysis, polysaccharide storage myopathies, and ingestion of ionophores or toxic plants. The clinical history is an important feature of the diagnostic process in that typically the horses are full-time pastured, not being exercised and the outbreaks occur in the autumn. A notable feature of AM is a dark chocolate-colored urine, increased serum creatine kinase, and increased cardiac troponin-I [25]. Atypical myopathy has no specific treatment. Horses receiving supportive care have about a 70% mortality rate [26].

Toxicities Leading to Myocardial Failure

Toxicities such as ionophore toxicity, yew plants (*taxus sp.*), oleander (*nerium oleander*), and white snakeroot (*Eupatorium rugosum*) can lead to sudden death in horses from ventricular dysfunction and arrhythmias.

Ionophore toxicity is typically introduced by cross-contamination of cattle food into the equine food source. Compounds such as monensin, lasalocid, or salinomycin are often added to cattle rations to promote growth, or poultry feeds as a coccidiostat. A dose-dependent relationship exists for morbidity and if the amount of ionophore ingested can be determined it is helpful. Food samples should always be collected for analysis. Ionophore toxicity results in VPCs, ventricular tachycardia, and/or sudden death. Dilated, rounded, and a poorly contractile left ventricle as seen with dilated cardiomyopathy is the echocardiographic hallmark of ionophore toxicity and may lead to CHF. Cardiac troponin-I serum concentration may be a useful test in suspected cases of ionophore toxicity and may be elevated. Horses affected with ionophore toxicity need supportive care for several months after exposure as the full effects can be delayed. Because of potential legal complications, owners of horses with suspected ionophore toxicity should keep accurate and detailed records of the horse's medical care.

White snakeroot toxicity can occur in any grazing stock in the eastern and midwest parts of north America. The plant was originally classified as *Eupatorium rugosum,* but in recent years botanists have renamed it *Ageratina altissima,* and it can also lead to heart failure in horses. White snake root can be found in nearly all states east of the Rocky Mountains and a few provinces of Canada. After grazing on the herby shrub, livestock will show sign of neurologic disease, including ataxia, tachypnea, muscle tremors and arched posturing. The toxin also damages the myocardium, leading to fatal ventricular arrhythmias. One distinct clinical pathologic feature that can be noted in the blood of affected animals is markedly elevated creatine–kinase levels and elevated troponin-I. Unfortunately, the only therapy is supportive and the prognosis is poor to grave.

Although not a true toxicity, deficiencies in Vitamin E and selenium can also be associated with myocardial failure.

References

1 Rose, R.J. (1983) An evaluation of heart rate and respiratory rate recovery for assessment of fitness during endurance rides, in *Equine Exercise Physiology* (eds S.G.B. Persson, A. Lindholm and L.B. Jeffcott). Granta Editions, Cambridge. pp. 505–509.

2 Stadler, P, Kinkel, N. and Deegen, E. (1994) A comparison of cardiac stroke volume determination using the thermodilution method and PW Doppler echocardiography for the evaluation of systolic heart function. *Deutsche Tierarztliche Wochenschrift*, **101**, 312–315.

3 Poole, D.C. and Erikson, H.H. (2004) Heart and vessels: function and response to training, in *Equine Sports Medicine and Surgery*, 2nd Edition (eds K. Hinchcliff, A. Kaneps and R. Geor). Saunders, Philadelphia.

4 Young, L.E., Rogers, K. and Wood, J.L.N. (2008) Heart murmurs and valvular regurgitation in thoroughbred racehorses: epidemiology and associations with athletic performance. *Journal of Veterinary Internal Medicine*, **22**, 418–426.

5 Young, L.E. and Wood, J.L. (2000) Effect of age and training on murmurs of atrioventricular valvular regurgitation in young thoroughbreds. *Equine Veterinary Journal*, **32**, 195–199.

6 Patterson, D.E., Detweiler, D.K. and Glendening, S.A. (1965) Heart sounds and murmur of the normal horse. *Annals of the New York Academy of Science*, **127**, 242–305.

7 Boon, J. (2011) *Veterinary Echocardiography*, 2nd Edition. Wiley-Blackwell, Oxford.

8 Phillips, W., Giguere S., Franklin R.P. *et al.* (2003) Cardiac troponin I in pastured and racing thoroughbred horses. *Journal of Veterinary Internal Medicine*, **17**, 597–599.

9 Johnson, A., Jesty, S.A, Gelzer, A.R.M. *et al.* (2007) ECG of the month. *Journal of the American Veterinary Medical Association*, **231**, 706–708.

10 Holbrook, T.C., Birks, E.K., Sleeper, M.M. *et al.* (2006) Endurance exercise is associated with increased plasma cardiac troponin I in horses. *Equine Veterinary Journal Supplement*, **36**, 27–31.

11 Durando, M., Reef, V.B., Kine, K. and Birks, E.K. (2006) Acute effects of short duration maximal exercise on cardiac troponin I in healthy horses. *Equine and Comparative Exercise Physiology*, **4**, 217–223.

12 Nostell, K. and Haggstrom, J. (2008) Resting concentrations of cardiac troponin I in fit horses and effect of racing. *Journal of Veterinary Cardiology*, **10**, 105–109.

13 Gardner, S.Y., Atkins, C.E., Sams, R.A. *et al.* (2004) Characterization of the pharmacokinetic and pharmacodynamics properties of the angiotensin-converting enzyme inhibitor, enalapril in horses. *Journal of Veterinary Internal Medicine*, **18**, 231–237.

14 Reef, V.B, Bonagura, J., Buhl, R. *et al.* (2014) Recommendations for management of equine athletes with cardiovascular abnormalities. *Journal of Veterinary Internal Medicine*, **28**, 749–761.

15 Marr, C. and Bowen, M. (2010) *Cardiology of the Horse*, 2nd Edition. Elsevier, London.

16 Reef, V.B, Reimer, J.M. and Spencer, P.A. (1995) Treatment of atrial fibrillation in horses: new perspectives. *Journal of Veterinary Internal Medicine*, **9**, 57–67.

17 van Loon, G., Blissitt, K.J., Keen, J.A. and Young, L.E. (2004) Use of intravenous flecainide in horses with naturally-occurring atrial fibrillation. *Equine Veterinary Journal*, **36**, 609–614.

18 Taylor, D.H. and Mero, M.A. (1967) The use of an internal pacemaker in a horse with Stokes-Adams Syndrome. *Journal of the American Veterinary Medical Association*, **151**, 1172–1176.
19 Marr, C.M., Reef, V.B., Brazil, T.J. *et al.* (1998) Aorto-cardiac fistulas in seven horses. *Veterinary Radiography and Ultrasound*, **39**, 22–31.
20 Valberg, S. and Mickelson, J.R. *Glycogen Branching Enzyme Deficiency (GBED) in Horses.* College of Veterinary Medicine, University of Minnesota, St Paul. http://www.cvm.umn.edu/umec/lab/gbed/home.html.
21 Hardy, J., Robertson, J.T. and Reed, S.M. (1992) Constrictive pericarditis in a mare: attempted treatment by partial pericardiectomy. *Equine Veterinary Journal*, **24**, 151–154.
22 Votion, D-M. (2012) The story of equine atypical myopathy: a review from beginning to a possible end. *International Scholarly Research Network.* Article ID 281018.
23 van der Kolk, J.H., Wijnberg, I.D, Westerman, C.M., *et al.* (2010) Equine-acquired multiple acyl-CoA dehydrogenase deficiency (MADD) in 14 horses associated with ingestion of maple leaves (*Acer psuedoplantus*) covered with European tar spot (*Rhytisma acerinum*). *Molecular Genetics and Metabolism*, **101**, 289–291.
24 Unger-Torroledo, L., Straub, R., Lehmann A.D. *et al.* (2010) Lethal toxin of *Clostridium sordellii* is associated with fatal equine atypical myopathy. *Veterinary Microbiology*, **144**, 487–492.
25 Verheyen, T., Decloedt, A., De Clercq, D. and van Loon, G. (2012) Cardiac changes in horses with atypical myopathy. *Journal of Veterinary Internal Medicine*, **26**, 1019–1026.
26 Votion, D.M. and Serteyn, D. (2008) Equine atypical myopathy: a review. *Veterinary Journal*, **178**, 185–190.
27 Escudero, A., Gonzalez, J.L. *et al.* (2009) Electrocardiographic parameters in the clinically healthy Zamorano-leones donkey. *Research in Veterinary Science*, **87**, 458–461.

18

Ruminant and Camelid Cardiology

Mark W. Harmon

Approach to the Cardiac Patient

Ruminants and camelids with cardiac disease often present for evaluation of nonspecific complaints such as decreased muscle mass or milk production, increased respiratory rate or effort, and decreased exercise tolerance. As with any patient, it is important to take a systematic approach when evaluating these species for cardiac disease. Crucial information includes the signalment of the animal, and the onset, duration, and progression of the chief complaint. Other essential information to be collected includes diet and dietary supplements, housing environment, reproductive status, deworming program, history of other illnesses, and presence of any other animals with similar signs [1].

Although camelids are actually considered pseudoruminants, for the purposes of this chapter, all further references to ruminants should be assumed to include camelids except where otherwise specified.

Physical Examination

A complete and thorough physical examination, taking a nose-to-tail approach is the foundation of any cardiovascular examination. Knowledge of the normal parameters in a given species is necessary to determine what is abnormal. Normal heart rate parameters for common ruminants are provided in Table 18.1.

Evaluation of mucous membranes is useful for indications of abnormalities in cardiac perfusion and changes in the red cell mass. Normal mucous membranes should be moist, pink, and have a capillary refill time of less than two seconds. Pale mucous membranes may indicate anemia, or decreased cardiac output. Hyperemic mucous membranes may occur secondary to sepsis with peripheral vasodilation, or occasionally, states of hyperdynamic cardiac output. Prolongation in the capillary refill time is usually indicative of diminished cardiac output, and in particular shock. A capillary refill time of greater than 3 s is an indication for aggressive fluid resuscitation.

Normal jugular veins should appear flat. Jugular vein pulsations that extend higher than the lower one-third of the neck are abnormal. Distention of the jugular veins or increased jugular vein pulsation may be indicative of right heart abnormalities or sometimes arrhythmias. Common causes of right heart failure in ruminants include cor pulmonale (right heart failure secondary to pulmonary hypertension), pericardial

Cardiology for Veterinary Technicians and Nurses, First Edition. Edited by H. Edward Durham, Jr.

Table 18.1 Normal heart rate ranges for the common ruminants.

Animal	Normal heart rate range (bpm)
Cattle	
Adult	40–80
Calf	100–140
Sheep	
Adult	60–120
Lamb	120–160
Goat	
Adult	70–110
Kid	120–160
Llama	
Adult	60–90
Cria	80–120

disease (pericardial effusion, or traumatic reticulopericarditis), and infectious or toxic myocarditis. Evaluation of the jugular veins in camelids is difficult due to their normal anatomical depth.

Subcutaneous ventral edema is a common clinical sign of heart failure in ruminants. So-called brisket edema appears as a soft tissue swelling between the forelegs. It will often extend all along the ventral abdomen to include the udder or prepuce. Although much more common with right heart failure, subcutaneous ventral edema can occur with left heart failure as well. However, peripheral limb edema in ruminants is more likely to be secondary to vasculitis or lymphatic obstruction than heart disease [1].

Evaluation of arterial pulse rate and quality is important. The arterial pulse rate should match the ausculted heart rate. For this purpose, the facial artery is convenient to palpate while simultaneously ausculting the heart. The perception of pulse strength is based upon the difference between systolic and diastolic pressures. Hyperkinetic pulses are caused by either an increased systolic pressure, decreased diastolic pressure, or both. Common causes of hyperkinetic pulses include sepsis, fever, and pain resulting in hyperdynamic cardiac function. Another important consideration for hyperkinetic pulses is the presence of aortic valve regurgitation or a patent ductus arteriosus. Regurgitation of blood into the left ventricle, or flow through the ductus arteriosus, widens the pulse pressure by decreasing diastolic arterial pressure and results in a hyperdynamic pulse. Conversely, hypokinetic pulses are caused by a decrease in the difference between these systolic and diastolic pressures. This can be caused by a diminution in cardiac output, or systemic arterial vasodilation such as occurs in shock.

Auscultation is important to perform to evaluate for the presence of abnormal heart sounds including murmurs, arrhythmias, and the presence of split heart sounds. Due to the slower heart rates of most adult ruminants, it is normal to hear three or even all four heart sounds. Respiratory auscultation should be carefully performed by listening in all four quadrants of the chest on both sides of the thorax. Abnormalities that the examiner may find on physical examination include muffled heart sounds that may indicate pericardial effusion, or muffled lung sounds that may indicate pleural effusion. Pleural effusion is sometimes identified by the presence of a fluid line, which is identified by normal to increased lung sounds dorsally, with a marked diminution in lung sounds ventrally. Pleural effusion would be expected to cause the combination of both muffled heart and lung sounds. In contrast, pericardial effusion would be expected to result in muffled heart sounds with normal lung sounds. Readers are encouraged to review Chapter 3 on cardiovascular physical examination for a more in-depth description of these findings.

Pericardial effusion associated with gas-forming microbes may cause a "washing-machine murmur" associated with the accumulation of fluid, gas, and fibrin being sloshed around inside the pericardium by the contracting heart. Sometimes the presence of gas may be suggested by "plinking noises" similar to water flowing through a small fountain. The examiner should be careful to be far enough forward on the thorax so as not to confuse normal gut sounds with pericardial sloshing.

Diagnostic Tools

With few exceptions, all of the commonly performed diagnostic tests that are utilized in small animal patients can be used in ruminants suspected of having cardiovascular disease. Important limitations to consider include the size of the patient which will affect the ease of using some of these modalities, and the cost-effectiveness of the diagnostic test relative to the value of the animal.

Radiographs

In smaller ruminants and in younger patients, thoracic radiography can be an invaluable component of the cardiovascular evaluation. Radiographs allow the clinician to evaluate the size and shape of the cardiac silhouette relative to the thorax; the appearance of the lung fields including pulmonary parenchyma, airways, and pulmonary vasculature; assess for pleural effusion; intrathoracic masses; and the integrity of the diaphragm. Radiographs can be attempted in larger ruminants; however, their increased girth may limit how effectively the X-ray beam can penetrate the thoracic cavity. An alternate imaging modality to consider, though rarely employed, is CT scanning.

Electrocardiography

In spite of the relative antiquity of this modality, no other diagnostic test has superseded the electrocardiogram (ECG) for accurate diagnosis of rhythm disturbances. The ECG in large animals is most commonly recorded using a base-apex lead configuration. This is performed by attaching the positive lead (red) over the left apex of the heart at the level of the costochondral junction in the fifth intercostal space, and attaching the negative lead (white) in the right jugular furrow [1]. This creates a vector across the major axis of the heart. The ground lead (black) can be attached anywhere, and is helpful for improving signal quality. Depending upon how frequently an arrhythmia occurs, it may be necessary to record several minutes of ECG data, or to attempt recordings at multiple times. Alternatively, ambulatory or telemetry electrocardiography may be more feasible for recording arrhythmias that occur less frequently.

Ruminants have a ventricular conduction system that penetrates extensively from the endocardium to the epicardium causing nearly instantaneous depolarization of the entire mass of the left and right ventricles. Consequently, changes in the QRS complex morphology are not particularly useful for diagnosis of chamber enlargement. Thus, the primary utility of the ECG in these species is the diagnosis of rhythm disturbances.

Echocardiography

Echocardiography is extremely useful for diagnosing the specific nature of cardiac abnormalities. Echocardiography allows the evaluator to determine the cause of a murmur (valve dysfunction, septal defect, or physiologic), and to assess systolic and diastolic myocardial function. Additional information that may be obtained includes the presence of pericardial effusion, or changes in the appearance of the myocardium that can be consistent with neoplasia, or chronic fibrosis. Younger animals can often be scanned in lateral recumbency, similar to a small animal patient, which will facilitate obtaining a good imaging window. Larger animals must be scanned while standing. Normal echocardiographic values have been published for some bovine breeds (Table 18.2).

Congenital Cardiac Disease

Congenital cardiac disease is an important cause of failure to thrive in young ruminants. Indications of cardiac disease may include weakness, respiratory distress, cyanotic mucous membranes, exercise intolerance, poor nursing, and diminished rate of weight gain. Although any congenital malformation is possible, there are only a few that are seen with any frequency.

Ventricular Septal Defect

Ventricular septal defect (VSD) is the most common congenital cardiac disease reported in ruminants. In cattle, the most common location for a VSD is in the perimembranous region just below the aortic and tricuspid valves [2]. In llamas, the most common location for a VSD is in the apical region (referred to as a "muscular" VSD) (Figure 18.1) [3]. The typical murmur of a VSD is a loud, harsh, plateau-shaped murmur with its point of maximal intensity on the right side of the thorax. A murmur of relative pulmonic stenosis may be heard on the left side of the thorax. This murmur is explained by the increased volume seen by the right heart due to the VSD. Although the pulmonic valve is structurally normal, it is functionally stenotic relative to the increased volume.

The clinical signs associated with VSD are dependent on its size [2, 3]. A relatively small VSD with normal left and right ventricular systolic pressures will result in a very noisy murmur, but little to no overt cardiovascular clinical signs. A large VSD may allow pressures in the two chambers to equilibrate and therefore there may not be an obvious murmur, but the patient will be severely compromised. Patients with a large VSD are at risk of developing congestive heart failure from volume overload of the lungs and left atrium and ventricle. Although one might expect a VSD to cause right heart failure, the

Table 18.2 Adult cow reference ranges.

Parameter	Generic	Jersey	Holstein-Friesian
		X ± SD	
HR	47.8 ± 5.90	71.0 ± 6.0	72.3 ± 4.5
N	15	10	12
M-Mode			
RVd (cm)	3.04 ± 0.56	2.45 ± 0.53	2.27 ± 0.76
RVs (cm)		1.32 ± 0.63	1.14 ± 0.43
LVd (cm)	7.54 ± 0.80	7.7 ± 0.7	8.7 ± 1.0
LVs (cm)	3.97 ± 1.1	4.2 ± 0.53	4.2 ± 0.8
% FS	43.5 ± 5.80	44.7 ± 8.3	46.5 ± 9.5
Vcf (circ/s)	0.87 ± 0.14		
VSd (cm)	2.24 ± 0.26	2 ± 0.4	2.2 ± 0.51
VSs (cm)		3.6 ± 0.5	3.4 ± 0.5
LVWd (cm)	2.00 ± 0.19	1.2 ± 0.3	1.5 ± 0.4
LVWs (cm)		1.5 ± 0.5	1.4 ± 0.5
AO (cm)	6.00 ± 0.40		
LA (cm)	4.80 ± 0.57		
LV EF		0.85 ± 0.09	0.79 ± 0.15
EPSS		0.45 ± 0.48	0.62 ± 0.23
Two-dimensional			
PAd (cm)		4.2 ± 0.27	5.5 ± 0.8
AOd (cm)		5 ± 0.26	6.4 ± 0.62
PA:AO		0.85 ± 0.07	0.86 ± 0.09
AO S d(cm)		5.7 ± 0.34	7.94 ± 0.56
Aod—cs (cm)		5.15 ± 0.31	7.05 ± 1.17
LADs (cm)		10.9 ± 0.5	12 ± 1.2
Doppler			
AO VTI (cm)		30.4 ± 3.41	
CO (L/min)		56.5 ± 8.44	
CI (ml/kg/min)		123.2 ± 5.7	
Two-dimensional guided		Yes	Yes

HR, heart rate; d, diastole; s, systole; RV, right ventricle; LV, left ventricle; FS, fractional shortening; Vcf, velocity of circumferential fiber shortening; circ, circumference; VS, ventricular septum; LVW, left ventricular wall; AO, aorta; LA, left atrium; EF, ejection fraction; EPSS, E point to septal separation; PA, pulmonary artery diameter; AO S, aortic sinus diameter; AO cs, aortic cross-sectional diameter; LAD, left atrial diameter; VTI, velocity time integral; CO, cardiac output; CI, cardiac index.
Source: Data from Boon, J. (2011) *Veterinary Echocardiography*, 2nd Edition.Wiley-Blackwell, Ames.

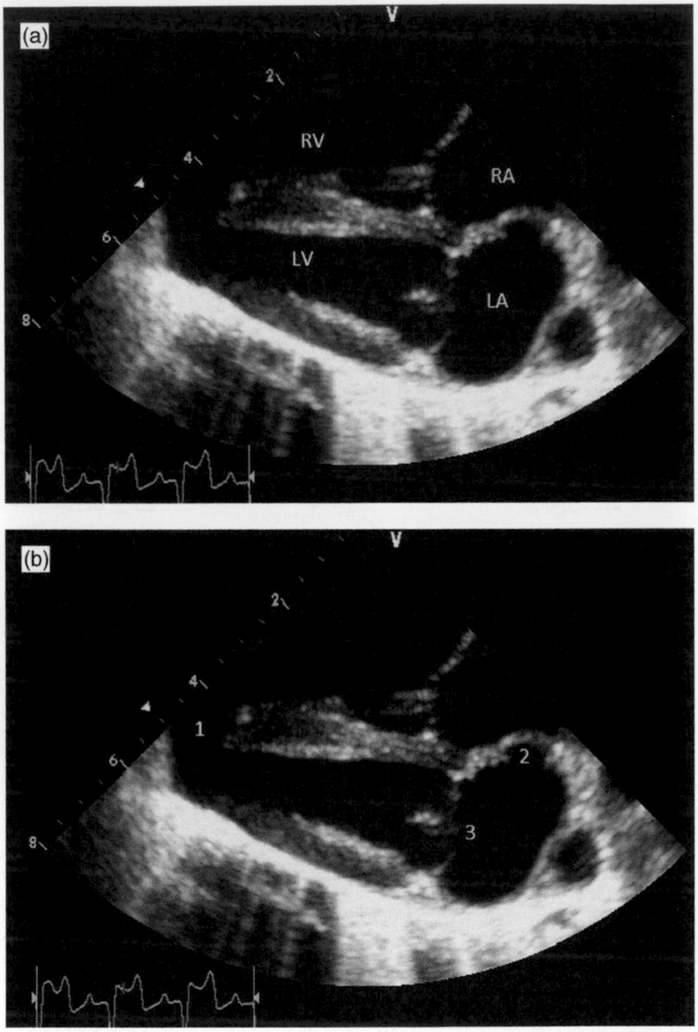

Figure 18.1 (a) Right parasternal long axis four-chamber view from a 5-day old alpaca cria that was initially presented for lethargy, anorexia, and weight loss. RA, right atrium; LA, left atrium; RV, right ventricle; LV, left ventricle. (b) The same echocardiographic image with labeled abnormalities. A large muscular ventricular septal defect (1) is present at the cardiac apex. The interatrial septum is protruding toward the right atrium. This appearance is secondary to a patent foramen ovale (2). The mitral valve leaflets can also be seen prolapsing into the left atrium consistent with mitral valve dysplasia (3).

right ventricle is merely acting as a conduit for blood flow from the left heart to the lungs. Unless pulmonary hypertension develops secondary to the increased blood flow, the right heart will be unaffected by a VSD.

Pulmonary hypertension with congenital cardiac disease can occur from persistence of fetal physiology, meaning that the high prenatal pulmonary resistance fails to decrease at birth. In this instance, the shunt flow of a VSD is always from the right ventricle to the left ventricle. Alternatively, an increase in pulmonary vascular resistance can come from a reactive change secondary to the increased flow from a left to right shunt. In this instance, the increased flow stimulates vasoconstriction of the precapillary arterioles in an effort to protect the microcirculation from being overwhelmed. Over time, this stimulates remodeling (intimal hyperplasia and medial hypertrophy) that becomes irreversible if the shunt persists. Right heart failure that is secondary to pulmonary hypertension is referred to as *cor pulmonale* (see below).

Prognosis with a VSD is determined echocardiographically measuring the velocity of flow across the defect with continuous-wave Doppler. The ultrasound machine converts the measured velocity to a pressure gradient using the Bernoulli equation (pressure gradient $= 4 * V^2$((see Chapter 6). A velocity of $\geq$4 m/s (pressure gradient $\geq$64 mmHg) is typically associated with a good prognosis and an asymptomatic patient. A velocity between 3 and 4 m/s results in a more variable prognosis with some patients remaining asymptomatic and others developing heart failure. A velocity <3 m/s is indicative of a very hemodynamically significant shunt and heart failure is quite likely in these patients.

Tetralogy of Fallot

Tetralogy of Fallot is the most common cause of cyanotic heart disease in the neonatal ruminant. It is a complex congenital defect that results from a defect in the formation of the conal septum (the region below the pulmonic valve). This causes pulmonic valve stenosis with resultant right ventricular hypertrophy. Malformation of the conal septum prevents closure of the interventricular foramen, resulting in a VSD. The interventricular septum is part of the normal support structure for the aortic root and in its absence the aorta deviates rightward and overrides the VSD. If an atrial septal defect is also present, then this combination is known as a pentalogy of Fallot [2]. Tetralogy of Fallot is diagnosed by demonstrating the four features echocardiographically. Although this disease can be potentially palliated surgically, prognosis is poor in animals that are symptomatic.

Branch Pulmonic Arterial Stenosis

Branch pulmonic arterial stenosis appears to be a relatively common cause of innocent murmurs in young crias. The disease appears to be similar to peripheral pulmonary artery stenosis in human infants. It occurs due to physiologic narrowing and acute angulation of the pulmonary arteries as they branch from the main pulmonary artery. These murmurs are typically gone by 2 months of age [3]. In an asymptomatic cria with a murmur $\leq$3/6, it is reasonable to wait until after 8 weeks of age to perform an echocardiogram to see if the murmur resolves spontaneously.

Patent Ductus Arteriosus

The ductus arteriosus is a normal fetal vascular structure that connects the aorta and the pulmonary artery. In the fetus, the placenta is the organ of oxygenation, and the lungs only need enough blood flow to stimulate their normal growth and development. *In utero*, the ductus arteriosus shunts blood from the pulmonary artery to the aorta (right-to-left shunt). When the neonate is born and the lungs inflate, the pulmonary vascular resistance drops markedly and the shunt flows from the aorta to the pulmonary artery (left to right). The increased oxygen tension in the ductus normally stimulates the contraction of smooth muscle resulting in closure of the ductus. Inadequate amounts of smooth muscle will allow the ductus to remain patent and shunting to persist. The characteristic murmur of a patent ductus arteriosus (PDA) is a continuous or "washing-machine" murmur caused by flow from the high pressure aorta (120/80 mmHg) to the low pressure pulmonary artery (25/10 mmHg). Normally the ductus is functionally closed by 4 days of life. If a continuous murmur is ausculted after this time, an echocardiogram should be performed. A small PDA is hemodynamically inconsequential; however, a large PDA will most likely result in left-sided congestive heart failure.

A small percentage of PDAs will reverse direction and shunt from the pulmonary artery to the aorta. Right-to-left PDAs are rare and challenging to diagnose. The blood flow velocity with a right-to-left shunt is often low and therefore may not cause an audible loud murmur. The hallmark of right-to-left PDAs is differential cyanosis – the presence of pink mucous membranes cranially, and cyanotic mucous membranes caudally. This is due to normally oxygenated blood being delivered to the head via the brachicephalic trunk and left subclavian artery. The PDA shunts blood distal to these structures and delivers a mixture of venous and arterial blood to the caudal portions of the body. A right-to-left PDA is diagnosed by performing a contrast echocardiogram (see Chapter 6) and visualizing the presence of bubbles in the abdominal aorta.

Ectopia Cordis Cervicalis

Ectopia cordis cervicalis occurs when the heart develops partially or completely outside the thorax. The cause is incompletely understood but results from failure of midline mesoderm and ventral body wall formation during embryonic development. Most commonly the heart is found in the cervical region, but there are reports of the heart being found in the abdomen or pectoral region. Concurrent defects are common and have included other cardiac abnormalities, torticollis, and malformations of the ribs and sternum [2]. Prognosis is generally poor, although there is at least one report of an affected cow giving birth at the age of three [4].

Acquired Heart Disease

Acquired cardiac disease in adult ruminants is most often of an infectious or toxic etiology. However, other etiologies including neoplastic, idiopathic, degenerative, and genetic disorders must also be considered depending on the patient's signalment.

Endocarditis

In cattle, tricuspid valve endocarditis is most commonly reported, though any of the four valves may be affected. The most common organisms isolated are *Streptococcus, Pasteurella, Actinobacillus,* and *Arcanobacterium*. Most commonly endocarditis occurs without an obvious antecedent event; however, chronic foot abscesses, rumenitis, mastitis, or other septic processes may lead to recurrent bacteremia which increases the risk of a valvular infection [2].

There are few reports describing endocarditis in camelids, but one study found a higher incidence of mural thrombotic lesions than valvular [5, 6]. In this study, no infectious cause could be consistently identified and it was theorized that camelids may manifest endocarditis similar to humans with chronic nonbacterial thrombotic endocarditis [5]. In other camelid endocarditis reports, the bacterial organisms found included *Escherichia coli*, *Corynebacterium pseudotuberculosis* (dromedary camel), *Actinobacillus suis* (alpaca), *Clostridium perfringens* (llama), and *Listeria monocytogenes* (alpaca) [6].

Although some animals are asymptomatic, infectious endocarditis is generally associated with signs of lethargy, anorexia, decreased milk production in dairy cattle, and loss of muscle mass [2]. Jugular distension and pulsations are common findings with tricuspid endocarditis in cattle. Similarly, there may be evidence of brisket and ventral subcutaneous edema, limb edema, and ascites (rare). The respiratory rate and effort are frequently increased, and harsh lung sounds on auscultation are common. A murmur is usually present on cardiac auscultation. The murmur may be systolic or diastolic depending on the valve affected, but regurgitation is a more common complication than stenosis. Arrhythmias, particularly atrial fibrillation, are common with endocarditis. Other arrhythmias that may be noted include atrial premature complexes, ventricular premature complexes, and ventricular tachycardia. Other abnormalities that are common include fever, hematuria, pyuria, and shifting limb lameness. Lameness can be the result of septic tenosynovitis or immune-mediated inflammation. Camelids are often sternally recumbent [5, 6].

Definitive diagnosis of endocarditis requires identification of a likely organism on blood culture coupled with other supporting evidence; however, blood cultures are often negative if previous empiric antibiotic therapy has been attempted. Echocardiographically, endocarditis usually appears as irregular vegetative nodules on the valve leaflets. However, some organisms are more destructive than proliferative and the evidence of a growth may be minimal. Clinical pathologic changes can include mild anemia, thrombocytopenia, neutrophilia (sometimes with a left shift), increased globulin concentrations, mild elevations in hepatic enzymes, hematuria, and pyuria. In addition to blood, cultures of urine, joint fluid, and transtracheal wash fluid may increase the likelihood of identifying an infectious organism [9].

Treatment of endocarditis is initially with empiric broad-spectrum bactericidal antibiotics. In cattle, penicillin and beta-lactam drugs are frequently first-line therapy due to the high incidence of gram-positive infections. Results of a bacterial culture and sensitivity should be used to more specifically target the etiologic agent. The best results are obtained with long-term intravenous antibiotics. However, there are numerous challenges associated with treating infective endocarditis. The organisms tend to be densely packed and slowly growing and therefore agents which have good penetration into poorly vascular regions are preferred. The addition of rifampin in combination with another antibiotic may improve outcome. Anticoagulant therapy with subcutaneous heparin and low-dose aspirin may help prevent thrombotic complications, and reduce growth of the vegetations [2].

Long-term prognosis with endocarditis is poor. It is difficult to completely sterilize the lesions and recurrences are common. Even in cases where the infection is eradicated, often the valve is so badly damaged that heart failure is an inevitable sequela.

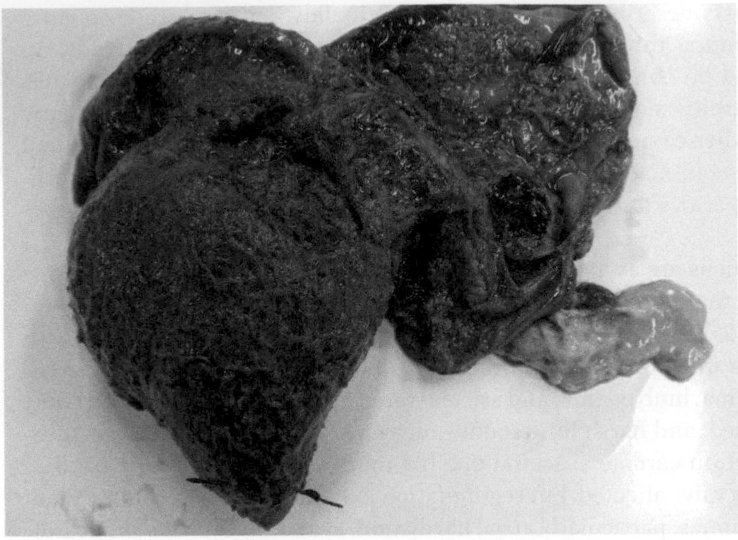

Figure 18.2 A bovine heart with the pericardium reflected toward the cardiac base and caudally. A thick layer of fibrin can be seen covering the entire epicardial surface. The cause of fibrinous pericarditis in this animal was traumatic reticuloperitonitis, as evidenced by the metallic wire penetrating the left ventricular apex. Photo courtesy of Dr Gayle Johnson.

Pericarditis

Pericarditis is most commonly reported in cattle; reports in other ruminant species are uncommon. Similarly, it is uncommon in camelids although there is a report of a llama affected by pericarditis that was attributed to bovine tuberculosis [7]. In cattle, pericarditis may be primary (idiopathic aseptic inflammation, which is rare) or secondary to a number of processes, such as a penetrating foreign body or external wound, septicemia, or extension of a pre-existing pneumonia, pleuritis, or neoplasia. A common cause in cattle is secondary to traumatic reticuloperitonitis (also known as "hardware disease"). In this situation, a metallic foreign body is ingested and subsequently perforates the reticulum. Continuous contractions of the ruminant stomach can cause migration of the foreign body cranially to perforate the diaphragm and then the adjacent pericardium [2, 8]. The resultant inflammation of the pericardial sac is often accompanied by the accumulation of fluid in the pericardial space (pericardial effusion) that may also have strands of fibrin (Figure 18.2).

Clinical signs are variable and highly dependent on both the rate and volume of pericardial effusion that develops. The parietal pericardium surrounding the heart is a distensible structure and with slowly developing effusions can accommodate small volumes without significant hemodynamic effects. More rapidly developing or large volume effusions are more likely to be symptomatic. These animals are often presented for decreased or absent appetite or decreased milk production. Affected cattle are often reluctant to move and stand with abducted elbows and an abnormal distribution of their weight [2, 8]. Common physical examination findings include tachypnea with or without an expiratory grunt, tachycardia, fever, and muffled heart sounds. Auscultation of the lungs may reveal decreased lung sounds ventrally if accompanied by pleuritis. Infection of the pericardium with gas-producing anaerobes may lead to both gas and fluid in the pericardial space. This can give rise to a "washing-machine" murmur heard on cardiac auscultation [1, 2]. If the pressure in the pericardial space exceeds that of the right heart, systemic venous return is decreased and signs of right-sided heart failure (jugular venous pulsation, poor arterial pulse quality, brisket edema) may be present. Evaluation of the gastrointestinal tract can reveal decreased or absent ruminal contractions, rumen bloat, and scant feces [8]. Direct compression of the xyphoid or ventral chest may elicit a pain response; however, interpretation of this test can be complicated due to differing pain thresholds among the ruminant species [8, 9].

Radiographs may reveal a metallic foreign body, gas in the pericardial space, or an enlarged cardiac silhouette [3]. Fibrinogen is elevated in the majority of pericarditis cases [9]. Changes present on an electrocardiogram are inconsistent but may include decreased R wave amplitudes (less than 1.5 mV in a base-apex lead), electrical alternans, or changes in the ST segment. The most useful diagnostic technique is echocardiography. Visualization of an echo-free or hypoechoic space between the parietal pericardium and the heart is diagnostic for pericardial effusion. Often fibrin strands can be seen in the effusion. Cardiac tamponade may also be documented if the effusion is impairing the diastolic function of the right heart. Fluid analysis of the pericardial effusion is typically consistent with a suppurative exudate and a mixed population of gastrointestinal flora may also be identified. Idiopathic effusions reported in cattle tend to be hemorrhagic in appearance. Although not commonly performed, jugular venous catheterization can be used to measure elevations in the central venous pressure and right atrial pressure [2].

Treatment of cattle affected with pericarditis is generally unrewarding and prognosis is poor, especially if signs of right heart failure have developed. These animals can develop constrictive pericardial disease due to the inflammation decreasing the distensible nature of the parietal pericardium or left-sided congestive heart failure due to the involvement of the epicardium and myocardium. Treatment is usually aimed at salvage or short-term survival until calving. Pericardiocentesis, ideally with the guidance of echocardiography, can be performed to decrease the pressure in the pericardial space and enhance venous return to the right side of the heart. If ultrasonographic guidance is not available, the ideal spot for pericardiocentesis is usually the left fifth intercostal space dorsal to the olecranon and above the level of the lateral thoracic artery. If treatment is attempted, a pericardial catheter should be placed at the time of initial pericardiocentesis to allow for serial drainage, lavage, and instillation of antibiotics. Broad-spectrum antimicrobial coverage should be instituted given the wide variety of bacteria found in the gastrointestinal tract. Nonsteroidal anti-inflammatory drugs or corticosteroids (barring evidence of septicemia) may also be beneficia [2]. Preventive measures can be taken to address some causes of pericarditis. Traumatic reticuloperitonitis can be effectively prevented through the routine administration of magnets. Additionally, routine vaccination for respiratory disease should be performed.

Cardiomyopathy

The only cardiomyopathy of significance in ruminants is dilated cardiomyopathy. Cardiomyopathy is rare in camelids, but there are cases of both dilated cardiomyopathy and an asymmetrical hypertrophic cardiomyopathy reported [3, 10]. Cardiomyopathy can be primary or secondary as detailed below. Clinical signs may include failure to thrive, tachycardia, and arrhythmias. Secondary cardiomyopathies include myocarditis which usually include a fever. All conditions listed below carry a guarded to poor prognosis once animals are symptomatic, but animals may be able to be salvaged for breeding purposes [2].

Primary Cardiomyopathy

An inherited cardiomyopathy has been described in cattle with the red Holstein gene and in polled Herefords with the curly hair coat gene [2]. Severe left ventricular dysfunction is often present (with or without right ventricular dysfunction) along with enlargement of the left atrium. As juveniles, many of these animals will progress into congestive heart failure. A juvenile cardiomyopathy of llamas has been reported but is not well characterized [3]. Breeding of animals suspected to have an inherited cardiomyopathy is not recommended.

Secondary Cardiomyopathy

There are numerous causes of secondary cardiomyopathy described for ruminants. Nutritional muscular dystrophy, also called "white muscle disease", occurs secondary to vitamin E, selenium, or copper deficiencies or excessive molybdenum or sulfates (secondary copper deficiency). The typical myocardial lesions found are white streaks of hyaline degeneration, necrosis, and infiltration by mononuclear cells. This condition is not well documented in llamas or alpacas, but has been reported in Arabian camels [3].

Infectious and toxic causes of myocarditis, listed in Table 18.3, may also be considered as a secondary cardiomyopathy. Bacterial causes of myocarditis may be from local infections (pericarditis, endocarditis) or from septicemia [2]. Sarcosporidiosis is the most common myocardial parasite of camels, but its significance in llamas and alpacas is unknown [3].

Echocardiographic examination of the patient with myocarditis typically reveals dilated ventricles with decreased systolic function and dilated atria. Atrial and ventricular arrhythmias are common with myocarditis. Cardiac troponin I (cTnI) is a subcellular myocardial protein that is normally found in very low concentrations in the peripheral circulation. It is a sensitive indicator of acute myocardial injury and is often elevated in patients with myocarditis [11].

Treatment is aimed at addressing the underlying cause if possible. In animals with severe toxemia and complicated arrhythmias, corticosteroids may be beneficial although their use is controversial [2]. Congestive heart failure should be treated as detailed below.

Neoplasia

Cardiac neoplasia is not common in ruminants or camelids; however, the most common primary cardiac tumor of cattle is lymphosarcoma which has a predilection for infiltrating the right atrial and right ventricular myocardium [2, 3]. Clinical signs are usually absent or nonspecific and include anorexia, weight loss, and fever. Cardiac lymphosarcoma can lead to tachycardia, arrhythmias, and heart murmurs which may progress to congestive heart failure.

Clinicopathologic examination is not a reliable means of diagnosis, and the lack of leukemic changes does not rule out lymphosarcoma. Definitive diagnosis requires

Table 18.3 Selected causes of myocarditis in ruminants and camelids.

Bacteria	
	Borrelia burgdorferi (Lyme disease)
	Clostridium chauvoei
	Mycobacterium spp.
	Staphylococcus aureus
	Streptococcus equi
Viruses	
	Foot-and-mouth disease (picornavirus)
Parasites	
	Cysticercosis
	Sarcocystis
	Sarcosporidiosis (camels)
	Toxoplasmosis
Toxins	
	Coffeeweed (*Senna* spp.)
	Death Camas (*Zygadenus* spp.)
	Gossypol
	Ionophores (monensin, lasalocid, salinomycin)
	Oleander (*Nerium* spp.)
	Phalaris spp.
	Yew (*Taxus* spp.)

histopathologic examination of the tumor tissue. Lymphosarcoma in cattle is most common with the adult (greater than 4 years old) or the enzootic form of bovine leukosis virus. It is rarely seen with the thymic form of lymphosarcoma that tends to affect younger cows [2].

Pulmonary Hypertension and Cor Pulmonale

Brisket disease (also known as high mountain disease or high altitude disease) is a primary lung disease that secondarily affects cardiac function, a condition called cor pulmonale [2]. The response of the pulmonary vasculature to hypoxia is vasoconstriction which is a compensatory attempt to shunt blood from underventilated areas to regions of higher perfusion. When hypoxia is diffuse, the resulting vasoconstriction causes pulmonary hypertension. The inciting cause of hypoxia is commonly increased altitude, although bronchopneumonia and lungworm infections may also lead to the development of pulmonary hypertension. The resultant increase in afterload to the right ventricle leads to cardiac remodeling and eventually, right-sided heart failure. Cattle exposed to locoweed (*Oxytropis* spp. and *Astragalus* spp.) are more sensitive to the effects of altitude and are more likely to develop right-sided heart failure [2].

Brisket disease is almost exclusively a disease of cattle. Camelids have developed several adaptations to aid the tolerance of chronic hypoxia that may be seen in their native mountainous environments in South America. Alveolar hypoxia does not significantly affect pulmonary vascular resistance in these species which explains why camelids are relatively resistant to the development of hypoxic pulmonary hypertension [3].

Subcutaneous edema, especially of the submandibular and ventral regions, distended jugular and/or superficial abdominal veins and dyspnea/tachypnea are common physical examination findings. A murmur of tricuspid insufficiency or pulmonic regurgitation may be ausculted, as well as a split S2 due to early closure of the pulmonic valve [2]. For cattle not affected by altitude, radiographs may show evidence of bronchopneumonia, bronchiectasis, or bronchitis. Transtracheal washes or fecal sedimentations may be useful for determining a nonaltitude related etiology. Electrocardiographic changes include increased P wave amplitude indicative of right atrial enlargement ("P pulmonale") and a right axis deviation of the mean electrical axis indicative of right ventricular hypertrophy. Changes that may be found on echocardiography include right atrial enlargement, right ventricular hypertrophy, and dilation of the main pulmonary artery. The velocity of tricuspid regurgitation, if present, can be used to determine the severity of pulmonary hypertension.

Prior to the development of right-heart failure, pulmonary hypertension and cor pulmonale can be reversed by removing the cattle from high altitude or addressing the primary lung disease. Oxygen supplementation is beneficial in these animals. Once heart failure develops, the prognosis is guarded to poor even with treatment. Preventive measures include routine vaccination for pulmonary disease, avoiding overcrowding situations, and preventing exposure to locoweed [2].

Treatment of Congestive Heart Failure

Prognosis for congestive heart failure in ruminants and camelids is guarded to poor. Common medical therapies in these species include oxygen supplementation, diuretics (furosemide), and digoxin if systolic dysfunction has been documented. If effusion has been identified, removal may help to alleviate some signs of dyspnea. Digoxin, a cardiac glycoside with positive inotropic and negative chronotropic effects, has poor oral bioavailability in ruminants and is limited to the intravenous route. Hydration abnormalities, acid-base disturbances, and electrolyte imbalances should be addressed prior to starting digoxin therapy. Serum digoxin levels may be measured 3–5 days after initiating therapy, with ideal peak and trough levels in the range of 1–2 ng/mL. Use of digoxin is contraindicated in the treatment of ionophore toxicity. Both atrial and ventricular arrhythmias may be managed with quinidine [2]. Pharmacokinetic and pharmacodynamic studies in ruminants and camelids are lacking, so care should be taken using the conventional therapies mentioned above.

Atrial Fibrillation

Atrial fibrillation is one of the most common arrhythmias encountered in large animal patients. Typically, this arrhythmia is secondary to a concurrent disease process such as foot rot, pneumonia, myocarditis, or endocarditis. Electrolyte and acid-base disturbances are common in these species, the most common being metabolic alkalosis. In cattle, atrial fibrillation is commonly seen with gastrointestinal disease (e.g. displaced abomasum) and presenting complaints of anorexia and decreased milk production are common [1,2]. The arrhythmia and clinical signs can be paroxysmal or persistent. Examination findings include pulse deficits with highly variable pulse quality, an irregularly irregular rhythm, tachycardia, and other findings attributable to the primary disease process. With gastrointestinal disease, the degree of tachycardia is thought to reflect severity of the underlying disease. Confirmation of the rhythm is accomplished with electrocardiography. Anti-arrhythmic therapy is rarely warranted in ruminants with atrial fibrillation. With proper treatment of the underlying cause, these animals usually spontaneously convert back to a normal rhythm [2].

References

1 McGuirk, S.M. and Reef, V.B. (2008) Alterations in cardiovascular and hemolymphatic systems, in *Large Animal Internal Medicine*, 4th Edition (ed. B.P. Smith). Mosby, St Louis. pp. 83–95.

2 Reef, V.B. and McGuirk, S.M. (2008) Diseases of the cardiovascular system, in *Large Animal Internal Medicine*, 4th Edition (ed. B.P. Smith). Mosby, St Louis. pp. 453–489.

3 Margiocco, M.L., Scansen, B.A. and Bonagura, J.D. (2009) Camelid cardiology. *Veterinary Clinics of North America: Food Animal Practice*, **25**, 423–454.

4 Onda, K., Sugiyama, M., Niho, K. et al. (2011) Long-term survival of a cow with cervical ectopia cordis. *Canadian Veterinary Journal*, **52**, 667–669.

5 Firshman, A.M., Wünschmann, A., Cebra, C.K. et al. (2008) Thrombotic endocarditis in 10 alpacas. *Journal of Veterinary Internal Medicine*, **22**, 456–461.

6 McLane, M.J., Schlipf, J.W. Jr, Margiocco, M.L. and Gelberg, H. (2008) Listeria associated mural and valvular endocarditis in an alpaca. *Journal of Veterinary Cardiology*, **10**, 141–145.

7 Barlow, A.M., Mitchell, K.A. and Visram, K.H. (1999) Bovine tuberculosis in llama (Lama glama) in the UK. *Veterinary Record*, **145**, 639–640.

8 Abdelaal, A.M. *et al.* (2009) Clinical and ultrasonographic differences between cattle and buffaloes with various sequelae of traumatic reticuloperitonitis. *Veterinarni Medicina*, **54**, 399–406.

9 Divers, T.J. and Peek, S.F. (2007) The clinical examination, in *Rebhun's Diseases of Dairy Cattle*, 2nd Edition. Saunders, Philadelphia. pp. 56–58.

10 Van Alstine, W.G. and Mitsui, I. (2010) Sudden death associated with hypertrophic cardiomyopathy in an alpaca (Llama Pacos). *Journal of Veterinary Diagnostic Investigation*, **22**, 448–450.

11 Varga, A., Schober, K.E., Holloman, C.H. et al. (2009) Correlation of serum cardiac troponin I and myocardial damage in cattle with monensin toxicosis. *Journal of Veterinary Internal Medicine*, **23**, 1108–1116.

12 Boon, J. (2011) *Veterinary Echocardiography*, 2nd Edition. Wiley-Blackwell, Oxford.

Appendix: Commonly Used Cardiovascular Drugs

Drug name	Drug classification	Uses/indications	Side effects	Supplied veterinary preparations	Supplied human preparations
Acepromazine	Phenothiazine sedative	Sedation/tranquilization	Vasodilation, hypotension, rare penile retractor muscle paralysis in stallions, prolapse of membrana nictitans	*Injectable*: 10 mg/mL 50 mL *Tablet*: 5, 10, 25 mg in 100 and 500 tablet bottles	None
Aminophylline /theophylline	Phosphodiesterase inhibitor Bronchodilator	Bronchodilation	Nausea, vomiting, insomnia, nervousness, increased gastric secretion, diarrhea, polyphagia, polydipsia, polyuria	None	*Injectable*: 250 mg/mL in 10 or 20 mL vial *Tablet*: 100 mg and 200 mg *Time released*: 100, 125, 200, 300, 400 mg tab/cap
Amiodirone	Class 3 anti-arrhythmic	Treats ventricular arrhythmia	*Gastrointestinal*: vomiting, anorexia CONTRAINDICATED: atrioventricular block and bradycardia	None	*Injectable*: 50 mg/mL in 3 mL ampule/vial *Tablet*: 100, 200 and 400 mg
Amlodipine	Calcium channel blocker	Vasodilator, treats systemic hypertension	Hypotension, inappetence Rarely: azotemia, lethargy, hypokalemia, reflex tachycardia, weight loss	None	*Single agent tablet*: 2.5, 5, 10 mg. Also available combined with benazepril

(continued)

Cardiology for Veterinary Technicians and Nurses, First Edition. Edited by H. Edward Durham, Jr.

Appendix: (*continued*)

Drug name	Drug classification	Uses/indications	Side effects	Supplied veterinary preparations	Supplied human preparations
Atenolol	ß-adrenergic receptor blocker	Treats tachyarrhythmias, systemic hypertension, obstructive cardiomyopathy	Bradycardia, lethargy, inappetence, depression, impaired AV node conduction, reduced systolic function, worsening congestive heart failure, hypotension, hypoglycemia, syncope, diarrhea NOTE: this drug should not be suddenly discontinued. Patients should be weaned gradually from the drug	None	*Injectable*: 5 mg/mL × 10 mL ampule *Tablet*: 25, 50, 100 mg
Atropine	Anticholinergic	Bradycardia, reduce salivation, differentiate between vagally and non-vagally mediated bradyarrhythmia, pre-anesthetic medication, Tx : organophosphate toxicity	*Cardiovascular*: tachycardia, bradycardia (initially or at low dose), hypertension, hypotension, arrhythmias *Gastrointestinal*: dry mouth, decreased GI motility, dysphagia, constipation, vomiting, thirst *Central nervous system*: drowsiness, ataxia, seizure, respiratory depression *Ocular*: pupil dilation, photophobia, cycloplegia NOTE: contraindicated in patients with narrow angle glaucoma, ileus, urinary obstruction	*Injectable*: 1/20 g (0.54 mg/mL) × 100 mL, 15 mg/mL × 100 mL *Ophthalmic ointment*: 10 mg/g (1.0%) in 3.5 g tube	*Injectable*: 0.05 mg/mL × 5 mL syringe, 0.1 mg/mL × 5 and 10 mL syringes, 0.3 mg/mL × 1 mL and 30 mL vial, 0.4 mg/mL × 1 mL ampule, 0.4 mg/mL in 1, 20, 30 mL vial, 0.5 mg/mL in 1 or 30 mL vial and a 5 mL syringe, 0.8 mg/mL × 0.5 and 1 mL ampule, 0.8 mg/mL in 0. 5 mL syringe, 1 mg/mL in 1 mL ampule/syringe and 10 mL syringe *Tablet*: 0.4 mg *Ophthalmic drops*: 0.5%, 1% 2% unit dose droppers of 2, 5, 10 mL bottles *Ointment*: 5 mg/g and 10 mg/g in 3.5 g tubes

Benazapril	Angiotensin-converting enzyme inhibitor	Treats congestive heart failure, systemic hypertension, protein-losing nephropathy, chronic renal failure	*Gastrointestinal*: vomiting, diarrhea, anorexia *Cardiovascular*: hypotension, hyperkalemia, renal dysfunction	UK only: tablet: 2.5, 5, 20 mg	*Tablet*: 5, 10, 20, 40 mg
Bupenorphine	Opioid agonist-antagonist	Sedation, analgesia	Rare respiratory depression	None	*Injectable*: 0.3 mg/mL in 1 mL ampule *Sublingual tablet*: 2 mg or 8 mg
Butorphanol tartrate	Partial μ agonist	Sedation, analgesia	Sedation, ataxia, anorexia, diarrhea, respiratory depression	*Injectable*: 0.5, 2.0, 10.0 mg/mL × 10 mL. 10 mg/mL also comes in 50 mL vial *Tablet*: 1, 5, 10 mg × 100	*Injectable*: 1 mg/mL in 1 or 2 mL vial. 2 mg/mL in 1, 2 and 10 mL vial *Nasal spray*: 10 mg/mL
Carvedilol	α- and β-adrenergic receptor blocker	Treats tachyarrhythmias, systemic hypertension, obstructive cardiomyopathy	Bradycardia, lethargy, inappetence, depression, impaired AV node conduction, reduced systolic function, worsening congestive heart failure, hypotension, hypoglycemia, syncope, diarrhea. NOTE: this drug should not be suddenly discontinued. Patients should be weaned gradually from the drug	None	*Tablet*: 3.125, 6.25, 12.5, 25 mg *Extended release tablet*: 10, 20 40, 80 mg

(continued)

Appendix: (*continued*)

Drug name	Drug classification	Uses/indications	Side effects	Supplied veterinary preparations	Supplied human preparations
Digoxin	Cardiac glycoside	Positive inotrope, treats congestive heart failure and supraventricular tachyarrhythmias	Vomiting, diarrhea, anorexia, weight loss, arrhythmias, worsening congestive heart failure, delayed atrioventricular nodal conduction	None	*Injectable*: 0.1 mg/mL × 1 mL ampule, 0.25 mg/mL × 2 mL ampule *Tablet*: 0.125 and 0.25 mg *Capsule*: 0.05, 0.1, and 0.2 mg *Elixir*: 0.05 × 60 mL bottle
Diltiazem	Calcium channel blocker	Treats systemic hypertension, hypertrophic cardiomyopathy, supraventricular tachyarrhythmias	Hypotension, inappetence Rarely: azotemia, lethargy, hypokalemia, bradycardia, reflex tachycardia, weight loss	None	*Injectable*: 5 mg/mL in 5, 10, and 25 mL vial, 25 mg single use syringe *Tablet*: 30, 60, 90 and 120 mg *Extended release*: 60, 90, 120, 180 240 300, 360, and 420 mg
Dobutamine	Parenteral β-adrenergic agonist. USED as constant rate infusion	Cardiovascular support, positive inotrope	Cardiac ectopy, hypertension, tachycardia	None	*Injectable*: 12.5 mg/mL in 25 mL vial

Dopamine	Adrenergic/dopaminergic inotrope. USED as constant rate infusion	Cardiovascular support, positive inotrope	Nausea, vomiting, cardiac ectopy, tachycardia, hypotension, hypertension, dyspnea, vasoconstriction. NOTE: extravasation will cause tissue necrosis and sloughing. SHOULD EXTRAVASATION OCCUR: treat with 5–10 mg phentolamine in 10–15 mL saline and infiltrate area	None	*Injectable*: 40, 80, and 160 mg/mL × 5, 10, 20 mL vials, or 5 mL ampule, or 5 and 10 mL syringes
Enalapril	Angiotensin-converting enzyme inhibitor	Control vascular volume in congestive heart failure, protein-losing nephropathy	*Gastrointestinal*: vomiting, diarrhea, anorexia *Cardiovascular*: hypotension, hyperkalemia, renal dysfunction	*Tablet*: 1, 2.5, 5, 10, and 20 mg	*Tablet*: 2.5, 5 10 and 20 mg *Injectable*: 1.25 mg/mL × 1 or 2 mL vial
Esmolol	β-adrenergic receptor blocker	Rapid, short-acting, negative inotrope	Bradycardia, lethargy, inappetence, depression, impaired AV node conduction, reduced systolic function, worsening congestive heart failure, hypotension, syncope NOTE: this drug should not be suddenly discontinued. Patients should be weaned gradually from the drug	None	*Injectable*: 10 mg/mL × 10 mL vial, 20 mg/mL × 5 mL vial and 100 bag, 250 mg/mL in 10 mL ampule

(*continued*)

Appendix: (*continued*)

Drug name	Drug classification	Uses/indications	Side effects	Supplied veterinary preparations	Supplied human preparations
Furosemide	Loop diuretic	Diuretic in all species	Iatrogenic polyuria/polydipsia, dehydration, prerenal azotemia, hypotension, electrolyte imbalances (esp. K^+, Ca^{++}, Mg^+, Na^+). Increases risk of digoxin toxicity, increased risk of hypotension used in combination with ACE-I	*Injectable*: 50 mg/mL × 50 mL and 100 mL vial *Tablet*: 12.5 mg and 50 mg *Oral liquid*: 10 mg/mL × 60 mL	*Injectable*: 10 mg/mL × 2, 4, or 10 mL vial (multidose vial available in 10 mL) *Tablet:* 20, 40, or 80 mg *Oral liquid*: 10 mg/mL × 60 or 120 mL, 40 mg/5 mL × 500 mL
Hydralazine	Vasodilator	Reduce afterload in congestive heart failure, treats hypertension	Hypotension, reflex tachycardia, sodium/water retention, vomiting, diarrhea	None	*Injectable*: 20 mg/mL × 1 mL vial *Tablet*: 10, 25, 50, and 100 mg
Lidocaine	Class 1b anti-arrhythmic	Local anesthetic, anti-arrhythmic	Seizure, tremors, ataxia, nausea, vomiting. CONTRAINDICATED in complete atrioventricular block	*Injectable*: 20 mg/mL × 100, 250 mL vial	*Injectable*: 5, 10, 20, 40 mg/mL in 5, 10, 20, 30 and 50 mL vials
Mexilitine	Class 1b anti-arrhythmic	Oral treatment of ventricular arrhythmias	Gastrointestinal upset, vomiting, diarrhea, trembling, dizziness, ataxia, depression CONTRAINDICATED in atrioventricular blocks	None	*Capsule*: 150, 200, 250 mg

Pimobendan	Phosphodiesterase inhibitor, positive inotrope and vasodilator (inodilator)	Adjunctive therapy for congestive heart failure, treats pulmonary hypertension	Gastrointestinal upset, anorexia, lethargy, diarrhea, dyspnea, azotemia, weakness/ataxia. Other adverse reactions reported are consistent with worsening congestive heart failure or arrhythmias	*Tablet*: 1.25, 2.5, 5 and 10 mg chewable tablet	None
Procainamide	Class 1a anti-arrhythmic	Anti-arrhythmic (primarily ventricular)	Gastrointestinal upset, vomiting, anorexia, diarrhea, hypotension, negative inotropy, widened QRS, atrioventricular blocks	None	*Injectable*: 500 mg/mL × 2 mL vial *Tablet*: 250, 375, 500 mg capsules. 375, 500 mg tablet *Extended release tablet*: 250, 500, 750, 1000 mg
Propranolol	β-adrenergic receptor blocker (non-selective)	Anti-arrhythmic (primarily supraventricular)	Bradycardia, lethargy, inappetence, depression, impaired AV node conduction, reduced systolic function, worsening congestive heart failure, hypotension, bronchoconstriction, syncope. NOTE: this drug should not be suddenly discontinued. Patients should be weaned gradually from the drug	None	*Injectable*: 1 mg/mL in 1 mL vial *Oral solution*: 4 mg/mL and 8 mg/mL in 500 mL bottle *Tablet*: 10, 20, 40, 60, 80, and 90 mg *Extended release tablet*: 60, 80, 120, 160 mg capsules

(*continued*)

Appendix: (*continued*)

Drug name	Drug classification	Uses/indications	Side effects	Supplied veterinary preparations	Supplied human preparations
Sotalol	Class 3 anti-arrhythmic, β-adrenergic receptor blocker	Anti-arrhythmic (primarily ventricular)	Decreased systolic function, pro-arrhythmic, vomiting, nausea, dyspnea/bronchospasm, fatigue/dizziness	None	*Tablet*: 80, 120, 160, 240 mg
Spironolactone	Aldosterone antagonist	Potassium-sparing diuretic. Adjunct treatment for congestive heart failure	Hyperkalemia, hyponatremia, dehydration, increased blood urea nitrogen in renal patients, vomiting, anorexia, lethargy, ataxia	None	*Tablet*: 25 50, 100 mg
Tocainide	Class 1b anti-arrhythmic	Anti-arrhythmic (primarily ventricular)	Seizure, tremors, ataxia, nausea, vomiting, hypotension, bradycardia, tachycardia, arrhythmias, worsening congestive heart failure	None	*Tablet*: 400, 600 mg
Torsemide	Loop diuretic	Treats congestive heart failure	Iatrogenic polyuria/polydipsia, dehydration, prerenal azotemia, hypotension, electrolyte imbalances (esp. K^+, Ca^{++}, Mg^+, Na^+), increases risk of digoxin toxicity, increased risk of hypotension used in combination with ACE-I	None	*Tablet*: 5, 10, 20, 100 mg *Injectable*: 10 mg/mL × 2 and 5 mL ampules

Information referenced from: Plumb, D.C. (2008) *Veterinary Drug Handbook*, 6th Edition. Wiley-Blackwell, Oxford.

Index

Cardiology for Veterinary Technicians and Nurses, First Edition. Edited by H. Edward Durham, Jr.

Printed and bound by CPI Group (UK) Ltd, Croydon, CR0 4YY
27/10/2024
14580246-0002